The SAGES Manual

Second Edition

The SAGES Manual

Fundamentals of Laparoscopy, Thoracoscopy, and GI Endoscopy

Second Edition

Carol E.H. Scott-Conner, MD, PhD, MBA

Professor of Surgery, Department of Surgery,
University of Iowa Hospitals and Clinics, Iowa City, Iowa

Editor

With 311 Illustrations

With a Foreword by David W. Rattner, MD

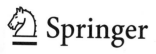 Springer

Carol E.H. Scott-Conner, MD, PhD, MBA
Professor of Surgery
Department of Surgery
University of Iowa Hospitals and Clinics
Iowa City, IA 52242
USA

Library of Congress Control Number: 2005923808

ISBN: 10: 0-387-23267-2
ISBN: 13: 978-0387-23267-6

Printed on acid-free paper.

Printed in the United States of America.   (BS/MVY)

9 8 7 6 5 4 3 2 1

springeronline.com

Foreword

SAGES (The Society of American Gastrointestinal and Endoscopic Surgeons) has made resident education a priority for most of its 25-year history. In the 1990s, when there was need for additional training in minimally invasive surgery, SAGES responded by developing multiple courses for residents and fellows to fill in the gaps left by the spotty penetration of minimally invasive surgery in some training programs. SAGES resident programs have been attended by more than one thousand trainees and helped educate future surgeons to safely incorporate laparoscopic surgery into their practices. While a variety of atlases and textbooks of laparoscopic surgery had been published in the mid-1990s, none had focused on the residents' need for a daily guide that could be carried in a white coat pocket for immediate reference. In 1998, the first edition of *The SAGES Manual* was published. This pocket-sized manual was the first text specifically designed to help residents understand both the indications and techniques for laparoscopic and flexible endoscopic procedures and immediately became a "best seller." Since publication of *The SAGES Manual* seven years ago, new minimally invasive surgical techniques have been introduced, the indications for traditional minimally invasive surgical procedures have expanded and hence the time has come to update the manual.

Dr. Carol E.H. Scott-Conner has once again done a terrific job in selecting the subjects to be covered and enlisting leaders in the Society to write about areas of their own expertise. Perusing the table of contents one is struck by the number of new chapters that Dr. Scott-Conner has added. This reflects the substantial changes that have occurred in minimally invasive surgery—a field that was viewed as mature in 1998 when the original manual was published! The second edition addresses some areas that were controversial in 1998 but are now mainstream, such as laparoscopy in pregnancy and laparoscopic colectomy for cancer. The burgeoning area of laparoscopic bariatric surgery has been significantly expanded. Laparoscopic pediatric surgery is another rapidly growing area that is given significant coverage in this second edition of *The SAGES Manual.* Areas that still remain controversial, such as hand-assisted surgery and the role of robotics in minimally invasive surgery are included. Areas that probably should be considered unproven, such as laparoscopic esophageal resection and endoluminal therapies, are included so that residents can be familiar with potential future directions that minimally invasive surgery may take. In spite of these exciting developments, it is sobering to realize that chapters on avoiding complications in laparoscopic cholecystectomy are still necessary as bile duct injuries continue to occur.

The SAGES Manual is a comprehensive notebook-style reference covering basic material that all residents should master while completing surgical training. In the near future, it is likely that competence-based testing will replace the traditional multiple-choice format. High-stake examinations such as SAGES Fundamentals of Laparoscopic Surgery (FLS) will test both the fund of knowledge contained in *The SAGES Manual*, as well as the ability to apply that knowledge to both patient scenarios and task performance. In the new millennium SAGES remains committed not only to providing the highest quality resident education, but also demonstrating that this effort promotes the competent practice of minimally invasive surgery.

David W. Rattner, MD
SAGES President 2004–2005
Boston, Massachusetts

Preface

How do you know it is time to create a second edition of a book? In the case of *The SAGES Manual*, the decision was easy. Is it by number of copies sold? Not really. True, *The SAGES Manual* has gone through multiple printings and has been translated into several languages, but success alone does not mandate the kind of comprehensive revision offered here. We created this substantially expanded and enhanced second edition because of the rapid advance of technology and its successful integration into practice and the training environment. Almost every chapter has been revised, new material has been added, and some chapters have new authors.

The most visible difference is the inclusion of a third section on thoracoscopy. Six new chapters in this section provide detailed information that will be useful to both general and cardiothoracic surgeons. The bariatric surgery section has been significantly expanded. New chapters have been added on robotic surgery and several new endoscopic procedures. If you own an old, dog-eared copy of *The SAGES Manual*, you will feel comfortable with this new edition, but you will also find much that is new.

As with the first edition, it is our hope that you will find this manual a guide and a companion, a way to keep SAGES experts with you in your practice.

Carol E.H. Scott-Conner
Iowa City, Iowa

Contents

Part 1 Laparoscopy

I General Principles

V   Laparoscopic Gastric Surgery

**VI   Laparoscopic Procedures on the Small Intestine,
Appendix, and Colon**

Part 2   Flexible Endoscopy

III   Small Bowel Enteroscopy

IV   Endoscopic Retrograde Cholangiopancreatography

Part 3   Thoracoscopy for the Gastrointestinal Surgeon

Contributors

Gina L. Adrales, MD, Assistant Professor, Department of Surgery, Medical College of Georgia, Augusta, GA 30912, USA

Mohan C. Airan, MD, FACS, Chairman, Department of Surgery, Good Samaritan Hospital, Downers Grove, IL 60515, USA

Charles H. Andrus, MD, FACS, Vice-Chairman, Department of Surgery, San Joaquin General Hospital, French Camp, CA 95213, USA

Gintas Antanavicius, MD, General Surgical Resident, Department of Surgery, The Western Pennsylvania Hospital, Pittsburgh, PA 15224, USA

Keith N. Apelgren, MD, Professor, Department of Surgery, Michigan State University, Lansing, MI 40912, USA

Maurice E. Arregui, MD, FACS, Director, Fellowship in Advanced Laparoscopy, Endoscopy and Ultrasound, Department of General Surgery, St. Vincent Hospital, Indianapolis, IN 46260, USA

Ahmad Assalia, MD, Deputy Director, Department of Surgery B, Rambam Medical Center, Haifa, Israel

Mirza K. Baig, MD, Clinical Fellow, Department of Colorectal Surgery, Cleveland Clinic Florida, Weston, FL 33331, USA

Christopher Baird, MD, Clinical Fellow, Department of Pediatric Cardiothoracic Surgery, Children's Hospital of Boston, Boston, MA 02115, USA

George Berci, MD, FACS, Senior Director, Minimally Invasive Surgery Center, Department of Surgery, Cedars Sinai Medical Center, Los Angeles, CA 90048, USA

David M. Brams, MD, Senior Staff Surgeon, Department of General Surgery, Lahey Clinic Medical Center, Burlington, MA 01805, USA

Bipan Chand, MD, Staff Surgeon, Department of General Surgery, Cleveland Clinic Foundation, Cleveland, OH 44195, USA

John A. Coller, MD, Senior Colon and Rectal Surgeon, Lahey Clinic; Assistant Clinical Professor of Surgery, Tufts University School of Medicine, Burlington, MA 01805, USA

Michael J. Conlin, MD, Associate Professor, Department of Surgery and Urology, Oregon Health and Science University, Portland, OR 97201, USA

Daniel R. Cottam, MD, Fellow, Minimally Invasive Surgery, Department of Surgery, Division of Minimally Invasive Surgery, Magee Women's Hospital, University of Pittsburgh, Pittsburgh, PA 15213, USA

Joseph Cullen, MD, Professor, Department of Surgery, University of Iowa, Iowa City, IA 52246, USA

Myriam J. Curet, MD, Associate Professor, Department of Surgery, Stanford University Medical Center, Stanford, CA 64305, USA

Alfred Cuschieri, FRSE, MD, ChM, FRCS, F.Med.Sci, Professor, Department of Surgery and Molecular Oncology, University of Dundee, Ninewells Hospital and Medical School, Dundee, Tayside, Scotland DD1 9SY

Eric J. DeMaria, MD, FACS, Professor, Department of General Surgery, Virginia Commonwealth University, Richmond, VA 232219, USA

Ketan M. Desai, MD, General Surgery Resident, Department of Surgery, Washington University School of Medicine, St. Louis, MO 63110, USA

Karen Deveney, MD, Professor and Program Director, Department of Surgery, Oregon Health and Science University, Portland, OR 97239, USA

Daniel J. Deziel, MD, Professor of Surgery, Department of General Surgery, Rush University Medical Center, Chicago, IL 60612, USA

James P. Dolan, MD, Staff Surgeon, General and Laparoscopic Surgery, Department of Surgery, USAF Keesler Medical Center, Biloxi, MS 39534, USA

Brian J. Dunkin, MD, Associate Professor, Department of Surgery, University of Miami, Miami, FL 33136, USA

David Duppler, MD, Staff Surgeon, Fox Valley Surgical Associates, Appleton Medical Center, Appleton, WI 54911, USA

David W. Easter, MD, FACS, Professor, Department of Surgery, University of California San Diego, San Diego, CA 92103, USA

Adolfo Z. Fernandez, Jr., MD, Medical Director, Bariatric Surgery Program, Department of General Surgery, Wake Forrest University Baptist Medical Center, Winston-Salem, NC 27157, USA

Hiran Fernando, MD, FRCS, FACS, Associate Professor, Department of Cardiothoracic Surgery, Boston Medical Center, Boston, MA 02118, USA

Peter F. Ferson, MD, Professor, Department of Surgery, University of Pittsburgh School of Medicine, Pittsburgh, PA 15213, USA

Aaron S. Fink, MD, Chief, Perioperative and Surgical Care, Atlanta VAMC, Professor, Department of Surgery, School of Medicine, Emory University, Decatur, GA 30033, USA

Robert J. Fitzgibbons, Jr., MD, FACS, Professor, Department of Surgery, Chief, Division of General Surgery, Creighton University School of Medicine, Omaha, NE 68131, USA

Thomas R. Gadacz, MD, FACS, Chair Bonnier, Professor, Department of Surgery, Section of Gastrointestinal Surgery, Medical College of Georgia, Augusta, GA 30912, USA

Michel Gagner, MD, FRCSC, FACS, Professor, Department of Surgery, Weill Medical College of Cornell University, New York-Presbyterian Hospital, New York, NY 10021, USA

Ali Ghazi, MD, Beth Israel Medical Center, New York, NY 10003, USA

Frederick L. Greene, MD, Chairman, Department of General Surgery, Carolinas Medical Center, Charlotte, NC 28203, USA

Norman B. Halpern, MD, FACS, Retired, Department of Surgery, University of Alabama, University Station, Birmingham, AL 35294, USA

Giselle G. Hamad, MD, FACS, Medical Director, Minimally Invasive General Surgery and Bariatrics, Department of Surgery, Mage Women's Hospital, University of Pittsburgh, Pittsburgh, PA 15213, USA

Stan C. Hewlett, MD, Baptist-Princeton, Department of Surgery, Birmingham, AL 35211, USA

Harry S. Himal, MD, FACS(C), FACS, Associate Professor, Department of Surgery, University of Toronto, Toronto, Ontario MST 3A9, Canada

Alberto de Hoyos, MD, Assistant Professor, Director, Center for Minimally Invasive Thoracic Surgery, Department of Cardiothoracic Surgery, Northwestern Memorial Hospital, Chicago, IL 60611, USA

John G. Hunter, MD, Professor and Chair, Department of Surgery, Oregon Health and Science University, Portland, OR 97239, USA

Sayeed Ikramuddin, MD, Associate Professor, Department of Surgery, University of Minnesota, Minneapolis, MN 55455, USA

Todd A. Kellogg, MD, Assistant Professor, Department of Surgery, University of Minnesota, Minneapolis, MN 55455, USA

Chris Kimber, MBBS, FRACS, Department of Surgery, Ninewells Hospital and Medical School, Dundee, Scotland DD1 9SY, UK

Andreas Kirakopolous, MD, Fellow, Center for Minimally Invasive Surgery, The Ohio State University, Columbus, OH 43210, USA

Jason Lamb, MD, Director, West Penn Center for Lung and Thoracic Disease, Western Pennsylvania Hospital; Assistant Professor, Department of Surgery, Temple University, Pittsburgh, PA 15224, USA

Rodney J. Landreneau, MD, Director, Comprehensive Lung Center, Division of Thoracic and Foregut Surgery and the Minimally Invasive Center, University of Pittsburgh Medical Center, Shadyside Medical Center, Pittsburgh, PA 15215, USA

Gerald M. Larson, MD, Professor, Department of Surgery, University of Louisville, Louisville, KY 40292, USA

Thom E. Lobe, MD, Blank Children's Hospital, Des Moines, IA 50309, USA

James D. Luketich, MD, Professor and Chief, Department of Surgery, Division of Thoracic and Foregut Surgery, University of Pittsburgh Medical Center, Pittsburgh, PA 15213, USA

Bruce V. MacFadyen, Jr., MD, Professor and Chairman, Chief of General Surgery, Section of Gastrointestinal Surgery, Medical College of Georgia, Augusta, GA 30912, USA

Anne T. Mancino, MD, FACS, Associate Professor, Associate Program Director, Department of Surgery, University of Arkansas for Medical Sciences; Central Arkansas Veterans Health Care System, Little Rock, AR 72205, USA

Aloke K. Mandal, MD, PhD, Assistant Professor, Department of Surgery, Division of Liver and Pancreas Transplantation, Oregon Health and Science University, Portland, OR 97239, USA

Jeffrey M. Marks, MD, Assistant Clinical Professor, Department of Surgery, Case Western Reserve University, Mayfield Heights, OH 44139, USA

John J. Meehan, MD, Assistant Professor, Department of General Surgery, Division of Pediatric Surgery, University of Iowa, Iowa City, IA 52246, USA

John D. Mellinger, MD, FACS, Associate Professor, Department of Surgery, Medical College of Georgia, Augusta, GA 30912, USA

W. Scott Melvin, MD, Associate Professor, Department of Surgery, Ohio State University, Columbus, OH 43210, USA

Muhammed Ashraf Memon, MBBS, DCH, FRCSI, FRCSEd, FRCSEng, Consultant General, Upper GI and Laparoscopic Surgeon, Whiston Hospital, Prescot, Merseyside L35 5DR, UK

Amanda Metcalf, MD, Professor, Department of Surgery, University of Iowa, Iowa City, IA 52242, USA

Scott H. Miller, MD, FACS, Vice Chairman, Department of Surgery, Condell Medical Center, Libertyville, IL 60048, USA

Richard M. Newman, MD, Co-director, Minimally Invasive Surgery Center of Excellence, St. Francis Hospital and Medical Center, Hartford, CT 06105, USA

Nihn T. Nguyen, MD, Chief, Professor of Gastrointestinal Surgery, Department of Surgery, University of California, Irvine Medical Center, Orange, CA 92868, USA

Margret Oddsdöttir, MD, Professor and Chief, Department of Surgery, Landspitali University Hospital, Hringbraut, Reykjavik 101, Iceland

Raymond P. Onders, MD, Associate Professor, Director of Minimally Invasive Surgery, Department of Surgery, Case Western Reserve University, University Hospitals of Cleveland, Cleveland, OH 44106, USA

† *Claude H. Organ, Jr., MD, MS (surg.), FACS, FRCSSA, FRACS, FRCS, FRCS (Ed.)*, Emeritus Professor, Department of Surgery, University of California San Francisco—East Bay, Oakland, CA 94602, USA

Emma Patterson, MD, FRCSC, FACS, Director, Bariatric Surgery, Department of Surgery, Legacy Health System, Portland, OR 97210, USA

Joseph B. Petelin, MD, FACS, Clinical Associate Professor, Department of Surgery, University of Kansas School of Medicine, Shawnee Mission, KS 66204, USA

Jeffrey H. Peters, MD, Professor and Chairman, Department of Surgery, University of Rochester, Rochester, NY 14627, USA

D. Mario del Pino, MD, Fellow, Minimally Invasive Surgery, Department of Thoracic Surgery, Presbyterian Hospital, Pittsburgh, PA 15213, USA

Jeffrey L. Ponsky, MD, Director, Department of Endoscopic Surgery, Vice Chairman of the Division of Health, Cleveland Clinic, Cleveland, OH 44195, USA

Robert V. Rege, MD, Chairman, Department of Surgery, University of Texas Southwestern Medical Center, Dallas, TX 75390, USA

Bassem Y. Safadi, MD, Assistant Professor, Department of Surgery, Stanford University; VA Palo Alto Health Care, Palo Alto, CA 94304, USA

---

† Deceased

Barry Salky, MD, Chief, Laparoscopic Surgery, Department of Surgery, Mount Sinai Medical Center, New York, NY 10029, USA

Ricardo Santos, MD, Clinical Instructor, Department of Surgery, University of Pittsburgh Medical Center, Pittsburgh, PA 15232, USA

Philip R. Schauer, MD, Professor and Chief, Minimally Invasive General Surgery, Director, Bariatric Surgery, Department of Surgery, Cleveland, Clinic Lerner College of Medicine, Cleveland, OH 44195, USA

Bruce David Schirmer, MD, Professor, Department of Surgery, University of Virginia Health System, Charlottesville, VA 22908, USA

Benjamin E. Schneider, MD, Instructor, Department of Surgery, Beth Israel Deaconess Medical Center, Harvard Medical School, Boston, MA 02215, USA

Carol E.H. Scott-Conner, MD, PhD, MA, Professor, Department of Surgery, University of Iowa Hospitals and Clinics, Iowa City, IA 52242, USA

Irwin B. Simon, MD, JD, Associate Clinical Professor, Department of Surgery, University of Nevada School of Medicine, Las Vegas, NV 89128, USA

C. Daniel Smith, MD, FACS, Chief, General and Gastrointestinal Surgery, Department of Surgery, Emory University School of Medicine, Atlanta, GA 30322, USA

Nathaniel J. Soper, MD, Professor, Vice Chair of NMH Clinical Affairs, Director, Minimally Invasive Surgery, Department of Surgery, Northwestern University Feinberg School of Medicine, Northwestern Memorial Hospital, Chicago, IL 60611, USA

Steven C. Stain, MD, Professor and Chair, Department of Surgery, Meharry Medical College, Nashville, TN 37208, USA

Thomas A. Stellato, MD, MBA, Professor and Chief, Department of Surgery, Division of General Surgery, Case Western Reserve University School of Medicine, University Hospitals of Cleveland, Cleveland, OH 44106, USA

Gregory Van Stiegmann, MD, Professor and Head, GI, Tumor and Endocrine Surgery, University of Colorado Health Sciences Center, Denver, CO 80262, USA

Choichi Sugawa, MD, Professor of Surgery, Director of Endoscopy, Department of Surgery, Wayne State University Hospital, Detroit, MI 48201, USA

Lee L. Swanstrom, MD, Clinical Professor, Department of Minimally Invasive Surgery, Oregon Health and Science University, Legacy Health System, Portland, OR 97210, USA

Zoltan Szabo, PhD, FICI, Director, MOET Institute, San Francisco, CA 94114, USA

Mark A. Talamini, MD, Professor and Chair, Department of Surgery, University of California San Diego, San Diego, CA 92103, USA

David S. Tichansky, MD, Assistant Professor, Department of Surgery, University of Tennessee Health Science Center, Memphis, TN 38163, USA

L. William Traverso, MD, Attending Surgeon, Department of General Surgery, Virginia Mason Clinic, Seattle, WA 98072, USA

Edmund K.M. Tsoi, MD, Associate Clinical Professor, Department of Surgery, University of California San Francisco—East Bay, Oakland, CA 94602, USA

Gary C. Vitale, MD, Professor, Department of Surgery, University of Louisville, Louisville, KY 40292, USA

Morris Washington, MD, FACS, Attending Physician, Department of Surgery, CentraState Medical Center, Freehold, NJ 07728, USA

Eric G. Weiss, MD, Program Director, Department CRS, Chairman, Graduate Medical Education, Director, Surgical Endoscopy, Cleveland Clinic Florida, Weston, FL 33331, USA

Steven D. Wexner, MD, Chief of Staff, Department of Colorectal Surgery, Cleveland Clinic Hospital, Weston, FL 33331, USA

Carlos M. Zavaleta, MD, Surgeon, Department of Surgery, University of Louisville, Louisville, KY 40292, USA

Part 1 Laparoscopy

Laparoscopy
I—General Principles

1. Equipment Setup and Troubleshooting

Mohan C. Airan, M.D., F.A.C.S.

A. Room Layout and Equipment Position

1. **General considerations** include the size of the operating room, location of doors, outlets for electrical and anesthetic equipment, and the procedure to be performed. Time spent in positioning the equipment and operating table is well spent. Come to the operating room sufficiently early to assure proper setup, and to ascertain that all instruments are available and in good working order. This is particularly important when a procedure is being done in an operating room not normally used for laparoscopic operations, or when the operating room personnel are unfamiliar with the equipment (e.g., an operation performed after hours).

2. **Determine the optimum position and orientation for the operating table.** If the room is large, the normal position for the operating table will work well for laparoscopy.

3. **Small operating rooms** will require diagonal placement of the operating table and proper positioning of the laparoscopic accessory instrumentation around the operating table.

4. **An equipment checklist** helps to ensure that all items are available and minimizes delays once the patient has arrived in the operating room. Here is an example of such a checklist. Most of the equipment and instruments listed here will be needed for operative laparoscopy. Additional equipment may be needed for advanced procedures. This will be discussed in subsequent sections.

   a. Anesthesia equipment
   b. Electric operating table with remote control if available
   c. Two video monitors
   d. Suction irrigator
   e. Electrosurgical unit, with grounding pad equipped with current monitoring system
   f. Ultrasonically activated scissors, scalpel, or other specialized unit if needed
   g. Laparoscopic equipment, generally housed in a cart on wheels:
      i. Light source
      ii. Insufflator
      iii. Videocassette recorder (VCR), other recording system, tapes
      iv. Color printer (optional)

        v. Monitor on articulating arm
       vi. Camera-processor unit

h. C-arm x-ray unit (if cholangiography is planned) with remote monitor

i. Mayo stand or table with the following laparoscopic instrumentation:
        i. #11, #15 scalpel blades and handles
       ii. Towel clips
      iii. Veress needle or Hasson cannula
      iv. Gas insufflation tubes with micropore filter, if desired
       v. Fiberoptic cable to connect laparoscope with light source
      vi. Video camera with cord
     vii. Cords to connect laparoscopic instruments to the electro-surgical unit, with various adapters for all instruments needed
    viii. 6-in. curved hemostatic forceps
     ix. Small retractors (Army-Navy or similar pattern) for umbilical
      x. Trocar cannulae (size and numbers depend on the planned operation, with extras available in case of accidental contamination)
     xi. Laparoscopic instruments
        Atraumatic graspers
        Locking toothed jawed graspers
        Needle holders
        Dissectors: curved, straight, right-angle
        Bowel grasping forceps
        Babcock clamp
        Scissors: Metzenbaum, hook, microtip
        Fan retractors: 10 mm, 5 mm
        Specialized retractors, such as endoscopic curved retractors
        Biopsy forceps
        Tru-Cut biopsy-core needle
     xii. Monopolar electrocautery dissection tools
        L-shaped hook
        Spade-type dissector/coagulator
    xiii. Ultrasonically activated scalpel (optional)
        Scalpel
        Ball coagulator
        Hook dissector
        Scissors dissector/coagulator/transector
    xiv. Endocoagulator probe (optional)
     xv. Basket containing:
        Clip appliers
        Endoscopic stapling devices
        Pretied suture ligatures
        Endoscopic suture materials
        Extra trocars

j. Robot holder if available

B. Room and Equipment Setup

1. **With the** operating **table positioned**, and all equipment in the room, reassess the configuration. Once the patient is anesthetized and draped, it is difficult to reposition equipment. Consider the room size (as previously discussed), location of doors (particularly if a C-arm is to be used), and the quadrant of the abdomen in which the procedure will be performed. Figure 1.1 shows a typical setup for a laparoscopic cholecystectomy or other procedure in the upper abdomen.

2. **Set up the equipment** before bringing the patient into the operating room. A systematic approach, starting at the head of the table, is useful.

   a. There should be sufficient space to allow the anesthesiologist to position the anesthesia equipment and work safely.

   b. Next, consider the position of the monitors and the paths that connecting cables will take. Try to avoid "fencing in" the surgeon and assistants. This is particularly important if surgeon and assistant need to change places or move (for example, during cholangiography).

   c. The precise setup must be appropriate to the planned procedure. The setup shown is for laparoscopic cholecystectomy or other upper abdominal procedures. Room and equipment setups for other laparoscopic operatings are discussed with each individual procedure in the chapters that follow (Chapters 12 to 46). A useful principle to remember is that the laparoscope must point toward the quadrant of the abdomen with the pathology, and the surgeon generally stands opposite the pathology and looks directly at the main monitor.

   d. If a C-arm or other equipment will need to be brought in during the procedure, plan the path from the door to the operating table in such a manner that the equipment can be positioned with minimal disruption. This will generally require that the cabinet containing the light source, VCR, insufflator, and other electronics be placed at the side of the patient farthest from the door. Consider bringing the C-arm into the room before the procedure begins.

   e. Additional tables should be available so that water, irrigating solutions, and other items are not placed on any electrical units where spillage could cause short circuits, electrical burns, or fires.

3. **Check the equipment** and ascertain the following:

   a. There should be two full carbon dioxide cylinders in the room. One will be used for the procedure, and the second is a spare in case the pressure in the first cylinder becomes low. The cylinder should be hooked up to the insufflator and the valve turned on. The pressure gauge should indicate that there is adequate gas in the cylinder. If the cylinder does not appear to fit properly, **do not**

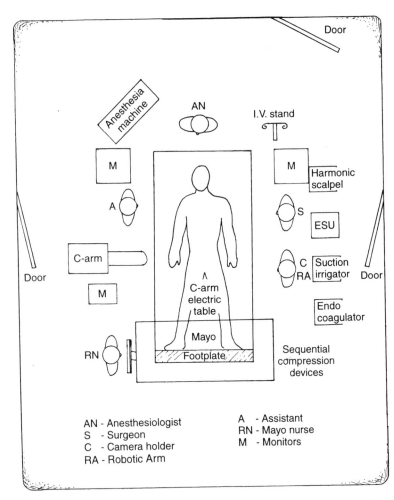

Figure 1.1. **Basic room setup.** This is the typical setup for laparoscopic chole-cystectomy. The room must be sufficiently large to accommodate all of the equip-ment (see Fig. 1.2 for setup for smaller room). A similar setup can be used for hiatus hernia repair or other upper abdominal surgery. In these cases, one 21-in. or larger monitor can be used in the center where the anesthesiologist usually sits, with the anesthesiologist positioned to the side. The position of the surgeon (S), camera holder (C), and the assistant (A) depends on the procedure that is planned. The best position for the monitor is opposite the surgeon in his line of sight. A C-arm, if used, should be placed perpendicular to the operating table. A clear pathway to the door facilitates placement of the C-arm, and should be planned when the room is set up.

force it. Each type of gas cylinder has a unique kind of fitting, and failure to fit properly may indicate that the cylinder contains a different kind of gas (e.g., oxygen).

b. If the carbon dioxide cylinder needs to be changed during a procedure:

   i.   Close the valve body with the proper handle to shut off the gas (old cylinder)

   ii. Unscrew the head fitting

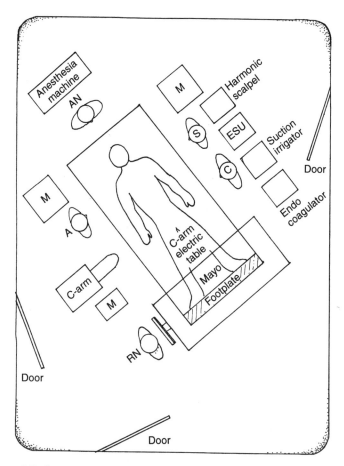

Figure 1.2. **Laparoscopic cholecystectomy, small operating room.** The monitors, anesthesia machine, and relative position of surgeon and first assistant have been adapted to the diagonal operating table placement.

      iii. Replace the gasket in the head fitting with a new gasket, which is always provided with a new tank of gas

      iv. Reattach the head fitting so that the two prongs of the fitting are seated in the two holes in the carbon dioxide gas tank valve body

      v. Firmly align and tighten the head fitting with the integral pointed screw fisture

      vi. Open the carbon dioxide gas tank valve body, and pressure should be restored to the insufflator.

  c. Look inside the back of the cabinet housing the laparoscopic equipment. Check to be certain that the connections on the back of the units are tightly plugged in (Fig. 1.3).

4. **Attention to detail** is important. The following additional items need careful consideration, and can be checked as the patient is brought into the room and prepared for surgery:

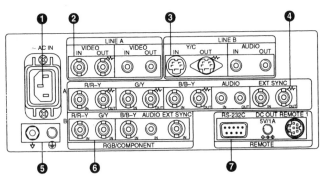

(The ⌁ mark indicates automatic termination.)

Figure 1.3. **Connections on rear panel.** The actual configuration of connections on the rear panels varies, but there are some general principles that will help when tracing the connections. The video signal is generated by the camera box. A cable plugs into the "video out" port of the camera box and takes the video signal to the VCR or monitor by plugging into a "video in" port. A common arrangement takes the signal first to the VCR, and then from the "video out" port of the VCR to the "video in" port of the monitor. (see Chapter 9, Documentation). Some cameras have split connectors that must be connected to the proper ports. Once connected, these should not be disturbed. The surgeon should be familiar with the instrumentation, as connections frequently are loose or disconnected. The last monitor plugged in should have an automatic termination of signal port to avoid deterioration of the picture quality.

a. Assure table tilt mechanism is functional, and that the table and joints are level and the kidney rest down.

b. Consider using a footboard and extra safety strap for large patients.

c. Position patient and cassette properly on operating table for cholangiography.

d. Notify the radiology technologist with time estimate.

e. Assure proper mixing and dilution of cholangiogram contrast solution for adequate image.

f. Assure availability of Foley catheter and nasogastric tube, if desired.

g. Assure all power sources are connected and appropriate units are switched on. Avoid using multiple sockets or extension cords plugged into a single source, as circuits may overload.

h. Check the insufflator (see Chapter 2, Access to Abdomen). Assure that insufflator alarm is set appropriately.

i. Assure full volume in the irrigation fluid container (recheck during case).

j. Assure adequate printer film and video tape if documentation is desired.

k. Check the electrosurgical unit; make sure the auditory alarm of the machine is functioning properly and the grounding pad is appropriate for the patient, properly placed, and functioning.

5. **Once you are gowned and gloved**, connect the light cable and camera to the laparoscope. Focus the laparoscope and white balance it. Place the laparoscope in warmed saline or electrical warmer. Verify the following:

a. Check Veress needle for proper plunger/spring action and assure easy flushing through stopcock and/or needle channel.

b. Assure closed stopcocks on all ports.

c. Check sealing caps for cracked rubber and stretched openings.

d. Check to assure instrument cleaning channel screw caps are in place.

e. Assure free movements of instrument handles and jaws.

f. If Hasson cannula to be used, assure availability of stay sutures and retractors.

C. Troubleshooting

Laparoscopic procedures are inherently complex. Many things can go wrong. The surgeon must be sufficiently familiar with the equipment to troubleshoot and solve problems. Table 1.1 gives an outline of the common problems, their cause, and suggested solutions.

Table 1.1. Common problems, causes, and solutions.

Problem	Cause	Solution
1. Poor insufflation/loss of pneumoperitoneum	Carbon dioxide tank empty	Change tank
	Open accessory port stopcock(s)	Inspect all accessory ports—close stopcock(s)
	Leak in sealing cap or stopcock	Change cap or cannula
	Excessive suctioning	Allow abdomen to reinsufflate
	Instrument cleaning channel screw cap missing	Replace screw cap
	Loose connection of insufflator tubing at source or at port	Tighten connection
	Hasson stay sutures loose	Replace or secure sutures
2. Excessive pressure required for insufflation (initial or subsequent)	Veress needle or cannula tip not in free peritoneal cavity	Reinsert needle or cannula
	Occlusion of tubing (kinking, table wheel, inadequate size tubing, etc.)	Inspect full length of tubing, replace with proper size as necessary
	Port stopcock turned off	Assure stopcock is opened
	Patient is "light"	More muscle relaxant
3. Inadequate lighting (partial/complete loss)	Loose connection at source or at scope	Adjust connector
	Light is on "manual-minimum"	Go to "automatic"
	Bulb is burned out	Replace bulb
	Fiberoptics are damaged	Replace light cable
	Automatic iris adjusting to bright reflection from instrument	Reposition instruments, or switch to "manual"
	Monitor brightness turned down	Readjust setting

Problem	Cause	Solution
4. Lighting too bright	Light is on "manual-maximum"	Go to "automatic"
	"Boost" on light source activated	Deactivate "boost"
	Monitor brightness turned up	Readjust setting
5. No picture on monitor(s)	Camera control unit or other components (VCR, printer, light source, monitor) not on	Make sure all power sources are plugged in and turned on
	Cable connector between camera control unit and/or monitors not attached properly	Cable should run from "video out" on camera control unit to "video in" on primary monitor; use compatible cables for camera unit and light source
		Cable should run from "video out" on primary monitor to "video in" on secondary monitor
6. Poor-quality picture		
a. Fogging, haze	Condensation on lens of cold scope entering warm abdomen	Gently wipe lens on viscera; use antifog solution, or warm water; it is preferred not to wipe the lens on the viscera or the end of the telescope may get hot; gently wiping on liver or uterine surface is preferable
	Condensation on scope eyepiece, camera lens, coupler lens	Detach camera from scope (or camera from coupler); inspect and clean lens as needed
	Moisture in camera cable connecting plug	Use compressed air to dry out moisture (don't use cotton-tip applicators on multiprong plug)
b. Flickering electrical interference	Poor cable shielding	Replace video cable between monitors
	Insecure connection of video cable between monitors	Reattach video cable at each monitor

Continued

Table 1.1. Common problems, causes, and solutions. (*Continued*)

Problem	Cause	Solution
c. Blurring, distortion	Incorrect focus	Adjust camera focus ring
	Cracked lens, internal moisture	Inspect scope and camera, replace as needed
7. Inadequate suction/ irrigation	Occlusion of tubing (kinking, blood clot, etc.)	Inspect full length of tubing; if necessary, detach from instrument and flush tubing with sterile saline
	Occlusion of valves in suction/irrigator device	Detach tubing, flush device with sterile saline
	Not attached to wall suction	Inspect and secure suction canister connectors, wall source connector
	Irrigation fluid container not pressurized	Inspect compressed gas source, connector, pressure dial setting
8. Absent/inadequate cauterization	Patient not grounded properly	Assure adequate patient grounding pad contact, and pad cable–electro-surgical unit connection
	Connection between electrosurgical unit and pencil not secure	Inspect both connecting points
	Foot pedal or hand-switch not connected to electrosurgical unit	Make connection

D. Selected References

SAGES Continuing Education Committee. Laparoscopy Troubleshooting Guide. Santa
    Monica, CA: SAGES, 1995.
Sony Corporation. Rear panel diagram for Trinitron color video monitor, 1995.

2. Access to Abdomen

Nathaniel J. Soper, M.D.

A. Equipment

Two pieces of equipment are needed to gain access to the abdomen: an insufflator and a Veress needle (or Hasson cannula, see Section C).

1. Insufflator

Turn the insufflator on and check the carbon dioxide (CO_2) cylinder to ascertain that it contains sufficient gas to complete the procedure. If there is any doubt, bring an extra CO_2 container into the operating room. In any event, always keep a spare tank of CO_2 immediately available.

Check the insufflator to assure it is functioning properly. Connect the sterile insufflation tubing (with in-line filter) to the insufflator. Turn the insufflator to high flow (>6 L/min); with the insufflator tubing not yet connected to a Veress needle, the intra-abdominal pressure indicator should register 0 (Fig. 2.1).

Lower the insufflator flow rate to 1 L/min. Kink the tubing to shut off the flow of gas. The pressure indicator should rapidly rise to 30 mm Hg and flow indicator should go to zero (Fig. 2.2). The pressure/flow shutoff mechanism is essential to the performance of safe laparoscopy. These simple checks verify that it is operating properly.

Next, test the flow regulator at low and high inflow. With the insufflator tubing connected to the insufflator and the Veress needle (before abdominal insertion), low flow should register 1 L/min and at high flow should register 2 to 2.5 L/min; measured pressure at both settings should be less than 3 mm Hg. A pressure reading 3 mm Hg or higher indicates a blockage in the insufflator tubing or the hub or shaft of the Veress needle; if this occurs, replace the needle. Maximal flow through a Veress needle is only about 2.5 L/min, regardless of the insufflator setting, because it is only 14 gauge. A Hasson cannula has a much larger internal diameter and can immediately accommodate the maximum flow rate of most insufflators (i.e., >6 L/min).

During most laparoscopic procedures, the pressure limit should be set at 12 to 15 mm Hg; intra-abdominal pressures higher than this limit can diminish visceral perfusion and vena caval return.

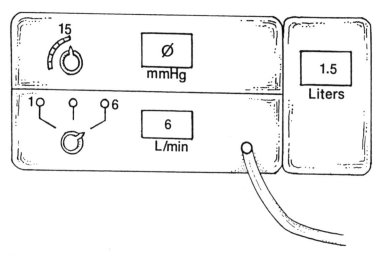

Figure 2.1. **Insufflator testing.** With insufflator tubing open (i.e., not connected to Veress needle) and flow rate set at 6 L/min, the intra-abdominal pressure reading obtained through the open insufflation line should be 0 mmHg.

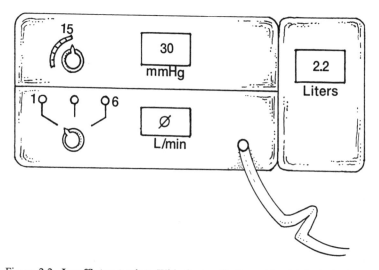

Figure 2.2. **Insufflator testing.** With the insufflation tubing kinked, the intra-abdominal pressure should rapidly rise (e.g., 30 mmHg), thereby exceeding the preset 15 mmHg pressure set point. The flow of CO_2 should immediately cease (0 L/min) and an alarm should sound.

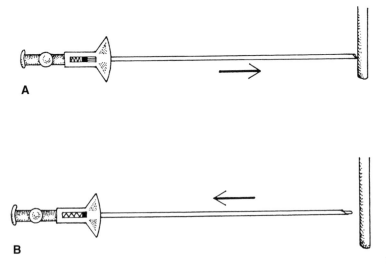

Figure 2.3. **Testing retractable tip of disposable Veress needle.** A. Blunt tip retracts as it contacts resistance (e.g., a knife handle). B. When the needle is pulled away from the point of resistance, the blunt tip springs forward and protrudes in front of the sharp edge of the needle.

2. Veress Needle

Both disposable and reusable (nondisposable) Veress needles are available. The former is a one-piece plastic design (external diameter, 2 mm; 14 gauge; length, 70 or 120 mm), whereas the latter is made of metal and can be disassembled. Check the Veress needle for patency by flushing saline through it. Then occlude the tip of the needle and push fluid into the needle under moderate pressure to check for leaks. Replace a disposable Veress needle if it leaks; check the screws and connections on a reusable Veress needle.

Next, push the blunt tip of the Veress needle against the handle of a knife or a solid, flat surface to be certain that the blunt tip will retract easily and will spring forward rapidly and smoothly (Fig. 2.3). A red indicator in the hub of the disposable needle can be seen to move upward as the tip retracts.

B. "Closed" Technique with Veress Needle

1. Umbilical Puncture

Place the supine patient in a 10- to 20-degree head-down position. If there are no scars on the abdomen, choose a site of entry at the superior or inferior border of the umbilical ring (Fig. 2.4). There are several ways to immobilize the umbilicus and provide resistance to the needle. The inferior margin of the umbilicus can be immobilized by pinching the superior border of the umbilicus between the thumb and forefinger of the nondominant hand and rolling the superior margin of the umbilicus in a cephalad direction. Alternatively, in the anesthetized patient, a small towel clip can be placed on either side of the upper margin of the umbilicus; this makes it a bit easier to stabilize the umbilicus and lift it upward.

Next, make a stab incision in the midline of the superior or inferior margin of the umbilicus. With the dominant hand, grasp the shaft (not the hub) of the Veress needle like a dart and gently pass the needle into the incision—either at a 45-degree caudal angle to the abdominal wall (in the asthenic or minimally obese patient) or perpendicular to the abdominal wall in the markedly obese patient. There will be a sensation of initial resistance, followed by a give, at two points. The first point occurs as the needle meets and traverses the fascia and the second as it touches and traverses the peritoneum (Fig. 2.5). As the needle enters the peritoneal cavity, a distinct click can often be heard as the blunt-tip portion of the Veress needle springs forward into the peritoneal cavity.

Connect a 10-mL syringe containing 5 mL of saline to the Veress needle. There are five tests that should be performed in sequence to confirm proper placement of the needle.

    a.   Aspirate to assess whether any blood, bowel contents, or urine enter the barrel of the syringe.

    b.   Instill 5 mL of saline, which should flow into the abdominal cavity without resistance.

    c.   Aspirate again. If the peritoneal cavity has truly been reached, no saline should return.

    d.   Close the stopcock and disconnect the syringe from the Veress needle, then open the stopcock and observe as any fluid left in the hub of the

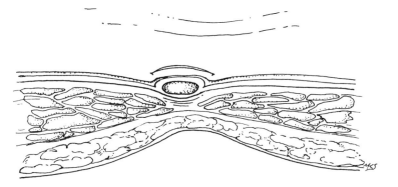

Figure 2.4. Site of Veress needle insertion at superior crease of umbilicus; stab incision has been made. Transverse oblique section at superior crease of umbilicus; the peritoneum is closer to the skin at the umbilicus and is more densely adherent to the umbilicus than at any other site along the abdominal wall.

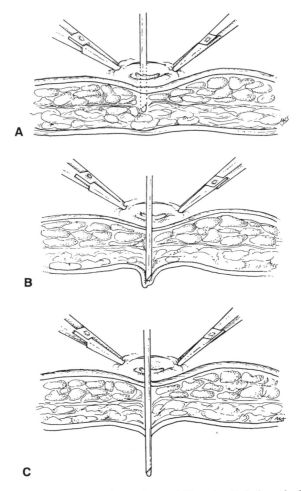

Figure 2.5. A. Veress needle inserted at umbilicus (sagittal view; the blunt tip retracts as it encounters the fascia of the linea alba). B. As the sharp edge of the needle traverses the fascia, the blunt tip springs forward into the preperitoneal space and then retracts a second time as it encounters the peritoneum. C. Blunt tip springs forward as Veress needle passes across the peritoneum to enter the abdominal cavity.

syringe falls rapidly into the abdominal cavity (especially if the abdominal wall is elevated slightly manually). This is the so-called drop test. If free flow is not present, the needle either is not in the coelomic cavity, or it is adjacent to a structure.

e.   Finally, if the needle truly lies in the peritoneal cavity, it should be possible to advance it 1 to 2 cm deeper into the peritoneal cavity without encountering any resistance. Specifically, the tip indicator or the hub of the needle should show no sign that the blunt tip of the needle is retracting, thereby indicating the absence of fascial or peritoneal resistance. Similarly, resistance to the needle tip may be caused by impingement on intra-abdominal viscera or adhesions.

Always be cognizant of anatomic landmarks when placing the needle, and carefully stabilize the needle during insufflation. Minimize side-to-side and back-and-forth movements of the needle to avoid inadvertent injuries.

After ascertaining that the tip of the Veress needle lies freely in the peritoneal cavity, connect the insufflation line to the Veress needle. Turn the flow of CO_2 to 1 L/min, and reset the indicator on the machine for total CO_2 infused to 0. The pressure in the abdomen during initial insufflation should always register less than 10 mm Hg (after subtracting any pressure noted when the needle was tested by itself and with the insufflator) (Fig. 2.6).

If high pressures are noted or if there is no flow because the 15 mm Hg limit has been reached, gently rotate the needle to assess whether the opening in the shaft of the needle is resting against the abdominal wall, the omentum, or the bowel. The opening is on the same side of the needle as the stopcock. If the abdominal pressure remains high (i.e., needle in adhesion, omentum, or preperitoneal space), withdraw the needle and make another pass of the Veress needle. If necessary, repeat this process several times until you are certain that the needle resides within the peritoneal cavity. Do not continue insufflation if you are uncertain about the appropriate intraperitoneal location of the tip of the Veress needle. Multiple passes with the Veress needle are not problematic, provided the error is not compounded by insufflating the "wrong" space.

One of the first signs that the Veress needle lies freely in the abdomen is loss of the dullness to percussion over the liver during early insufflation. When the needle is correctly placed, the peritoneum should effectively seal off the needle around the puncture site; if CO_2 bubbles out along the needle's shaft during insuf-

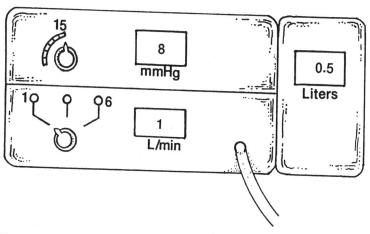

Figure 2.6. Initial insufflation readings: proper inflow at beginning of CO_2-Veress needle insufflation.

flation, suspect a preperitoneal location of the needle tip. During insufflation, a previously unoperated abdomen should appear to expand symmetrically, and there should be loss of the normal sharp contour of the costal margin.

Monitor the patient's pulse and blood pressure closely for a vagal reaction during the early phase of insufflation. If the pulse falls precipitously, allow the CO_2 to escape, administer atropine, and reinstitute insufflation slowly after a normal heart rate has returned.

After 1 L of CO_2 has been insufflated uneventfully, increase the flow rate on the insufflator to ≥6 L/min (Fig. 2.7). When the 15 mm Hg limit is reached, the flow of CO_2 will be cut off. At this point approximately 3 to 6 L of CO_2 should have been instilled into the abdomen (Fig. 2.8). When percussed, the abdomen should sound as though you are thumping a ripe watermelon.

2. Alternate Puncture Sites

Prior abdominal surgery mandates care in selection of the initial trocar site, and may prompt consideration of use of the open technique (see Section C). If the previous incisions are well away from the umbilicus, the umbilical site may still be used, with either a closed or open technique.

A midline scar in the vicinity of the umbilicus increases the risk that adhesions will be tethering intra-abdominal viscera to the peritoneum at that level. In this situation, the closed technique may still be used, but it is safer to use an alternate insertion site. This site should be well away from the previous scar and lateral to the rectus muscles, to minimize the thickness of abdominal wall traversed and avoid the inferior epigastric vessels.

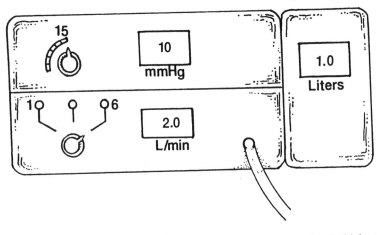

Figure 2.7. After 1 L has been insufflated, the set flow is increased to the highest rate.

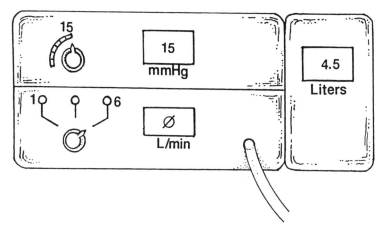

Figure 2.8. At 15 mm Hg intra-abdominal pressure, 3 to 6 L of CO_2 will usually have been insufflated; the registered flow should then fall to 0.

In general, patients with prior low vertical midline scars should be approached through a trocar placed at the lateral border of the rectus muscle in either the left or right upper quadrant (Fig. 2.9). With previous upper vertical midline incision or multiple incisions near the midline, the right lower quadrant site may be appropriate. Alternatively, it is possible to perform an open technique with the Hasson cannula.

Upper abdomen. In the upper abdomen, the subcostal regions are good choices. Carefully percuss the positions of the liver and spleen to avoid inadvertent injury to these organs, and decompress the stomach with a nasogastric or orogastric tube.

Lower abdomen. The right lower quadrant, near McBurney's point, is preferable to the left because many individuals have congenital adhesions between the sigmoid colon and anterior abdominal wall. Decompress the bladder when using a closed insertion technique at, or caudad to, the umbilicus.

3. Placement of Trocar

A wide variety of trocars are available in both disposable and reusable forms. Most have sharp tips of either a tapered conical or pyramidally faceted configuration. Several new disposable trocar designs incorporate unique design features such as direct serial incision of the tissue under visual control, or serial dilatation of the Veress needle tract. This section describes blind entry with the basic sharp trocar, with or without a "safety shield."

Always inspect the trocar to ensure that all valves move smoothly, that the insufflation valve is closed (to avoid losing pneumoperitoneum), and that any

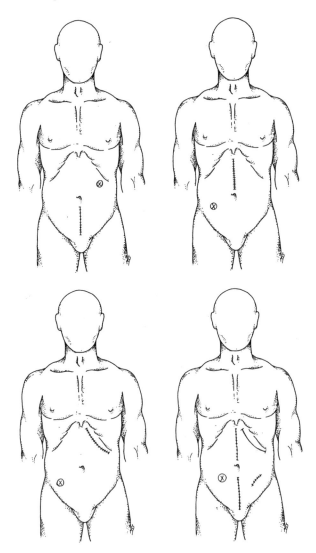

Figure 2.9. Optional trocar sites in previously operated abdomen. Consider the open-cannula technique.

safety shields work properly. Make sure you are familiar with the trocar; with the variety of designs available, it is not uncommon to be handed a different device (especially if it is less costly!).

Once you have attained a full pneumoperitoneum, remove the Veress needle. Most surgeons augment the pneumoperitoneum by lifting up on the fascia or abdominal wall to provide additional resistance against which to push the trocar. In a slender individual, the distance to the viscera and retroperitoneal structures is slight, and it is prudent to aim the trocar down into the pelvis. In an obese patient, this is less a problem and the trocar may be passed in a more direct path. There should be moderate resistance as the trocar is inserted. Excessive resistance may indicate that the trocar is dull or the safety shield (if one is present) has not released, or that the skin incision is too small. The resistance suddenly decreases when the peritoneum is entered. Open the stopcock briefly to confirm intraperitoneal placement by egress of CO_2. Insert the laparoscope and visually confirm entry. Connect the insufflator tubing and open the valve to restore full pneumoperitoneum. Subsequent trocars may be placed under direct vision.

If the trocar has been placed preperitoneally, it is rarely possible to redirect it. Time is often saved in this situation by converting to an open technique for placement of the initial trocar.

C. "Open" Technique with Hasson Cannula

The open (e.g., Hasson) cannula provides the surgeon with an alternative, extremely safe method to enter the abdomen, especially in a patient who has previously undergone intra-abdominal procedures. In these patients in particular, the blind insertion of a trocar would be fraught with the potential for injury to the abdominal viscera. Some surgeons use the open cannula routinely in all patients for placement of the initial umbilical trocar.

The open cannula consists of three pieces: a cone-shaped sleeve, a metal or plastic sheath with a trumpet or flap valve, and a blunt-tipped obturator (Fig. 2.10). On the sheath or on the cone-shaped sleeve, there are two struts for affixing two fascial sutures. The cone-shaped sleeve can be moved up and down the sheath until it is properly positioned; it can then be tightly affixed to the sheath. The two fascial sutures are then wrapped tightly around the struts, thereby firmly

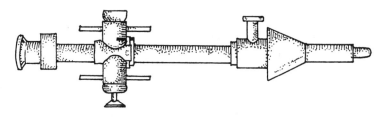

Figure 2.10. Open (Hasson) cannula, reusable type.

seating the cone-shaped sleeve into the fasciotomy and peritoneotomy. This creates an effective seal so the pneumoperitoneum will be maintained.

Make a 2- to 3-cm transverse incision at the selected entry site (in the quadrant of the abdomen farthest away from any of the preexisting abdominal scars or in the periumbilical skin crease if there has been no prior midline surgery). Dissect the subcutaneous tissue with scissors, and identify and incise the underlying fascia (Fig. 2.11). Exposure is usually facilitated by the use of small **L**- or **S**-shaped retractors. Gently sweep the preperitoneal fat off the peritoneum in a very limited area. Grasp the peritoneum between hemostats and open sharply. This incision should be just long enough to admit the surgeon's index finger. Confirm entry into the abdominal cavity visually and by digital palpation, to ensure the absence of adhesions in the vicinity of the incision. Place a #0 absorbable suture on either side of the fascial incision. Some surgeons place the fascial sutures first, use these to elevate the fascia, and then incise the fascia and peritoneum under direct vision.

Insert the completely assembled open cannula through the peritoneotomy with the blunt tip of the obturator protruding. When the obturator is well within the abdominal cavity, advance the conical collar of the open cannula down the sheath until it is firmly seated in the peritoneal cavity. Secure the collar to the sheath with the setscrew. Next, twist or tie the two separate fascial sutures around the struts on the sheath or collar of the open cannula, thereby fixing the cannula in place. Connect the CO_2 line to the sidearm port of the cannula and withdraw the blunt-tipped obturator. Establish pneumoperitoneum with the insufflator set at high flow. Increase intra-abdominal pressure to 12 to 15 mm Hg.

With facility, it is possible to establish pneumoperitoneum just as fast (or faster) with the open technique as can be done with Veress needle and "closed" trocar passage. Indeed, many surgeons consider this to be the safest way to establish pneumoperitoneum.

If a Hasson cannula is not available, a standard laparoscopic cannula can be placed by an open technique. For this maneuver, place two concentric pursestring monofilament sutures in the midline fascia and make an incision into the free peritoneal cavity through the center of the purse strings. Keep both sutures long, and pass the tails of each suture through a 3-cm segment of a red rubber catheter, thereby creating two modified Rummel tourniquets. Place a standard laparoscopic sheath (with the sharp-tipped trocar removed), cinch the pursestring sutures against the sheath, and secure by placing a clamp on the red rubber catheter. At the conclusion of the operation, close the fascia by simply tying the sutures.

D. Avoiding, Recognizing, and Managing Complications

1. **Bleeding from abdominal wall**
   a. **Cause and prevention.** This problem usually manifests itself as a continuous stream of blood dripping from one of the trocars, and/or as blood seen on the surface of the abdominal viscera or

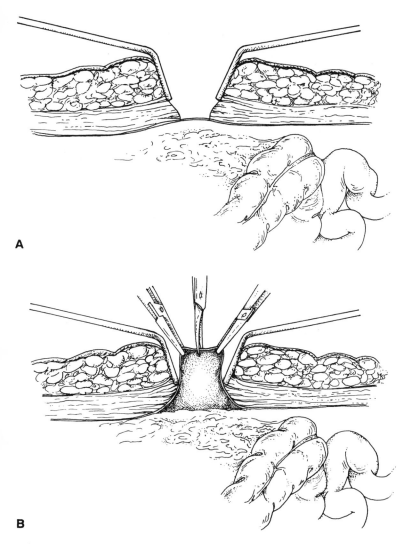

Figure 2.11. A. Retractors expose peritoneum. B. Peritoneum is elevated and sharply incised. Two fascial sutures are secured to the struts on the sheath of the open cannula. The cone-shaped sleeve is then pushed firmly into the incision and the setscrew is tightened, thereby fixing the sleeve to the sheath of the open cannula. The sutures are wound tightly around the struts on the sheath, thereby securing it in place and sealing the incision.

omentum. Less commonly, delayed presentation as a hematoma of the abdominal wall or rectus sheath may occur. This source of bleeding is usually the inferior epigastric artery or one of its branches. Abdominal wall hemorrhage may be controlled with a variety of techniques, including application of direct pressure with the operating port, open or laparoscopic suture ligation, or tamponade with a Foley catheter inserted into the peritoneal cavity (Fig. 2.12).

b.   **Recognition and management.** To determine the point at which the vessel is injured, cantilever the trocar into each of four quadrants until the flow of blood is noted to stop. Then place a suture

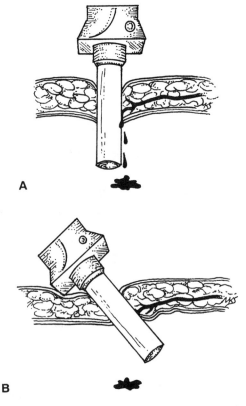

Figure 2.12.   A. Bleeding from a trocar site. B. Cantilevering the sheath into each quadrant to find a position that causes the bleeding to stop. When the proper quadrant is found, pressure from the portion of the sheath within the abdomen tamponades the bleeding vessel, thus stopping the bleeding. A stitch can then be passed under laparoscopic guidance.

in such a manner that it traverses the entire border of the designated quadrant. Specialized devices have been made that facilitate placement of a suture, but are not always readily available. The needle should enter the abdomen on one side of the trocar and exit on the other side, thereby encircling the full thickness of the abdominal wall. This suture can either be passed percutaneously using a large curved #1 absorbable suture as monitored endoscopically, or using a straight Keith needle passed into the abdomen and then back out using laparoscopic grasping forceps. The suture, which encircles the abdominal wall, is tied over a gauze bolster to tamponade the bleeding site.

2. **Visceral injury**
   a. **Cause and prevention.** Careful observation of the steps enumerated just will minimize the chance of visceral injury. However, placement of the Veress needle is a blind maneuver, and even with extreme care puncture of a hollow viscus is still possible.
   b. **Recognition and management.** If aspiration of the Veress needle returns yellowish or cloudy fluid, the needle is likely in the lumen of the bowel. Due to the small caliber of the needle itself, this is usually a harmless situation. Simply remove the needle and repuncture the abdominal wall. After successful insertion of the laparoscope, examine the abdominal viscera closely for significant injury.

      If, however, the laparoscopic trocar itself lacerates the bowel, there are four possible courses of action, depending on the surgeon's experience: formal open laparotomy and bowel repair or resection; laparoscopic suture repair of the bowel injury; laparoscopic resection of the injured bowel and reanastomosis; minilaparotomy, using an incision just large enough to exteriorize the injured bowel segment for repair or resection and reanastomosis (similar to the technique of laparoscopic-assisted bowel resection). If possible, leave the trocar in place to assist in identifying the precise site of injury.

3. **Major vascular injury**
   a. **Cause and prevention.** Major vascular injury can occur when the sharp tip of the Veress needle or the trocar nicks or lacerates a mesenteric or retroperitoneal vessel. It is rare when the open (Hasson cannula) technique is used.
   b. **Recognition and management.** If aspiration of the Veress needle reveals bloody fluid, remove the needle and repuncture the abdomen. Once access to the abdominal cavity has been achieved successfully, perform a full examination of the retroperitoneum to look for an expanding retroperitoneal hematoma.

      If there is a central or expanding retroperitoneal hematoma, laparotomy with retroperitoneal exploration is mandatory to assess for and repair major vascular injury. Hematomas of the mesentery and those located laterally in the retroperitoneum are generally innocuous and may be observed. If during closed insertion of the initial trocar there is a rush of blood through the trocar with associated hypotension, leave the trocar in place (to provide some tamponade of hemorrhage and assist in identifying the tract) and immediately perform laparotomy to repair what is likely to be an injury to the aorta, vena cava, or iliac vessels.

E. References

Baadsgaard SE, Bille S, Egeblad K. Major vascular injury during gynecologic laparoscopy: report of a case and review of published cases. Acta Obstet Gynecol Scand 1989;68:283–285.

Chapron CM, Pierre F, Lacroix S, Querleu D, Lansac J, Dubuisson J-B. Major vascular injuries during gynecologic laparoscopy. J Am Coll Surg 1997;185:461–465.

Deziel DJ, Millikan KW, Economou SG, Doolas A, Ko ST, Arian MC. Complications of laparoscopic cholecystectomy: a national survey of 4,292 hospitals and an analysis of 77,604 cases. Am J Surg 1993;165:9–14.

Oshinsky GS, Smith AD. Laparoscopic needles and trocars: an overview of designs and complications. J Laparoendosc Surg 1992;2:117–125.

Riza ED, Deshmukh AS. An improved method of securing abdominal wall bleeders during laparoscopy. J Laparoendosc Surg 1995;5:37–40.

Soper NJ. Laparoscopic cholecystectomy. Curr Probl Surg 1991;28:585–655.

Soper NJ, Odem RR, Clayman RV, McDougall EM, eds. Essentials of Laparoscopy, St. Louis: Quality Medical Publishing, 1994.

Wolfe WM, Pasic R. Instruments and methods. Obstet Gynecol 1990;75:456–457.

3. Abdominal Wall Lift Devices

Edmund K.M. Tsoi, M.D.
Claude H. Organ, Jr., M.D.

A. Types of Abdominal Wall Lifting Device

Although pneumoperitoneum provides exposure and access for laparoscopic surgery, it is associated with potential complications and restricts instrument design because of the constraints of working in a sealed environment. Various investigators have sought alternative ways to obtain exposure by a variety of abdominal wall lifting devices. These devices provide vertical upward forces to lift the anterior abdominal wall, creating a space similar to that produced by pneumoperitoneum. Virtually every open procedure can be performed with minimally invasive techniques using these devices, which thus may serve as a bridge between open and conventional laparoscopic techniques. In this section, three types of abdominal lifting devices are described, and the technique for using one type of device (planar lift) is given in detail. References at the end of the chapter give further information about the other techniques mentioned in the text.

1. **Low-pressure pneumoperitoneum and "sequential" lifting devices.** Before the current standard of 15 mm Hg was adopted, laparoscopists used pressures as high as 30 mm Hg. Recognizing the detrimental cardiopulmonary effects of such elevated pressures, the first abdominal wall lifting devices were developed to allow exposure without elevated intra-abdominal pressure. These devices were placed after exposure was obtained, and were variously employed with low-pressure pneumoperitoneum.

    a. A **T-shaped** instrument was described in 1991 by Gazayerli. This was designed to be inserted into a trocar port to elevate a small portion of the abdominal wall, thus providing an increased ceiling in obese patients, or allowing exposure without cardiopulmonary compromise in patients unable to tolerate more than 8 mm Hg. Low-pressure pneumoperitoneum was generally needed.

    b. A **U-shaped** retractor was described in 1992 by Kitano et al. Once the retractor is in place, the pneumoperitoneum can be evacuated and the procedure completed without insufflation.

    c. Banting and associates introduced a **falciform lift** device in 1993. Consisting of a long, curved 4-mm trocar to which a flexible polyethylene tube is attached, the device is inserted through a stab wound in the left upper quadrant lateral to the falciform ligament. Under direct visual guidance, the trocar,

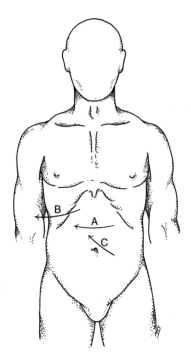

Figure 3.1. Diagram demonstrating the placement of flexible tubing or wire in combination with low-pressure pneumoperitoneum: (A) Banting et al. (1993), (B) Inoue et al. (1993), (C) Go et al. (1995). These techniques can be adapted using readily available materials and hence should be part of the laparoscopist's armamentarium.

together with the tubing, is passed beneath the falciform ligament to exit in the right upper quadrant. A similar design by Inoue et al., which is inserted from the supraumbilical area to the right upper quadrant, is reported to provide comparable exposure to intra-abdominal pressure of 15 mm Hg. Go and colleagues placed a Kirschner wire at the subcostal region for lifting to reduce the amount of pneumoperitoneum needed for adrenalectomy (Fig. 3.1). In 1997, Angelini and colleagues reported a new abdominal lifter, which is designed to be used with or without pneumoperitoneum. The authors suggested that by combining the use of an optical trocar and subcutaneous abdominal wall retraction, both pneumoperitoneum-related side effects and trocar injuries can be reduced.

2. **Gasless devices** are designed to provide the requisite exposure without utilizing pneumoperitoneum, even in the initial stages of exposure.

   a. In 1991, a Japanese team led by Nagai used an abdominal wall wire lifting system to perform laparoscopic cholecystectomy without pneumoperitoneum. In this system, Kirschner wires are placed in the subcutaneous tissue of the abdomen to act as a handle for lifting. Small winching devices connected by an L-shaped bar fixed to the side rail of the operating table are connected to the Kirschner wires to elevate the abdominal wall. An alternate wire lifting method reported by Hashimoto and associates in 1993 used two 30-cm stainless steel wires connected to a Kent retractor (Fig. 3.2). Subsequent refinements in the design of these wire lifting systems have simplified and extended their use to a wide variety of advanced laparoscopic procedures.

   b. **Planar lifting devices.** Chin and Moll developed a planar lifting technique to elevate the abdominal wall (see Chin et al., 1994). Unlike the wire lifting devices, the planar lifting device is widely available around the world; it can elevate the abdominal wall with minimal trauma and can be used in heavier patients. Because this device has gained wide acceptance, the technique of its use will

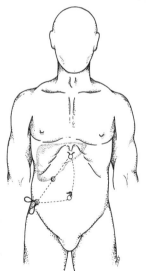
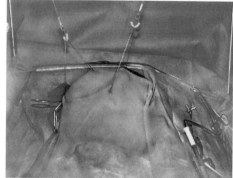

Figure 3.2. Hashimoto's subcutaneous lift method. (Reprinted with permission from Tsoi EKM, Organ CH Jr, eds., Abdominal Access in Open and Laparoscopic Surgery. New York: Wiley-Liss, 1996.).

be described in detail (Section B). The advantages and disadvantages of this device are summarized in Table 3.1.

c. **Conventional retractors** (Richardson, Army-Navy, and abdomainl wall retractors), used in strategically placed small incisions, can provide the necessary exposure for selected procedures performed under laparoscopic guidance with laparoscopic instruments. Examples of such procedures include laparoscopic cholecystectomy performed through the "minimal stress triangle" described by Tyagi et al. This corresponds to the subxiphoid regions and is bounded by the medial costal margins of the sixth to eighth ribs (Fig. 3.3). Similar approaches have been used for other procedures, including tube gastrostomy construction and closure of Hartmann's procedure. Using a modified conventional body wall retractor, video-assisted minilaparotomy had been used to perform donor nephrectomy.

Table 3.1. Advantages and disadvantages of planar abdominal wall lifting devices.

Advantages	Disadvantages
• Minimally invasive	• Exposure is less than ideal in the lateral gutters
• Avoids cardiopulmonary side effects associated with pneumoperitoneum	• Exposure is poor in patients with a muscular abdominal wall, such as highly conditioned athletes, or who are morbidly obese
• Operates in an isobaric environment (a "sealed environment" not needed)	• Abdominal contents can shift with mechanical ventilation
• Conventional as well as laparoscopic instruments can be used by surgeon interchangeably	• The abdominal lifting devices can be an obstacle for the surgeon during the conduct of the operation
• High-volume suction device and a large volume of irrigation solution can be used to maintain a clear operating field	
• Tactile examination of intra-abdominal contents is possible	
• Less contamination risk for the surgical team since the operating field is semienclosed in an isobaric environment where abdominal fluids will not be forced out of the abdomen by CO_2 insufflation	

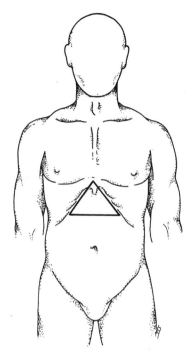

Figure 3.3. Boundaries of "minimal stress triangle" described by Tyagai et al. Incisions placed within this triangle are well tolerated.

B. Technique for Planar Lifting Device

The use of the most widely available device, both intra- and extra-peritoneally, is briefly described here. For further information, consult the references at the end of this section.

1. **Intraperitoneal exposure**
   a. Secure the abdominal wall lifter (Laparolift, Origin Medsystems, Lathrop Engineering, San Jose, CA) to a side rail before draping the patient. Prep the abdomen in the usual sterile fashion. Drape the abdominal wall lifter with a transparent plastic cover before the abdomen is draped.
   b. Initial access for the abdominal procedure is made in the peri-umbilical area.
   c. Make a small incision in the abdomen to allow the placement of the lifting device.
   d. Both fan-shaped and donut-shaped devices are available.

e. Open the device within the abdomen (Fig. 3.4).

f. Connect the planar lifting device to the Laparolift (Fig. 3.5). The Laparolift is then activated to raise the abdominal wall to provide exposure equivalent to 15 mm Hg of pneumoperitoneum.

g. Place the laparoscope into the abdomen through the periumbilical incision.

h. Insert additional instruments through trocars or small incisions (generally < 2 cm long). Through these incisions, both conventional laparoscopic instruments or extralong traditional instruments for open surgery may be used. A clear operating field can be maintained with traditional high-volume suction and copious irrigation without the fear of losing exposure.

2. **Extraperitoneal exposure**

a. Obtain initial access into the extraperitoneal space via a small incision (<2 cm).

b. Enter the extraperitoneal space by using a muscle-splitting technique.

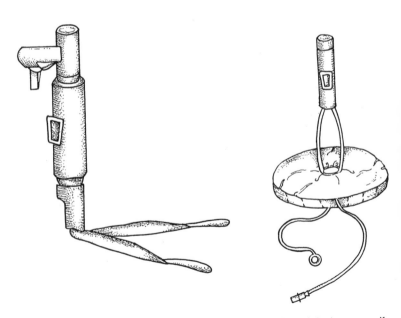

Figure 3.4. Both a fan-shaped and an inflatable donut-shaped device are available. Each is inserted into the abdomen in a collapsed configuration, then expanded within the peritoneal cavity.

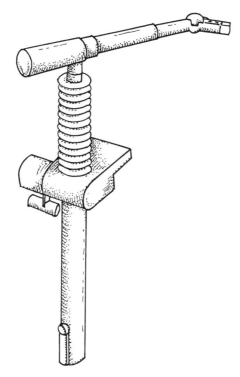

Figure 3.5. The Laparolift is a powered articulating arm that attaches to the operating table. The arm lifts up on the lifting device, providing upward displacement of the anterior abdominal wall and producing retraction.

    c.   Place a dissecting balloon into this newly created space to create an operating field.

    d.   Place the abdominal wall retractor into the extraperitoneal space through this incision. Connect the abdominal wall retractor to the lifter and elevate the abdominal wall to a maximum pressure equivalent to 15 mm Hg pneumoperitoneum.

    e.   Insert the laparoscope.

    f.   Place inflatable laparoscopic bowel retractors into the extraperitoneal space to push the peritoneum (together with the abdominal viscera) away from the operating field.

3.   **A wide variety of procedures** have been performed with the planar abdominal wall lift device (Table 3.2).

Table 3.2. Intra- and extraperitoneal procedures.

Intraperitoneal procedures	Extraperitoneal procedures
• Diagnostic laparoscopy	• Aortic surgery
• Gastrostomy	• Inguinal herniorrhaphy
• Gastrojejunostomy	• Retroperitoneal lymph node dissection
• Gastric resection	• Retroperitoneoscopic assisted spine surgery
• Nissen fundoplication	• Bladder neck suspension
• Closure of perforated viscus	
• Adrenalectomy	
• Appendectomy	
• Colectomy and colostomy	
• Derotation of volvulus	
• Cholecystectomy, and common bile duction exploration	
• Liver biopsy and resection	
• Pancreatic pseudocysts	
• Hysterectomy and myomectomy, tubal ligation, salpingo-oophorectomy	
• Closure of diaphragmatic hernia	
• Peritoneal dialysis catheter management	

C. Selected References

Angelini L, Lirici MM, Papaspyropoulos V, et al. Combination of subcutaneous abdominal wall retraction and optical trocar to minimize pneumoperitoneum-related effects and needle and trocar injuries in laparoscopic urgery. Surg Endosc 1997;11: 1006–1009.

Banting S, Shimi S, Velpen GV, et al. Abdominal wall lift: low pressure pneumoperitoneum laparoscopic surgery. Surg Endosc 1993;7:57–59.

Barr LL. Minimally invasive tube gastrostomy. Surg Laparosc Endosc 1997;7(4):285–287.

Chin AK, Eaton J, Tsoi EKM, et al. Gasless laparoscopy using a planar lifting technique. J Am Coll Surg 1994;178:401–403.

Gazayerli MM. The Gazayerli endoscopic retractor model I. Surg Laparosc Endosc 1991;1:98–100.

Go H, Takeda M, Imai T, et al. Laparoscopic adrenalectomy for Cushing's syndrome: comparison with primary aldosteronism. Surgery 1995;117:11–17.

Hashimoto D, Nayeem AS, Kajiwara S, et al. Laparoscopic cholecystectomy: an approach without pneumoperitoneum. Surg Endosc 1993;7:54–56.

Inoue H, Muraoka Y, Takeshita K, et al. Low pressure pneumoperitoneum using newly design devised flexible abdominal wall retractor. Surg Endosc 1993;7:133 (abstr).

Kitano S, Tomikawa M, Iso Y, et al. A safe and simple method to maintain a clear field of vision during laparoscopic cholecystectomy. Surg Endosc 1992;6:197–198.

Nagai H. Subcutaneous lift system (SCLS) for laparoscopic surgery. In: Tsoi EKM, Organ CH Jr, eds. Abdominal Access in Open and Laparoscopic Surgery. New York: Wiley-Liss, 1996;99–128.

Nagai H, Inaba T, Kamiya S, et al. An new method of laparoscopic cholecystectomy: an abdominal wall lifting technique without pneumoperitoneum. Surg Laparosc Endosc 1991;1:126 (abstr).

Navarra G, Occhionorelli S, Marcello D, et al. Gasless video-assisted reversal of Hartmann's procedure. Surg Endosc 1995;9:687–689.

Yang, SC, Retroperitoneoscopy assisted live donor nephrectomy: The Yonsei experience. J Urol 2001;165;1099–1102.

Tsoi EKM, Organ CH Jr, eds. Abdominal Access in Open and Laparoscopic Surgery. New York: Wiley-Liss, 1996.

Tyagi NS, Meredith MC, Lumb JC, et al. A new minimally invasive technique for cholecystectomy: subxiphoid "minimal stress triangle" microceliotomy. Ann Surg 1994;220(5):617–625.

Vazquez RM, Gireesan GT. Balloon-assisted endoscopic retroperitoneal gasless (BERG) technique for anterior lumbar interbody fusion (ALIF). The Northwestern experience. 2003;17(2):268–272.

Vogt DM, Goldstein L, Hirvela ER. Complications of CO_2 pneumoperitoneum. In: Tsoi EKM, Organ CH Jr, eds. Abdominal Access in Open and Laparoscopic Surgery. New York: Wiley-Liss, 1996;75–98.

4. Generation of Working Space: Extraperitoneal Approaches

David M. Brams, M.D.

A. Indications

Extraperitoneal endoscopic surgery (EES) was first described by Bartel in 1969. Wickham and Miller described the use of carbon dioxide (CO_2) and videoscopic control in 1993. Gaur introduced balloons for retroperitoneal dissection in 1993, and Hirsch and coworkers described the use of a trocar mounted balloon for extraperitoneal dissection in 1994. There are both advantages and disadvantages to this approach (Table 4.1).

Procedures in which EES has been utilized include the following:

1. Totally extraperitoneal (TEP) inguinal herniorrhaphy (see Chapter 40)
2. Retroperitoneal endoscopically assisted spine surgery
3. Renal surgery
4. Adrenalectomy (see Chapter 39.2)
5. Varicocele ligation
6. Pelvic lymph node dissection (see Chapter 38)
7. Bladder suspension
8. Aortoiliac surgery
9. Lumbar sympathectomy

B. Anatomic Considerations

Knowledge of anatomic landmarks is essential to orientation in the extraperitoneal space. The retroperitoneum can be divided into three spaces:

1. The retropubic space (space of Retzius) is the space between the pubic bone and the bladder. This space is obliterated by prior retroperitoneal urologic surgery such as retropubic prostatectomy.
2. The space of Bogros is lateral and cephalad to the space of Retzius.
3. The lumbar retroperitoneal space is the posterior continuation of the space of Bogros bounded by the vena cava and aorta medially, the psoas dorsally, the colon ventrally, and transversalis fascia laterally. This space contains the kidney, adrenal, ureter, and Gerota's fascia.

Table 4.1. Advantages and disadvantages of extraperitoneal endoscopic surgery.

Advantages	Disadvantages
• Decreased risk of bowel injury • Decreased problems with bowel retraction • Less postoperative ileus	• Small working space • Orientation can be confusing • Inadvertent entry into peritoneum causes loss of working space
• Closure of peritoneum not required when mesh implanted retroperitoneally • Less adverse hemodynamic effects from retroperitoneal insufflation	• Retractors often needed to displace peritoneal sac • Prior extraperitoneal dissection is a contraindication to this approach

C. Access to the Extraperitoneal Space

There are three basic ways to gain access to the extraperitoneal space.

1. The **open approach**
   a. Make a 2-cm incision overlying the space to be developed.
   b. Bluntly dissect down to the preperitoneal space and develop this space.
   c. Place a Hasson cannula or a structural balloon trocar (U.S. Surgical, Norwalk, CT).
   d. Continue dissection with laparoscope or balloon dissector (see dissection, below).
2. Use of a **lens-tipped trocar**
   a. Make a 12-mm skin incision over the desired location.
   b. Place a 0-degree laparoscope into a lens-tipped trocar.
   c. Use this to penetrate the layers of the abdominal wall under direct vision.
   d. Once the correct plane is achieved, place a Hasson cannula or structural balloon trocar and continue dissection (see Section D).
3. **Dulocq technique**
   a. Insert a Veress needle suprapubically through the fascial layers into the preperitoneal position. The needle will traverse two palpable points of resistance (the anterior rectus sheath and transversalis fascia).
   b. Insufflate 1 L of CO_2.
   c. Make a skin incision lateral to the midline.
   d. Insert a 10-mm trocar, directed caudad, until the gas-filled space is entered.
   e. Place the laparoscope into the trocar and use it to dissect the space while insufflating CO_2.
   f. The major **disadvantage** is that this procedure is relatively "blind" and risks visceral and vascular injury as well as

penetration of the peritoneum. If this technique is used to develop the lumbar retroperitoneal space, fluoroscopic control with ureteral and nephric imaging is essential.

D. Dissection of Extraperitoneal Space

Just as there are several techniques for obtaining access, there are several methods of dissection of the extraperitoneal space to create working room.

1. **Operating laparoscopes** have a 5-mm instrument channel (in a 10-mm laparoscope). These allow dissection under direct vision during insufflation of CO_2.

2. Alternatively, a **30-degree laparoscope** can be used alone to open the space by sweeping tissue away while insufflating CO_2.

3. **Balloon dissection** is the most popular, if most expensive, method of developing the extraperitoneal space. It *may* be beneficial, particularly early in the surgeon's experience with this procedure.

    a. Insert an air-inflated, trocar-mounted clear plastic dissection balloon into the space to be developed.

    b. Place a 0-degree laparoscope into the balloon and inflate the balloon while identifying landmarks (Fig. 4.1). Identify blood

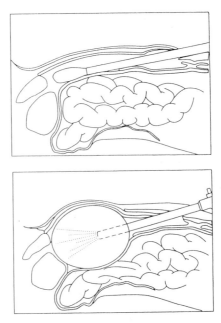

Figure 4.1. Balloon used to dissect extraperitoneal space. (Reproduced with permission from Tsoi EKM and Organ CH Jr, eds. Abdominal Access in Open and Laparoscopic Surgery. New York: Wiley-Liss, 1996.)

               vessels, such as the inferior epigastrics, and avoid injury by controlled insufflation.

    c.   Spherical balloon dissectors are most useful.

    d.   Kidney-shaped balloon dissectors are available for lateral dissection in bilateral hernia repair.

4.   Insert additional trocars under direct vision after creating the initial space. Develop and enlarge the extraperitoneal space with blunt dissection and atraumatic graspers, "peanut" dissection, and cautery scissors. A 30-degree laparoscope can facilitate exposure.

5.   Avoid subcutaneous emphysema by maintaining a tight seal between skin and fascia.

E. Maintenance of Extraperitoneal Space

There are several ways to maintain an extraperitoneal working space.

1.   Insufflation to 12 to 15 mm Hg CO_2 will maintain a working space.

2.   Planar abdominal wall-lifting devices (Laparolift, Origin Medsystems, Menlo Park, CA), allow gasless extraperitoneal endoscopy using conventional instruments (see Chapter 3).

3.   In TEP hernia repairs, the structural balloon trocar (U.S. Surgical, Norwalk, CT) replaces a Hasson cannula and displaces peritoneum posteriorly while providing a seal between skin and fascia and providing access for the laparoscope (Fig. 4.2).

4.   Peritoneal retraction devices are necessary to displace the peritoneal sac for lumbar and iliac extraperitoneal laparoscopy. Instruments such as the Laparofan (U.S. Surgical, Norwalk, CT) can be used in a gasless or gas extraperitoneal laparoscopic procedure.

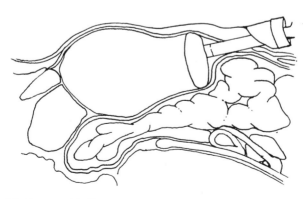

Figure 4.2. Structural balloon trocar provides access for gas insufflation and laparoscope while the peritoneum is retracted posteriorly.

F. Potential Problems

1. **Peritoneal holes** allow CO_2 to leak, creating a pneumoperitoneum that decreases the extraperitoneal space. Close peritoneal holes with a pretied suture ligature or by suturing them shut.

2. **Penetration into the peritoneal cavity** during access or dissection may necessitate a transabdominal laparoscopic or open procedure.

3. **Venous bleeding** can be controlled with cautery and will usually stop spontaneously in the limited extraperitoneal space.

4. Cautery, clips, harmonic scalpel or suture ligation can also be used to control **arterial hemorrhage**. Suction and irrigation should be available.

5. **Prior retroperitoneal dissection** obliterates the potential space and is a contraindication to the extraperitoneal approach.

6. **Prior intra-abdominal surgery** will fuse the peritoneum to the abdominal wall. Begin the dissection away from old scars and leave dissection of these areas for last. This will diminish the risk of peritoneal violation.

7. This procedure is more difficult in **obese patients**, as excess adipose tissue in the extraperitoneal space will obscure planes and landmarks.

8. In retroperitoneal approaches to the kidney and adrenal, **laparoscopic ultrasound** can be used to help identify structures.

G. Selected References

Arregui ME, et al. Laparoscopic mesh repair of inguinal hernia using a pre-peritoneal approach: a preliminary report. Surg Laparosc Endosc 1992;2:53–58.

Bartel M. Die Retroperitoneskopie. Eine endoskopische Methode zur Inspektion und bioptischen Untersuchung des Retroperitonealen. Zentralbl Chir 1969;94:377–383.

Coptcoat MJ. Overview of extraperitoneal laparoscopy. Endosc Surg 1995;3:1–2.

Eden CG. Alternative endoscopic access techniques to the retroperitoneum. Endosc Surg 1995;3:27–28.

Farinas LP, et al. Cost containment and totally extraperitoneal laparoscopic herniorrhaphy. Surg Endosc 2000;19:37–40.

Gaur DD. Laparoscopic operative retroperitoneoscopy. Use of a new device. J Urol 1993;148:1137–1139.

Himpens J. Techniques, equipment and exposure for endoscopic retroperitoneal surgery. Semin Laparosc Surg 1996;3(2):109–116.

Hirsch IH, Moreno JG, Lotfi MA, et al. Controlled balloon dilatation of the extraperitoneal space for laparoscopic urologic surgery. J Laparoendosc Surg 1994;4:247–251.

McKernan JG, Laws HL. Laparoscopic repair of inguinal hernias using a totally extraperitoneal prosthetic approach. Surg Endosc 1993;7:26–28.

Tsoi EKM, Organ CH Jr, eds. Abdominal Access in Open and Laparoscopic Surgery. New York: Wiley-Liss, 1996.

Wickham JEA, Miller RA: Percutaneous renal access. In: Payne SR, Webb DR, eds. Percutaneous Renal Surgery. New York: Churchill Livingstone, 1983;33–39.

5. Hand-Assisted Laparoscopic Surgery

Benjamin E. Schneider, M.D.

A. Background

Hand-assisted laparoscopic surgery (HALS) or handoscopic surgery was described in the 1990s as a means of overcoming obstacles presented by laparoscopic procedures. Surgeons first introduced the gloved hand into the abdomen via a mini laparotomy to improve depth perception, regain tactile sensation, aid in tissue extraction, and reduce operative time. This method relied upon tight apposition of the abdominal wall tissues against the surgeon's forearm to maintain pneumoperitoneum. Difficulty with air leak and the inability to advance or withdraw the hand without sudden loss of pneumoperitoneum led necessarily to the development of hand-assist devices.

B. Indications

HALS may be useful when a large fascial defect is required for tissue extraction, tactile feedback is required, or the laparoscopic approach is not progressing and otherwise would require conversion to an open procedure. The advantages and disadvantages of HALS are listed in Table 5.1. For some procedures, the nondominant hand is the gentlest retracting device available. HALS has been applied to procedures in all the following areas:

1. Nephrectomy
2. Colorectal surgery
3. Splenectomy
4. Gastroesophageal surgery
5. Gynecology
6. Aortoiliac surgery
7. Pancreatic surgery
8. Hepatic resection

Applications to specific procedures are discussed and illustrated in the chapters that follow.

C. Devices

A number of hand port devices are commercially available. Among the commonly used devices reported in the literature are:

Table 5.1. Advantages and disadvantages of hand-assisted laparoscopic surgery.

Advantages	Disadvantages
• Allows for tactile sensation	• Hand encroaches upon intra-abdominal working space
• Specimen retrieval and anastomosis may be performed through hand port site	• May reduce benefit of laparoscopic procedure secondary to larger hand port
• Rapid control of bleeding by direct pressure	• Large incision at risk for incisional hernia
• Improved depth perception and shortened learning curve	• Device-dependent air leak
• Avoidance of conversion to open approach	• Ergonomically unfavorable, leading to shoulder and forearm fatigue and strain
• Reduced operative time	• May increase cost

GelPort (Applied Medical, Rancho Santa Margarita, CA)
Lapdisc (Ethicon Endosurgery, Cincinnati, OH)
HandPort System (Smith & Nephew, Inc., London, England)
Dexterity Pneumo Sleeve device (Dexterity Inc., Roswell, GA)
Omniport (Advanced Surgical Concepts, Dublin, Ireland)
Intromit Device (Medtech Ltd, Dublin, Ireland)

D. Technical Tips for HALS

Strategic placement of the hand port is critical to avoid obstruction of the laparoscopic view and to improve ergonomics. Concepts crucial to HALS success include the following:

1. Remember the concept of triangulation and place the incision in a location that allows the nondominant hand to assist much like a standard laparoscopic instrument.
2. For procedures involving dissection in several abdominal quadrants, placement of the port centrally or in the midline will improve the range over which the hand may function.
3. For procedures centered upon a single quadrant, place the hand port at the periphery.
4. For certain cases, consider placing the hand port so that the incision is oriented to facilitate conversion to an open approach or for specimen extraction.
5. The necessary incision is typically 7 to 8 cm in length, corresponding to the surgeon's glove size.
6. Use a darker colored glove to reduce reflective glare in the operative field.

Figures 26.7 and 26.8 show the application of one system to facilitate HALS gastrectomy.

G. Selected References

Darzi A. Hand-assisted laparoscopic colorectal surgery. Surg Endosc 2000;14:999–1004.

HALS Study Group. Hand-assisted laparoscopic surgery vs standard laparoscopic surgery for colorectal disease: a prospective randomized trial. Surg Endosc 2000; 14:896–901.

Hanna GB, Elamass M, Cuschieri A. Ergonomics of hand-assisted laparoscopic surgery. Semin Laparosc Surg 2001;8:92–95.

Leahy PF, Bannenberg JJ, Meijer DW. Laparoscopic colon surgery: a difficult operation made easy. Surg Endosc 1994;8:992.

Meijer DW, Bannernberg JJ, Jakimowicz JJ. Hand-assisted laparoscopic surgery. Surg Endosc 2000;14:891–895.

Southern Surgeon's Club. Handoscopic surgery: a prospective multicenter trial of a minimally invasive technique for complex abdominal surgery. Arch Surg 1999;134: 477–485.

Targarona EM, et al. Hand-Assisted Laparoscopic Surgery. Arch Surg 2003;138:133–141.

Wolf JS Jr, Moon TD, Nakada SY. Hand assisted laparoscopic nephrectomy: comparison to standard laparoscopic nephrectomy. J Urol 1998;160:22–27.

6. Principles of Laparoscopic Hemostasis

Richard M. Newman, M.D.
L. William Traverso, M.D.

Hemostasis has been a key issue from the beginning of laparoscopic general surgery. Precise visualization during laparoscopy can be attained only in a bloodless field. Hemostasis must be attained at the first attempt because the limitations of access and a small visual field make a second chance much more risky. Prevention of bleeding requires the timely and appropriate use of technology, much of it newly modified for the laparoscopic approach. We present a variety of major hemostatic modalities that can be used during laparoscopic surgery. Monopolar electrosurgery is emphasized because it is employed during most operations. A practical section on the laparoscopic control of active bleeding is included.

A. Mechanical Methods of Hemostasis

1. Endoscopic clip appliers were developed to facilitate ligation of small (2–5 mm) structures such as ducts and vessels. Metallic (titanium) clips are most often used. The common disposable clip appliers contain up to 20 clips and are available in a 10-mm diameter instrument or more recently a 5-mm instrument. High-quality reusable clip appliers available from several manufacturers allow the surgeon to considerably decrease costs, but these instruments have to be reloaded after each clip is fired.

Clip application requires visualization of both sides of the clip to ensure adequate tissue purchase and to prevent inadvertent clipping of nontarget tissues. The theoretic risk of clip migration into duct and vascular structures has prompted the advent of absorbable clips usually made of polyglycolic acid polymers (Dexon or Vicryl). These clips have identical ligation properties but may pose less threat to adhesion formation or migration.

Inadvertent mechanical ischemic necrosis can occur from metallic clips placed in close proximity to bile duct or bowel wall, resulting in stricture or perforation. These complications can be prevented by better visualization of the structures prior to placing the clip or not relying on a clip when a loop ligature would be more applicable.

2. Linear stapling devices are used primarily for anastomotic purposes, but these instruments are of vital use to prevent major hemostatic complications. Endoscopic linear cutters that deploy two or three parallel rows of hemostatic staples (height = 2.5 mm vascular or 3.5 mm intestinal applications) on each side of a simultaneously produced linear incision are available to facilitate *hemostatic* division of tissue. The tissue is atraumatically crushed between the stapler and its opposing anvil before firing. With effective cutting lengths from 30 to 60 mm, larger vessels or highly vascularized tissues such as in the lung or bowel mesentery can be controlled and divided in one motion. Inspection of both sides of the device is mandatory prior to firing unintended structures to prevent damage to and to ensure that the entire target tissue is within the active area as indicated in marks or numbers on the side of the device. Depending on the manufacturer, the shaft diameters of these linear cutters vary from 12 to 18 mm. Appropriately large trocars must be strategically placed to allow opening of the active portion of these instruments within the desired operative field.

   3.   **Pretied suture loops** with slip knots have a limited use in *primary* hemostasis because the vessel or vascular pedicle must first be divided, grasped, and then encircled with the loop. This leaves a bleeding structure for a period of time while being encircled by the loop. However, the loops are extremely useful to secure bleeding vessels after transection. The bleeding structure is grasped, and the field irrigated. An atraumatic grasper is passed through another port, and passed through the loop of the suture ligature. The first grasper is then released, and the second grasper grasps the stump of the bleeding structure. The loop is snugged down over the shaft of the instrument, securing the bleeder. More information about specific strategies is given in Section D.

   4.   **Simple ligatures** need to be nothing more than a long suture (at least 42 in.) that is passed around a clearly dissected vessel. Care must be taken to employ an instrument to act as a fulcrum and prevent "sawing" of the tissue or vessel as the ligature is being passed and redelivered out the entry port (for an extracorporeally tied knot). If an intracorporeal knot is planned, the suture material should be fashioned about 6 in. long (length of a scalpel handle is a convenient reference). Further details on knot tying are given in Chapter 7, Principles of Tissue Approximation).

   5.   **Suturing** in laparoscopic surgery has been used primarily for tissue approximation. When tissue approximation will result in hemostasis, suturing is a valuable adjunct. An obvious example is the use of figure-of-eight suture to secure a bleeding vessel.

B. General Principles of Energy-Induced Hemostasis

   Even before the laparoscopic revolution, surgeons relied on energy sources, rather than mechanical means such as sutures and clips, to aid in hemostasis in the operating room. Electricity, ultrasonic waves and laser energy have been the energy sources most often employed. These modalities all function by the same mechanism, i.e., an energy source is delivered to tissue, resulting in hemostasis via a predictable pattern of **thermal tissue destruction**. The temperature attained in the tissues may predict the changes observed:

   1.   **At 45°C**, collagen uncoils and may reanneal, allowing apposed edges to form covalent bonds and fuse.

2. **At 60°C**, irreversible protein denaturation occurs and coagulation necrosis begins. This is characterized by a blanching in color.
3. **At 80°C**, carbonization begins and leads to drying and shrinkage of tissue.
4. **From 90° to 100°C**, cellular vaporization occurs and vacuoles form and coalesce, leading to complete cellular destruction. The surgeon observes a plume of gas and smoke that represents water vapor.
5. **Above 125°C**, complete oxidation of protein and lipids leads to carbon residue or eschar formation.

Variations in the rate of tissue heating and the degree of thermal spread accounts for the differences seen between the various energy sources. A basic understanding of how each energy source functions, as well as its limitations and potential complications, allows the surgeon to make careful choices of operative settings and avoid potential problems.

C. Energy Sources Used in Laparoscopy

1. Electrical Energy

Electrosurgery has evolved into the gold standard of energy sources for achieving laparoscopic hemostasis because of familiarity, cost, and versatility. The **active electrode** is a conductor connected directly to the **electrosurgical unit (ESU)** generator. The **return electrode** is a conductor that accepts current from the active electrode and returns it to the ESU, thus completing the electrical circuit. The configuration of the active and return electrode determines the path of current or "mode" during electrosurgery.

a. **In monopolar electrosurgery**, current from the active electrode (hook, spatula, or any instrument tip such as insulated scissors) is allowed to return through the patient to a large return electrode (grounding plate). The path taken by the current is unpredictable, but generally diffuses over a large-enough volume of tissue outside the immediate surgical field.
b. **In bipolar electrosurgery** the active electrode can be intermittently apposed to the return electrode (usually in a forceps-type arrangement). Electrical current passes between the electrodes to complete the circuit, and flow of current beyond the surgical field is minimal.

Bipolar coagulators have been employed for some time by gynecologists in performing laparoscopic tubal ligations. More recently, bipolar vessel sealing devices such as the Liga-Sure (Balleylab, Boulder CO) have become available. The unique feature of this type of device is the automatic generator feedback control that allows for high current and low voltages. The high current melts the collagen and elastin within the tissue bundles and creates a seal that allows the effected tissue to be divided hemostatically. As the resistance in the tissues changes with desiccation, the generator adjusts the pulsed energy up to the appropriate level. The bipolar vessel sealing device is approved by the U.S. Food and Drug Administration for vessels up to 7 mm in diameter.

Monopolar electracautery is used for most applications in laparoscopic surgery. The ESU can produce two general types of current, depending on the waveform:

a. **Cutting current (continuous wave, high frequency, lower voltage)** produces focal and rapid tissue heating and a cutting effect. Heating occurs so rapidly that there is minimal associated coagulation necrosis and therefore no hemostasis.

b. **Coagulating current (pulsed waveform, low frequency, high voltage)** produces a slower heating that causes protein denaturation. Hemostasis occurs via coagulative necrosis in and around the target tissue. In laparoscopic surgery, owing to its limited visual field, the control of even the smallest amount of bleeding is desirable; therefore, pure cutting is rarely employed. Often the cutting mode is turned completely off by the surgeon and all laparoscopic electrosurgery is performed with the pulsed coagulation current.

Since laparoscopic surgery requires cutting as well as coagulation, how can monopolar electrosurgery accomplish bloodless division of tissues using pure coagulating current? The answer is through current density. Reducing the surface area of the active electrode increases current density. This produces a cutting effect as is illustrated by a comparison of Figures 6.1 and 6.2.

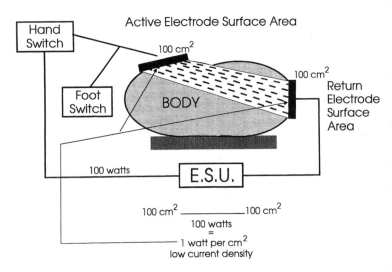

Figure 6.1. Low current density is depicted schematically by showing an active electrode with a large surface area (low density of current in the larger surface area). The amount of current going through the patient at this electrode is only 1 Watt/cm². Heating that may occur here is low and will not result in coagulation or cutting. (Airan and Ko, 1995.)

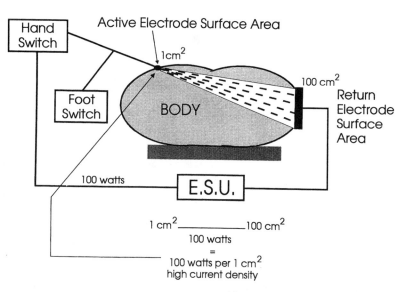

Figure 6.2. High current density: the active electrode has been decreased to 1 cm², raising the current density at this site to 100 W/cm². Now there will be a rapid rate of temperature rise—quickly with a thin-wire electrode (cutting results) and less quickly with a broad electrode (coagulation will result). (Airan and Ko, 1995.)

Although any instrument can act to deliver a high current density with monopolar electrosurgery the following familiar example of a hook or **L**-shaped electrode will further illustrate the concept of current density:

A cutting effect is achieved when the tip of the **L**, with its small surface area and thus high current density, is applied to Glisson's capsule at the side of the gallbladder to produce a cutting effect utilizing coagulation current (Fig. 6.3). Care must be taken when a pointed electrode is used in this regard because this high-current-density situation can lead to powerful cutting with little control. Puncture of the gallbladder could result at this point.

Coagulation or desiccation can be achieved by using the outer side of the L with its greater surface area and thus lower current density (Fig. 6.4). The use of the active electrode in this manner leads to slower tissue heating and controlled tissue division; and a coagulation effect as the gallbladder is freed from the liver bed. The same effect may be obtained by use of a spatula tip, or the side of a scissors blade connected to electrocautery.

Fulguration is achieved with high power and low current density at the target tissue. This is done by using the outer side of the **L** or other blunt-shaped electrode, but at the same time increasing the distance from a specific bleeding point (liver bed in the example). The increased distance allows further

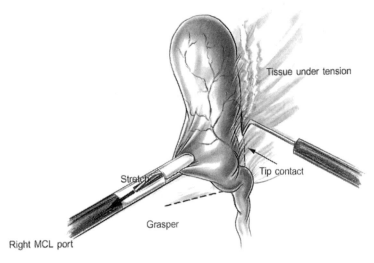

Figure 6.3. Using a coagulation current (low current and high voltage) to achieve a cutting effect by placing the tissue on tension and using the tip of the thin-wire electrode, resulting in a high current density. (Airan and Ko, 1995.)

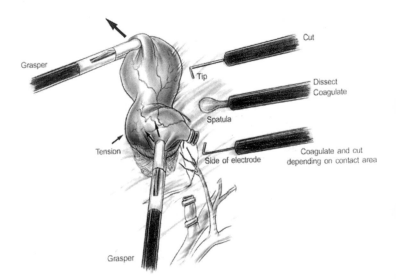

Figure 6.4. By using just coagulation current, different tools can vary the contact area (and the contact density) to achieve cutting or coagulation. The current is constant and only the contact density changes, resulting in the "art" of bloodless electrosurgical dissection with little energy loss for coagulation. (Airan and Ko, 1995.)

dissipation of the current density, as the current must arc from the active electrode to the liver bed. The result is superficial tissue heating, producing a carbonized eschar and hemostatic coagulum.

These physical principles can be used to predict potential areas of danger as discussed in the next section.

Complications of monopolar electrosurgery. Early attempts to utilize electrosurgery for laparoscopic applications were associated with specific complications. To complete the monopolar circuit, electrical current will take the lowest resistance pathway back to the return electrode. This may result in injuries if current density is sufficiently high. Factors that contribute to this include insulation failure, direct coupling, and capacitive coupling.

1. Insulation failure. Laparoscopic instruments and electrosurgical electrodes are insulated to prevent electrical current from contacting surrounding structures. Even a break in insulation too small to be noted by the casual observed can allow electrical current to leak or arc to a metal trocar or to an adjacent viscus such as the colon. Current pathway and density are unpredictable in this situation. Often the tissue effects of this current are out of the visual field of the operator. This obvious source of patient injury can be minimized by routine inspection of the insulation covering all electrosurgical instruments. Current leakage detectors can be used to test adequacy of insulation. Modern ESUs have automatic leakage detection that results in system shut off.

2. Direct coupling. This phenomenon occurs when one conductive material touches or arcs to another one. Some surgeons use the direct coupling effect to coagulate tissue grasped in one instrument by touching it with a different active electrode. Caution must be employed, since this potentially can lead to current directed toward nontarget structures. The laparoscopic visual field must ensure that no conductive part of any instrument is in contact with nontarget structures prior to ESU activation.

3. Capacitive coupling. This phenomenon will explain many of the otherwise inexplicable injuries reported to have occurred during laparoscopic monopolar electrosurgery. It occurs when a conductor has intact insulation but passes through an noninsulated conductor such as a metal trocar, operative laparoscope, or metal suction–irrigation tip. Electromagnetic forces produce a coupled current on the outside conductor, resulting in transfer of energy to unintended structures outside the visual field. The high voltages that are produced when activating the electrode without tissue contact or when the power setting is increased during fulguration may produce capacitively coupled currents strong enough to produce injury. One way to limit these injuries of types is to use all-metal (conductive) trocar systems. The large conductive surface area dissipates energy via the abdominal wall to the return electrode, preventing a capacitor from forming around the metal instrument. In plastic (nonconductive) trocar systems, the trocar itself does not generate capacitively coupled currents; however, metal suction irrigation tips and operative laparoscopes do, and because the current cannot escape safely through nonconductive trocar to the abdominal wall, it must find its way back to the return electrode through nontarget tissue, potentially injuring it. In hybrid systems, such as metal trocars with plastic abdominal wall stabilizers, capacitively coupled currents on the metal trocar cannot get back to the return electrode safely via the abdominal wall and must go through another unpredictable and potentially dangerous route. Knowledge and attention to the physics behind electrosurgery help the surgeon to prevent potentially dangerous situations.

2. Argon Beam Coagulator

An argon beam coagulator uses electrical circuitry essentially similar to monopolar electrosurgery. The difference is that ionized, pressurized argon gas completes the circuit between the active electrode and the target tissue, resulting in denaturation of surface tissue proteins and formation of a shallow eschar. At the same time, argon gas pressure displaces oxygen from the combustion area so that heat is confined to a lower temperature range. This pressurized gas beam also displaces blood and fluid away from the bleeding source and allows for more precise fulguration.

Some studies have shown that this energy source saves time and minimizes blood loss in common laparoscopic applications like cholecystectomy. The significantly limited cutting ability, lack of tactile feedback, and concerns about gas embolism limit routine use. The argon beam coagulator may have a role in advanced procedures requiring solid organ parenchyma dissection via a minimally invasive approach.

3. Ultrasonic Energy

Ultrasonically activated "scissors" and related instruments use high frequency (>20,000 Hz) to induce mechanical vibration at the cellular level. The result is localized heat generation from friction and shear, producing a predictable pattern of thermal destruction. The first surgical use of ultrasonic mechanical energy was in the form of the **cavitational ultrasonic aspirator** (CUSA Technologies, Salt Lake City, UT), Ultrasonic waves from the CUSA (23,000 Hz) cause cavitational fragmentation of parenchyma, which the apparatus then aspirates from the field. The more resistant vessels and ducts remain and are clipped and divided. Though helpful in open solid-organ surgery, CUSA has limited laparoscopic applications.

The modern laparoscopic **ultrasonic scalpel** became available in 1992. It was developed to provide precise hemostatic cutting and coaptive coagulation, but it also provided a lower risk of lateral thermal injury associated with electrocautery and laser. The ultrasonic scalpel functions by providing electrical energy to a piezoelectric ceramic element that expands and contracts rapidly (55,500 Hz). This mechanical energy is transduced to an imperceptibly moving blade that oscillates to produce heat secondary to friction and shear when coupled to tissue.

In general, lower power causes slower tissue heating and thus more coagulation effect. Higher power setting and rapid cutting is relatively nonhemostatic. In these regards ultrasonic energy is similar to other forms of energy-induced hemostatic modalities. Aside from the power setting, hemostatic tissue effect can be enhanced by blade configuration and tissue traction in a manner analogous to electrode design for electrosurgery (i.e., the broader the blade, the more coagulation effect).

Blade configuration has a significant effect on device performance.

a. **A single blade or hook type of blade** is used much as one uses the familiar monopolar electrosurgical appliances. The activation of the blade creates localized heating and hemostatic cutting of tissues where tension and countertension (supported tissues) can be created. The cutting effect on tissue not under tension is minimal. Cutting speed is inversely proportional to hemostasis. Coagulation can be achieved with a lower power setting and utilizing the broader side of the activated blade. This allows slower tissue heating that denatures protein to form a hemostatic coagulum.

b. **Ultrasonic coagulating shears** were developed because of the difficulty of applying ultrasonic energy to unsupported tissues. The shears have one ultrasonically activated blade that can be rotated to expose the tissue to a sharp edge, a rounded edge, or a flat edge. A nonactivated pad opposes the active blade and acts as an anvil to hold tissue, enabling the creation of frictional and shearing forces necessary for cutting and coagulating.

In the cutting mode, tissue is compressed against the **sharp blade** edge and cut when the shears are activated. Hemostasis is minimal. In the hemostatic cutting/coagulation mode, moderately to highly vascular tissues are grasped to oppose tissue between one of two blade shapes—the **rounded** or the **flat** blade and the tissue pad. The frictional energy developed between the blade and pad produces coaptive coagulation of vessels in the shears. For vascularized adipose tissue, the **rounded** blade with a medium power setting usually suffices. A larger vessel of around 2 mm would require the **flat edge** of the activated blade on a low power setting to slowly coagulate the vessel. As coagulation occurs, added pressure can be applied opposing the tissue to the anvil, and this will facilitate cutting the coagulated vessel. The opened, activated blade of the coagulating shears can also be used alone as a single blade.

In the single-blade mode, ultrasonic cutting and coagulation offer little advantage over electrosurgery for routine laparoscopic applications. The real advantage to the coagulation shears is the hemostatic division of unsupported vascular tissues with the coagulating shears. This versatile tool can grasp, bluntly dissect, sharply cut, and coagulate. This technology adds efficiency (with less instrument exchanges) and could reduce costs (by not using expensive disposable clips or staplers). This technology has enjoyed recent application during minimally invasive surgery for division of the short gastric vessels, the mesentery, or the tissues around the adrenal gland.

Because energy (heat production) is localized in ultrasonic wave production, the risk of lateral thermal injury is minimized. There are no electrical grounding devices required and coupling is not a problem. The laparoscopic use of ultrasonic energy appears to be a safe and versatile energy source that has a specialized role to the advanced laparoscopic surgeon. This role may expand as the costs for this technology decrease and the units become more widely available and more familiar to the surgical community.

D. Laparoscopic Prevention and Management of Active Hemorrhage

Develop an operative plan that includes visualizing and identifying all structures prior to division. Avoid bluntly avulsing adhesions and adipose tissue; contained small vessels tend to retract into the divided tissue and are difficult to control. Safe application of energy to the area of the vascular structure to be divided, prior to its division, helps to prevent uncontrolled hemorrhage. If one is unsure about the vascularity of a structure, it is better to mechanically occlude it with a clip prior to its division or at least to have enough of the structure dissected free to allow manual control if bleeding is observed after division.

Even with the most careful dissection and hemostatic techniques, laparoscopic surgeons will occasionally encounter active bleeding. Often this leads to panic, culminating in conversion to an open procedure, or, worse, the dangerous and random application of energy and/or clips in the direction of the presumed bleeding point. It is far better to have a plan for bleeding before it occurs. The following stepwise guidelines for the control of active hemorrhage emphasize visualization. When bleeding is encountered and not easily controlled by electrocautery, the surgeon should:

1. Try to visually identify the bleeding source without moving any instrument that is providing retraction.
2. Avoid the "redout" that occurs when even small amounts of blood obscure the laparoscope's view.
3. Suction with a large-bore suction cannula (10 mm, if available). Irrigation, while helpful in identifying slow bleeding sites, should be minimized in active bleeding because it adds to blood/liquid pool and potentially can splatter onto the laparoscope and limit visualization.
4. Apply a 5-mm atraumatic grasper to the bleeding point when identified. A maneuver specifically for uncontrolled bleeding from the cystic artery may be useful—use the gallbladder infundibulum grasped by the instrument through the right upper quadrant trocar to apply direct pressure over the actively bleeding area. This allows the surgeon to stop the bleeding temporarily by tamponade, aspirate blood from the field, clean the laparoscope, and place new instruments or trocars to control the cystic artery. (This maneuver was first described by S. T. Ko and M. C. Airan, personal communication.)
5. **If the vessel cannot be controlled under direct vision in step 4, the surgeon should convert to an open procedure.**
6. If the bleeding point is controlled with a grasper, the next step is to evaluate the trocar situation. Simply put, there must be enough trocars to control the bleeding and to introduce a clip applier or suture ligature. Most commonly, a clip will be used to control the bleeding. A trocar must be available that can accommodate a clip applier, without removing any instruments that are providing retraction. It is better to add a trocar than to compromise by moving instruments and risk losing control of the bleeder. The added port should be placed at least 15 cm away from the bleeding site in a vector that will allow torque-free

clipping and at right angles to the laparoscope (so that the placement of a clip can be easily observed).
7.   Place a clip precisely on both sides of the atraumatic grasper with care not to torque or displace the controlling grasper.
8.   Irrigate and evaluate. If it is not certain whether the clips are providing secure hemostasis or whether they have injured surrounding structures, the procedure should be converted to open exploration.

E. Selected References

Airan MC, Ko ST. Electrosurgery techniques of cutting and coagulation. In: Arregui ME, Fitzgibbons RJ Jr, Katkhouda N, McKernan JB, Reich H, eds. Principles of Laparoscopic Surgery. New York: Springer–Verlag, 1995;30–35.

Hunter JG. Laser or electrocautery for laparoscopic cholecystectomy. Am J Surg 1991;161:345–349.

Hunter JG, Trus TL. Lasers and argon beam in endoscopic surgery. In: Toouli J, Gossot D, Hunter JG, eds. Endosurgery. New York: Churchill Livingstone, 1996;103–109.

Matthews BD, Pratt BL, Backus CL, et al. Effectiveness of ultrasonic coagulating shears, Liga-Sure Vessel Sealer, and surgical clip. Application in biliary surgery: a comparative analysis. Am Surg 2001;67:901–906.

Melzer A. Endoscopic instruments—conventional and intelligent. In: Toouli J, Gossot D, Hunter JG, eds. Endosurgery. New York: Churchill Livingstone, 1996;69–95.

Tucker RD, Voyles CR. Laparoscopic electrosurgical complications and their prevention. AORN J 1995;62:51–71.

Voyles CR. Education and engineering solutions for potential problems with laparoscopic monopolar electrosurgery. Am J Surg 1992;164:57–62.

7. Principles of Tissue Approximation

Zoltan Szabo, Ph.D., F.I.C.S.

A. Laparoscopic Suturing and Intracorporeal Knot Tying: General Principles

Although the benefits to the patient of laparoscopic suturing are considerable, demands placed on the surgeon are high. For the patient, care is improved by a greater precision of repair, because of better access and minimized access trauma. These results are accomplished by a surgeon confronted with the technical challenge of performing intracorporeal maneuvers using optical equipment, illumination, and video that present a less-than-ideal visual image, as well as limited movement because of the use of awkward instrumentation. These challenges can be overcome by performing a mental choreography of step-by-step maneuvers, and by working slowly, precisely, and patiently to master this new skill.

In laparoscopic tissue approximation, intracorporeal suturing and knot tying are the preferred methods because they are highly adaptable, flexible, economical, and use commercially available equipment. In deep crevices and other situations, intracorporeal knotting is possible but extracorporeal knotting may be preferred. In either instance, learning to suture requires special attention to the setup, visual perception, eye–hand coordination, and motor skill. These factors are described and illustrated individually.

1. **Position of the surgeon** in relation to the instruments and intended suture line determines the challenge and result. Visual path, coaxial alignment, and triangulation of camera and operating ports are crucial aspects of the setup. Positioning of the laparoscopic and instrument ports has the same function as in open surgery. The camera is positioned midway between two instrument ports; this setup mimics the normal relationship between the eyes and two hands. The three ports should be shifted in unison when the surgeon attempts to suture in a different location. The port positioning, relative to the proposed suture line, provides the proper angle of access and a fulcrum for the instruments (Fig. 7.1).

2. **Visual perception** is a significant factor because the operative field is viewed indirectly through a closed-circuit video system. A three-chip camera and high-resolution 19-in. monitor, viewed from a distance of no more than 5 to 6 ft, are used. One of the challenges of this procedure is the magnification of a small operative field, inversely proportional to the magnification power and which is requires a proportionate reduction of the speed and range of instrument movement to maintain control. The visualization is affected by:

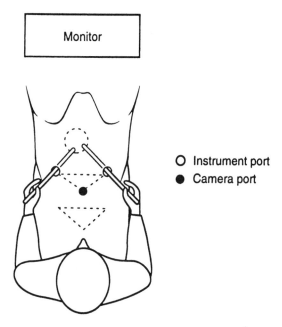

Figure 7.1. Position of the surgeon for visual path coaxial alignment. Note the triangulation of camera and operating ports, which corresponds to triangulation of the surgeon's eyes and two hands. The surgeon, target tissue, suture line, and monitor are aligned.

    a. Use of optical instrument (laparoscope)
    b. Flat two-dimensional (2D) image on the video monitor
    c. Ability of the surgeon to adjust to the new viewing perspective
The following factors are present with this visualization setup:
    a. Details are magnified and become more appreciable, but the visual field becomes proportionately smaller and depth of the field more shallow.
    b. At higher magnification, the image becomes better defined with an improved, three-dimensional (3D) effect.
    c. The surgeon must readjust eye–hand coordination and adapt to the speed of instrument movement.
    d. Visual health, 20/20 vision, corrected by regular visits to the optometrist, as well as well-rested eyes, determine the success of a flawless procedure. Visual memory and a trained eye are the ideal cognitive instruments.
  3. **Eye–hand coordination:** Movements in laparoscopic surgery should be slower than in open surgery. Seeing one's movements magnified on a screen shows how quickly instruments are perceived to move, even at a normal pace. By slowing the pace of movement, control is restored

and sufficient visual information gathered, but operating time is increased. Eliminating unnecessary movements and tightly choreographing the procedure are of assistance in achieving the most efficient use of time. Choreographed movements increase precision and eliminate unnecessary movements. A proper formal training course and supervised practice improve the overall success and efficiency of these procedures.

4. **Motor skill** determines the performance of a successful surgical procedure. Balance and coordination of perception, decision making, and motor skill orchestrate the ideal procedure. The motor skills one has developed over a lifetime in everyday practice are distorted because laparoscopic surgery requires adjustment to a magnified field. Magnification and the use of foot-long instrumentation create an imbalance, compensated for by a special approach referred to commonly as principles of microsurgery. Familiarity with open microsurgery eases the transition from open, traditional surgery to laparoscopic surgery.

B. Equipment and Instrumentation

1. **Video equipment.** High-standard optical and video components are preferred owing to the greater visual acuity necessary to visualize the tissue layers accurately and track needle and suture movements.

2. **Suturing instruments** have various designs. The handle can have either a pistol grip or an in-line, coaxial handle, with or without a ring to hold it securely (the ringless handle affords greater maneuverability). The **assisting grasper**, used by the nondominant hand, handles the tissue and is more curved and pointed. The **needle driver**, used by the dominant hand, handles the needle and suture material and is short and powerful, with a curved and blunt tip.

3. **Trocars** should be slightly longer than the thickness of the abdominal wall, with a preferred diameter of 5 to 10 mm. Trocars that are too long interfere with instrument mobility and function by preventing the opening of the instrument jaws and minimizing movement in the abdomen.

4. **Geometry of the needle tip** controls the characteristics of the tissue penetration and size and shape of the tunnel cut. To minimize tissue trauma, ease of penetration is important in laparoscopic surgery. Stronger, sturdier needles are required to penetrate thicker tissue layers; smaller, thinner needles are required to penetrate delicate tissues. A needle tip with a high tapering ratio, or "taper cut" tip, penetrates tissue layers more readily.

5. Suture material is selected based upon favorable tissue response, handling characteristics, and visibility, and for its particular attributes such as absorbability, strength, and tissue reaction. Pitch-black or fluorescent white sutures are preferred, rather than colorless sutures, because visibility is limited in laparoscopic surgery. The handling characteristics of the 2-0 and 3-0 silk are optimal for folding and bending

memory. Alternatives such as monofilament polypropylene, polydiox-anone, and nylon can be too stiff to readily knot intracorporeally.

6. **Needle handling and passage.** Bicurve geometry affects the handling and scooping characteristics of the needle and can be adapted easily to particular tissues and their access requirements. In difficult situations, one should take the time necessary to reexamine simple movements to execute them efficiently. Entrance and exit bites and knot tying are the main movements repeated during tissue approximation. In this technique, the needle follows the tip in passing through tissue layers with the least amount of trauma and effort if the tissue resistance, needle tip, grasping point, and direction of force are assembled on the same axis. The directions of (1) the needle tip and (2) the needle-driving force must be identical; the optimal direction for both is 90°, head-on against tissue resistance (Fig. 7.2). If these directions are dissimilar, the needle will be deflected within the instrument jaws.

7. **A high level of concentration** is integral to performing even simple needle-driving maneuvers when one is working in a magnified field. Indirect tissue manipulation further complicates this.

8. **Needle driver design.** The length of the laparoscopic needle driver results in the transmission of reduced force from the surgeon's hands to the instrument jaws, and consequently diminished needle control as well. To compensate, surgeons seek instruments whose jaws are more powerful, and features such as the self-righting jaws may be of interest. As mentioned previously, needle control is accomplished by correctly directing the needle tip as well as the needle-driving force. Without awareness of these factors, application of increased force can easily result in tissue damage or a poorly constructed suture line. In addition, instruments designed to hold the needle more forcefully tend to be have a more cumbersome lock mechanism whose deployment can also play a role in increased tissue trauma. Finally, a self-righting design involves positioning the needle in one position, perpendicular to the instrument shaft. This is helpful when the suture line is aligned perpendicular to the resulting needle plane; when it is not, this

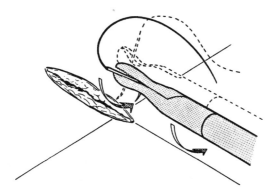

Figure 7.2. Pushing the needle head-on against tissue resistance.

feature can be counterproductive. Therefore, one should develop and learn needle-driving techniques that depend more on skill than on gadgetry.

C. Knot Tying

Both intracorporeal and extracorporeal knot tying techniques have an important role in laparoscopic surgery. For most purposes, intracorporeal knot tying is preferred. **Intracorporeal knots** are placed by a process that duplicates the methods used during open surgical procedures. Intracorporeal tying is faster and requires less suture. **Extracorporeal tying** involves knots designed to slip in only one direction; both categories of knotting methods are illustrated in Figures 7.3 and 7.4.

An **extracorporeal knot** is tied externally and slid down to the tissue with the aid of a knot pusher. This method requires long threads and, whereas extra-

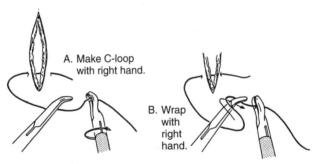

Figure 7.3. A. **Square and surgeon's knot. overhand flat knot.** (1) *Starting position*: Create a C-loop as the right instrument reaches over to the left side of the field, grasps the long tail, and brings it back to the right below the short tail. This loop must be in a horizontal plane; otherwise it will be difficult to wrap the thread. If a monofilament material is used, the right instrument can rotate the thread counterclockwise until it lies flat against the tissue. The right instrument holds the long tail, and the left instrument is placed over the loop. The short tail should be so long that it cannot be pulled out of the tissue accidentally, but not so long that its end requires additional effort to locate it. A large loop should be used to allow ample space to maneuver both instruments, and movements should be slowed to retrieve the short tail without disturbing the setup. Use the right instrument to wrap the long tail around the stationary tip of the left instrument. Rotate the right instrument forward (clockwise) to create an arch in the suture and assist the wrapping motion. Keep the jaws of the instruments retrieving the short tail closed until ready to grasp the tail. In the inset, the right instrument is shown wrapping the suture around the left instrument twice, which creates a surgeon's knot.

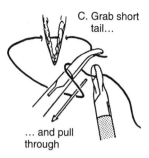

C. Grab short
tail...

... and pull
through

Figure 7.3. (2) *Grasping the short tail*: Both instruments should move together toward the short tail. This process prevents a tight noose from forming around the instrument, making it difficult to reach the short tail. Grasping the short tail near the end avoids formation of an extra loop (or "bow tie") when one is pulling the suture through.

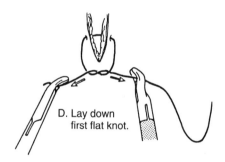

D. Lay down
first flat knot.

Figure 7.3. (3) **Completing the first flat knot.** Pull the short tail through the loop and hold it still, while the long tail continues to be pulled, parallel to the stitch, until the knot is cinched down. The end will be hard to find if the tail is too long. The left instrument then drops the short tail, and the right instrument keeps its grasp on the long tail. This illustrates the surgeon's knot that has been created.

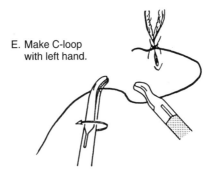

E. Make C-loop
with left hand.

Figure 7.3. B. **Second opposing flat knot.** (1) *Creating the reversed C-loop, wrapping the thread, and grasping the short tail.* The reversed **C-loop** is created as the right instrument is brought to the left side of the field under the short tail and rotated clockwise 180 degrees. The right instrument transfers the long tail to the left instrument. The right instrument is placed over the reversed C-loop and the left instrument wraps the thread around the right instrument. The tips of both instruments are moved in unison toward the short tail, which is grasped with the right instrument.

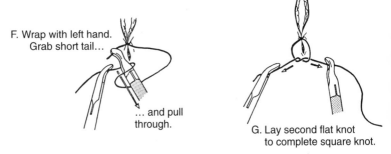

F. Wrap with left hand.
Grab short tail…

… and pull
through.

G. Lay second flat knot
to complete square knot.

Figure 7.3. (2) *Completing the second knot.* Pull the short tail through the loop; then pull both tails in opposite directions, parallel to the stitch, with equal tension. Verify that the knot is configured correctly as the knot cinches up.

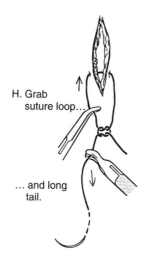

H. Grab
suture loop...

... and long
tail.

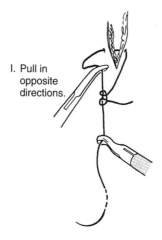

I. Pull in
opposite
directions.

Figure 7.3. C. **Slip knot for the square knot.** (1) *Starting position and pulling.* To convert the square knot (locking configuration) to a slip knot (sliding configuration), both instruments must grasp the suture on the same (ipsilateral) side. One instrument grasps the thread outside the knot and the other in the suture loop (between the knot and issue). Both instruments pull in opposite directions (perpendicular to the stitch). A snapping or popping sensation often can be felt, and the short tail may flip up. The knot now resembles a pretzel. If the conversion does not occur after several attempts, try the maneuver on the other side of the knot. Conversion is easier on monofilament suture.

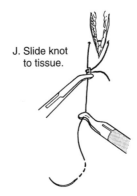

J. Slide knot
to tissue.

Figure 7.3. (2) *Pushing the slip knot.* The right instrument maintains its grasp on the tail and pulls tightly. The left instrument now assumes the role of a knot pusher and advances the knot to the tissue by sliding on the tail. A common error is caused by the surgeon inadvertently grasping the knot or tail, rather than solely pushing the knot forward.

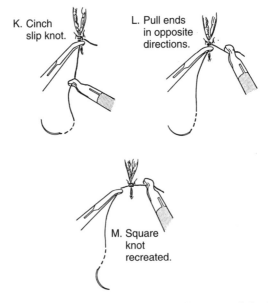

K. Cinch
slip knot.

L. Pull ends
in opposite
directions.

M. Square
knot
recreated.

Figure 7.3. (3) *Cinching down.* Cinch down the slip knot until the tissue edges have been approximated to the desired tension. Recenter the knot and recheck the tension. Before making additional overhand throws, reconvert the slip knot to a square knot as follows: both instruments regrasp the tails in opposite directions, parallel to the stitch in the same way as when the square knot was tried originally. An additional overhand knot is necessary on top, and is tied in the same manner as the first throw [Fig. 7.3.A(1)–(3)].

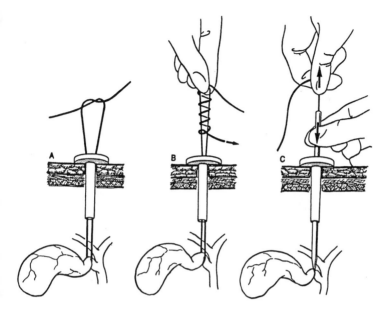

Figure 7.4. **Extracorporeal knot.** Bring a long suture into the laparoscopic field, leaving its tail outside the port. Place the stitch; then bring the needle end out through the same port. Create a Roeder knot by tying an overhand knot and then wrapping the suture tail back around both arms of the loop three times. Lock the suture by bringing the tail back through the large loop, between the last two twists of the wrap. Slide the knot down with a plastic applicator rod or knot pusher.

corporeal knotting appears to be a simpler approach, it requires a systematic and careful application to avoid traumatizing the tissues and contaminating or damaging the suture.

While other types of extracorporeal knots have now been introduced for laparoscopic surgery, the Roeder knot was the first and is widely used. It was developed around the turn of the century and incorporated into laparoscopic practice before intracorporeal knotting was developed. This knot is also used in commercially available, pretied suture ligatures; the method is described and illustrated in Figure 7.4. Another common method of extracorporeal knot tying uses a modified square knot, with each throw tied extracorporeally.

D. Suturing Techniques

Suturing and intracorporeal knotting are among the final challenges of a laparoscopic procedure, and the surgeon's skill and endurance. A surgeon's skill level can be measured to some degree, e.g., by the ability to tie a square knot correctly in 30 seconds or less. These techniques are a challenge that can be achieved with confidence and skill only after 20 to 40 hours of formal training (as observed by the author). Intracorporeal knotting can be the beginning and finishing points of continuous and interrupted suture lines.

Tissues should be prepared and positioned in anticipation of either interrupted sutures, continuous sutures, or a combination of both types, so minimal tension exists.

1. **Interrupted suturing.** When constructing a linear suture line, the factors involved in creating entrance and exit bites include length of incision or laceration, type of tissue layers to be approximated and their function, needle and thread combination selection, and length of suture.

   a. Place the instrument port positions so the laparoscope port is in line with the needle driver—parallel with the suture line—and the assisting grasper port is 45 to 90 degrees apart.

   b. Place the needle perpendicular to the suture line, with the ports at least 6 in. apart. The entrance and exit scooping motion should follow a 3 o'clock-to-9 o'clock direction relative to the surgeon's frontal plane.

   c. Interrupted stitches can be used with a suspension slip-knot technique if tension is present in the tissues or in instances of poor visibility or access. Evenly spaced stitches approximate the tissue precisely without tension.

2. **Continuous suturing.** This type of suture is more rapid, yet more difficult to accomplish correctly. The technique begins and ends with an anchoring knot, the last of which can be tied to the loop of the last stitch. Tissue edges must be identified by shifting the tension on the suture loops carefully as the approximation continues.

3. **Suture choice** is a necessary component, because monofilament and braided materials behave differently. Monofilament is stiff, springy, and slides smoothly through tissue. Braided material, which can drag through the tissue and lock unexpectedly, can be more cumbersome to work with because each stitch must be taut before proceeding to the next.

4. **Anastomosis.** Laparoscopic ductal anastomosis is a challenge that can be accomplished by using methods from microvascular anastomoses and duplication of open surgical techniques. It can be performed end to end, end to side, or side to side.

   a. End-to-end anastomosis is the preferred method for approximating ducts of equal caliber and wall thickness. The number of stitches, their configuration, and size of the bites are calculated depending on the function of the structure. Either interrupted or continuous sutures can be used. Interrupted sutures provide better precision and control; continuous sutures are performed more rapidly, but are less forgiving.

   b. Conduits with different lumina and wall thickness can be joined with end-to-side anastomosis in a less-invasive procedure.

   c. Side-to-side anastomosis is a practical method for conduits that lie side by side. This method of approximation is similar to the end-to-side anastomosis.

E. Tissue Gluing

Tissue adhesives can be used in combination with other techniques as an aid that provides a hemostatic or hydrostatic seal. Fibrin and other glues have been used but have not gained popularity for tissue approximation because they need anchoring or primary stitches to secure the tissue edges. As the boundaries of laparoscopic surgery expand, there will be more possibilities for, and developments in, tissue approximation. However, the traditional concept of hand suturing and square/surgeon's knot method of securing two suture ends will undoubtedly remain the most popular, as it has already endured centuries of trials.

F. Stapling

As a method of tissue approximation, stapling borrows the same principle as used in open surgery, but is technically more demanding and more expensive. Some general principles are discussed in Chapter 6, and details are given in Chapters 12 to 46, II–IX, which describe procedures in which stapling is used routinely.

Despite the use of staplers in laparoscopic procedures, the ability for surgeons to place stitches and tie knots should not be compromised. Staplers may lead to complications, and the surgeon must be aware of tissue ischemia if a procedure is inadequate. Proper mastery and knowledge of these techniques, with many prior successful practice runs, is essential for their use.

G. Selected References

Bowyer DW, Moran ME, Szabo Z. Laparoscopic suturing in urology: a model for vesicourethral anastomosis following radical prostatectomy. Min Invas Ther 1993;4(2):165–170.

Buncke HJ, Szabo Z. Introduction to microsurgery. In: Grabb WC, Smith JW, eds. A Concise Guide to Plastic Surgery. Boston: Little, Brown, 1980;653–659.

Cuchieri A, Szabo Z. Tissue Approximation in Endoscopic Surgery. Oxford: Isis Medical Media, 1995.

Guthrie CC. Blood vessel surgery and its application: a reprint. Pittsburgh: University of Pittsburgh, 1959;1–69.

Szabo Z. Laparoscopic suturing and tissue approximation. In: Hunter JG, Sackier JM, eds. Minimally Invasive Surgery. New York: McGraw-Hill, 1993;141–155.

Wolfe BM, Szabo Z, Moran ME, Chan P, Hunter JG. Training for minimally invasive surgery: need for surgical skills. Surg Endosc 1993;93–95.

8. Principles of Specimen Removal

Daniel J. Deziel, M.D.

A. General Considerations

A major advantage of laparoscopic surgery, small incisions, must be balanced with the need to remove and preserve specimens that may be larger than the laparoscopic port site. Specimens vary in dimensions, physical characteristics (hollow versus solid), and ease of extraction. Special considerations apply to specimens that may be infected or malignant, where improper removal may lead to wound infection or tumor dissemination. The best method for removal depends on the size, location, and nature of the specimen and whether there is a need to preserve the specimen intact for pathologic evaluation.

B. Routes of Specimen Removal

Ideally the site selected for specimen removal should be along the path of least resistance that produces the least pain, prevents contamination, and provides the best cosmesis. If a specimen cannot be removed from the abdominal cavity immediately after it has been resected, it must be secured in a position that will permit ready identification and retrieval later. Several potential routes for removal of abdominal and pelvic specimens are listed in Table 8.1 and will be considered individually here.

1. **Small specimens** can be removed directly through an appropriate cannula (usually 10 mm or larger) with or without a reducing sleeve. Use a toothed grasper to secure the specimen as it is retrieved under direct laparoscopic visualization and control. Open the valve mechanism of the cannula to allow the specimen to pass through unimpeded, if a reducing sleeve is not used.

2. Specimens originally **larger than the size of the cannula** can be retrieved **at the port site** by several methods:

   a. Reduce the size of the specimen while it is still within the peritoneal cavity; that is, remove contents of hollow structures (fluid, stones) or cut up solid structures. This technique permits removal without enlarging the incision. The major disadvantages include the risk of losing portions of the specimen and contamination of the peritoneal cavity. This method may be appropriate for the removal of specimens such as lymph node packets and benign solid tumors of moderate size.

   b. Exchange the existing cannula for a **larger cannula** at the port site (20–40 mm), by placing it over a blunt probe with a tapered introducer. This method protects the wound from direct contact with the specimen. A major disadvantage is that the specialized cannulae are not

Table 8.1. Routes for removal of abdominal and pelvic specimens.

- Port sites
- Separate abdominal wall incisions
- Transanal (if colon resection performed)
- Transvaginal (via culpotomy incision)

always available. This method is sometimes used for removal of specimens such as an inflamed appendix, gallbladder, fallopian tube, and ovary.

c. **Exteriorize portions of the specimen** and then remove the contents so that the specimen can be pulled through the port site. This is most commonly used for removal of the gallbladder following laparoscopic cholecystectomy. Hold the specimen firmly against the end of the cannula as both are pulled out together under laparoscopic visualization. Grasp a portion of the gallbladder outside of the abdomen with clamps and open the gallbladder. Aspirate fluid, and remove stones (fragmenting them if necessary) with stone forceps or ring forceps. This technique avoids enlarging the incision and requires no special equipment. However, it risks wound contamination and is tedious if the stones are multiple or large.

d. **Enlarge the incision at a port site.** This is perhaps the simplest, most efficient, and most commonly used method in many circumstances. It works particularly well at umbilical or other midline port sites since only a single fascial layer requires division. Either stretch the fascia or elevate it with a right-angled clamp and divide it with scissors or a scalpel. Perform this maneuver under direct laparoscopic visual control, with the specimen held in a relaxed manner (**not** taut against the abdominal wall) to avoid puncturing the specimen. This is frequently the best method of removing a large, stone-filled gallbladder. This is also the typical method for removing larger organs such as the colon and spleen.

The length of incision necessary in these cases varies but is usually only several centimeters. When the port site incision is not midline, use a muscle spreading technique to avoid dividing abdominal wall musculature. During colectomy the colon is often exteriorized through an extended port site incision prior to complete resection. After resection the anastomosis can be constructed extracorporally. These are considered "laparoscopically assisted" operations.

A disadvantage of this technique is the loss of pneumoperitoneum that occurs during specimen extraction. To reestablish the pneumoperitoneum, completely close the incision if that port site is no longer needed. Alternatively, close or tighten the fascia around a cannula. Another disadvantage of incision enlargement for specimen retrieval is the increased discomfort that patients may have at that site. Regardless, this is often the most practical method.

3. **Separate abdominal wall incision.** In some situations it may be most practical to remove the specimen through a separate abdominal wall incision that does not incorporate any of the existing port sites. These incisions can generally be limited to a few centimeters in length, and a muscle-splitting technique can be used for nonmidline sites. Examples of this technique include removal of the right or left colon through transverse incisions lateral to the rectus in the right or left abdomen, respectively, removal of the sigmoid colon through a suprapubic or left lower abdominal incision, and removal of an intact spleen through a low midline or Pfannenstiel incision. During colon resection the site of incision can be gauged by holding the mobilized specimen up to the abdominal wall; this location may or may not correspond to an existing cannula site.

4. **Transanal route.** Transanal extraction has been used for some laparoscopic low anterior colon resections. This route can be considered when the lower limit of transection is near or below the pelvic brim and the specimen is not too bulky. Place the specimen in a bag. Slowly dilate the anus and pass a ring forceps or similar instrument transanally. Grasp the bag and gently pull it through the rectal stump and anus. During laparoscopic abdominoperineal resection the specimen is readily delivered through the perineal incision in a similar manner.

5. **Transvaginal route.** Another alternative to abdominal incision for intact removal of larger specimens is an incision in the posterior vaginal fornix (cul de sac), which is termed culdotomy or posterior colpotomy. This has most frequently been used for removal of ovarian masses or the uterus during laparoscopic-assisted vaginal hysterectomy and occasionally for other solid organs.

C. Retrieval Bags

Use of a specimen retrieval bag minimizes the risk of contamination and specimen loss. This is particularly important when the specimen may be malignant, infected, leaking or friable. Commercially manufactured bags and retrieval devices are available for this purpose but sterile gloves, glove fingers, condoms, or other containers may suffice. The important features to consider in selecting a retrieval bag are its strength, size, aperture, maneuverability, ease of deployment and retrieval, and porosity. Bags are typically made of polyurethane or of nylon with a polyurethane coating. Nylon bags are more resistant to tearing and are preferred for removing larger specimens that must be fragmented in the bag, such as the spleen or kidney.

The precise technique of specimen retrieval in a bag varies according to the specific specimen and bag employed but there are several common principles.

1. **Bag insertion.** Roll the bag tightly and insert it through an appropriately located cannula. Depending upon the size of the bag, either insert it directly through the cannula, through a reducing sleeve, or through the port incision with the cannula removed. A special two-pronged introducer facilitates insertion of larger bags. Coat the outside of the bag with water-soluble lubricant to make it slide easily.

2. **Bag deployment.** Pull the bag gently out of the cannula or sleeve. Use two graspers, placed through other cannula sites, to unroll it. Grasp

the edges of the bag and open the mouth by pulling in opposite directions. Use a third instrument, if necessary, to help open the bag by moving along the front edge in a circular direction. A commonly used commercial device consists of a bag with a flexible metal ring at its mouth, contained in a plastic sheath. The sheath is introduced through a cannula and the device deployed by advancing a plunger. A flexible ring automatically holds the bag open. Once the specimen is contained, a ring is pulled to close the bag.

3. **Specimen entrapment.** This is generally the most difficult step, particularly for large organs. Hold the mouth of the bag open with two, or preferably three (to allow triangulation of the opening), graspers. Manipulate the open bag so it lies behind the specimen, with the mouth facing the surgeon. Allow sufficient working distance for comfortable manipulation. For example, when retrieving the spleen, the closed end of the bag is positioned toward the diaphragm. Advance the grasper holding the specimen all the way to the depth of the bag. The specimen should enter the bag, and the entire specimen must fit within the bag prior to closure. Manipulating large organs can be difficult and care must be taken not to rupture the specimen. Wherever possible, grasp connective tissue around the organ rather than the organ itself. In some instances it may be useful to leave a portion of the organ attached (e.g., ligaments attaching the spleen to the diaphragm) and to divide this attachment only when the rest of the specimen has been maneuvered into the bag. Proper positioning of the patient may also facilitate entrapment (i.e., Trendelenburg, reverse Trendelenburg, rotation).

4. **Bag closure.** Commercial bags are usually equipped with a drawstring that must be tightened. Close small plastic bags, glove fingers, or condoms with a preformed endoscopic ligature.

5. **Bag extraction.** Keep the bag under constant laparoscopic visual control as it is pulled to the cannula site. Withdraw the bag and cannula (if still in place) through the abdominal wall as a unit. Small bags may be directly removed through a 10- to 12-mm port site. Usually the bag is partially pulled through the abdominal wall and secured externally. The bag and contained specimen are removed by either enlarging the port site, as described above, or by reducing the specimen in size by fragmentation (e.g., spleen or kidney) or removing portions (e.g., gallstones). Resist the temptation to pull hard, and use care to avoid puncturing or tearing the bag.

D. Specimen Fragmentation/Morcellation

Morcellation or fragmentation is an appropriate method for removing large solid specimens when it is not necessary to preserve the gross architecture of the organ for pathology. Classic examples include the spleen removed for immune thrombocytopenic purpura or the kidney removed for benign parenchymal disease. Fragmentation is contraindicated for the removal of known or potentially malignant tumors.

Place the specimen in a sturdy, nonporous retrieval bag. Partially external-ize the bag and open it. Break up the specimen and remove it piecemeal using ring forceps, clamps, suction catheters, or a commercial tissue morcellator. Maintain direct laparoscopic visualization of the sac and take care to avoid rupture of the sac and peritoneal spillage.

E. Complications of Specimen Retrieval

Attention to the technical details of specimen retrieval is critical to avoidance of some potentially vexing and devastating problems. The principal complications related to removal of laparoscopic specimens are self evident and include:

1. **Internal specimen loss.** This is less likely to happen if adequate time and care are taken during removal. Confining manipulations to a region of the abdomen where the specimen can be easily retrieved if dropped, or tagging it with a long suture, are two precautions that can safeguard against loss if the specimen is dropped.
2. **Specimen rupture** (consequences of which can include infection, splenosis, tumor dissemination, and inadequate pathologic assess-ment). This can be avoided by individualizing the technique of speci-men removal, considering the size of the specimen and its physical characteristics, and handling it gently.
3. **Wound infection.** Grossly infected specimens (e.g., a perforated appendix) should be placed in specimen bags rather than pulled through the abdominal wall.
4. **Tumor implantation at port site.** The mechanism of this complica-tion is not fully understood. Common sense suggests that malignant or potentially malignant specimens (e.g., thick-walled gallbladders) should be placed in specimen bags rather than pulled directly through the abdominal wall.
5. **Visceral injury** (due to entrapment during extraction). This can be avoided by maintaining constant visual laparoscopic control. Large specimen bags may obscure visualization of the area behind the bag and extra care must be taken during bag extraction. Awareness of the potential for this complication, and a bit of extra vigilance, should prevent its occurrence.
6. **Incisional hernia.** All trocar sites must be closed in an appropriate fashion to avoid this complication.

F. Selected References

Hernandez F, Rha KH, Pinto PA, et al. Laparoscopic nephrectomy: assessment of morcellation versus intact specimen extraction on postoperative status. J Urol 2003;170:412–415.

MacFadyen Jr BV, Ponsky JL, eds. Operative Laparoscopy and Thoracoscopy. Philadelphia: Lippincott-Raven, 1996.

Petelin JB. Technologies and techniques for telescopic surgery. In: Hunter JG, Sackier JM, eds. Minimally Invasive Surgery. New York: McGraw-Hill, 1993.

Tsin DA, Colombero LT. Laparoscopic leash: a simple technique to prevent specimen loss during operative laparoscopy. Obstet Gynecol 1999;94:628–629.

Way LW, Bhoyrul S, Mori T, eds. Fundamentals of Laparoscopic Surgery. New York: Churchill Livingstone, 1996.

9. Documentation

Daniel J. Deziel, M.D.

A. General Considerations

Modern video technology converts the optical image from a laparoscopic lens to an electronic signal that can be displayed, transmitted, and recorded. Electronic images can be archived in a variety of formats as videos or as still images. These recorded images are invaluable ways to convey information for clinical, scientific, educational, and medicolegal purposes. New formats for video imaging and laparoscopic documentation will continue to become available as technology develops. Cost, equipment, storage requirements, and general availability of a particular format are important practical considerations. Digital imagines, signal processing, and recording technology are replacing standard analog systems.

B. Components of Video Imaging

The basic components for laparoscopic imaging are the telescope, light cable, light source, camera head, video signal box, video cable, and monitor. In modern practice, additional recording components, such as videocassette recorders, photo printers, or digital capture devices, are usually appended. For best image quality these components should be arranged in a distributed configuration (Figs. 9.1 and 9.2).

The development of the Hopkins rod–lens system used in modern laparoscopes was key to allowing photographic and video documentation. Light is transmitted through a series of glass rods with lenses at the ends rather than through air, as in previous lens systems. This provides improved light transmission with higher resolution, a wider viewing angle, and a larger image than previously available. The problem of insufficient illumination for laparoscopic documentation was overcome by the development of the high-intensity halogen (150 W), metal halide (250 W), and xenon lamps (300 W). Light is transmitted from the lamp to the laparoscope through cables. There are two types of cable: fiberoptic and fluid. Fiberoptic cables are flexible but do not transmit a precise light spectrum. Fluid cables transmit more light and a complete spectrum but are more rigid. Fluid cables require soaking for sterilization and cannot be gas sterilized.

Integrated video endoscopes became available in the early 1990s. These systems have a silicon chip mounted directly behind the objective lens of the scope. There is no lens system in the shaft. The signal is transmitted directly to the camera located on the video cart. Other newer designs include flexible video laparoscopes and three-dimensional laparoscopes.

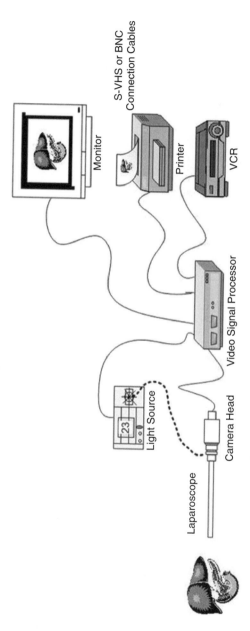

Figure 9.1. Standard video setup utilizing a distributed approach to the video signal array. (From Schwaitzberg, 2004, with permission.)

80   D.J. Deziel

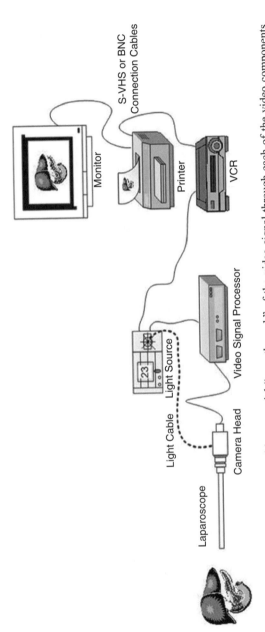

Figure 9.2. Standard video setup with sequential "pass-through" of the video signal through each of the video components. This arrangement degrades the signal at each step of the chair. (From Schwaitzberg, 2004, with permission.)

The basis of laparoscopic cameras is the solid-state silicon computer chip or charge-coupled device (CCD). This consists of an array of light-sensitive silicon elements. Silicon emits an electrical charge when exposed to light. These charges can be amplified, transmitted, displayed, and recorded. Each silicon element contributes one unit (referred to as a pixel) to the total image. The resolution or clarity of the image depends upon the density of pixels or light receptors on the chip. High-resolution cameras may contain 450,000 pixels.

Regardless of camera capability and wiring format, the clarity of the image depends on the resolution capability of the monitor. Standard consumer-grade video monitors have 350 lines of horizontal resolution; monitors with about 700 lines are preferred for laparoscopic surgery. High-definition television monitors have more than 1100 lines of resolution in a wide-screen format. Computer monitors provide higher resolution than video monitors. Computer monitors operate at a higher scan frequency, and resolution is based on the number of pixels per area. Current applications include telemedicine, robotic assisted surgery, and virtual reality simulators. Eventually, computer monitors may replace video monitors for standard operating room use.

The importance of the operator and of maintenance personnel for obtaining a quality video image cannot be underestimated. Besides assuring proper electronics, the operator must attend to mechanical details such as lens cleaning, focusing, and framing. No improvements in electronic signal processing can overcome the limitation of a scope that is damaged or a lens that is fogged, smeared, or out of focus. The ocular (proximal) and objective (distal) lenses of the laparoscope as well as the camera lens must be checked. The objective lens can be cleaned internally with irrigation and externally by wiping with cotton gauze soaked in warm water (not saline), then wiping with dry gauze before applying antifogging solution. It is imperative that the cannulas be clean and that no tissue be in the way during introduction of the scope.

C. Types of Video Signal

Video signals can be analog or digital. The video systems initially used in laparoscopic surgery and elsewhere grew out of television broadcast technology. Television analog systems read and transmit an image using scanning lines. In digital systems, a row of silicon elements on the CCD chip replaces the scanning line. The number of scanning lines represent the numbers of lines of information that can be transmitted and displayed on a monitor. The standard NTSC (National Television Systems Committee) format used in North America and Japan consists of 525 lines scanning at a rate of 30 frames per second. Systems used in other parts of the world (PAL, or phase-alternating line, and SECAM, or séquentiel couleur et mémoire) use 625 or 819 lines at 25 frames per second. Computer-enhanced high-definition television (HDTV) systems may have more than 1100 scanning lines and can incorporate five or six times more information than standard television and video formats. By comparison, the human eye can distinguish the equivalent of some 1600 scan lines, and the resolution of 35 mm photographic film is about 2300 scan lines.

Standard television and simple video signals are **composite** signals, meaning that all of the image information is carried over a single channel. These signals are subject to a certain amount of degradation during transmission and processing. Dividing the signal into **components** that are transmitted over separate channels provides a higher quality image. Super VH (S-VHS or S-Video or Y/C) splits the signal into separate components for brightness (luminance = Y) and color (chrominance = C). An RGB signal divides the color into red, green, and blue components that are transmitted over separate channels. A fourth channel is for image synchronization. Modern laparoscopic cameras have multiple output slots on the camera box that permit the operator to select the type of signal output. In addition to analog outputs, a number of digital outputs are available. These are generally reserved for recording devices and are not recommended for monitoring live surgical procedures. Obviously the monitor or recording equipment receiving the signal must be compatible in order to reconstruct the information.

Image quality can be improved by digital processing of the CCD signal. The original image is captured as an analog signal. This signal is transmitted as a continuous electronic waveform that is subject to interference and distortion. Digital systems convert the analog signal into binary code, which better preserves the original information and lessens distortion during reconstruction. Unlike analog images, digital recordings retain the quality of the original when duplicated or copied. Digital recordings can also be enhanced and modified for other applications in ways that analog images cannot.

D. Recording Media

There are multiple options for documenting laparoscopic procedures as either continuous recordings or still pictures. Videotapes obtained by attaching a videocassette recorder to the imaging system have been standard for continuous documentation. A variety of videotape formats are available: 0.5-in. VHS and 8 mm are acceptable but inferior in quality to 0.5-in. S-VHS, 0.75-in. U-Matic, Betacam, and high-8 mm. Digital videotape recorders (Mini DV, DVCAM, DVCPro) provide higher quality than analog recordings. The Y/C component signal of the S-VHS format provides better resolution than the single-channel composite signal of VHS systems. S-VHS machines can also record and play either S-VHS or conventional VHS tapes. Digital capture of still and video images has superseded older analog formats. Newer generation digital devices can store image and video files on CD, DVD, or memory cards. Digitally captured material can be edited, stored, and exported with much greater ease than analog types.

E. Selected References

Berber E, Siperstein AE. Understanding and optimizing laparoscopic video systems. Surg Endosc 2001;15:781–787.

Kouramba J, Preminger GM. Advances in camera, video and imaging technologies in laparoscopy. Urol Clin North Am 2001;28:5–14.

Schwaitzberg SD. Imaging systems in minimally invasive surgery. In: Soper N, Swanstrom L, Eubanks S, eds. Mastery of Endoscopic and Laparoscopic Surgery. 2d ed. Philadelphia: Lippincott Williams & Wilkins, 2004.

10.1 Laparoscopy During Pregnancy

Myriam J. Curet, M.D., F.A.C.S.

A. Indications for Laparoscopic Surgery During Pregnancy

The field of laparoscopic general surgery has exploded since the first laparoscopic cholecystectomy was performed in the late 1980s. Initially, pregnancy was considered an absolute contraindication to laparoscopic surgery. Recent clinical reports have demonstrated the feasibility, advantages, and potential safety of laparoscopic cholecystectomy in the pregnant patient. However, concerns about the effects of a carbon dioxide (CO_2) pneumoperitoneum on mother and fetus persist, resulting in controversy and concern.

Nongynecologic surgery is required in 0.2% of all pregnancies.

1. The safest time to operate on the pregnant patient is during the second trimester when the risks of teratogenesis, miscarriage, and preterm delivery are lowest. The incidence of spontaneous abortion is highest in the first trimester (12%), decreasing to 0% by the third. During the second trimester there is a 5%–8% incidence of preterm labor and premature delivery which increases to 30% in the third trimester. In addition, the risk of teratogenesis seen in the first trimester is no longer present during the second trimester. Finally, the gravid uterus is not yet large enough to obscure the operative field, as is the case during the third trimester.

2. The most common indications for operation on the pregnant patient are acute appendicitis and biliary tract disease.

   a. **Acute appendicitis** occurs in 1 out of 1500 pregnancies. Accurate diagnosis becomes more difficult as the pregnancy progresses: a correct preoperative diagnosis is given for 85% of patients evaluated in the first trimester of pregnancy, but accuracy is only 30%–50% in the third. The usual hallmarks of acute appendicitis such as abdominal pain, accompanying gastrointestinal symptoms and leukocytosis may already be present in a normal third-trimester pregnancy, obscuring the correct diagnosis. In addition, the description and location of the pain may change significantly as the uterus enlarges. The morbidity and mortality seen in the pregnant patient with acute appendicitis results from a delay in diagnosis and treatment. This delay leads to a 10 to 15% perforation rate. Fetal mortality has been shown to increase with perforation from 5% to 28%, while premature delivery can be as high as 40% in this situation. Therefore, the pregnant patient suspected of having acute appendicitis should be treated as if she were not pregnant. Immediate exploration after appropriate resuscitation is mandated regardless of gestational age.

b. **Biliary tract disease**: Gallstones are present in 12% of all pregnancies, and a cholecystectomy is performed in 3 to 8 of 10,000 pregnancies.

    i. An uncomplicated **open cholecystectomy** in a pregnant patient should be accompanied by a 0% maternal mortality, 5% fetal loss, and 7% preterm labor.

    ii. Complications such as **gallstone pancreatitis** or **acute cholecystitis** will increase maternal mortality to 15% and fetal demise to 60%.

    iii. Patients with **uncomplicated biliary colic** should be treated medically with nonfat diets and pain medications until after delivery. Patients who present in the **first timester** of pregnancy with crescendo biliary colic or persistent vomiting should be medically managed if possible until they are in the second trimester. Pregnant patients in the **second trimester** of pregnancy who present with the foregoing complications of biliary tract disease will need operative treatment during the second trimester after appropriate resuscitation. Patients with these complications who present in the third trimester of pregnancy should be treated conservatively until after delivery if possible or at least until a gestational age of 28 to 30 weeks, to maximize fetal viability.

B. Advantages and Feasibility of Laparoscopic Surgery During Pregnancy

Potentially, laparoscopic surgery in the pregnant patient should result in the proven advantages of laparoscopy seen in the nonpregnant patient: decreased pain, earlier return of gastrointestinal function, earlier ambulation, decreased hospital stay, and faster return to routine activity. In addition, a decreased rate of premature delivery due to decreased uterine manipulation, decreased fetal depression secondary to decreased narcotic usage, and a lower rate of incisional hernias may be seen in the pregnant patient.

To date, over 320 laparoscopic cholecystectomies in pregnant patients have been reported in the literature. Average operative time was 68.5 minutes (30–106 minutes) and average length of stay was 1.9 days (1–7 days). There is one report of a maternal and fetal death and 5 additional fetal deaths, one of which occurred after conversion. Of 268 babies delivered at time of publication, 10 were premature and one was born with hyaline membrane disease at 37 weeks gestation. The remaining 257 were full, term and healthy. Seven of these experienced preterm labor, which was controlled with tocolytics.

Two studies have retrospectively compared pregnant patients undergoing open laparotomy to pregnant patients undergoing laparoscopic surgery and found that the latter resumed regular diet earlier, required less pain medication, and were hospitalized for a shorter time. These differences were statistically significant.

There have been 15 reports detailing 77 patients undergoing laparoscopic appendectomies. The average time in the operating room was 56 minutes (30–85 minutes), with mean length of stay of 3.7 days (1–11 days). There have been 4 fetal deaths reported: 2 secondary to uterine infection misdiagnosed preoperatively as appendicitis and one due to pneumoamnion after uterine puncture with Veress needle. Four patients delivered prematurely, while 58 patients delivered healthy infants at term. Four of these experienced preterm labor, which was controlled with tocolytics.

C. Disadvantages and Concerns About Laparoscopic Surgery During Pregnancy

Concerns about laparoscopic surgery in the pregnant patient center on three areas:

1. Increased intra-abdominal pressure can lead to decreased inferior vena caval return resulting in **decreased cardiac output**. The fetus is dependent on maternal hemodynamic stability. The primary cause of fetal demise is maternal hypotension or hypoxia, so a fall in maternal cardiac output could result in fetal distress.
2. The increased intra-abdominal pressure seen with a pneumoperitoneum could lead to **decreased uterine blood flow** and **increased intrauterine pressure**, both of which could result in fetal hypoxia.
3. Carbon dioxide is absorbed across the peritoneum and can lead to **respiratory acidosis** in both mother and fetus. Fetal acidosis could be potentiated by the decreased vena caval return.

One clinical study has reported 4 fetal deaths following laparoscopic surgery. Three occurred during the first postoperative week and the last 4 weeks postoperatively. The causes of death are unknown but might be related to prolonged operative time. The operative times in these 4 patients was 106 minutes in comparison to the average of 55 minutes seen in the other studies. The laparoscopic procedure was performed for pancreatitis in 3 of these women and a perforated appendix in the fourth. It is possible that fetal loss was the result of the inflammatory process itself rather than the laparoscopy per se. There is a 4% fetal mortality rate for all reported laparoscopic cholecystectomies; it compares favorably with a 5% fetal mortality rate seen with open procedures.

Animal studies raise several concerns about the effects of a CO_2 pneumoperitoneum on the mother and fetus. Because of the complexity of the maternal–fetal unit, it is useful to summarize these individually:

1. In pregnant baboons, a CO_2 pneumoperitoneum held at 20 mm Hg pressure for 20 minutes resulted in increased pulmonary capillary wedge pressure, pulmonary artery pressure, and central venous pressure. The mothers developed a respiratory acidosis despite controlled ventilation and an increase in respiratory rate. One fetus developed severe bradycardia, which responded to desufflation.

2. In pregnant ewes, no change in maternal placental blood flow was seen after 2 hours of 13 mm Hg pressure. However, maternal and fetal respiratory acidosis developed. Fetal tachycardia, fetal hypertension, an increase in intrauterine pressure, and a decrease in uterine blood flow were also seen in pregnant ewes undergoing a CO_2 pneumoperitoneum at 15 mm Hg.

3. Maternal respiratory acidosis and severe fetal respiratory acidosis are common findings in all studies utilizing a CO_2 pneumoperitoneum in pregnant animals. Changes in respiratory rate did not completely correct the problems. Despite these problems, one study demonstrated that the ewes delivered fullterm healthy lambs following intra-abdominal insufflation to 15 mm Hg pressure with CO_2 for one hour.

4. The physiologic changes exhibited by the pregnant ewe and fetus during insufflation with CO_2 are not present with nitrous oxide. Fetal tachycardia, hypertension, and acidosis, as well as maternal acidosis, are not present when a nitrous oxide pneumoperitoneum is used in animal studies. Use of nitrous oxide as an insufflating gas in the pregnant woman has yet to be evaluated, but may prove to be safer than CO_2.

D. Guidelines

The following practices should be followed when one is performing laparoscopic surgery in the pregnant patient to minimize adverse effects on the fetus or mother. More information is given in the SAGES Guidelines for Laparoscopic Surgery During Pregnancy (see Appendix).

1. Obtain an **obstetric consultation** for the perioperative management of the patient.

2. Be aware of the **cardiovascular and pulmonary physiologic changes** seen with pregnancy, including relative anemia, increased cardiac output and heart rate, increased oxygen consumption, increased tidal volume, and compensatory respiratory alkalosis.

3. Pregnant patients are at **increased risk of aspiration** because of decreased lower esophageal sphincter pressure and delayed gastric emptying.

4. Place the patient in the **left lateral decubitus position** as with open surgery to prevent uterine compression of the inferior vena cava. Minimizing the degree of reverse Trendelenburg position may also further reduce possible uterine compression of the vena cava.

5. **Use antiembolic devices** to prevent deep venous thrombosis. Stasis of blood in the lower extremities is common in pregnancy. Levels of fibrinogen and factors VII and XII are increased during pregnancy leading to an increased risk of thromboembolic events. These changes, coupled with the decreased venous return seen with increased intra-abdominal pressure and the reverse Trendelenburg position used during laparoscopic surgery, significantly increase the risk of deep venous thrombosis.

6. An **open Hasson technique** for gaining access to the abdominal cavity is safer than a closed percutaneous puncture. Several authors have inserted a Veress needle in the right upper quadrant without complications, but the potential for puncture of the uterus or intestine still exists, especially with increasing gestational age and has been reported in 4 cases.
7. **Maintain the intra-abdominal pressure as low as possible** while still achieving adequate visualization. A pressure of less than 12 to 15 mm Hg should be used until concerns about the effects of high intra-abdominal pressure on the fetus are answered.
8. Continuously **monitor maternal end-tidal CO_2** and maintain it between 25 and 30 mm by changing the minute ventilation. Promptly correcting any evidence of maternal respiratory acidosis is critical, as the fetus is typically slightly more acidotic than the mother.
9. Use **continuous intraoperative fetal monitoring** if the fetus is viable. If fetal distress is noted, release the pneumoperitoneum immediately. The use of monitoring if the fetus is not viable is controversial, but is recommended by this author because desufflation may reverse fetal distress, preventing serious problems. If intraoperative monitoring is not used, then fetal heart tones should be documented pre- and post-operatively. Transabdominal ultrasound fetal monitoring may not be effective because the establishment of the pneumoperitoneum may decrease fetal heart tones, so intravaginal ultrasound may be necessary for intraoperative monitoring.
10. If intraoperative cholangiography is to be performed, **protect the fetus**.
11. **Minimize operative time.** Several studies have demonstrated a correlation between the duration of a CO_2 pneumoperitoneum and an increase in portial pressure of arterial CO_2.
12. **Tocolytic agents** should not be administered prophylactically but are appropriate if there is any evidence of uterine irritability or contractions.
13. **Trocar placement**
    a. **Biliary tract disease.** Place a Hasson trocar above the umbilicus. Place the remaining ports under direct visualization in the usual locations.
    b. **Appendicitis/diagnostic laparoscopy.** Place a Hasson trocar in the subxiphoid region. Insert the camera and locate the appendix or other inflammatory process. Insert the remaining trocars in locations appropriate to the pathology. For appendicitis, this will usually be the right upper quadrant at the costal margin and in the right lower quadrant. Ocasionally, an additional port might need to be placed just above the uterus. If the uterus is too large and appendectomy cannot be performed laparoscopically, then laparoscopic visualization of the appendix may help determine the best location for the open incision.

In conclusion, animal studies indicate that a CO_2 pneumoperitoneum causes fetal acidosis, which may not be corrected by changes in maternal respiratory status. These intraoperative findings do not appear to have any long-term adverse effects on the fetus. The pregnant patient clearly benefits from laparoscopic surgery and should be offered this option as long as the foregoing guidelines are followed.

E. Selected References

Abuabara SF, Gross GW, Sirinek KR. Laparoscopic cholecystectomy during pregnancy is safe for both mother and fetus. J Gastrointest Surg 1997;1:48–52.

Affleck DG, Handrahan DL, Egger MJ, Price RR. The laparoscopic management of appendicitis and cholelithiasis during pregnancy. Am J Surg 1999;178:523–529.

Amos JD, Schorr SJ, Norman PF, et al. Laparoscopic surgery during pregnancy. Am J Surg 1996;171:435–437.

Barnard JM, Chaffin D, Drose S, Tierney A, Phernetton T. Fetal response to carbon dioxide pneumoperitoneum in the pregnant ewe. Obstet Gynecol 1995;85:669–674.

Curet MJ. Special problems in laparoscopic surgery: previous abdominal surgery, obesity and pregnancy. Surg Clin North Am 2000;80:1093–1110.

Curet MJ, Allen D, Josloff RK, et al. Laparoscopy during pregnancy. Arch Surg 1996a;131:546–551.

Curet MJ, Vogt DM, Schob O, et al. Effects of CO_2 on pneumoperitoneum in pregnant ewes. J Surg Res 1996b;63:339–344.

Hunter JG, Swanstrom L, Thornburg K. Carbon dioxide pneumoperitoneum induces fetal acidosis in a pregnant ewe model. Surg Endosc 1994;4:268–271.

Kammerer WS. Nonobstetric surgery during pregnancy. Med Clin North Am 1979; 63:1157–1163.

McKellar DP, Anderson CT, Boynton CJ, Peoples JB. Cholecystectomy during pregnancy without fetal loss. Surg Gynecol Obstet 1992;174:465–486.

Melnick DM, Wahl WL, Kalton VK. Management of general surgical problems in the pregnant patient. Am J Surg 2004;187:170–180.

Motew M, Ivankovich AD, Bieniarz J, Albrecht RF, Zahed B, Scomegna A. Cardiovascular effects and acid-base and blood gas changes during laparoscopy. Am J Obstet Gyncol 1973;113:1002–1012.

Reedy MB, Galan HL, Bean JD, Carnes A, Knight AB, Kuehl TJ. Laparoscopic insufflation in the gravid baboon: maternal and fetal effects. J Am Assoc Gynecol Laparoscopist 1995;2:399–406.

Soper NJ, Hunter JG, Petri RH. Laparoscopic cholecystectomy in the pregnant patient. Surg Laparosc Endosc 1994;4:268–271.

10.2 Previous Abdominal Surgery

Norman B. Halpern, M.D., F.A.C.S.

A. General Considerations

Previous intra-abdominal operation may have only trivial impact on the performance of a subsequent laparoscopic procedure or may render laparoscopy not only unwise, but impossible. This wide spectrum of influence is related to the substantial variation in patients' tendencies to form postoperative adhesions. The laparoscopic surgeon should not be intimidated by the potential difficulties posed by such adhesions, but should approach the circumstances with an awareness of the strategies and tactics that have been utilized routinely and successfully during decades of traditional (open) operations. The influence of previous abdominal incision on choice of access for induction of pneumoperitoneum was discussed briefly in Chapter 4, and is considered more fully here.

B. Preoperative Analysis and Planning

During preoperative planning, first consider the **geographical relationships of the previous and the intended operations**. For example, the most commonly performed general surgical laparoscopic procedure is cholecystectomy, usually upon women. Since many women have previously undergone transabdominal hysterectomy, infraumbilical body wall adhesions may interfere with periumbilical cannula placement, although the remainder of the cholecystectomy may be entirely uneventful. Unfortunately, however, adhesions are not always limited to the precise area of the incision, but may occupy a much greater expanse of the peritoneal membrane than the cutaneous scar would suggest.

Next, determine **whether the old scar has healed properly or has developed a herniation**. If weakness is detected, the operative plan should include hernia repair. Since laparoscopic techniques for incisional hernia repair have not been widely applied, a suitable approach would be a combined operation. If the hernia is located remotely from the laparoscopic field, then a conventional herniorrhaphy could precede the laparoscopy. If the hernia is in the general area of the anticipated laparoscopy (e.g., an upper midline hernia in a patient being considered for laparoscopic cholecystectomy), it may be preferable to utilize that weakened incision for an open procedure with repair at the time of closure.

Finally, consider **patient positioning, operating table tilt and roll capabilities, and accessories** (ankle straps, footboard) and assure that the benefits of gravity and shifting tissue–organ relationships may be exploited if necessary.

C. Access to the Peritoneal Cavity

Carefully plan the steps to achieve intra-abdominal access. Make the initial entry at a reasonable distance from any obvious scars. Possible access sites relative to common scars are illustrated in Chapter 2 (Fig. 2.9).

1. Some surgeons utilize an alternate-site Veress needle puncture technique (e.g., the left subcostal region). For most, the Hasson cannula is a straightforward and possibly safer means, and some surgeons use this technique routinely. With practice, this will be found to be an expeditious means for entering any quadrant by making a miniature muscle-splitting incision in the subcostal, hypogastric, flank, or other region. Just as with open operations, however, bowel that happens to be adherent immediately under the chosen site of entry will be damaged by any blind cutting, spreading, or cauterization. If there is any question as to adherent underlying tissue, the initially chosen site may need to be abandoned and another one selected.

2. A small-caliber "needle scope" can be passed into the peritoneal cavity through this alternate site; the abdomen is then inspected for adhesions and secondary sites are chosen.

3. **Achieving appropriate working distance** is another reason for judicious selection of the entry site. Avoid ending up too close to any tissue of interest. There must be a comfortable working distance available to the surgeon to properly manipulate instruments, either for lysing the interfering adhesions or for performing the primary procedure. Secondary cannulas must then be placed with these considerations in mind, also.

D. Managing Adhesions

Once the peritoneal cavity has been reached safely, the **presence and extent of any adhesions** will become apparent. The surgeon must resist the common tendency to excessively eliminate adhesions. Only those adhesions that truly interfere with visualization of the area of interest or would prevent the placement of subsequent cannulas under vision should be dealt with. At times, the end of the telescope can be very easily manipulated around the edge of a sheet of omentum, suspended from the elevated body wall like a curtain, or fenestrated areas can be used as windows through which the scope can be advanced toward the operative area. If these maneuvers are not applicable, then adhesion lysis must be begun.

Safe lysis of adhesions requires a **combination of skillful technique and attention to visual cues**. If the line of tissue adherence can be recognized, it will provide the most expeditious path to follow, with the least chance of causing significant bleeding or visceral injury. Principles of traction/countertraction are essential components of this phase of the operation, and the surgeon may occasionally need to experiment with varying directions of pull on the tissues to clearly display the boundary lines. For body wall adhesions, the combination of gravity pulling the tissues down while the distended abdominal wall moves in the opposite direction sometimes provides adequate stretch to allow the dissection to be done with only one working instrument. Frequently, however (and especially with viscera-to-viscera adherence), an assisting grasper is required, with its cannula being carefully positioned according to principles mentioned previously.

E. Instrument Considerations

The best tool to be used for adhesion lysis is determined by the circumstances and the characteristics of the adhesions and surrounding tissues. Naturally weak areas of areolar tissues appear "foamy" and can be swept away using techniques resembling finger dissection. Rounded graspers, the blunt edges of the scissors blades, and even the suction-irrigator all accomplish the same result with these types of adhesions. For more firmly adherent structures, however, scissors may be the next choice. If the fusion of the tissues has not resulted in very much neovascularity, then as long as the proper plane of dissection is followed, adding cautery current to the scissors' action is not helpful.

Use of **the cautery tool** requires diligence and respect for the potential tissue damage that may result from uncontrolled electrical energy. In addition, the surgeon's expectations for hemostasis must be realistic, using coaptive coagulation (pinching while applying current) for some vessels, but clips or ligatures for larger ones. Techniques for utilizing J- or L-shaped cautery devices commonly involve a hook-pull-burn sequence, but if the surgeon places sturdy traction on the tissues, and then gently sweeps or caresses with the elbow of the wire, a more precise and delicate separation of tissues will follow, as if the traction is actually performing the dissection, and the current is merely weakening the adherence. Although bipolar electrocautery instruments and Harmonic scalpel (Ultracision, Ethicon Endo-Surgery, Cincinnati, OH) devices are commercially available, their actual use and availability is probably somewhat limited in comparison to conventional monopolar instrumentation.

The loss of natural proprioceptive processes cannot be eliminated but can be minimized by careful attention to instrument design and function. The acceptability of the "feel" of a dissecting or grasping instrument is determined partly by personal preference. For example, some surgeons find rotatable instrument shafts to be very useful; however, others dislike the added bulk and the change in balance produced by the rotating mechanism. Other design features such as length, shaft flexibility, overall weight, and handle configurations must each be considered as a surgeon is determining whether adequate dexterity exists and whether careful tissue handling will be accomplished. It is particularly important for the closing and spreading movements of the jaws to be smooth and effortless; otherwise it will be impossible to sense how much force is being applied to the tissues.

The use of an angled lens laparoscope (e.g., a 30-degree laparoscope) is sometimes extremely helpful. Observing adhesions and abnormal tissue relationships from more than a single vantage point renders new, safer, or more productive dissection pathways apparent. Remember that although such lenses are conventionally thought of as "looking down," there may be great advantages to looking "up" or from a "sideways" perspective.

F. Complications

No operative procedure is risk free. If an operation requires more than the usual efforts for tissue dissection or organ manipulation, there likely will be **an increased opportunity for mishaps**, so the surgeon must develop a keen sense of vigilance for any potentially dangerous situations.

1. **Bleeding**
   a. **Cause and prevention.** Although not life threatening, any additional blood loss during a laparoscopic procedure not only can be time-consuming to control, but can add to the frustration and mental fatigue associated with an already difficult operation. In addition, if tissues become blood stained, ability to recognize structures may be impaired, and illumination is less effective. Careful, painstaking dissection is the best preventive measure.
   b. **Recognition and management.** Minimization of blood loss will be favorably influenced by rigorous attention to tissue planes, by careful observation of tissue characteristics, and by appropriate precautionary use of electrocautery or other hemostatic maneuvers. Such maneuvers, however, may cause injuries to adjacent structures if hurriedly applied, especially during efforts to control active bleeding. Remember that simple pressure—even with the scissors blades that created the problem—is an immediately available solution to consider when confronted with a spurting vessel. (See Chapter 6, Principles of Laparoscopic Hemostasis, for a discussion of management strategies.)
2. **Visceral injury**
   a. **Cause and prevention.** Injury to the viscera can result from excessive traction, as well as cutting, burning, or ligating misidentified structures. As previously described, careful controlled dissection in a bloodless field, with identification of all structures as the dissection progresses, is crucial to prevent these injuries.
   b. **Recognition and management.** With solid-organ injury (liver, spleen), bleeding is the immediate, as well as the obvious, consequence. Management of these injuries is primarily directed at obtaining hemostasis. Injuries to hollow viscera may be subtle and apparent only because of the appearance of luminal contents. The decision to perform a laparoscopic repair, as contrasted to open conversion, should be influenced by the characteristics of the tissues and associated injury, as well as the surgeon's experience and capabilities. A "delayed" intestinal perforation, manifesting itself as postoperative peritonitis, may very well be an intraoperative injury that was undetected. For that reason, prior to removing the laparoscope, the mandatory final step of the

operation should be a methodical inspection of all intra-abdominal areas that had been subjected to adhesion lysis, tissue manipulation, or actions to control bleeding.

G. Selected References

Caprini JA, Arcelus JA, Swanson J, et al. The ultrasonic localization of abdominal wall adhesions. Surg Endosc 1995;9:283–285.

Chang FH, Chou HH, Lee CL, Cheng PJ, Wang CW, Soong YK. Extraumbilical insertion of the operative laparoscope in patients with extensive intraabdominal adhesions. J Am Assoc Gynecol Laparosc 1995;2:335–337.

Chopra R, McVay C, Phillips E, Khalili TM. Laparoscopic lysis of adhesions. Am Surg 2003;69:966–968.

Golan A, Sagiv R, Debby A, Glezerman M. The minilaparoscope as a tool for localization and preparation for cannula insertion in patients with multiple previous abdominal incisions or umbilical hernia. J Am Assoc Gynecol Laparosc 2003;10:14–16.

Halpern NB. The difficult laparoscopy. Surg Clin North Am 1996;76:603–613.

Halpern NB. Access problems in laparoscopic cholecystectomy: postoperative adhesions, obesity, and liver disorders. Semin Laparosc Surg 1998;5:92–106.

Patel M, Smart D. Laparoscopic cholecystectomy and previous abdominal surgery: a safe technique. Aust NZ J Surg 1996;66:309–311.

Schirmer BD, Dix J, Schmieg RE, et al. The impact of previous abdominal surgery on outcome following laparoscopic cholecystectomy. Surg Endosc 1995;9:1085–1089.

Sigmar HH, Fried GM, Gazzon J, et al. Risks of blind versus open approach to celiotomy for laparoscopic surgery. Surg Laparosc Endosc 1993;3:296–299.

Weibel MA, Majno G. Peritoneal adhesions and their relation to abdominal surgery: a post mortem study. Am J Surg 1973;126:345–353.

Wongworowat MD, Aitken DR, Robles AE, Garberoglio C. The impact of prior intra-abdominal surgery on laparoscopic cholecystectomy. Am Surg 1994;60:763–766.

11. Robotics in Laparoscopic and Thoracoscopic Surgery

Andreas Kirakopolous
W. Scott Melvin, M.D., F.A.C.S.

A. Introduction

Every aspect of modern surgery is currently under technology-influenced transformation, including the following:

- **Training**: configuration and implementation of virtual reality simulators
- **Diagnosis**: development of noninvasive diagnostic imaging modalities and micro-sized sensors
- **Exchange of medical information and consultation**: World Wide Web and telemedicine/telementoring
- **Surgeon–patient interface**: computer-enhanced and telerobotic surgery

Behind these changes is revolutionary progress in computer science in conjunction with robotic systems development. After a long period in which research focused mainly on industrial robots, research groups turned their attention to building machines able to interface with humans in unstructured domains and to intelligently perform their assigned tasks. The introduction of robotics in the field of minimally invasive surgery came as no surprise, as the increased precision and improved quality associated with industrial robots stimulated the application of robots and computer systems in modern health-care systems.

This chapter gives an overview and introduction to these emerging technologies and their applications.

B. Robotics Overview

1. Historical Evolution

Czech writer Karel Čapek introduced the term *robot* in a play he wrote in 1920 called *RUR* (Rossum's Universal Robots), first performed in 1923. It is derived from the Czech word *roboto* meaning "compulsory labor."

Modern robots have been developed through a process that in the very first stages involved the configuration of numerous automated tools used mainly as industrial machinery addressing the demand for increased productivity and improved quality and product performance. From the initial attention devoted more toward flexible automation, the research shifted toward the development of systems that could operate in accordance to, or even without, human intervention, and interact in real time with dynamic environments. Today's robotic systems are mechanical systems controlled by computer processors and equipped with sensors and motors. Appropriate computer algorithms based on sophisticated software utilize environmental information and the operator input provided by sensors to determine appropriate motor movements to the associated mechanical system.

The application of robotics in the field of minimally invasive surgery represents the state of the art in surgery. The revolution began with the introduction of laparoscopic surgery, which changed the perception and the practice of surgery for both the patient and the surgeon. However, the ever-increasing complexity of the laparoscopic procedures and, especially, the performance of advanced laparoscopic operations, posed some serious demands on both the equipment and the personnel in the operating room. The goal of these sytems is to relieve the limitations found in standard laparoscopic surgery, including two-dimensional perception of the operative field, an unstable camera platform, nonarticulated instruments inserted through fixed points resulting in limited movement, natural hand tremor, and difficult fine motor activity.

These inherent shortcomings gave impetus for the introduction and development of robotic systems in minimally invasive surgery. Additionally, one of the initial concepts for the introduction of robotics in surgery was to develop the capability for operating remotely. The capability to perform a surgical procedure over a distance, transferring surgical expertise to a remote site (space station, developing country) seemed to be quite intriguing.

Advances in robotic engineering and computer technology soon allowed the development of several prototypes that eventually became commercially available. Current applications of robotics include surgical assistance, dexterity enhancement, systems networking, and image-guided therapy. Dexterity is enhanced by an interposed microprocessor between the surgeon's hands and the tip of the surgical instrument that allows downscaling of the gross hand movements and the physical hand tremor.

2. Current Status

The most advanced of today's robotic systems (Zeus^{TM} and daVinci^{TM}) make use of a master–slave telemanipulator where all robotic movements are dictated from the surgeon through the use of an "on line" input device. The surgeon remains in control of the procedure while the movements of the instrument handles ("master unit") are transformed into electronic signals filtered and transmitted in real time to the motorized robotic arm ("slave unit") that controls the instrument tips. The term *computer-enhanced telesurgery* is the most descriptive term of the active functions of these devices. The different systems available today allow various operative tasks to be accomplished, with different levels of interface between the surgeon and the system established.

So far, the advantages that have been correlated with the initial use of the computer-enhanced robotics systems in surgical practice include the following:

- Allowance for increased degrees of freedom of movement, leading to significant improvement of intraabdominal instrument articulations
- Better visual control of the operative field due to three-dimensional (3D) view and the "immersing effect" to the surgeon
- Filtering, modulation, and downscaling of the amplitude of the surgical motions resulting in more precise, hand-tremor-free operative manipulations
- Ability to operate at a distance from the patient

3. Definitions

- A robot is defined as (1) A mechanical device that sometimes resembles a human and is capable of performing a variety of often complex human tasks on command or by being programmed in advance. (2) A machine or device that operates automatically or by remote control.
- B. Davies (2000) describes a surgical robot as "a powered, computer controlled manipulator with artificial sensing that can be reprogrammed to move and position tools to carry out a wide range of surgical tasks."

Under the guise of these two definitions, multiple tasks can be undertaken by the surgical robot or computer-assisted devices.

- Computer-assisted surgery is a term that should include most of the active functions of these devices. In some situations robots act autonomously and would be truly robotic, not computer-assisted interventions.
- Current systems are, in fact, either surgical assistants or computer-enhanced telemanipulators.

C. Current Clinical Applications

Robotic surgery encompasses a variety of different types of interaction that extend from the passive use of a robotic machine to computer-enhanced telemanipulators and even to truly robotic systems.

1. Image-Guided Robotic Systems

The various image-guided robots designed for targeting tissues and holding surgical instruments for biopsies and other relatively simple and linear uses exemplify the passive use of robots. The term "passive" implies that the surgeon provides the physical energy to manipulate the surgical tool. A system called PAKY, developed at Johns Hopkins University for the percutaneous access of the kidney, has been found to offer an unquestionable improvement in needle

placement accuracy and total procedure time, while reducing the radiation exposure to both patient and urologist. Another system has been designed to perform
transperineal prostate biopsies under ultrasound guidance. A compatible with
magnetic resonance imaging techniques has been developed needle insertion
manipulator for stereotactic neurosurgery. The **NeuroMate**^{TM} (Integrated Surgical Systems, Sacramento, CA), is an image-guided, computer-controlled robotic
system designed for stereotactic functional brain surgery.

2. Computer-Assisted Surgery

Active use of robotic systems involves the achievement of motion using non-
human-powered devices and, specifically, a computer. Active-use robots have
been designed to be used as assistants under mechanical or voice guidance.
AESOP (Automated Endoscopic System for Optimal Positioning, Computer
Motion, Goleta, CA), the first surgical robot that received the approval of the
federal Food and Drug Administration (FDA), fits perfectly into this category.
This device is a robotic laparoscopic camera holder that responds specifically to
voice commands, and it has two useful features: the surgeon can at any time take
manual control of the system, and the robot can return to a memorized position
on command. The system abolishes the need for a surgical assistant, provides
stability of view, and offers savings in time and personnel required for the laparoscopic operation.

HERMES (Computer Motion, Goleta, CA) is also a voice-activated system
that adjusts various parameters of the operating room environment (lighting,
camera, insufflator, phone). A recent study highlighted the high acceptance of
the system from both physician and nursing personnel due to the more smooth
and interruption-free environment created. An example of a freestanding laparoscopic camera manipulator is the **EndoAssist** (Armstrong Healthcare Ltd., High
Wycombe, England), a device controlled by infrared signals from a headset worn
by the operator. In a recent randomized, controlled trial (Aiono et al., 2002), the
use of the EndoAssist was correlated with a statistically significant and potentially clinically significant operative time reduction and a short learning curve.

3. Computer-Enhanced Robotic Telesurgery

The prefix *tele* in term "telesurgery" and "telemanipulator" implies distance
between the surgeon and the patient. In this setting the surgeon sits at a dedicated workstation and uses either joysticks or more sophisticated devices to
control the motion of the robotic arms at the bedside of the patient. The interposition of a computer allows for scaling of the surgeon's motions, while the
presence of a camera attached to the robot offers a 3D view of the actions of the
manipulators.

There are currently two commercially available telemanipulator robotic
systems. **Zeus** (Computer Motion, Goleta, CA, Z2P system) incorporates three

interactive arms: one, voice activated, controls the laparoscope, two robotic arms manipulate the instruments. There is also a remotely located workstation with an interface for the manipulation of the instruments and the perception of force feedback. The 3D illusion of the operative field is accomplished using active eyewear that allows a three-dimensional image. The system allows 5 degrees of freedom of movement within the abdominal cavity.

The **da Vinci** system (Intuitive Surgical, Sunnyvale, CA), the only computer-enhanced robotic system with FDA approval, includes the remotely located control console and the surgical arm unit that holds and manipulates the instruments. The instruments are capable of delivering 7 degrees of freedom of movement, while a cable-driven **EndoWrist** device adds another 3 degrees of freedom. The EndoWrist instruments allow for an impressively complete range of motion of the instrument tips, facilitating tissue dissection, optimal needle positioning, and direct suturing comparable to open surgery. Additionally, the **da Vinci** system incorporates a magnified 3D display of the operative field through the ingenious integration of the view offered by a two-channel endoscope. A primary feature, also, of this robotic system is the complete "immersion" of the surgeon to the endoscopic operative field without any external or operative cues, enabling for intuitive hand–eye coordination and superb depth perception.

4. True Robotic Surgery

True robotic surgery is accomplished with such advanced devices as **ROBODOC** (Integrated Surgical Systems, Sacramento, CA), designed for orthopedic surgery; this device can be programmed to perform primary or revision total hip or knee replacement. The task is facilitated by a preoperative planning workstation called **ORTHODOC** that simulates the surgery using the actual computed tomographic (CT) scan of the patient. Using the CT scans of the patient along with models of the virtual prosthesis, the surgeon is able to provide all the necessary preoperative data for the robotic surgery.

5. "Computer-Enhanced" Telesurgery: Operative Procedures

The clinical usefulness of computer-enhanced telesurgery is under intense development. Many applications have been utilized, and feasibility has been reported in a variety of clinical scenarios and operative techniques using both Zeus and daVinci robotic systems.

a. Cardiac Surgery

During the last 10 years the demand for a minimally invasive cardiac surgery has been met by the introduction of the beating heart surgery that eliminates the need for cardiopulmonary bypass and by decreasing the size of the incision so that some procedures can be performed through small incisions and limited thoracotomies. However, the development of a total endoscopic cardiac procedure proved extremely difficult, mainly owing to the inherent limitations of the laparoscopic technique in the microsurgical environment. The introduction of computer-enhanced robotic systems addressed many of the physical limitations of traditional endoscopic surgery in the microsurgical setting and allowed the performance of various procedures such as:

- Harvesting of the left internal thoracic artery
- Total endoscopic coronary artery bypass grafting (TECABG)
- Mitral valve repair and replacement
- Repair of atrial septal defects.

However these procedures are applicable only to very carefully selected patients, and the current worldwide experience with robotic heart surgery is largely retrospective and uncontrolled. A recent, controlled pilot study has documented the safety and the efficiency of robotically assisted TECABG in a small group of patients, with a 1-year follow up. Equally encouraging results have also been reported from various centers in Europe, but all studies agree that the use of robotic technology in cardiac surgery is still in its infancy. Additional enabling technology is needed to overcome the challenges posed by totally endoscopic off-pump multivessel coronary artery bypass surgery, and further controlled clinical trials are warranted for the development of the appropriate criteria for proper patient selection. Thousands of cardiac surgical procedures have been performed worldwide.

b. General Surgery

The feasibility of computer-enhanced robotic surgery (daVinci) in non-cardiac procedures was reported in a study that described the initial clinical experience of U.S. four centers. The vast majority of the procedures were intra-abdominal, including the following:

- Various antireflux procedures (69)
- Cholecystectomies (36)
- Heller myotomies (26)
- Bowel resections (17)
- Donor nephrectomy (15)
- Left internal mammary artery mobilization (14)
- Gastric bypasses (7)
- Splenectomies (7)
- Adrenalectomies (6)
- Exploratory laparoscopies (3)
- Pyloroplasties (4)
- Gastrojejunostomies (2)
- Distal pancreatectomy
- Duodenal polypectomy
- Gastric mass resection
- Lysis of adhesions

The study concluded that the clinical results of robotic assisted surgery compared favorably with those of conventional laparoscopy with respect to mortality, complications, and length of stay.

Antireflux surgery has been extensively evaluated by Melvin et al. (2001) in a prospective trial comparing the results of computer-enhanced robotic fundoplication and traditional laparoscopic antireflux procedures. With 20 patients in each arm of the study, there was little difference in clinical outcomes. Operative times were longer with the robot, but decreased as experience was gained. The study concluded that computer-assisted laparoscopic antireflux surgery is safe, but at the current level of development, offers little advantage over standard laparoscopic approaches.

Certain procedures such as Heller myotomy may be improved with the use of robotic devices. This assumption is based on the fact that computer-enhanced robotic devices, through the features of visual magnification, motion scaling, and fine tremor reduction, drastically improve manual performance in the microsurgical setting.

c. Urology

The feasibility of robotic assisted telesurgery in urologic laparoscopy is under investigation, and there are reports on nephrectomy, radical prostatectomy, pyeloplasty, and laparoscopic donor nephrectomy. There are significant advantages over standard laparoscopy in complex procedures such as prostatectomy. The experience with these advanced urological procedures is increasing rapidly at various centers throughout the world.

e. Pediatric Surgery

Chapter 46 discusses in detail the experience with pediatric robotic surgery.

D. Emerging Issues

The introduction of robotics to the field of minimally invasive surgery represents the way that cutting-edge technologies (computers and robotic engineering) have already started to affect the shape of surgery in the foreseeable future. However, being a new and developing concept, "robotic surgery" faces many challenges. Considering the difficulty of implementing robotics into this highly demanding field, we should address its current limitations.

- From the technological point of view, a major drawback of the current computer-enhanced robotic systems appears to be the lack of tactile feedback. As such, novel software programs need to be developed to incorporate force feedback seamlessly with the three-dimensional visual perception.
- To be practical, performance of telepresence surgery demands very-high-bandwidth communication channels and elimination of the transmission time delay.

Apart from the technological limitations, a serious issue regarding the clinical use of these robotic systems has to do with the assessment of their outcomes. Since computer-enhanced telesurgery is truly in its infancy, there are no randomized controlled studies demonstrating a clear-cut superiority in the clinical results associated with its use. While the technical superiority of these systems in the areas of motion and optics in comparison with standard laparoscopic instruments is taken for granted, the limited operative experience constitutes a serious drawback.

Moreover, the issues of credentialing and resident training appear to gain significant value as the use of robotic surgery is anticipated to expand. Skill for the novice may be acquired more rapidly with computer-assisted surgery, as shown by Melvin et al. (2002), who found that skill performance on a standardized test with the robotic system remains superior to that with standard laparoscopic instrumentation, even after training. However, the true learning curve for such complex devices has not been well demonstrated, and the encountered difference may be eliminated for the experienced surgeon.

A significant potential advantage of computer enhancement is the ability to increase the precision of surgery beyond that capable with the free hand. This would be most important in procedures requiring fine motor skills, high magnification, and microsurgical skills. Preliminary work with the existing devices has demonstrated the feasibility of using robotic devices for enhancement of open surgical procedures.

Merging imaging systems with computer-controlled operating systems may allow some significant benefits. This would potentially allow procedures to be performed without direct visualization. Another clear benefit would be the ability to simulate a patient-specific surgery and allow for preoperative planning and preoperative simulation to help reduce errors.

Continued technologic advances have allowed further minutarization of various devices. Future devices will allow intracorporeal flexible instruments and perhaps complex therapeutic interventions via existing body orifices. Telerobotic control and information system integration will allow these advanced procedures and technology to improve patient care outcomes.

E. Conclusion

The role of robotic surgery remains under development. However, it is certain that as technology advances, robotic technology will continue to change the patient–surgeon interface and improve patient outcomes.

F. References

Aiono S, Gilbert JM, Soin B, Finlay PA, Gordan A. Controlled trial of the introduction of a robotic camera assistant (EndoAssist) for laparoscopic cholecystectomy. Surg Endosc 2002;16:1267–1270.

Cadeddu JA, Stoianovici D, Chen RN, Moore RG, Kavoussi LR. Stereotactic mechanical percutaneous renal acess. J Endourol 1998;12:121–126.

Davies B. A review of robotics in surgery. Proc Inst Mech Eng 2000;214(H):129–140.

Lavallee S, Brunie L, Mazier B, et al. Image guided operating robot: a clinical application in stereotactic surgery. In: Taylor R, et al., eds. Computer Integrated Surgery. Cambridge, MA: MIT Press, 1996;77–98.

Luketich JD, Fernardo HC, Buanaventura PO, Christie NA, Grondin SC, Schauer PR. Results of a randomized trial of HERMES-assisted vs non-HERMES-assisted laparoscopic antireflux surgery. Surg Endosc 2002;16:1264–1268.

Massamune K, Kobayashi E, Masutani Y, et al. Development of an MRI-compatible needle insertion manipulator for stereotactic neurosurgery. J Image Guid Surg 1995; 1:242–248.

Melvin WS, Krause RK, Needleman JB, Wolf WR, Ellisson EC. Computer assisted "robotic" Heller myotomy: initial case report. J Lapar Advanc Surg Techniques 2001;11(4):251–253.

Melvin WS, Needleman JB, Krause RK, Schneider C, Ellisson EC. Computer-enhanced vs. standard laparoscopic antireflux surgery. J Gastroint Surg 2002;6:11–16.

Prasad SM, Ducko CT, Stephenson ER, Chambers CE, Ralph J. Prospective clinical trial of robotically assisted endoscopic coronary grafting with 1-year follow-up. Ann Surg 2001;233(6):725–732.

Rovetta A, Sala R. Robotics and telerobotics applied to a prostate biopsy on a human patient. Proceedings of the second International Symposium on Medical Robotics and Computer–Assisted Surgery, Baltimore, 2000;104.

Talamini M, Chapman W, Melvin S, Horgan S. A prospective analysis of 211 robotic assisted surgical procedures. Surg Endosc 2002;16(suppl 1):S205.

Laparoscopy
II—Diagnostic Laparoscopy and Biopsy

12. Emergency Laparoscopy

Steven C. Stain, M.D., F.A.C.S.A.

A. General Considerations

The entire peritoneal cavity can be visualized by the laparoscope, and diagnostic laparoscopy is an effective modality for determining pathology within the abdominal cavity. The decision to perform diagnostic laparoscopy is based on clinical judgment, weighing the sensitivities and specificities of other modalities (computed tomographic (CT) scan, ultrasound, diagnostic peritoneal lavage, mesenteric arteriography) versus the relative morbidity of minimally invasive laparoscopy. Although some centers have experience in performing laparoscopy in the emergency room or intensive care unit, most surgeons have reserved laparoscopy for the operating room. Once a surgical diagnosis has been made, laparoscopic therapeutic options are based upon the expertise of the surgeon. Equally important is the ability to exclude disease processes requiring surgical intervention, sparing the patient the potential morbidity of a negative celiotomy.

The **indications for emergency laparoscopy** can be grouped into those related to abdominal pain of uncertain etiology and those related to trauma resulting in intra-abdominal injury (Table 12.1). The therapies for individual conditions once identified are described elsewhere in this text.

B. Abdominal Pain

1. The most common indication for emergent abdominal operation or diagnostic laparoscopy is **suspected appendicitis**. Laparoscopic appendectomy is part of the modern surgeon's armamentarium, and diagnostic laparoscopy provides an excellent opportunity to establish and treat the diagnosis of appendicitis, but it also can diagnose other pathology mimicking the signs and symptoms of appendicitis. This enthusiasm of diagnostic laparoscopy for suspected appendicitis, which can accurately establish a diagnosis, should be weighed against the accuracy of thin-section CT scanning.
2. Diagnostic laparoscopy may be most appropriate for women of childbearing age, the group that historically has had the highest rates of negative appendectomy. In such patients, the differential diagnosis of appendicitis versus gynecologic pathology may be difficult, and laparoscopy can establish a precise diagnosis, and therapy if indicated. The gynecologist may be consulted preoperatively, or intraoperatively

Table 12.1. Indications for emergency laparoscopy.

Abdominal pain	• Right lower quadrant pain (rule out gynecologic pathology) • Right upper quadrant pain (rule out Fitz-Hugh-Curtis syndrome) • Peritonitis • Mesenteric ischemia • Intra-abdominal abscess, not amenable to image-guided drainage • Acalculous cholecystitis • Small bowel obstruction • Fever of unknown origin • Gastrointestinal hemorrhage of unexplained etiology
Trauma	• Blunt abdominal trauma • Penetrating trauma ■ Exclude peritoneal penetration ■ Evaluate diaphragm

if necessary. The technique of laparoscopic appendectomy is described in Chapter 30; but it is the policy of most surgeons to complete the appendectomy (if possible), even if alternate diagnoses are found at operation. Salpingitis is readily identified by visualization of inflamed fallopian tubes. A tubo-ovarian abscess may warrant gynecologic consultation. In women of reproductive age with right upper quadrant pain and negative radiologic studies, the diagnosis of Fitz-Hugh-Curtis syndrome should be entertained. Laparoscopy provides the opportunity to confirm the diagnosis and divide the perihepatic adhesions.

3. Small bowel obstruction due to adhesions is generally diagnosed radiologically, but may be treated laparoscopically (Chapter 28). Preoperative CT scan may provide information about the location of the obstructing adhesion and direct the exploration.

4. In certain patients with symptoms suggestive of peritonitis despite non-diagnostic radiologic studies, laparoscopy can accurately exclude surgical pathology, direct the placement of the appropriate surgical incision, or provide access for treatment (perforated duodenal ulcer, small bowel obstruction, Meckel's diverticulitis, etc.).

5. Emergency laparoscopy may be indicated for certain critically ill patients in the intensive care unit, especially those with sepsis of unknown etiology, whose instability would make a trip to the CT scan suite or operating room hazardous. Diagnostic laparoscopy can exclude surgical pathology or identify ischemic bowel, acalculous cholecystitis, or perforated viscus as the source.

6. Infrequently, diagnostic laparoscopy may be employed in patients with fever of unknown origin. In the patient presenting with vague

abdominal signs and fever, especially if there is a history of foreign travel or recent immigration, the diagnosis of tuberculosis or brucellosis should be considered. Laparoscopy can assist with confirming these diagnoses.

C. Method of Diagnostic Laparoscopy for Abdominal Pain

Emergency diagnostic laparoscopy requires a skill set different from that for a therapeutic laparoscopy for a known diagnosis (e.g., appendicitis or cholecystitis). If no pathology is found, the surgeon must be confident that he or she was able to exclude pathology requiring definitive surgical treatment. One must feel comfortable exposing solid organs and manipulating bowel for a thorough exploration. **It should never be considered a failure to resort to celiotomy for complete exploration or definitive therapy.**

Although it is feasible to perform diagnostic laparoscopy in the intensive care unit or the emergency department, diagnostic laparoscopy is best performed in the operating room.

Several principles of technique facilitate the procedure.

1. Unless prior abdominal surgery suggests otherwise, the laparoscope should be inserted at the umbilicus. In cases of abdominal distension, the open insertion of a Hasson cannula is safer.
2. Both a 30-degree laparoscope and a 0-degree laparoscope should be available. The 30-degree scope will be especially useful to "see around corners" and visually approach bowel or viscera from different angles for optimal maneuvering or dissection. A **10-mm laparoscope** provides better light and view, although a 5-mm scope may adequate. Remember the important objective of complete exploration, if the anticipated pathology is not readily identified.
3. Maximal working area is available when the surgeon stands on the side of the patient that is opposite the anticipated pathology. It may be advantageous to move from side to side if necessary to gain access to all four quadrants of the abdomen.
4. Two video monitors should be available, preferably mobile units, to locate the most favorable positions for the surgeon and assistant.
5. A second, or third, trocar will be necessary to manipulate, palpate, and move viscera for a thorough exploration. While 5-mm trocars are often adequate for laparoscopic instruments necessary for bowel manipulation, placement of 10-mm trocars may provide increased opportunity to relocate the laparoscope for improved visualization. Alternatively, a 5-mm laparoscope may be used for the alternate views.
6. If pathology is identified that requires a therapeutic intervention (e.g., appendectomy, patch of perforated ulcer), it can be performed by conversion to celiotomy, or laparoscopic treatment (refer to the appropriate chapter).

D. Laparoscopy for Trauma

The proper role of laparoscopy for injured patients is contingent upon the expertise of the surgeon, available instrumentation, and the diagnostic algorithm adopted for blunt or penetrating trauma. The established priorities provided by advanced trauma life support (airway, breathing, circulation) must be adhered to.

Patients with **blunt abdominal trauma** and obvious indications for celiotomy (hypotension, increasing abdominal girth, and other signs of hemorrhage) should have open exploration. There are few indications for emergency diagnostic laparoscopy for blunt trauma. Focused abdominal sonography for trauma (FAST) scans are indicated for unstable patients, and CT scan provides reliable definition of solid viscus injury of stable patients after blunt trauma. Laparoscopy may be appropriate for patients with a **"seat belt sign"** in whom suspicion of bowel injury exists. These patients have a 15% to 35% incidence of significant injury and warrant further investigation. A thorough diagnostic laparoscopy can identify bowel injury or exclude intra-abdominal pathology. Laparoscopy in head-injured patients should be performed with caution, as abdominal insufflation leads to increased intracranial pressure.

The evaluation of patient with **penetrating abdominal trauma** is evolving. Most centers perform celiotomy for all patients with gunshot wounds, however laparoscopy can be utilized to reliably exclude peritoneal violation in patients with anterior or flank tangential injuries. Laparoscopic evaluation of posterior gunshot wounds (posterior to the midaxillary line) is not appropriate. The majority of stab wounds do not require therapeutic celiotomy. The diagnostic evaluations used most frequently for stable patients are observation by serial physical examinations, CT scan, or ultrasonography. The application of local wound exploration and diagnostic peritoneal lavage appears to be decreasing. Several centers have reported their experience with diagnostic laparoscopy for anterior abdominal stab wounds as a valuable tool to exclude peritoneal violation, and select patients for early discharge.

Laparoscopy has an important role for **thoracoabdominal stab wounds**, especially on the left, that may have violated the diaphragm, and occult injury may present years later with diaphragmatic hernia and intestinal strangulation. These patients have up to a 24% incidence of diaphragm injury. No other modality (short of abdominal exploration) can reliably exclude diaphragm injury. Isolated diaphragm injuries can be repaired laparoscopically or by open exploration.

E. Method of Laparoscopy for Trauma

Hemodynamically unstable patients with abdominal injury require exploration. Emergency laparoscopy can be performed in the emergency room or operating room. Because trauma patients are assumed to have full stomachs, general endotracheal anesthesia in the operating room is preferred, and the surgical team should be prepared to convert to open celiotomy. The purpose of laparoscopy for trauma is to **exclude or confirm intra-abdominal injury**.

Appropriate use of diagnostic laparoscopy for trauma may reduce the incidence of nontherapeutic celiotomies that may occur with diagnostic peritoneal lavage or CT scan.

Application of the modality in the diagnostic algorithm adopted requires consideration of the technical expertise of the surgeon, the available resources in the hospital, and the relative strengths and weaknesses of other diagnostic tests available.

For penetrating trauma, diagnostic laparoscopy can be used to exclude peritoneal violation or to diagnose enteric injury. CT scan provides better information about the severity of solid organ injury because the entire organ is imaged, whereas laparoscopy allows only a surface view. It may be difficult to adequately evaluate the entire spleen with laparoscopy owing to overlying omentum.

Some principles to guide the exploration are as follows:

1. The patient should be placed supine, with a standard trauma prep, from clavicles to pelvis to allow for access for open exploration if necessary.

2. Always review the chest x-ray prior to general anesthesia with positive pressure ventilation. Penetrating wounds to the chest may result in a pneumothorax, which can be **converted to a tension pneumothorax** from abdominal insufflation and a diaphragm injury. An occult pneumothorax (not recognized by chest x-ray) may also lead to a tension pneumothorax with positive pressure ventilation or peritoneal insufflation.

3. Generally, the laparoscope (10 mm) should be inserted through the umbilicus. Mobile monitors should be positioned opposite the surgeon and assistant. The operating room table should allow Trendelenburg, reverse Trendelenburg, and side-to-side tilting of the table.

4. **A stab wound entrance site must be closed** (simple skin closure) to allow creation of the pneumoperitoneum. If no peritoneal injury is identified, one can assume there has not been peritoneal violation, and therefore no intra-abdominal injury.

5. Peritoneal violation from a stab wound **does not mandate open exploration**. If peritoneal violation has occurred, complete exploration is necessary to exclude injury, and additional trocars will be needed. Five-millimeter trocars will suffice, and utilizing atraumatic bowel graspers, the colon should be inspected and the small bowel should be run.

6. Diagnostic laparoscopy from a gunshot wound is generally performed to exclude peritoneal violation. Because the energy associated with ballistic injury, and the variability of the paths of bullets, peritoneal violation by a gunshot wound warrants open exploration.

7. In the case of blunt abdominal trauma, the bleeding can be characterized by a standard grading system (Table 12.2). Generally, grade 2 or 3 hemoperitoneum requires open celiotomy. Depending upon the mechanism of injury, the surgeon may choose to observe patients with grade 1 hemoperitoneum. Grade 0 is a normal examination.

The complications of laparoscopy for trauma include the complications of anesthesia and laparoscopy, but also some that are unique to the trauma patient.

Table 12.2. Grading system for hemoperitoneum observed at diagnostic laparoscopy.

- **Grade 0**: No blood is seen within the peritoneal cavity.
- **Grade 1**: Small flecks of blood on the bowel or small amounts of blood in the paracolic gutters. Blood does not recur when aspirated. No bleeding sight is seen.
- **Grade 2**: Blood is seen between loops of bowel and in the paracolic gutter. Blood recurs after aspiration.
- **Grade 3**: Frank blood is aspirated from the Veress needle, or the intestines are noted to be floating on a pool of blood.

1. Blunt trauma patients may have sustained closed head injury. It has been demonstrated that both pneumoperitoneum and reverse Trendelenburg position lead to increased intracranial pressure with potentially serious consequences.
2. Hypothermia may be exacerbated with insufflation of cold carbon dioxide gas, leading to worsening of acidosis.
3. Pneumothorax, from occult pulmonary injury or peritoneal insufflation through a diaphragm injury, may occur.
4. Physiologic changes, such as acidosis, cardiac depression, arrhythmias, and gas absorption causing subcutaneous emphysema, may have more profound consequences in the trauma patient.

F. Selected References

Bender JS, Talamini MA. Diagnostic laparoscopy in critically ill intensive care patients. Surg Endosc 1992;6:302–304.

Berci G, Sackier JM, Paz-Partlow M. Emergency laparoscopy. Am J Surg 1991;161:355–360.

Chandler DF, Lane JS, Waxman KS. Seatbelt sign following trauma is associated with increased incidence of abdominal injury. Am Surg 1997;885–888.

Decadt B. Sussman L, Lewis MPN, et al. Randomized clinical trial of early laparoscopy in the management of acute non-specific abdominal pain. Br J Surg 1999;1383–1386.

Eachempati SR, Barie PS. Minimally invasive and noninvasive diagnosis and therapy in critically ill and injured patients. Arch Surg 1999;1189–1196.

Forde KA, Treat MR. The role of peritoneoscopy (laparoscopy) in the evaluation of the acute abdomen in critically ill patients. Surg Endosc 1992;6:219–221.

Halverson A, Buchanan R, Jacobs K, et al. Evaluation of mechanism of increased intracranial pressure with insufflation. Surg Endosc 1998;266–269.

Murray JA, Demetriades D, Asensio JA, et al. Occult injuries to the diaphragm: prospective evaluation of laparoscopy in penetrating injuries to the left lower chest. J Am Coll Surg 1998;626–630.

Paw P, Sackier JM. Complications of laparoscopy and thoracoscopy. J Intensive Care Med 1994;9:290–304.

Sackier JM. Second-look laparoscopy in the management of acute mesentery ischemia. Br J Surg 1994;81:1546.

Schob OM, Allen DC, Benzel E, et al. A comparison of the pathophysiologic effects of carbon dioxide, nitrous oxide, and helium pneumoperitoneum on intracranial pressure. Am J Surg 1996;248–253.

Simon RJ, Rabin J, Kuhls D. Impact of increased use of laparoscopy on negative laparotomy rates after penetrating trauma. J Trauma 2002:297–302.

Sosa JL, Sims D, Martin L, Zeppa R. Laparoscopic evaluation of tangential abdominal gunshot wounds. Arch Surg 1992;127:109–110.

13. Elective Diagnostic Laparoscopy and Cancer Staging

Frederick L. Greene, M.D., F.A.C.S.

A. Diagnostic Laparoscopy

The laparoscope has become an important tool in the diagnosis of benign and malignant conditions in the abdominal cavity. This modality should be utilized in conjunction with conventional imaging techniques such as computed tomography (CT), percutaneous ultrasound, magnetic resonance imaging (MRI), positron emission tomography (PET) and other radiologic and nuclear medicine studies to differentiate between benign and malignant processes as well as to assess the degree of potential metastatic disease in the abdominal cavity. The laparoscope may also be used to identify the underlying cause of unexplained ascites.

1. Indications for Elective Diagnostic Laparoscopy

Patients with underlying malignancy may have either primary or metastatic malignant disease within the abdomen. Common lesions such as carcinoma of the esophagus, stomach, pancreas, and colorectum are reasons to consider diagnostic laparoscopy for full preoperative assessment (Table 13.1). Frequently, melanoma of the trunk or extremities may metastasize to the small bowel, causing unexplained bleeding or chronic intermittent small bowel obstruction. A patient with these findings may benefit from a laparoscopic examination. Other indications for laparoscopic staging include the full assessment of patients with Hodgkin lymphoma to plan appropriate chemotherapy and/or radiation therapy.

The laparoscope may be utilized for general inspection of the abdominal cavity and as a method of obtaining tissue from solid organs such as liver or lymph nodes (Table 13.2). Imaging studies give only indirect evidence of underlying disease and, therefore, the laparoscope may be used for directed biopsy, obtaining cytolologic specimens along with peritoneal lavage, or fine-needle aspiration techniques. In some parts of the world, infectious diseases (such as tuberculosis or parasitic infestation) causing abdominal problems may be more prevalent than cancer, and laparoscopic examination assists in the differential diagnosis of these entities. Diagnostic laparoscopy is also beneficial for patients with chronic abdominal pain who have had limited abdominal procedures in the

Table 13.1. Indications for laparoscopic staging of abdominal tumors.

- Preoperative assessment prior to major extirpation
- Documentation of hepatic or nodal involvement
- Confirmation of imaging studies
- Therapeutic decision making for Hodgkin lymphoma
- Full assessment of ascitic fluid

past. This is especially true in women who have undergone hysterectomy and who have chronic pelvic pain. The identification and lysis of adhesions may be beneficial in this group.

2. Technique of Elective Diagnostic Laparoscopy

After appropriate preoperative evaluation, diagnostic laparoscopy may be performed under either general or local anesthesia. General anesthesia is preferred for most cases, especially if cancer staging is to be performed. Diagnostic laparoscopy may be performed in the operating room (most common) or in a treatment area equipped for administration of anesthesia and with full resuscitative support. A proper table that allows the patient to be placed in both full Trendelenburg and reverse Trendelenburg positions during examination is essential. Appropriate time should be taken for a full examination of the upper and lower abdomen. This generally requires creating a pneumoperitoneum using carbon dioxide at 10 to 12 mm Hg.

A 10-mm laparoscope is preferred utilizing both 0-degree and 30-degree cameras for full visualization. Place the laparoscope through a midline subumbilical trocar site using a 10/11-mm trocar sleeve. Depending on the area to be examined, place one or two additional 5-mm trocars in each upper quadrant. These will be used for grasping forceps, palpating probes, and biopsy forceps.

Biopsy may be performed with cupped forceps passed through either a 5- or 10-mm trocar sleeve. Alternatively, cutting biopsy needles may be used to obtain liver or nodal tissue (Fig. 13.1). The needle biopsy may be performed

Table 13.2. Techniques utilized during diagnostic or staging laparoscopy.

- Full abdominal and pelvic evaluation
- Division of gastrohepatic omentum
- Biopsy using cupped forceps or core needle
- Abdominal lavage for cytologic study
- Retrieval of ascitic fluid for cytology and culture
- Identification and removal of enlarged lymph nodes
- Laparoscopic ultrasound

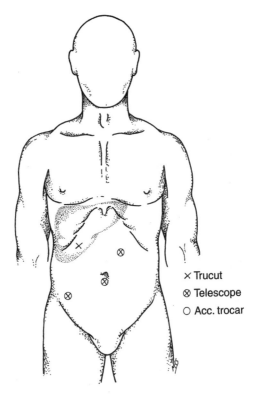

× Trucut
⊗ Telescope
○ Acc. trocar

Figure 13.1. Trocar and needle placement for liver biopsy. The biopsy needle may be passed through a trocar or percutaneously through the abdominal wall.

percutaneously under laparoscopic guidance, or the biopsy needle may be passed through one of the 5-mm trocar sheaths. It is important to **perform biopsy cleanly** without crushing tissue, since this might reduce the opportunity for pathologic review.

Specific areas of biopsy depend on the nature of the lesion and the tumor undergoing staging, and several malignancies will be discussed individually in the sections that follow. For example, in patients with lower esophageal and gastric cancer, the liver must be closely inspected and biopsies should be performed on any lesions on the surface of the liver. In addition, the gastrohepatic and gastrocolic omental areas may be divided to allow for evaluation of nodal tissue in these areas. Lymph nodes should be removed intact, if possible, to achieve better histologic identification. In assessing the patient with pancreatic cancer, the duodenum may be mobilized by means of Kocher maneuver.

Biopsies may be performed on retroduodenal tissue and lymph nodes may be assessed as follows. The gastrocolic omentum should be divided and the superior pancreatic area should be to observe for evidence of local or regional pancreatic cancer. In addition, lavage with 500 mL of saline should routinely be performed to obtain fluid for cytologic investigation. The operating table should be angled into various positions to allow for the disbursement of the lavage fluid. The fluid should be totally removed and sent to the cytology laboratory to be centrifuged and evaluated for malignant cells. Staging for pancreatic cancer prior to the planning of a Whipple procedure should be a separate event to allow for the assessment of cytology results and any biopsy specimens taken during the procedure. The laparoscope may not completely aid in the examination of the retropancreatic region especially in the region of the superior mesenteric artery and vein. Additional techniques specifically utilizing intraoperative laparoscopic ultrasound may aid in this assessment.

B. Esophageal Carcinoma (Squamous and Adenocarcinoma)

The majority of esophageal cancers occur in the middle and distal third and are predominantly squamous cell. An increase in the incidence of adenocarcinoma of the distal esophagus, recently seen in association with Barrett's changes, is believed to be related to reflux esophagitis. The classic approach to esophageal cancer management has been esophagectomy with reconstruction using either the stomach or the colon as an interposed organ. Because of the recent advances in esophageal cancer management using chemotherapy and radiation, postoperative or neoadjuvant therapy may be important in many of these patients. In addition, nodal involvement in carcinoma of the esophagus occurs in the mediastinal area as well as in the celiac region and may be advanced even when imaging studies fail to show nodal disease. Patients with advanced esophageal cancer, although amenable to palliation, may not benefit from major extirpative surgery. In these cases radiation with placement of new expandable stents may give appropriate treatment and support quality of life.

Laparoscopic assessment of esophageal cancer is important to identify the group of patients that will not benefit by esophagectomy. Careful assessment of the liver as well as the celiac axis can identify occult nodes in these regions or small metastases that have not been apparent on preoperative imaging studies.

The technique of laparoscopy for the assessment of esophageal cancer utilizes three ports: an umbilical port for the laparoscope and two accessory ports, one in each subcostal region.

1. Begin the assessment of the abdomen by placing the patient in steep Trendelenburg position and inspecting the pelvic peritoneum, looking for small peritoneal metastases.

2. Next, place the operating table in a neutral position. Rotate it sequentially to the right and left decubitus positions (commonly termed "airplaning" the table) and look for ascites. Aspirate any fluid and send it for cytology.

3. Next, inspect the liver. The reverse Trendelenburg position, with the left side down, assists by allowing the liver to drop down out of the

subdiaphragmatic space. Look at all visible surfaces of the liver, using an angled (45-degree) laparoscope to facilitate inspection. Carefully assess the liver for any unusual adhesions or plaques, which may initially appear benign yet harbor small metastases. Perform a biopsy on any suspicious areas with cup forceps or cutting needle.

4.   Perform biopsies on any lesions seen on the peritoneum or omentum with cupped forceps also. Electrocautery is extremely useful, as bleeding may occur; diagnostic laparoscopic examination should not be undertaken without this capability.

5.   Next, examine the anterior wall of the stomach and the region of the esophageal hiatus (Fig. 13.2). Place the table in reverse Trendelenburg position and use a 30-degree laparoscope.

6.   Divide the gastrohepatic omentum to search for lymph nodes in the region of the subhepatic space and the lesser curvature extending up to the esophageal hiatus. Lymph nodes in the region of the left gastric and celiac vessels may be inspected by this technique. Pass the laparoscope into the lesser sac for full identification (Fig. 13.3). If frozen-section-positive nodes are found, place metal clips to facilitate planning of radiation therapy, if appropriate.

C. Gastric Cancer

Although the approach to cancer of the stomach is generally resection whether it be for cure or palliation, laparoscopic evaluation may be important in patients who present with advanced disease and are unresectable. Recently, there has been a trend of more patients with carcinoma of the cardia and proximal stomach than with the antral carcinomas previously seen. The assessment of the patient with gastric cancer is similar to that noted in esophageal cancer, and many of the same maneuvers are involved. Because of the generally poor results with radiation and chemotherapy in the management of gastric cancer, these patients may be candidates for palliative resection.

Recently, sentinel node techniques have been advocated for the enhancement of staging in gastric cancer. There may be additional roles for staging laparoscopy in this disease, as recognition of the nodal drainage patterns in gastric cancer is increased by radionuclide and vital staining.

D. Tumors of the Liver (Primary and Metastatic)

Laparoscopic assessment of primary hepatic tumors is ideal because many of these tumors involve the surface of the liver. The recent application of laparoscopic ultrasound has aided in the identification of tumors deep to Glisson's capsule. Although metastatic disease of the liver is the most common indication for laparoscopic assessment, given the worldwide incidence of hepatocellular

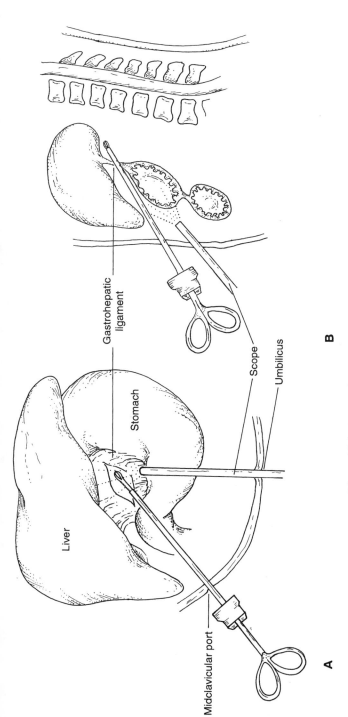

Figure 13.2. Approach to the esophageal hiatus.

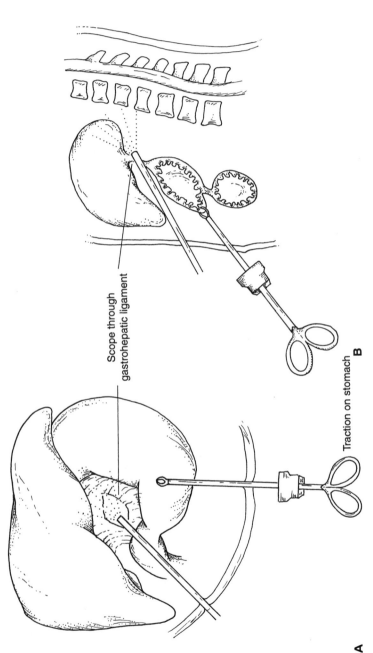

Figure 13.3. Laparoscope switched to right upper quadrant portal and passed into lesser sac through opening in avascular portion of gastrohepatic omentum. Traction on the stomach facilitates this maneuver.

cancer and the increase in hepatic tumors associated with chronic hepatitis, evaluation of hepatocellular cancer is becoming increasingly more important. Traditional imaging studies may underestimate involvement of the liver, and this becomes critically important when hepatic resection is being considered.

1. **A three-trocar technique** is used for hepatic assessment, with an umbilical trocar for the laparoscope, and accessory ports in the left and right upper quadrants. Peritoneal attachments to the liver may need division based on the anatomical findings in the specific patient (Fig. 13.4).

2. Hepatic lesions may have a variety of colors including white, gray, or yellow, and may be nodular or have a depressed center forming a "moon crater" or a "volcano" appearance. These lesions may also have increased vascularity, giving a hyperemic appearance.

3. Biopsy techniques using cutting needles or cup forceps are indicated. Electrocautery should be immediately available to achieve hemostasis. If a bleeding vessel is noted, it is generally just below the liver capsule and can be handled easily by combining pressure with the cautery tip at the time of applying cauterization.

4. In patients with hepatocellular cancer, diffuse lesions in both lobes of the liver as well as extrahepatic disease are obvious contraindications to primary resection. These patients may also have associated cirrhosis as a manifestation of chronic alcohol ingestion or hepatitis. Laparoscopy is important in the identification of the cirrhotic liver, which may also be a major contraindication to further resection.

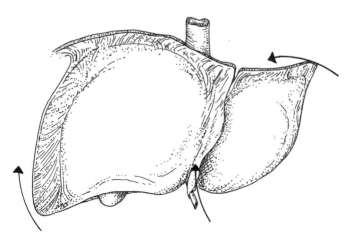

Figure 13.4. Schematic of peritoneal attachments of liver, which may need to be divided for full assessment of the hepatic surface. Generally this is not required, but the laparoscopist should be aware of the regional anatomy.

E. Pancreatic Carcinoma

Currently the most beneficial use of preoperative laparoscopic evaluation is in the management of patients with pancreatic cancer, which may aid in identifying patients in whom cancer cells are already disseminated throughout the abdomen, precluding curative resection. The identification of advanced nodal, peritoneal, or hepatic disease is important prior to undertaking celiotomy. This is especially true in patients with carcinoma of the body and tail, since these tumors generally are identified later in the course than in patients who have carcinomas of the head of the pancreas and present with early jaundice. Diagnostic laparoscopy is indicated when conventional imaging (helical CT, MRI) shows obvious disease or is suspicious for extrapancreatic tumors. The role for laparoscopic staging of all patients is unclear but advanced disease will be revealed when imaging studies show disease limited to the pancreas.

1. The goals of laparoscopic evaluation in pancreatic cancer are to **assess peripancreatic nodes** as well as **remote sites** that may harbor metastases.

2. Perform direct inspection of the pancreas by dividing the gastrocolic and gastrohepatic omental areas and by inserting the laparoscope into the **lesser sac**. Needle aspiration or biopsy of peripancreatic masses may be accomplished in this manner if a tissue diagnosis has not previously been obtained.

3. Pancreatitis and the development of adhesions in this area may render inspection of the lesser sac difficult. Gentle dissection of these adhesions by means of electrocautery may allow for excellent inspection of the pancreatic body and tail with opportunity for laparoscopically guided biopsy in a large number of patients.

4. The major purpose of laparoscopy is to look for superficial peritoneal and hepatic masses that have not been identified by conventional imaging studies. Using a combination of laparoscopy and CT or MRI of the abdomen, at least 90% of unresectible tumors can be identified, which benefits a large group of patients without the need for exploratory celiotomy.

5. Cytologic investigation of peritoneal washings should be performed if results of other examinations are negative. Carcinoma cells may be obtained from the free peritoneal cavity even when the peritoneum itself is grossly free of metastatic implants. Positive cytology indicates metastatic (M1) disease.

F. Staging of Other Malignancies, Including Hodgkin Lymphoma

Laparoscopic staging may also be utilized in patients with primary genitourinary malignancies including testicular tumors and prostate cancer. These are discussed in more detail in Chapter 38, Lymph Node Biopsy, Dissection, and

Staging Laparoscomy. Levels of serum tumor markers are used to delineate a subgroup of these patients that may benefit from preoperative laparoscopic assessment.

Patients with Hodgkin lymphoma may undergo limited staging laparoscopic procedures or complete laparoscopic staging (equivalent to staging laparotomy) including splenectomy. Hodgkin lymphoma may present as local, regional, or systemic disease. The traditional open-staging laparotomy includes wedge and needle biopsy of the liver, retroperitoneal and para-aortic nodal dissection, iliac nodal dissection, and splenectomy. Staging laparotomy has largely been supplanted by modern imaging techniques but still has a role in selected cases where therapeutic decisions require precise assessment of intra-abdominal disease. Staging laparoscopy for Hodgkin lymphoma combines several procedures (e.g., laparoscopic splenectomy) that are described in detail in other sections. A few remarks about the conduct of a staging laparoscopic examination for Hodgkin lymphoma may be helpful, however.

1. The **Hasson (open)** approach is preferred because tissue must be removed during the procedure (see Chapter 8, Principles of Specimen Removal).

2. Perform **a full abdominal evaluation**, and do a biopsy of any nodules on the surface of the **liver**. If, as is usually the case, the liver appears grossly normal, take a wedge biopsy of the liver (using either suture control or a laparoscopic stapler for hemostasis). Generally it will be most convenient to take this wedge from the lateral segment of the left lobe of the liver. Perform a deep cutting needle biopsy of the right lobe.

3. A **splenectomy** is still considered traditional in full staging for Hodgkin lymphoma and can be accomplished laparoscopically (see Chapter 37, Laparoscopic Splenectomy). Some protocols utilize a selective approach to splenectomy, based upon imaging studies and intraoperative findings, and this trend may continue.

4. Perform a careful inspection of the spleen in all patients. Identify the region of the tail of the pancreas and hilum of the spleen, and search for **splenic hilar lymph nodes**. Intraoperative ultrasound examination, discussed later in this section, is extremely helpful. The hilum of the spleen and region of the tail of the pancreas should be identified to assess nodes in this region.

5. Approach the **para-aortic lymph nodes** directly through the base of the transverse mesocolon. Prior study using lymphangiography may identify abnormal nodal regions that could be approached laparoscopically.

6. The nodes in the region of the **common iliac vessels** may be more easily approached and either sampled or totally removed for identification. See Chapter 38 for more information on the technique of node dissection in this region and in the pelvis.

7. Perform a careful assessment of the pelvis in young women and consider oophoropexy if pelvic irradiation is contemplated. Prior consultation with the radiation therapy department will determine whether this maneuver is needed. In addition, small clips could be placed in the region of the ovaries to guide the radiation oncologist in treatment

planning. Traditionally, oophoropexy may preserve ovarian function in 50% of patients receiving pelvic irradiation, but is less commonly needed with newer treatment protocols.

G. Laparoscopic Ultrasound in Cancer Staging

Laparoscopic cancer staging should include routine adjunctive laparoscopic ultrasound (LUS), which assists in identifying small lesions and directing biopsies. LUS examination uses either linear array or sector scan probes with rigid or flexible tips in frequencies ranging from 5 to 10 MHz. Color Doppler imaging may be available to discern venous or arterial blood flow. These probes allow high-resolution imaging of the liver, bile ducts, pancreas, abdominal vessels, and lymph nodes. Overall, the application of LUS in cancer staging increases the accuracy by approximately 5% to 25% in patients evaluated.

This section gives specific techniques for various anatomic regions and should be considered complementary to Sections B through F (which deal with specific malignancies).

1. **Liver.** Generally three trocars are used, including a 10/11-mm trocar in the right upper quadrant, an umbilical port for the laparoscope, and a left upper quadrant port (Fig. 13.5). Pass a flexible or rigid ultrasound probe over the right lobe, medial segment of the left lobe, and lateral segment of the left lobe to identify lesions in the hepatic parenchyma. The anterior and posterior surfaces may be scanned easily without mobilization of the liver.

   a. Contact between the ultrasound probe and the liver surface may be improved by lowering the pressure setting on the insufflator and allowing the pneumoperitoneum to partially collapse.

   b. Identify hemangiomas and differentiate these from metastatic lesions by their compressibility, elicited either by contact with the ultrasound probe directly or by palpation with an instrument. Small hemangiomas are usually hyperechoic.

   c. Small liver metastases are usually hypoechoic compared with normal liver parenchyma or isoechoic with a hypoechoic halo. Biopsy suspicious lesions with a cutting needle or biopsy forceps. Lesions as small as 3 mm may be identified by LUS.

2. **Biliary tract** (see also Chapter 14, Laparoscopic Cholecystectomy)

   a. Image the intrahepatic bile ducts, the bifurcation, and the proximal common bile duct by placing the probe on the anterior surface of segment IV of the liver. Use the umbilical and subcostal trocars alternately to obtain longitudinal and transverse scans. Bile duct dilatation, inflammatory bile duct thickening, and localized bile duct tumors of 1 cm or less may be seen.

   b. Image the **gallbladder** either through the liver or by placing the probe on the gallbladder itself.

   c. Tumors of the bifurcation or the proximal **common bile duct** are usually isoechoic in comparison to liver parenchyma. In some patients the falciform ligament prevents the appropriate applica-

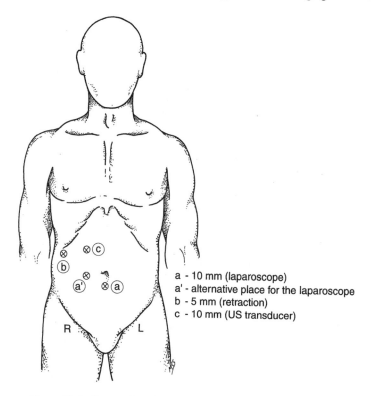

a - 10 mm (laparoscope)
a' - alternative place for the laparoscope
b - 5 mm (retraction)
c - 10 mm (US transducer)

Figure 13.5. Trocar sites for laparoscopic ultrasound examination.

tion of the laparoscopic ultrasound probe during the evaluation of tumors of the left hepatic duct and surrounding area. This may be resolved by scanning segment IV as well as segments II and III to the left of the falciform ligament.

3. **Pancreas and periampullary region**
   a. Visualize the pancreas, pancreatic duct, and common bile duct by placing the LUS probe on the stomach and duodenum. Tumors in this region are best imaged through the left and right subcostal trocars, which produce transverse or oblique sections of the pancreas.
   b. The portal venous system may also be imaged with LUS. The superior mesenteric vein is best evaluated from the left subcostal trocar, while the more obliquely oriented portal vein is best imaged from the right subcostal trocar. Vessels of the low-pressure portal system are easily compressed by the ultrasound probe, falsely implying stenosis when in fact the vessel is normal.

126   F.L. Greene

Tumor infiltration into the portal vein is characterized by loss of the hyperechoic interface between the vessel lumen and the tumor.

c. Adenocarcinomas of the pancreas as well as small cholangiocarcinomas and carcinomas of the papilla of Vater (approximately 1 cm) may be seen as a hypoechoic mass in comparison to normal pancreas. In contrast, neuroendocrine tumors of the pancreas and duodenal wall show higher echogenicity than adenocarcinomas.

d. Differentiation between pancreatic inflammation and tumor may be quite important. Generally inflamed pancreatic tissue is hypoechoic compared to normal pancreatic parenchyma.

4. **Lymph nodes.** LUS is an ideal technique for evaluating nodes without performing a formal node dissection. Ultrasound features suggesting benign nodes include a hyperechoic center, which represents hilar fat within the lymph node. If the image is more rounded and more hypoechoic with a loss of the hyperechoic center, metastasis must be assumed. There is overlap on occasion between benign and malignant features of nodes on ultrasound exam. Enlargement of lymph nodes by itself is not a characteristic of either benign or malignant lesions.

a. Nodes in the **hepatoduodenal ligament** and **celiac axis** are best seen through the left lobe of the liver or by direct approximation of the LUS probe directly on the hepatoduodenal ligament or celiac axis. Localization of these nodes will then allow for laparoscopic biopsy. This is especially helpful in the preoperative staging of gastric carcinoma, or during staging laparoscopy for Hodgkin lymphoma.

b. Tumors of the gastric cardia or distal esophagus have an isoechoic appearance on LUS. Nodal involvement especially in the **celiac and lesser curve areas** is apparent on LUS.

H. Selected References

Conlon KC, Dougherty E, Klimstra DS, Coit DG, Turnbull AD, Brennan MF. The value of minimal access surgery in the staging of patients with potentially resectable peripancreatic malignancy. Ann Surg 1996;223:134–140.

Feld RI, Liu J-B, Nazarian L. Laparoscopic liver sonography: preliminary experience in liver metastases compared with CT portography. J Ultrasound Med 1996;15:289–295.

Fleming ID, Cooper JS, Henson DE, eds. AJCC Cancer Staging Manual. 5th ed. Philadelphia: Lippincott-Raven, 1997.

Greene FL. Laparoscopy in malignant disease. Surg Clin North Am 1992;72:1125–1137.

Greene FL, Heniford BT. Minimally Invasive Cancer Management. New York: Springer-Verlag, 2001.

Greene FL, Rosin RD. Minimal Access Surgical Oncology. Oxford: Radcliffe Medical Press, 1995.

Hohenberger P, Conlon K. Staging Laparoscopy. Berlin: Springer-Verlag, 2002.

Hunerbein M, Rau B, Schlag PM. Laparoscopy and laparoscopic ultrasound for staging of upper gastrointestinal tumours. Eur J Surg Oncol 1995;21:50–54.

John TG, Greig JD, Carter DC, Garden OJ. Carcinoma of the pancreatic head and peri-ampullary region: tumor staging with laparoscopy and laparoscopic ultrasonography. Ann Surg 1995; 221:156–164.

John TG, Greig JD, Crosbie JL, Miles WF, Garden OJ. Superior staging of liver tumors with laparoscopy and laparoscopic ultrasound. Ann Surg 1994; 220:711–719.

Johnstone P, Rohde DC, Swartz SE, Fetter J, Wexner S. Port site recurrences after laparo-scopic and thoracoscopic procedures in malignancy. J Clin Oncol 1996; 14:1950–1956.

Pratt BL, Greene FL. Role of laparoscopy in the staging of malignant disease. Surg Clin North Am 2000;80:1111–1126.

Ramshaw BJ. Laparoscopic surgery for cancer patients. CA 1997;47:327–350.

Ravikumar TS. Laparoscopic staging and intraoperative ultrasonography for liver tumor management. Surg Oncol Clin North Am 1996;5:271–282.

Warshaw AL, Tepper J, Shipley W. Laparoscopy in the staging and planning of therapy for pancreatic cancer. Am J Surg 1986;151:76–80.

Watt I, Stewart I, Anderson D, Bell G, Anderson JR. Laparoscopy, ultrasound, and computed tomography in cancer of the esophagus and gastric cardia: a prospective comparison for detecting intra-abdominal metastases. Br J Surg 1989;76:1036–1039.

Laparoscopy
III—Laparoscopic Cholecystectomy and Common Duct Exploration

14. Laparoscopic Cholecystectomy

Karen Deveney, M.D.

A. Indications

The indications for cholecystectomy remain the same and should not be liberalized because the laparoscopic procedure is viewed as lower in morbidity than its open counterpart. Conditions for which the procedure is used include the following.

1. **Symptomatic cholelithiasis.** Ultrasound confirmation of gallstones in conjunction with a classic history is sufficient to make the diagnosis.
   a. The most common symptom pattern consists of episodic epigastric or right upper quadrant pain occurring several hours after meals.
   b. Patients with nonspecific symptoms, such as nausea, bloating, indigestion, and flatulence, are sometimes benefited by cholecystectomy; however, the more the symptoms differ from the classic pattern of biliary pain, the less likely the patient is to experience relief after cholecystectomy.

2. **Acute cholecystitis,** typically causing constant right upper quadrant discomfort accompanied by objective signs of right upper quadrant tenderness, with or without a Murphy's sign or a palpable mass: fever and leukocytosis are common but not necessary for cholecystitis to be present. Despite inflammation, laparoscopic cholecystectomy may be accomplished in most patients without conversion to an open procedure.
   a. **Calculus biliary tract disease** causes most acute cholecystitis, and stones are seen on ultrasound examination.
   b. **Acute acalculous cholecystitis** occurs in critically ill patients, those on prolonged total parenteral nutrition, and some immunosuppressed patients. The diagnosis is suggested by thickening of the gallbladder wall on ultrasound, pericholecystic fluid, or delayed emptying. Although laparoscopic cholecystectomy may be performed, percutaneous cholecystostomy is an alternative management option for critically ill patients.

3. Individuals with **asymptomatic cholelithiasis** may be appropriate candidates for laparoscopic cholecystectomy under **specific circumstances** such as candidacy for renal transplant.

4. Patients with episodes of right upper quadrant pain, which are "classic" for **biliary pain without evidence of cholelithiasis** on objective tests such as ultrasound or endoscopic retrograde cholangiopancereatography (ERCP) may also be referred for laparoscopic

cholecystectomy, but sustained resolution of symptoms is less likely in these patients. Biliary dyskinesia, determined by objective measurement of gallbladder emptying after fatty meal or cholecystokinin infusion, may be present in some of these patients.

5.   **Gallstone pancreatitis** occurs when small stones pass through the cystic duct. To prevent recurrence, cholecystectomy should be performed after the pancreatitis has resolved. Cholangiography is prudent to exclude small stones in the common duct.

Contraindications to laparoscopic cholecystectomy include the inability to tolerate general anesthesia, significant portal hypertension, and uncorrectable coagulopathy. The patient must be a suitable candidate for the equivalent open surgical procedure, since conversion to an open procedure may be necessary. Multiple prior operations (causing adhesions, see Chapter 10.2), inflammation from acute cholecystitis or pancreatitis, or unclear anatomy may preclude safe laparoscopic dissection and may require conversion to an open procedure. Conversion to an open procedure represents good judgment under these circumstances.

B. Patient Preparation, Position, and Room Setup

Preoperative evaluation should include verification of gallstones and assessment of common duct size by ultrasound, as well as liver function tests. An electrocardiogram (or even specialized cardiac tests) may be prudent to exclude the rare patient in whom cardiac ischemia masquerades as biliary colic. Serum amylase and lipase to exclude acute pancreatitis are ordered selectively.

1.   The operating table should be compatible with any radiographic equipment used for cholangiography (see Chapter 16), even if the routine use of this modality is not planned.

2.   Position the patient supine on the operating table. The arms may be extended, or may be tucked at the side. Tucking the right arm facilitates intraoperative cholangiography, since there is less impediment to positioning the C-arm.

3.   The surgeon stands at the left side of the patient. Some surgeons, especially in Europe, place the patient in the low lithotomy position and operate from between the patient's legs.

4.   Two monitors are used, placed on the right and left of the patient near the head. The typical room setup is shown in Figure 14.1.

5.   An orogastric tube is placed after induction of anesthesia. Most surgeons place sequential compression stockings to avoid venous stasis (it is important to note that there are insufficient data in the literature to support this). Some surgeons place a Foley catheter in the bladder.

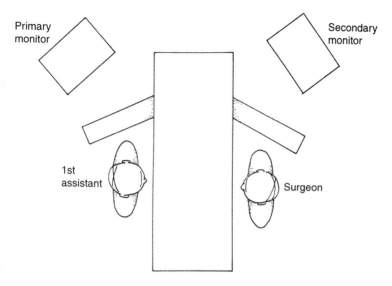

Figure 14.1. The most common patient and equipment positions; the cabinet containing the laparoscopic equipment should be placed on the side of the operating table opposite the main door, so that a C-arm or other radiographic equipment can be brought in if needed. Suction, cautery, and other ancillary equipment are similarly placed behind the monitor on the side away from the door.

C. Trocar Position and Choice of Laparoscope

1. Laparoscopic cholecystectomy usually is performed with four trocars: two 10-mm trocars (in the midepigastrium and umbilicus) and two 5-mm trocars along the right costal margin (Fig. 14.2). Some surgeons use a 5-mm camera and trocar in the epigastrium, and two- or three-port techniques have been described, but are not the norm.
   a. Place the first 10-mm trocar at the umbilicus, insert the laparoscope, and perform a general exploration of the abdomen.
   b. Although a 0-degree laparoscope can be used, a 30-degree laparoscope allows more flexibility in obtaining a complete view of all structures in the portal area and decreases the risk of injury to the ducts.
2. Place the patient in reverse Trendelenburg position and rotate the operating table with the left side down.
   a. Under laparoscopic visual control, place two 5-mm trocars along the right costal margin. The usual location is two fingerbreadths below the costal margin at the midclavicular and anterior axillary

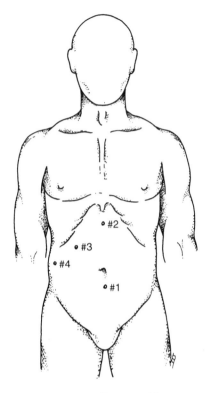

Figure 14.2. Trocar positions.

lines. These trocars should be approximately 8 to 10 cm apart. Exact position may need to be modified depending upon patient habitus and the location of the liver relative to the costal margin.

b. The fourth trocar will be the main operating trocar, so good placement is crucial. Some surgeons place graspers into the two lateral ports and manipulate the liver to estimate where Calot's triangle will be during dissection. The most usual location for the fourth trocar is epigastric, at least 10 cm from the laparoscope. The trocar is placed under laparoscopic visual control and should be directed to the right of the falciform ligament as it enters the abdominal cavity.

c. It is often possible to place the epigastric and two subcostal incisions along the line of an incision suitable for conversion to open procedure.

d. Modify these trocar positions slightly if the lithotomy position is used. Move the 10/11-mm epigastric trocar to the left upper quadrant, and place one of the 5-mm trocars to the right of the umbilicus. This facilitates two-handed operation from the lithotomy position.

D. Performing the Cholecystectomy

1. Pass two **atraumatic graspers** through the right subcostal trocars. Gently elevate the liver by passing these graspers beneath the visible liver edge. The gallbladder may be immediately apparent, or may be surrounded by omental adhesions.
2. Adhesions to the underside of the liver and gallbladder may contain omentum, colon, stomach, or duodenum, and hence must be dissected with care. It is prudent to use cautery as little as possible to avoid transmission of energy to the attached structures (which might result in delayed perforation of a viscus).
3. If the gallbladder is acutely inflamed and tense, decompress it before attempting to grasp it.
   a. Pass a Veress needle through the abdominal wall under laparoscopic visual control.
   b. Use the graspers, closed, to lift the liver and elevate the gallbladder.
   c. Stab the gallbladder with the Veress needle and connect the needle to suction.
   d. Remove the Veress needle and place the fundic grasper on the stab wound to hold it closed during retraction. Alternatively, use a suture ligature to close this small stab wound.
4. After the fundus of the gallbladder is exposed, the first assistant grasps the fundus with an atraumatic locking grasper passed through the most medial of the right subcostal ports. The assistant pushes the gallbladder over the liver toward the right shoulder, opening the subhepatic space and exposing the infundibulum of the gallbladder.
5. The surgeon or assistant then places a second atraumatic grasper on the gallbladder at its base. This grasper is generally also a locking grasper, although some surgeons will prefer a nonlocking grasper (particularly if a two-handed dissection technique is used).
   a. Throughout dissection, the direction of traction by this infundibular grasper is critical to prevent errors in identification of the ductal structures in this area.
   b. Retract the infundibulum laterally to expose Calot's triangle (Fig. 14.3).
   c. In the two-handed technique, the surgeon retracts the infundibulum with the left hand and dissects through the epigastric port with the right hand. Alternatively, the assistant may control both graspers and the surgeon maneuver the camera with the left hand.
6. Begin dissection directly adjacent to the gallbladder. Take down any additional adhesions to the base of the gallbladder sharply.
7. Identify the cystic duct where it enters the gallbladder. The gallbladder should be seen to funnel down and terminate in the cystic duct.

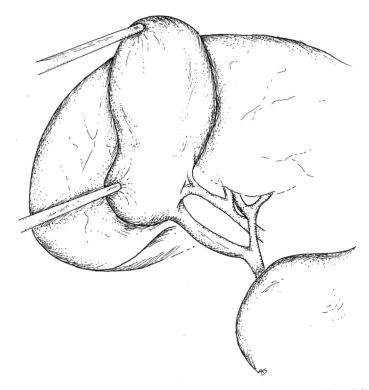

Figure 14.3. Retract the fundus of the gallbladder toward the right axilla and the infundibulum laterally to expose Calot's triangle. Retracting the infundibulum anteriorly or even upward tends to collapse Calot's triangle and increase the risk of ductal injury.

Move the infundibular grasper backward and forward, from side to side, so that the gallbladder–cystic duct junction may be carefully delineated.

8. Some surgeons incise the peritoneum extensively along the edge of the gallbladder and elevate the gallbladder to delineate the entire space medial to the gallbladder, leaving the cystic duct and artery intact until the gallbladder is almost completely separated from the liver bed.

9. Dissect the cystic duct free over an adequate length for cholangiography, if desired (see Chapter 18). Generally at least 1 cm of length is necessary.

10. A useful alternative technique is the "fundus-first" or "top-down" technique, useful for a severely inflamed gallbladder.
    a. After dissecting omental adhesions away from the gallbladder, the fundus is separated from the liver with a diathermy hook or dis-

secting forceps, leaving a peritoneal rim with which to grasp and retract the liver cranially. Alternatively, a malleable retractor can be placed through the lateral port to retract the liver cephalad.

b. The gallbladder is dissected away from the liver edge with a blunt dissecting forceps or cautery hook or spatula.

c. If a stone is impacted in Hartmann's pouch, it may be dislodged into the body of the gallbladder or removed by incising the pouch on the side away from the duct and removing the stone so that the entire circumference of the cystic duct–gallbladder junction can be viewed.

d. Cholangiogram should be performed before division of the cystic artery and cystic duct (see Chapter 18).

11. Place a clip as close to the gallbladder as possible and two similar clips on the cystic duct. Leave enough space between the sets of clips to make it possible to divide the duct with scissors. Take care not to retract the cystic duct so forcefully that the clips impinge on the cystic duct–common duct junction (Fig. 14.4).

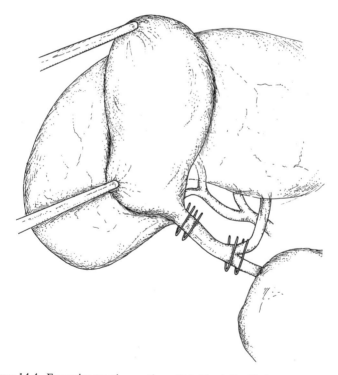

Figure 14.4. Excessive traction on the gallbladder infundibulum may "tent up" the common duct, increasing the likelihood that a clip will impinge on the duct and obstruct it.

12. Reposition the infundibular grasper to grasp the gallbladder adjacent to the cystic duct. Use this grasper to retract the gallbladder anteriorly and laterally so that the surgeon can expose the cystic artery by gentle spreading and dissecting with a Maryland dissector or laparoscopic right-angle clamp. The cystic artery will be noted to terminate by running onto the gallbladder, and visible pulsations may be observed. Generally 1 cm of length is necessary for safe division.

13. Divide the cystic artery with clips, leaving a minimum of two clips on the cystic artery stump. Division of the cystic artery will generally permit the gallbladder to be pulled farther away from the porta hepatis by traction on the infundibular grasper.

14. If the "fundus-first" technique has not been used, the remainder of the operation consists of dissection of the gallbladder from its bed, taking care to stay away from the porta hepatis and liver bed and to avoid perforating the gallbladder. The infundibular grasper is used to elevate the gallbladder and at a certain point it will become possible to use this grasper to push the gallbladder over the liver edge. Generally better exposure will be obtained if this maneuver is postponed until late in the dissection.

    a. Most surgeons use a hook cautery for this phase of the operation. The blunt edge of the hook can be used "cold," without cautery, as a dissector. Bands of connective tissue are hooked, placed on traction, and divided with cautery. Traction and countertraction facilitate the dissection.

    b. Some surgeons prefer cautery scissors or a spatula.

    c. Other energy sources such as laser or harmonic scalpel (Ultracision, Ethicon Endo-Surgery, Cincinnati, OH) may be used, but are generally unnecessary, less versatile, and more expensive than simple electrocautery (see Chapter 6, Principles of Laparoscopic Hemostasis).

15. When the gallbladder is dissected virtually free from the liver bed but a few strands remain, inspect the gallbladder bed and ducts for evidence of bleeding. Exposure of this region is more difficult often the gallbladder has been removed.

16. Irrigate with saline, but take care not to suction directly on the cystic duct or artery stumps to prevent clip dislodgment.

17. After achieving hemostasis, divide the remaining attachment of the gallbladder to the liver.

18. Place a gallbladder grasper through one of the 10-mm trocars and grasp the gallbladder at or near the cystic duct.

19. Remove the gallbladder from the abdomen.

    a. Consider using a specimen bag if the gallbladder is thick-walled (consider gallbladder carcinoma) or infected.

    b. Frequently bile or stones must be aspirated from the gallbladder before it can be withdrawn through the trocar site. Open the gallbladder outside the abdominal wall and suction bile from it.

    c. Crush and remove stones with stone forceps, ring forceps, or Kelly clamp. More details of specific extraction techniques are given in Chapter 8, Principles of Specimen Removal.

20. After the gallbladder has been removed, replace the epigastric trocar and inspect the surgical site for bleeding. Irrigate the surgical field, and aspirate the irrigant from the subphrenic space and other areas.
21. If a drain is desired, it can be placed through one of the lateral trocar sites.
    a. Pass an atraumatic grasper into the abdomen through the lateral trocar.
    b. Pass the "outside" end of the drain into the abdomen through the epigastric trocar.
    c. Grasp the "outside" end of the drain and pull it out of the abdomen, along with the trocar.
    d. Clamp the drain to avoid loss of pneumoperitoneum.
    e. Position the tip of the drain in the subhepatic space.
22. Remove the trocars and close the wounds in the usual fashion. Many surgeons inject the trocar sites with a long-acting local anesthetic to minimize pain and facilitate early discharge from hospital.

E. Selected References

Hunter JG. Avoidance of bile duct injury during laparoscopic cholecystectomy. Am J Surg 1991;162:71–76.

Lillemoe KD, Yeo CJ, Talamini MA, Wang BH, Pint HA, Gadacz TR. Selective cholangiography: current role in laparoscopic cholecystectomy. Ann Surg 1992;215: 669–676.

Martin IG, Dexter SPL, Marton J, et al. Surg Endosc 1995;9:203–206.

Mori T, Ikeda Y, Okamoto K, et al. A new technique for two-trocar laparoscopic cholecystectomy. Surg Endosc 2002;16:589–591.

Troidl H, Spangenberger W, Langen R, et al. Laparoscopic cholecystectomy: technical performance, safety and patient's benefit. Endoscopy 1992;24:252–261.

Voyles CR, Petro AB, Meena AL, Haick AJ, Koury AM. A practical approach to laparoscopic cholecystectomy. Am J Surg 1991;161:365–370.

15. Laparoscopic Cholecystectomy: Avoiding Complications

Joseph Cullen, M.D., F.A.C.S.

A. Hemorrhage

1. **Cause and prevention.** Bleeding during laparoscopic cholecystectomy can vary from inconsequential oozing to major hemorrhage.

   a. Bleeding can occur at a **trocar insertion** site and drip into the operative field. Obtain hemostasis in the skin before placing a trocar, and avoid any obvious vessels during insertion.

   b. Blunt dissection of adhesions from the gallbladder and liver can result in bleeding from **vessels in the omentum**. Cautious use of electrocautery when dividing omental adhesions prior to applying traction on the gallbladder, can be helpful in preventing this type of bleeding.

   c. Dissection in the **triangle of Calot** can result in sudden and often pulsatile bleeding. Careful and meticulous dissection in this area with accurate identification of the cystic artery and subsequent application of clips can often avoid this complication.

   d. One of the more difficult sources of bleeding is from the **gallbladder fossa**. If bleeding occurs in the area between the posterior wall of the inflamed gallbladder and liver bed, it should be controlled immediately rather than waiting until the entire operative field is obscured.

2. **Recognition and management**

   a. **Trocar site bleeding** may drip into the abdominal wall or run down instruments to drip into the operative site. There are several strategies for dealing with this kind of bleeding. Identify and gain temporary control by angling the trocar against the abdominal wall; when the trocar is pressed against the region of the bleeding, it will slow or stop. Injection of epinephrine solution (1: 10,000) in the vicinity of the bleeding site may stop the bleeding. If disposable trocars are being used, screwing in the anchoring device may compress and stop the bleeding. Finally, a suture ligature may be advanced through the abdominal wall, into the peritoneal cavity, and back out again, thus encompassing the bleeding site. Remember to double-check the area for hemostasis at the conclusion of the case. Remove the trocar under laparoscopic visual control and watch for recurrence of bleeding.

   b. When significant, unexpected bleeding occurs in the **triangle of Calot**, do not apply clips blindly. Indiscriminate application of clips in this area may injure the right hepatic artery, right hepatic duct, or common bile duct. If bleeding obscures the laparoscope, remove it and clean the lens. Do not hesitate to insert an additional trocar in the midline between the epigastric and umbilical ports, to provide an extra port for manipulation. Gently pushing the gallbladder against Calot's triangle by manipulating the fundic and infundibular graspers may provide temporary hemostasis while the situation is assessed and additional trocars inserted. Irrigate and aspirate the bleeding area to determine the exact area of bleeding. Grasp and elevate the bleeding vessel and perform any needed additional dissection around the area. Apply clips after precise isolation of the bleeding vessel. If bleeding continues or worsens, laparotomy should be performed.

c. Bleeding from the **gallbladder fossa** can usually be controlled by judicious use of electrocautery. If the cautery tip tends to dig into the liver, apply the metal tip of a suction irrigator to the liver and cauterize on the suction tip instead. Multiple, small areas of bleeding in this area can be controlled by application of oxidized cellulose or topical collagen hemostatic agents. If a bleeder retracts into the liver, a figure-of-eight suture ligature may be necessary. (See Chapter 6, Principles of Laparoscopic Hemostasis, for additional information.)

B. Gallbladder Problems

1. **Cause and prevention**

   a. The tensely **inflamed gallbladder** often proves difficult to grasp and hold. Preliminary needle decompression (see Chapter 14) is sometimes helpful. Stabilize the fundus of the gallbladder and pass a large-gauge needle percutaneously into the part of the gallbladder closest to the anterior abdominal wall. A Veress needle works well for this purpose. Connect the needle to suction and aspirate the contents. Close the hole with a grasping forceps or a pretied suture ligature. A large selection of laparoscopic forceps has been designed specifically for retraction of an inflamed and edematous gallbladder. Sometimes an endoscopic Babcock clamp is the best instrument.

   b. Despite care, **perforation of the gallbladder** still occurs frequently in the setting of acute cholecystitis. Perforation of during dissection can lead to contamination of the peritoneal cavity with potentially infected bile and gallstones. Tears in the gallbladder wall can also lead to further disruption of the wall, making subsequent dissection difficult. Preliminary decompression, as mentioned before, helps minimize contamination if it occurs.

   c. Gallbladders containing **large stones** or those with a thickened wall may also be difficult to remove from the abdominal cavity.

d. Occult **carcinoma of the gallbladder**, although rare, is occasionally found in the setting of long-standing chronic cholecystitis. Trocar site recurrence has been reported when laparoscopic cholecystectomy was performed in this setting. Some surgeons routinely request pathologic examination of the gallbladder mucosa with frozen section examination of any suspicious areas. The incidence of gallbladder carcinoma is increased in elderly patients with chronic cholecystitis and those with calcifications within the wall of the gallbladder. If preoperative ultrasound is suspicious, or the patient has a calcified gallbladder, consider open (rather than laparoscopic) cholecystectomy.

2. **Recognition and management**

a. When **acute cholecystitis** is encountered, partially decompress the tense, distended gallbladder by aspirating its contents through the fundus. Occlude the aspiration site by applying a grasping forceps over the opening or a pretied laparoscopic suture.

b. If disruption of the wall has occurred with **spillage**, copious irrigation and suctioning can remove the majority of stones and bile, while larger stones may be placed in a laparoscopic tissue pouch and removed. Placement of closed suction catheters may be indicated for extensive bile spillage. These drainage catheters can be introduced through a lateral cannula. The tip of the catheter is then held in place in the subhepatic space while the cannula is removed.

c. Gallbladders containing **large stones** may be placed in a retrieval bag to avoid spillage of stones if the gallbladder tears during attempted removal. Alternatively, the neck of the gallbladder may be pulled partially out of the abdomen and the stones within the gallbladder crushed and removed piecemeal. Gallbladders with thickened walls should be placed in a retrieval bag prior to removal; on rare occasion an occult carcinoma of the gallbladder will be found, and this method minimizes contamination of the trocar site. Finally, enlarging the skin and fascial incisions at the extraction site will usually suffice in completing the removal of the gallbladder from the abdomen. If the adjacent rectus muscles are not incised, enlarging the incision will add minimal additional postoperative pain or cosmetic defects. (See Chapter 8 for additional information.)

d. **Carcinoma of the gallbladder** is best recognized and dealt with at the time of the original operation. Maintain a high index of suspicion and request frozen section examination in doubtful cases. If carcinoma of the gallbladder is identified, consider conversion to open surgery, with excision of the gallbladder bed, regional lymphadenectomy (depending upon depth of penetration), and excision of trocar sites. Implantation of carcinoma of the gallbladder has been reported to occur as rapidly as one week after laparoscopic cholecystectomy and is not limited to the trocar used for specimen removal.

C. Postoperative Bile Leakage

1. **Cause and prevention.** Postoperative bile leaks or collections may be the result of common duct or right hepatic duct injury (discussed shortly), cystic duct stump leakage, or injury to an accessory bile duct. Severely edematous tissues from acute cholecystitis will result in failure of standard clips to completely occlude the cystic duct, resulting in postoperative bile leak. When dissection of the gallbladder is difficult in the setting of acute cholecystitis or when there is significant bile spillage, place a closed suction drain. This may prevent bile collections from minor leaks from the liver bed or aid in controlling cystic duct stump leaks.

2. **Recognition and management.** During operation, a number of conditions that predispose to bile leaks can be recognized, and if these are managed correctly, the complication can be avoided. If the cystic duct appears edematous and inflamed, both surgical clips and pretied laparoscopic sutures can be used to securely occlude the cystic duct. Bile leakage from small accessory ducts in the gallbladder may not be recognized at the time of laparoscopic cholecystectomy but may be the source of later bile leak. These accessory ducts should be suspected if the gallbladder fills with contrast during intraoperative cholangiography despite occlusion of the junction of the gallbladder and cystic duct. When this filling is noted at operation, these ducts should be recognized and clipped, ligated, or coagulated. Placement of closed suction drains are also recommended. When a collection is suspected, an ultrasound or computed tomography scan of the abdomen will establish the diagnosis and any collections may be aspirated and drainage established.

If a bile collection occurs, the biliary tree should be investigated by radionuclide scan and endoscopic retrograde cholangiopancreatography (ERCP). ERCP is useful in both the diagnosis and treatment. Cholangiography often demonstrates extravasation from the cystic duct stump. When a leak is noted, treatment consists of decreasing the pressure at the distal end of the common bile duct and may include passage of a nasobiliary drain, endoscopic sphincterotomy, or placement of a transpapillary stent. All these methods decrease the pressure in the duct and allow rapid closure in cases of both cystic duct stump leaks and accessory bile duct leaks. Early investigation of bile leaks with ERCP also allows prompt diagnosis of bile duct injury, facilitating early repair and increasing the chance of long-term success.

D. Bile Duct Injury

1. **Cause and prevention.** Injury to the ductal system usually occurs during the dissection at the triangle of Calot, exposing the cystic duct. Cephalad traction will often cause the cystic duct to lie in a straight line with the common bile duct, allowing the common duct to be mistaken for the cystic duct. To prevent this from happening, retract the infundibulum of the gallbladder laterally to fully expose the cystic duct and gallbladder from the common duct.

Excessive retraction of the gallbladder when the clips are applied to the proximal cystic duct may result in trapping a portion of the common duct in the clips. To prevent this, leave a longer cystic duct remnant. Dissect the cystic duct from the infundibulum of the gallbladder downward, incising the medial and lateral peritoneal attachments of the infundibulum to the liver. Remove all connective tissue and fat to clearly expose the junction of the cystic duct with the gallbladder. Avoid excessive use of electrocautery in the triangle of Calot, which may lead to late injury and strictures to the ductal system. Intraoperative cholangiography will outline the biliary anatomy and may avoid major ductal injuries (see Chapter 16, Cholangiography).

2. **Recognition and management.** Major injuries to the ductal system may be noted with continued dissection as bile leaks into the operative field, or later, when the patient presents with jaundice or an intra-abdominal bile collection.

When such injuries are recognized at operation, conversion to laparotomy is advised. If a significant portion of the ductal system has been excised, reconstruction with a hepaticojejunostomy is indicated. When only a small choledochotomy has been made, reconstruction over a T-tube may be attempted. A clean transection without tissue loss may require a ductal anastomosis over a T-tube. Patients with injury to the biliary system recognized several days later need cholangiography to adequately define the injury. If cholangiography reveals total occlusion or transection of the ductal system, immediate operative repair, usually by hepaticojejunostomy, is indicated. Injuries to the lateral wall of the common duct may be treated with external drainage of any intra-abdominal collections and biliary stenting.

E. Selected References

Airan M, Appel M, Berci G, et al. Retrospective and prospective multi-institutional laparoscopic cholecystectomy study organized by The Society of American Gastrointestinal Endoscopic Surgeons. Surg Endosc 1992;6:169–176.

Gadacz TR, Talamini MA. Traditional versus laparoscopic cholecystectomy. Am J Surg 1991;161:336–338.

McSherry CK. Laparoscopic cholecystectomy: time for critical analysis. Surg Endosc 1992;6:177–178.

Moosa AR, Easter DW, Van Sonnenberg E, et al. Laparoscopic injuries to the bile duct. Ann Surg 1992;215:203–208.

Ponsky JL. Complications of laparoscopic cholecystectomy. Am J Surg 1991;161:393–395.

Ponsky JL. Management of the complications of laparoscopic cholecystectomy. Endoscopy 1992;24:724–729.

Ponsky JL. Incidence and management of complications of laparoscopic cholecystectomy. Adv Surg 1994;27:21–40.

Rossi RL, Schirmer WJ, Baasch JW, et al. Laparoscopic bile duct injuries. Arch Surg 1992;127:596–602.

16. Laparoscopic Cholecystectomy: Cholangiography

George Berci, M.D., F.A.C.S.

A. Introduction

Routine intraoperative cholangiography (RIOC) (preferably utilizing fluoroscopy) is practiced by many surgeons and advocated by the author of this chapter for the following reasons:

1. RIOC allows immediate recognition of anatomy and anomalies or stones.
2. Discovery of partial or total transection of ducts or clip placement across the common bile duct (CBD), facilitating immediate repair, can be performed.
3. It allows removing a common duct stone during laparoscopic cholecystectomy, by either the transcystic duct or laparoscopic choledochotomy method (see Chapters 18 and 19).
4. It precludes unnecessary preoperative endoscopic retrograde cholangiopancreatography (ERCP) or endoscopic sphincterotomy.
5. Fluorocholangiography is an organic part of laparoscopic common duct exploration (see Chapters 18 and 19), allowing clearance of the common duct of stones during a single operative session.

The variety of anomalies and intraoperative hazards that may be detected by RIOC are shown in Figures 16.1 to 16.5.

B. Radiographic Equipment

Fluoroscopy is preferred for the following reasons:

1. It allows immediate observation of adequacy of filling using small increments of contrast to avoid obscuring small calculi and overlapping structures (e.g., the cystic duct drainage into the CBD).
2. It confers a tremendous savings in time; the anatomy or anomalies are immediately discovered but images are recorded and processed later, and the surgeon does not need to wait for films to be developed (and, all too often, find the film quality suboptimal, necessitating repeat studies).
3. Tiny calculi may be flushed from the common duct without duct exploration.

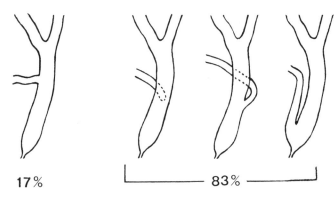

17%   ———— 83% ————

Figure 16.1. The textbooks state that the cystic duct enters the common duct along a relatively straight line in 75% of cases. The author has noted that this occurs in only 17% of operative cholangiograms; in the majority of cases, the cystic duct enters posterior, spiral, or parallel to the common duct.

The surgeon should be thoroughly familiar with the equipment and its operation, because after hours and on weekends, a fully trained technician may not available. In some states one must pass a simple fluoroscopy operator test. This is worthwhile, as the surgeon then has a license to operate the unit. Close collaboration with the Department of Radiology is advised; in some hospitals, it may be possible to transmit images via a simple coaxial cable to a radiologist, who can then watch as the cholangiogram is performed. An audio link allows communication between radiologist and surgeon. Such links are becoming more and more commonplace. The surgeon must, however, be familiar with basic radiographic anatomy of the biliary tree and be able to evaluate the images.

Equipment varies from totally dedicated, ceiling-mounted units in specialized operating room suites to the more common and mobile C-arm digital fluoroscope unit found in most hospitals. The image intensifier screen is typically 9/6 in. This means that under routine operation, the field size is 9 in., and that additional magnification can be attained by switching to a 6-in. field if needed.

The x-ray tube may be self-rectified or rotating anode. The latter is preferred because the beam penetrates obese patients better. The surgeon and assistants stand behind a mobile lead screen for protection. Use an extension tube on the cholangiogram catheter setup to allow greater distance (see later). Remember the inverse square law, which describes radiation intensity: dose diminishes as the square of the distance from the source. Therefore, a small additional distance from the x-ray tube greatly decreases the dose to surgeon and assistants. Radiation exposure is cumulative, and even small doses add up over a professional lifetime (Figs. 16.6 to 16.8).

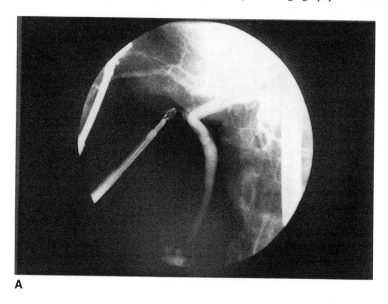

A

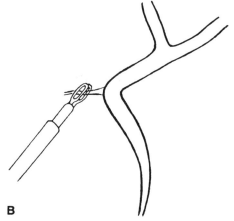

B

Figure 16.2. A. Slight traction on the cholangiograsper can tent the common duct, especially if the cystic duct is very short. In the two-dimensional view seen on the monitor, the common duct may be misinterpreted as the cystic duct and transected. The length of the cholangiograsper jaws is 10 mm. B. Schematic diagram of cholangiogram seen in A. It is very important to recognize the short cystic duct.

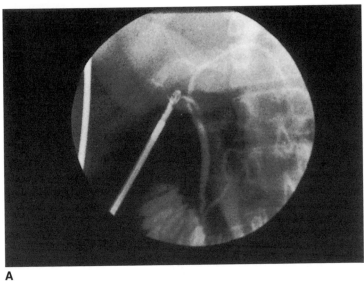

A

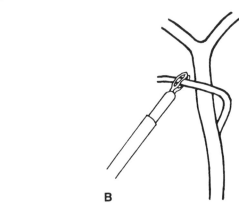

B

Figure 16.3. A. Very close spiral drainage of the cystic duct into the common duct. B. Schematic of cholangiogram.

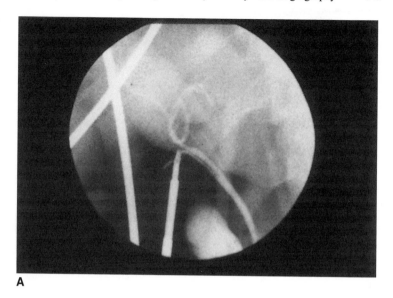

A

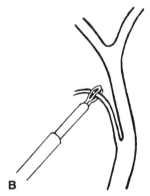

B

Figure 16.4. A. Close parallel run of cystic duct and common duct. Note how close the cholangiograsper jaw is to the common hepatic duct. B. Schematic diagram of cholangiogram. The cholangiograsper jaw is only 10 mm long; this gives some hint of distances and proximities.

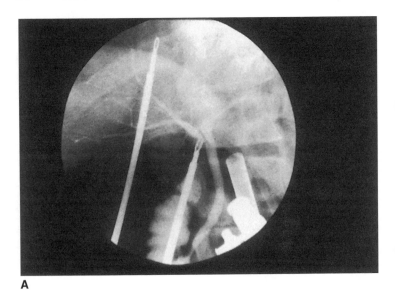

A

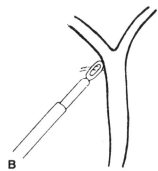

B

Figure 16.5. A. Dangerously short cystic duct draining directly into right hepatic duct. B. Schematic drawing of cholangiogram.

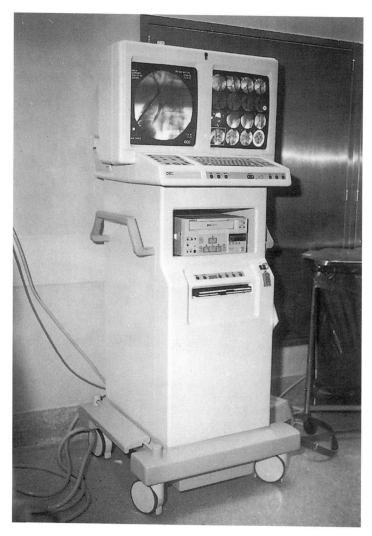

Figure 16.6. Mobile digitized C-arm fluoroscopy equipment. Left screen shows real-time full-size fluoroscopic image. Right screen shows stored images (frames) to be selected and printed. VHS recorder is seen below with the full-sized film camera.

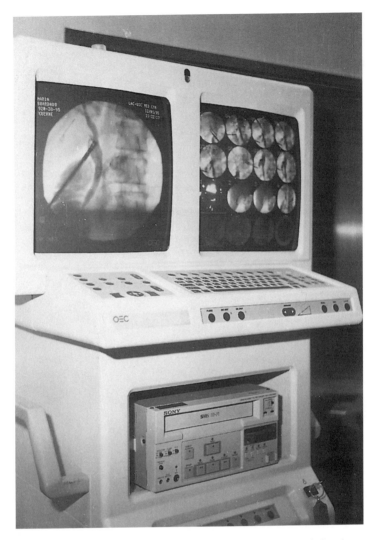

Figure 16.7. Close-up view of control panel. The functions for a cholangiogram are preprogrammed and only one button needs to be pushed. Modes are activated by a foot switch, as is VHS record. (OEC Co., Salt Lake City, UT.)

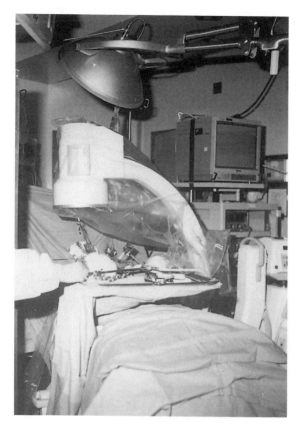

Figure 16.8. It is easy to position the sterile covered unit over the abdomen, and the required anatomy is immediately noted and corrected if necessary.

C. Cystic Duct Cholangiography

1. **The easy case.** In the patient with few adhesions, Calot's triangle is easily dissected and the cystic duct identified. It is crucial to see the duct entering the gallbladder, as mentioned in Chapter 15.
   a. Place a clip or ligature on the cystic duct at or near its termination upon the gallbladder.
   b. Clip the cystic artery as well. This ensures that the cholangiogram will be performed with all crucial structures clipped, minimizing the chance of ductal injury **after** cholangiography.

c. A large variety of cholangiocatheters are available, and selection is a matter of individual preference. The author prefers a blue 4-French ureteral catheter with black visual markers and an open-end tip. This is easy to manipulate and inexpensive.

d. Connect the catheter to a long extension tube with a Y connector. At the far end of the extension tube there should be two stopcocks and two syringes (Fig. 16.9).

e. Use a larger syringe for saline, and a smaller one for contrast medium. Have the scrub nurse mark the syringe containing contrast (with sterile marking tape, or a simple ligature of black silk).

f. Dilute the contrast medium. If you are using 60% contrast, dilute it 1 : 1. More dilute medium is less likely to obscure small stones within a dense dye column. Conversely, less dilute medium will show fine ductal detail better and may be preferred if stones are not a consideration.

g. Ensure that all air bubbles are removed from the system. Air bubbles can hide in the stopcocks, the Y connectors, or in the space between the syringe full of contrast and the extension tubing. Therefore, after the saline has been flushed through the system including the catheter, it is worthwhile to open the stopcock from the contrast syringe and push a full milliliter of saline back through the system into the contrast syringe to eliminate any air bubbles.

h. Make a small incision in the anterior wall of the cystic duct using a sharp pair of fine-tipped scissors. Try to judge the thickness of the duct and enter the lumen with a single cut. The cystic duct is

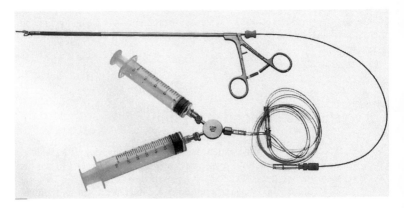

Figure 16.9. Cholangiograsper with 4-French ureteral catheter inserted, extension tubing, Y-shaped adapter, and two syringes of different sizes. (Karl Storz, Endoscopy-America, Culver City, CA.)

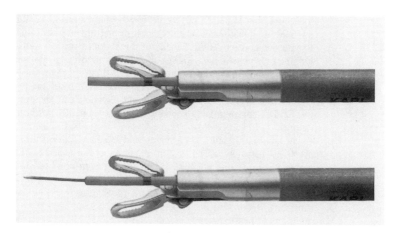

Figure 16.10. Cholangiograsper seen in close-up with protruding ureteral catheter (top). In case of difficult introduction, a guidewire is advanced and introduced into the cystic duct, followed by the catheter (bottom).

often thicker than expected, and making multiple cuts makes it harder to cannulate (as well as increasing the probability that the duct will be totally transected).

i. Use a flat grasper to milk the cystic duct toward the incision, to remove small stones and debris. Clear bile should flow, indicating an unobstructed passage into the proximal biliary tree. If a stone appears, remove it with a stone forceps.

j. Pass the cholangiograsper with its inserted catheter through the fourth trocar site (the one normally used to retract the infundibulum). This is generally done by the assistant, while the surgeon retracts the infundibulum of the gallbladder to provide slide tension on the cystic duct. Do not overstretch the cystic duct, as this will make the lumen collapse and render cannulation much more difficult.

k. The catheter should protude slightly (0.5–1 in.) from the end of the cholangiograsper jaws (Fig. 16.10).

l. Advance the catheter into the dochotomy with very small motions. Do not introduce too much of the catheter into the duct (1–2 cm is sufficient). Monitor the length of the catheter by watching the markings (one to two markings should go into the duct).

m. Open the cholangiograsper and slide it coaxially over the catheter, without introducing more catheter into the duct. Close the grasper to secure the catheter and secure a watertight closure of the dochotomy. Inject some saline to confirm placement.

n. Secure the grasper on the outside of the abdomen to avoid dislodgment. Remove the laparoscope. The infundibular grasper may be removed or left in situ. Place the fluoroscope in position and confirm that the field is centered. A marker on the abdomen is a great help to surgeon and technician in ensuring the field is approximately centered. Make a scout film without contrast.

o. Inject contrast medium very slowly and freeze a frame shortly after the first few drops are injected. Ascertain whether the catheter is in a good position. If the catheter is inserted too far, pull it back. Go very slowly with small increments and save several images during the procedure (6–8 films per cholangiogram). Record the images digitally or on tape.

2. **Management of problems**

a. **Inability to cannulate the cystic duct.** Ask the nurse to inject a small amount of saline as cannulation is attempted. This will open the lumen. If the catheter cannot be introduced after repeated attempts, the problem may be the spiral valves of Heister. In this case, introduce a small (0.35-in.) guidewire with a floppy end through the catheter. Slip the soft (floppy) end of the guidewire into the dochotomy and pass the catheter over the guidewire. Remove the guidewire before closing the cholangiograsper.

b. **Flaccid sphincter.** In this case, contrast material immediately passes out of the distal common duct into the duodenum and the upper biliary tree is not filled. Place the patient in the Trendelenburg position and ask the anesthesiologist to administer intravenous morphine to cause the sphincter to go into spasm. Do another cholangiogram. Sometimes additional contrast medium must be injected under sufficient pressure to fill the entire biliary tree because of spasm of the sphincter.

c. **Abnormal appearance of the sphincter.** Use the magnification function to observe the sphincter in greater detail (be sufficiently familiar with the equipment to do this!) and observe the sphincter for 5 or 10 seconds. By watching for sphincter motion a "pseudocalculus" may disappear (Fig. 16.11).

d. **Rounded lucencies: stones or air bubbles?** Slowly inject 2 to 3 mL of contrast under constant fluoroscopic control. Then withdraw the plunger to create a vacuum. Repeat this maneuver twice and observe the motion and appearance of the lucency. Bubbles move in synchrony with the column of contrast. Stones tend to adhere to the wall of the duct and do not move.

e. **Overfilled ductal system** or excess dye in the duodenum. Too much contrast on the film creates difficulties in interpretation. Wash out the duct with warm saline (to avoid sphincter spasm) and then do another cholangiogram (Fig. 16.12).

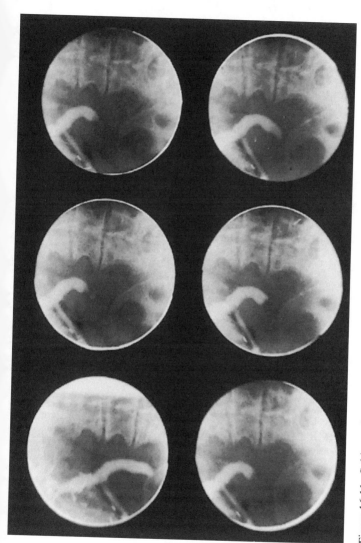

Figure 16.11. Sphincter function during the opening and closing cycles. The thumbprint configuration shown in middle figures can easily be misinterpreted as a stone. By observing the sphincter for a few seconds longer, one can easily see the opening and closing of the sphincter and interpret the image correct.

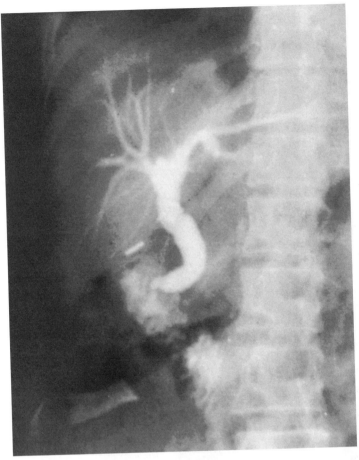

Figure 16.12. The ductal system is overfilled with contrast and no early filling stage is seen. The cystic duct drainage into the common duct is obscured by excess contrast.

D. Danger Signs

The surgeon should be able to recognize certain radiographic danger signs, which mandate immediate exploration:

1. Contrast material is seen in the distal CBD below the cystic duct but contrast extravasation is observed above this site: open the patient up immediately. There is a great probability that there is a **transection of the duct** (Fig. 16.13).

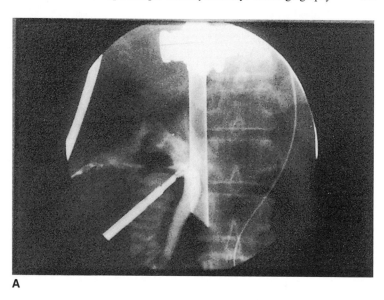

A

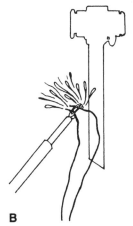

B

Figure 16.13. A. The distal duct is well seen but there is obvious extravasation of dye proximal. The duct was found to be transected. The injury was recognized and immediate repair performed. B. Schematic of cholangiogram.

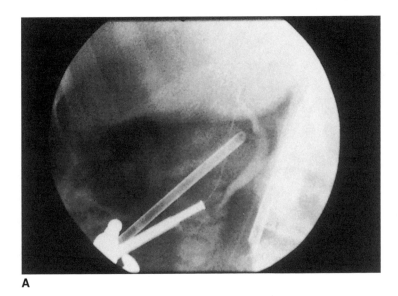

A

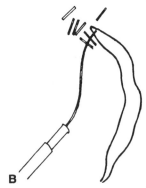

B

Figure 16.14. A. Distal duct is visible but no contrast material is seen in the proximal duct. A clip occluded the duct. If the proximal duct cannot be filled with contrast, open the patient immediately. B. Schematic of cholangiogram.

2. The distal duct is well filled with contrast but there is no filling of the proximal ductal system, and the situation does not change with repeated injection and the maneuvers just described. Convert to an open procedure because there is a chance that a clip (which you should see on films) or other manipulations caused the obstruction (Fig. 16.14).

E. Other Difficulties and Their Solution

There are a few additional tricks that every laparoscopic surgeon should be familiar with.

1. **Stone knowingly left behind.** Sometimes a stone is seen in the common duct and the decision is made not to do laparoscopic common duct exploration. If the equipment or expertise to perform laparoscopic common duct exploration is not available, or if a stone is difficult or impacted and cannot be removed, insert a guidewire through the cholangiocatheter. Pass the guidewire through into the duodenum under fluoroscopic guidance. Fix the other end of the guidewire at its exit site in the flank. This will greatly facilitate subsequent postoperative ERCP and sphincterotomy.

2. **Alternative methods of cholangiography.** There are other ways to perform a cystic duct cholangiogram. Sometimes these are easier than the method just described, particularly if it is difficult to get the correct alignment to introduce the catheter through one of the existing trocars, or if traction on both the infundibular and fundic graspers must be maintained to expose the cystic duct. In such a case, pass a straight or angled needle through the abdominal wall at the desired site and introduce the cholangiocatheter through the needle.

3. **Cholecystocholangiography.** At times, dissection in the cystic duct area is extremely difficult or appears hazardous and the surgeon decide must whether to convert to open surgery. Cholecystocholangiography is performed by needle puncture and injection of contrast directly into the gallbladder. When successful, it delineates the anatomy of the cystic duct and common duct.

   a. Tilt the patient to the right to avoid a contrast-filled gallbladder obscuring ductal anatomy.

   b. Puncture the gallbladder with the Veress needle connected to an extension tube filled with contrast.

   c. Place a clip near the infundibulum of the gallbladder as a marker.

   d. For this procedure, a large volume of contrast medium is needed. Instruct the nurse to prepare more than the usual 30 mL (100–200 mL may be needed).

   e. Inject slowly under continuous fluroroscopic guidance. Observe the location, relative to the clip on the infundibulum, where the cystic duct joins the gallbladder and then terminates on the common duct (Fig. 16.15).

   f. Subsequent decision making (to dissect further or to convert to an open procedure) can then be made rationally and with better information. At the end of the procedure, evacuate some of the contrast medium (now mixed with bile) and close the puncture site with a large clip or pretied ligature.

4. **Laparoscopic choledocholithotomy (LCL).** LCL is a logical extension of laparoscopic cholecystectomy. It requires more skill, teamwork, and equipment—but the patient can be treated and cured in one session. Operative (fluoro) cholangiography is an essential part of LCL

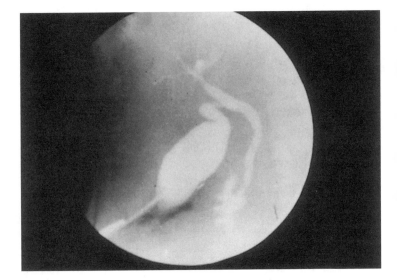

Figure 16.15. Cholecystocholangiogram. In the difficult case, direct needle puncture of the gallbladder with contrast injection can display the anatomy. In this example, the cystic duct drains directly into the common hepatic duct.

(for further details see Chapters 18 and 19 on laparoscopic common duct explorations).

5. **Preoperative ERCP.** If you routinely perform operative (fluoro) cholangiography, the overwhelming number of (negative) ERCPs can be eliminated. ERCP and E. Sphincterotomy are procedures with complications and additional costs involved. The indication for the preoperative ERCP is the high-risk patient with cholangitis, septicemia, and severe underlying disease.

F. Selected References

Berci G, Hamlin JA, eds. Operative Biliary Radiology. Baltimore: Williams & Wilkins, 1981.

Berci G, Hamlin JA. Operative cholangiography. In: Berci G, Hamlin JA, eds. Operative Biliary Radiology. Baltimore: Williams & Wilkins, 1981.

Berci G, Sackier J. Intraoperative cholangiography. In: Berci G, ed. Problems in General Surgery: Laparoscopic Surgery. vol 8. Philadelphia: Lippincott, 1991; 310–318.

Berci G, Shore JM, Hamlin JA, Morgenstern L. Operative fluoroscopy and cholangiography. The use of modern radiological techniques during surgery. Am J Surg 1977; 135:32–35.

Bergman JG, Vander Mays, Rauw AJ, et al. Long-term follow-up after endoscopic sphincterotomy. GI Endosc 1996;44:643.

Cohen SA, Siegel JH, Kasmin FE. Complications of diagnostic and therapeutic ERCP. Abdominal Imaging 1996;21:385.

Cotton PB, Lehman G, Vennes J, et al. Endoscopic sphincterotomy complications and their management. Special Report Gostrointest Endosc 1991;37:383.

Cullen JJ, Scott-Conner CEH. Surgical anatomy of laparoscopic common duct exploration. In: Berci G, Cushieri A, eds. Ducts and Ductal Stones. Philadelphia: WB Saunders, 1997;20–25.

Cuschieri A, Berci G. Training for laparoscopic surgery. In: Laparoscopic Biliary Surgery. London: Blackwell, 1982;1–217.

Cuschieri A, Berci G. The role of intraoperative fluorocholangiography during laparoscopic cholecystectomy. In: Berci G, Cuschieri A, eds. Bile Ducts and Ductal Stones. Philadelphia: WB Saunders, 1997.

Fletcher DR. Laparoscopic cholecystectomy: role of pre-operative and post-operative endoscopic retrograde cholangio-pancreatography and endoscopic sphincterotomy. Gastrointest Endosc Clin North Am 1993;3:249–259.

Freeman ML, Nelson DB, Sherman ST, et al. Complications of endoscopic biliary sphincterotomy. NJ Med 1996;825–909.

Hamlin JA. Radiological anatomy and anomalies of the extrahepatic biliary ducts. In: Berci G, Cuschieri A, eds. Bile Ducts and Ductal Stones. Philadelphia: WB Saunders, 1997.

Hicken NF, Best RR, Hunt HB. Cholangiography. Ann Surg 1936;103:210–215.

Katos GS, Tomplins RK, Turnipseed W, Zollinger R. Operative cholangiography. Arch Surg 1972;104:484–490.

Lee KH. Radiation safety considerations in fluoroscopy. In: Berci G, Cuschieri A, eds. Bile Duct and Ductal Stones. Philadelphia: WB Saunders, 1997.

Lillemoe D, Martin SA, Cameron J, et al. Major bile duct injuries during laparcholecystectomy. Ann Surg 1997;225:459–469.

Malley-Guy P. Television radioscopy during operations of the biliary passages. Surg Gynecol Obstet 1958;106:747–751.

Mirizzi PL. Operative cholangiography. Surg Gynecol Obstet 1932;65:702–710.

Soper NJ, Brunt LM. The case for routine operative cholangiography during laparoscopic cholecystectomy. Surg Clin North Am 1994;74:953–959.

Stewart L, Way LW. Bile duct injuries during laparoscopic cholecystectomy. Arch Surg 1995;130:1123–1133.

Stiegmann G, Goff, Manseur A, et al. Pre-cholecystectomy endoscopic cholangiography. Am J Surg 1992;163:227–232.

Strasberg SM, Hertl M, Soper NJ. An analysis of the problem of biliary injury during laparoscopic cholecystectomy. J Am Coll Surg 1995;180:101–125.

Traverso W, Hargrove K, Kozarek R. A cost effective approach to the treatment of CBD stones with surgical versus endoscopic techniques. In: Berci G, Cuschieri A, eds. Bile Ducts and Ductal Stones. Philadelphia: WB Saunders, 1997;154–160.

Woods MS, Traverso W, Kozarek R. Characteristics of biliary complications during laparoscopic cholecystectomy. Am J Surg 1994;167:27–30.

17. Laparoscopic Cholecystectomy: Ultrasound for Choledocholithiasis

Maurice E. Arregui, M.D., F.A.C.S.

A. Indications and Equipment

Laparoscopic ultrasound (LUS) is a safe, effective, sensitive, and specific technique for detecting stones in the common bile duct during laparoscopic cholecystectomy. It is also useful to rule out ligation or transection of the common bile duct. When sufficient experience is attained, it is an excellent substitute for digital fluorocholangiography. Additional information on other applications of laparoscopic ultrasound is given in Chapter 13, Elective Diagnostic Laparoscopy and Cancer Staging.

For ultrasound of the biliary tree, high-frequency probes in the 7- to 10-MHz range using solid state linear array transducers are optimal. Most probes fit through a 10-mm trocar. A deflectable tip is useful, but a rigid probe will suffice. Curved array or mechanical sector probes are options, but they do not provide optimal resolution and near-field detail for accurate diagnosis.

Color Doppler ultrasonography is a costly option that can distinguish bile ducts from vascular structures but does not substitute for a surgeon's knowledge of anatomy. Doppler without the dynamic color feature is a useful and much less expensive addition. For the most part, we find that color Doppler is seldom needed for the examination of the common bile duct. Others however find it quite useful. It is helpful for the novice sonographer.

B. Technique

1. Dissect and clip or ligate the cystic duct before performing laparoscopic ultrasound.
2. The ultrasound probe may be passed through a 10-mm epigastric trocar. From this access, the probe may be placed on the porta hepatis to obtain a transverse view of the biliary tree and portal structures.
3. The author prefers to place the probe through the 10-mm umbilical port. This gives a linear view of the portal structures, which is easier to interpret.
   a. Place a 5-mm laparoscope through the lateral right upper quadrant trocar to check the position of the ultrasound probe.

b. Place the probe over segment IV of the liver, directing the ultra-sound beam to the liver hilum (Fig. 17.1).

c. Identify the common hepatic duct through the liver parenchyma (Fig. 17.2) and follow the left and right hepatic ducts to their secondary and tertiary branchings.

d. Place the probe on the porta hepatis with the tip in the liver hilum (Fig. 17.3). The hepatic duct will be seen longitudinally. The hepatic artery is usually seen in transverse section between the bile duct and portal vein. Posterior to the portal vein is the caudate lobe of the liver, and deep to this is the inferior vena cava (Fig. 17.4).

e. A transverse view of the porta hepatis will give a classic "Mickey Mouse" view with the common bile duct seen as the one ear, the hepatic artery the other ear and the portal vein the face (Fig. 17.5).

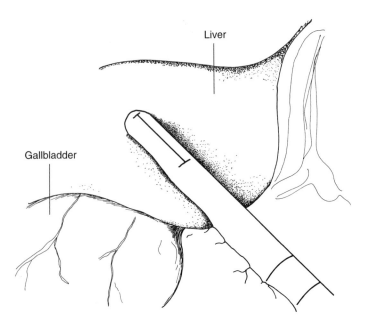

Figure 17.1. Probe over liver segment IV.

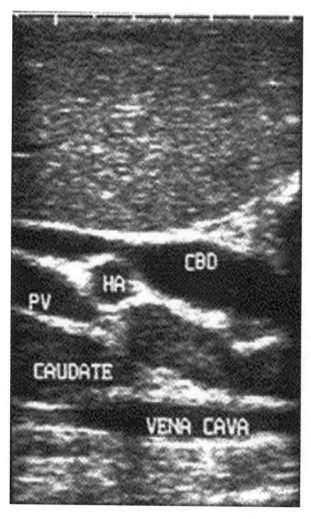

Figure 17.2. View through segment IV: CBD, common bile duct; HA, hepatic artery; PV, portal vein.

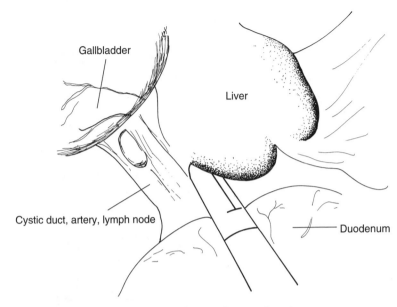

Figure 17.3. Probe over the porta hepatis.

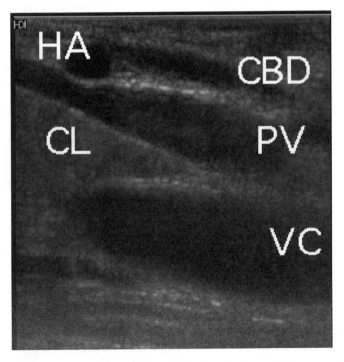

Figure 17.4. View through porta hepatis: HA, hepatic artery; CBD, common bile duct; PV, portal vein; CL, caudate lobe of liver; VC, vena cava.

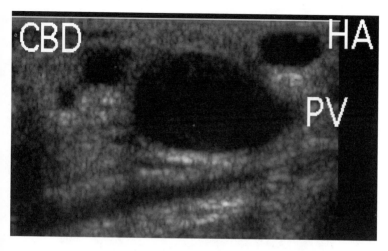

Figure 17.5. Transverse, or "Mickey Mouse," view of the portal structures: CBD, common bile duct; HA, hepatic artery; PV, portal vein.

f. The junction of the cystic duct with the hepatic duct is identified and the common duct distal to this is then measured with acoustic calipers.

g. Ultrasound following ligation or clipping of the cystic duct allows the surgeon to evaluate the common bile duct impingement or injury.

h. Follow the common duct to the head of the pancreas. Most stones are seen in the distal common bile duct (Fig. 17.6).

i. In many patients the fat overlying or a fatty pancreatic head obscures the ultrasound beam, making visualization of the distal common bile duct difficult. The duodenum provides a better acoustic window. Position the probe lateral to the duodenum with the ultrasound beam pointing toward the pancreas (Figs. 17.7 and 17.8). From this perspective, the common bile duct is seen transversely. Follow the common duct caudad until the pancreatic duct joins it (Fig. 17.9).

j. Follow both ducts to the ampulla.

k. If the distal bile duct is poorly seen, insert a cholangiocatheter into the cystic duct and infuse saline to distend the intrapancreatic bile duct, providing a better view.

l. A stone in the bile duct usually appears as a crescent-shaped hyperechoic structure with posterior shadowing (Fig. 17.6).

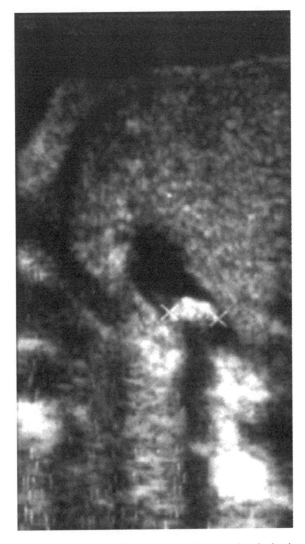

Figure 17.6. Common bile duct stone with posterior shadowing.

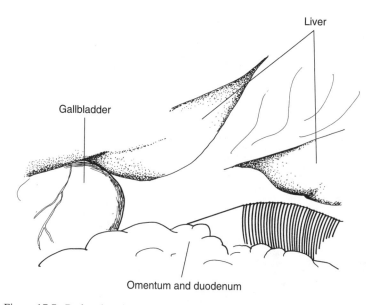

Figure 17.7. Probe placed transversely over the duodenum and pancreatic head.

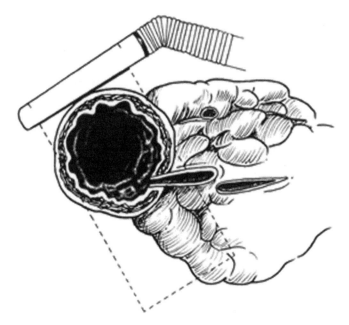

Figure 17.8. Illustration of probe placement over duodenum.

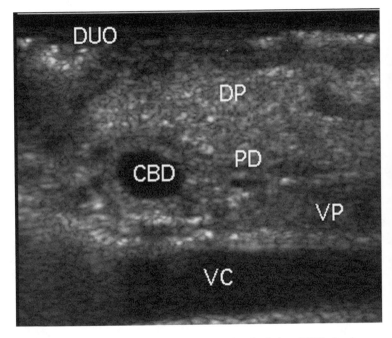

Figure 17.9. Transverse view through the duodenal window: DUO, duodenum; DP, dorsal pancreas; PD, pancreatic duct; CBD, common bile duct; VP, ventral pancreas; VC, vena cava.

C. Advantages

1.   It is quickly performed.
2.   It is repeatable.
3.   There is no radiation.
4.   It is less expensive.
5.   It is as sensitive as intraoperative cholangiography.
6.   It is more specific than intraoperative cholangiography.
7.   It give better anatomic information of the surrounding structures.

D. Disadvantages

1.   Bile duct anomalies are difficult to identify.
2.   Small common bile ducts are hard to see.
3.   The distal duct is not always seen clearly.
4.   A fatty pancreas or pancreatitis obscures the view.

Table 17.1. Learning curve shown in three different phases of our own experience: LUS, laparoscopic ultrasound; IOCG, intraoperative cholangiogram.

Phase	Number of patients		Specificity/Sensitivity (%)	
	LUS	IOCG	LUS %	IOCG %
I	140	140	76.5/100	100/96.7
II	78	78	100/100	100/98.6
III	142	67	95.7/100	95.2/100
Total	360	285	90/100	98.1/98.1

5. Duodenal diverticula with air can mimic a shadowing stone.
6. The equipment is not available to all.
7. There is a learning curve.
8. Artifacts can mimic stones.

C. Results in Clinical Practice

We have compared laparoscopic ultrasound images with images obtained by digital fluorocholangiography in 360 patients. Table 17.1 shows the improvement in the sensitivity and specificity over time. There were a total of five false negatives for ultrasound and one for digital fluorocholangiography. Four of the false negatives on ultrasound were in our first 140 patients. The last false negative was missed by ultrasound and digital fluorocholangiography. Others have shown that laparoscopic ultrasound for choledocholithiasis is as sensitive as intraoperative cholangiography and can be perfomed in less time (Table 17.2).

With experience, laparoscopic ultrasound can be as sensitive and specific as digital fluorocholangiography. It is more rapidly performed than either static x-ray imaging or digital fluorocholangiography. In our practice, it has replaced intraoperative digital fluorocholangiography.

Table 17.2. Several studies comparing laparoscopic ultrasound (LUS) with intraoperative cholangiography (IOCG).

Author	Year	Number of patients	Sensitivity (%)		Time (min)	
			LUS	IOCG	LUS	IOCG
Stiegman	1994	31	100	75	5.4	16.4
Thompson	1998	347	90	98.1	6.6	10.9
Birth	1998	518	83.3	100	7	16
Cathelin	2002	900	80	75	9.8	17.6
Halpin	2002	394/400	N/A	N/A	5.1	16.0

D. Selected References

Barteau JA, Castro D, Arregui ME, Tetik C. A comparison of intraoperative ultrasound vs cholangiography in the evaluation of the common bile duct during laparoscopic cholecystectomy. Surg Endosc 1995;9:490–498.

Birth M, Ehlers KU, Delinikolas K, Weiser HF. Prospective randomized comparison of laparoscopic ultrasonography using a flexible-tip ultrasound probe and intraoperative dynamic cholangiography during laparoscopic cholecystectomy. Surg Endosc 1998;12(1):30–36.

Catheline JM, Turner R, Paries J. Laparoscopic ultrasonography is a complement to cholangiography for the detection of choledocholithiasis at laparoscopic cholecystectomy. Br J Surg 2002;89(10):1235–1239.

Halpin VJ, Dunnegan D, Soper NJ, Laparoscopic intracorporeal ultrasound versus fluoroscopic intraoperative cholangiography: after the learning curve. Surg Endosc 2002;16(2):336–341.

Machi J, Siegel B. Ultrasound for Surgeons. 1st ed. New York: Igaku-Shoin, 1997.

Rothlin MA, Schlumpf R. Largiader F. Laparoscopic sonography: an alternative to routine intraoperative cholangiography? Arch Surg 1994;129:694–700.

Staren ED, Arregui ME. Ultrasound for the Surgeon. 1st ed. Philadelphia: Lippincott–Raven, 1997.

Stiegmann GV, McIntyre RC, Pearlman NW. Laparoscopic intracorporeal ultrasound: an alternative to cholangiography. Surg Endosc 1994;8(3):167–171.

Thompson DM, Arregui ME, Tetik C, Madden MT, Wegener M. A comparison of laparoscopic ultrasound with digital fluorocholangiography for detecting choledocholithiasis during laparoscopic choecystectomy. Surg Endosc 1998;12(7):929–932.

18. Laparoscopic Common Bile Duct Exploration: Transcystic Duct Approach

Joseph B. Petelin, M.D., F.A.C.S.

A. Indications, Contraindications, and Choice of Approach

1. **Indications.** The most common indication for laparoscopic common bile duct exploration (LCDE) is an **abnormal intraoperative cholangiogram**. Preoperative abnormalities that suggest a possible need for LCDE are listed in Table 18.1.
2. **Contraindications.** The most significant contraindication to LCDE is inability of the surgeon to perform the necessary maneuvers. Absence of any of the indications listed in Table 18.1, instability of the patient, and local conditions in the porta hepatis that would make exploration hazardous are also contraindications.
3. **Choice of approach.** There are two possible routes for LCDE. The **transcystic duct** approach is discussed in this section. LCDE may also be performed by laparoscopic **choledochotomy** (see Chapter 20).
    a. The transcystic approach is particularly useful when the cystic duct is ample in diameter and enters the common duct via a relatively straight, lateral approach.
    b. The factors that influence choice of approach are summarized in Table 18.2.
    c. Transcystic duct exploration is generally attempted before laparoscopic choledochotomy because it is both possible and highly successful in the majority of cases, and because it is less invasive than laparoscopic choledochotomy. In addition, transcystic duct exploration does not usually require facility with laparoscopic suturing techniques.

Table 18.1. Preoperative abnormalities suggesting that LCDE may be required.

Clinical history	Jaundice Pancreatitis
Liver function tests	$\uparrow$ Bilirubin
	$\uparrow$ Alkaline phosphatase
	$\uparrow$ γ-GTP
Ultrasound	Dilated bile ducts
	Choledocholithiasis
	Ductal obstruction
ERCP (or, rarely, transhepatic cholangiography)	Choledocholithiasis

ERCP, endoscopic retrograde cholangiopancreatography; GTP, glutamyl transpeptidase.

B. Patient Positioning, Equipment Needed, Room Setup

1. Position the patient supine with both arms tucked at the sides.
2. Reverse Trendelenburg position and rotation to a slight left lateral decubitus position are often helpful in displaying the porta hepatis; this consideration is more important for laparoscopic common bile duct exploration than for laparoscopic cholecystectomy because access to the cystic duct–common duct junction is often necessary.

Table 18.2. Factors influencing the approach to LCDE: note that negative factors have a more profound impact on choice of approach than positive or neutral ones.

Factor	Transcystic	Choledochotomy
One stone	+	+
Multiple stones	+	+
Stones ≤6 mm diameter	+	+
Stones >6 mm diameter	−	+
Intrahepatic stones	−	+
Diameter of cystic duct <4 mm	−	+
Diameter of cystic duct ≥4 mm	+	+
Diameter of common duct <6 mm	+	−
Diameter of common duct ≥6 mm	+	+
Cystic duct entrance—lateral	+	+
Cystic duct entrance—posterior	−	+
Cystic duct entrance—distal	−	+
Inflammation—mild	+	+
Inflammation—marked	+	−
Suturing ability—poor	+	−
Suturing ability—good	+	+

Table 18.3. Instruments, drugs, and supplies needed for transcystic duct exploration.

Glucagon, 1 to 2 mg (given intravenously by the anesthetist)
Balloon-tipped catheters
    4-French preferred over 3- and 5-French
Segura-type baskets
    Four-wire, flat, straight in-line configuration
Guidewire (0.035-in. diameter)
Mechanical "over-the-wire" dilators (7- to 12-French)
High-pressure "over-the-wire" pneumatic dilator
Intravenous tubing (for saline instillation through the choledochoscope)
Atraumatic grasping forceps (for choledochoscope manipulation)
Flexible choledochoscope with light source (≤3 mm o. d., with ≥1.1-mm
    working channel preferred)
  Second camera
  Second monitor (or picture-in-picture display on the primary laparoscopic
    monitor)
  Video switcher (for simultaneous same monitor display of
    choledochoscopic and laparoscopic images)
Waterpik (Teledyne Water Pik, Fort Collins, CO)
Electrohydraulic lithotripter
C-tube (transcystic)
Stent (straight, 7-French or 10-French)
Sphincterotome (for antegrade sphincterotomy)

---

3. The standard instruments used for laparoscopic cholecystectomy with intraoperative cholangiography are needed, and include forceps, scissors, dissecting instruments, cholangiographic accessories, and a fluoroscope. Specialized instruments, drugs, and supplies needed to perform common bile duct exploration are listed in Table 18.3.
4. Keep all this equipment on a separate cart that can be brought into the room for LCDE.
5. Place the specific items that are needed for a particular case on a separate sterile Mayo stand, located to the right of the surgeon near the patient's left shoulder.

C. Trocar Position and Choice of Laparoscope and Choledochoscope

1. Place the trocars in the standard laparoscopic cholecystectomy configuration.
    a. Place a 10-mm port at the umbilicus and insert a laparoscope.
    b. Place 5- to 10-mm ports under direct laparoscopic vision in the epigastrium just to right of the midline, in the right midclavicu-

lar line, and in the right anterior axillary line. If LCDE is contemplated preoperatively, place the epigastric port slightly more
inferior than for laparoscopic cholecystectomy alone. Otherwise,
suture closure of the cystic duct or common bile duct may be
awkward (suturing backward).
  c. The author routinely performs laparoscopic cholecystectomy
     with just three ports, and uses the last port mentioned only for
     laparoscopic common bile duct exploration.
2. The author prefers a **0-degree, 10-mm laparoscope** for visualization,
   but others favor a 30-degree, 10-mm laparoscope. The angled laparoscope is especially useful in obese patients, in whom the mesenteric
   and omental adipose tissue obscures visualization of the porta hepatis.
3. Many vendors supply flexible choledochoscopes. Several points
   should be kept in mind:
  a. Reusable scopes generally perform better than disposable scopes,
     but are expensive, fragile, and easily damaged.
  b. Become facile with the gentle maneuvers required for manipula-
     tion of the scope.
  c. Use atraumatic instruments to grasp or position the
     choledochoscope.

D. Preparation for LCDE

1. Generally, LCDE is performed in conjunction with laparoscopic cholecystectomy. Elevate the gallbladder and expose the cystic duct in the
   usual fashion (Chapter 16).
2. Obtain an image of the bile ducts to delineate the anatomy, confirm
   the presence of choledocholithiasis, and determine the number and
   location of stones.
  a. Either standard cystic duct cholangiography with fluoroscopy
     (see Chapter 16), or intraoperative ultrasound (see Chapter 17)
     may be used.
  b. Fluoroscopic imaging is the gold standard for intraoperative radi-
     ologic evaluation because it is faster and more detailed than other
     methods, and allows the surgeon to interact with the images in
     real time (e.g., scanning the ductal system by moving the C-arm
     while injecting contrast material).
3. Dissect the porta hepatis.
  a. Start the dissection of the triangle of Calot from just lateral to the
     neck of the gallbladder, and continue this dissection toward the
     cystic duct–common duct junction as the anatomy is further
     defined.
  b. Access to the cystic duct–common duct junction or the anterior
     surface of the common duct itself is often necessary for ductal
     exploration.
  c. Use the cholangiogram as a guide to the anatomy during this
     sometimes tedious dissection.

4. Determine whether the transcystic approach is appropriate or whether laparoscopic choledochotomy will be required (see Table 18.2).

E. Techniques for LCDE

The techniques for LCDE may be used with either the transcystic or laparoscopic choledochotomy access route.

1. **Irrigation techniques.** When very small stones (≤2-mm diameter), sludge, or sphincter spasm is suspected to be responsible for lack of flow of contrast into the duodenum, transcystic flushing of the duct with saline or contrast material is occasionally successful in clearing the duct.
    a. Glucagon (1–2 mg), administered intravenously by the anesthetist, may relax the sphincter of Oddi and improve the success rate.
    b. Monitor the progress (or lack thereof) fluoroscopically.
    c. This method is unlikely to work for stones 4 mm and larger.
2. **Balloon techniques.** Fogarty-type, low-pressure, balloon-tipped catheters are sometimes useful in clearing the ductal system of stones or debris. The technique described here is used for retrieval of stones from the distal common bile duct. Stones in the upper biliary tree may be retrieved under choledochoscopic guidance.
    a. A long 4-French catheter is passed through the 14-gauge sleeve used for percutaneous cholangiography.
    b. The insertion site for the sleeve is usually located 3 cm medial to the midclavicular port.
    c. Use forceps, introduced through the medial epigastric port, to guide the catheter into the cystic duct.
    d. Advance the catheter into the common duct, and pass it into the duodenum. Generally, the 10-cm mark on the catheter will have just entered the cystic duct when the tip enters the duodenum.
    e. Inflate the balloon and withdraw the catheter slightly until resistance is felt at the papilla. Confirm the location of the papilla by observing motion of the duodenum as the catheter is moved.
    f. Deflate the balloon, withdraw it an additional centimeter, and reinflate.
    g. Withdraw the catheter until the balloon exits the cystic duct orifice.
    h. Repeat this maneuver until no debris or stones exit from the cystic duct orifice.
3. **Basket techniques.** Baskets may be used to retrieve stones under fluoroscopic control, under choledochoscopic control, or freely without either visual monitoring method. Thus these methods are useful when unsuspected stones are encountered (e.g., when the duct exploration equipment is not already prepared), while the nursing team is preparing the choledochoscope. They are also useful in somewhat rare cases in which the patient's common bile duct is of such small diameter

(<5 mm) that choledochoscope passage would be difficult or hazardous.

a.   In the **fluoroscopic method**, insert the basket through a 14-gauge sleeve (an IV sheath), placed 3 cm medial to the midclavicular port.

    i.   Advance the basket through the cystic duct into the common bile duct with forceps inserted through the medial epigastric port (Fig. 18.1).

    ii. Under fluoroscopic guidance, identify and capture the stone in the contrast-filled common bile duct.

    iii. If too much contrast has drained from the ductal system after completion of the cholangiograms, it may be necessary to instill more contrast with the cholangiocatheter. This potentially cumbersome and time-consuming step is one of the disadvantages of this method.

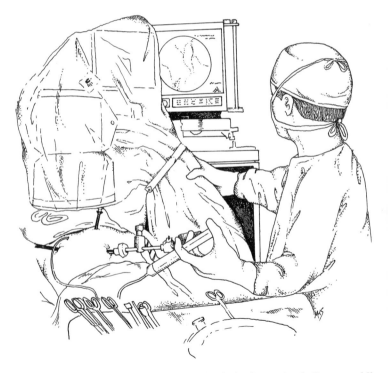

Figure 18.1. Cholangiography in preparation for basket retrieval of common bile duct stones under fluoroscopic guidance. Note location of monitors, surgeon, and instruments.

      iv. Another disadvantage of this method is the increased radiation exposure for the patient and the team during stone capture.

      v. In addition, it is often difficult or impossible to manipulate the forceps controlling the basket while the C-arm is in place because the fluoroscope impedes movement of the forceps introduced through the medial epigastric port.

  b. When the basket is used in conjunction with the **choledochoscope**, insert it through the working channel of the scope.

      i. Capture the stone under direct vision.

      ii. Remove the entire ensemble from the cystic duct; deposit the stone on the omentum.

      iii. Grasp and deliver the stone through the medial epigastric or other 10-mm port.

  c. Baskets may also be used without fluoroscopic or choledochoscopic guidance. This is an advanced technique and should be used by the novice only with great caution.

      i. Introduce the basket through the 14-gauge sleeve and guide it into the common duct through the cystic duct.

      ii. Open the basket as soon as the tip of the basket passes into the common bile duct.

      iii. Use forceps, introduced through the medial epigastric port, to advance the open basket to the distal portion of the common bile duct. This minimizes the risk of accidental perforation of the duct by the basket tip or accidental capture of the papilla (since it is the rounded contour of the basket, rather than the relatively sharp tip, that forms the leading edge).

      iv. After the basket has reached the distal duct, it is withdrawn proximally as the basket is closed. Incomplete closure of the basket handle usually signals stone capture.

      v. The basket may have to be passed back and forth in the duct several times before the stone is captured.

4. **Choledochoscopic techniques.** Capturing stones under direct vision has always given the greatest sense of safety and accuracy. While the surgeon may choose to look directly into the choledochoscope, it is much simpler to attach a video camera and view the image indirectly. Viewing the video image then either requires a third monitor, replacement of the image on the "slave" or secondary monitor, or, preferably, use of a video switcher to incorporate the image onto the same monitors used for the laparoscopic camera. This switcher should reside on one of the monitor towers for easy manipulation. In some integrated systems the switching controls are located on a sterile touch pad controlled by the surgeon. Simultaneous visualization of both images allows the surgeon to manipulate the controls of the choledochoscope as well as employing external manipulation with atraumatic forceps. Smaller-diameter (<3 mm) flexible choledochoscopes facilitate transcystic choledochoscopy. Even with the smallest scopes, the cystic duct must usually be dilated.

a. Adequate dilatation is usually possible if the initial cystic duct diameter is greater than 2.5 mm, and unlikely if it is not.

b. Dilatation may be carried out with either mechanical over-the-wire graduated dilators or pneumatic over-the-wire dilators. The former are inexpensive and found in most urology departments.

    i. Pass a guidewire through the midclavicular port into the cystic duct.

    ii. Guide a series of successively larger dilators over the guidewire and into the cystic duct and common duct, using forceps inserted through the medial epigastric port. Because these dilators exert a shearing-type force, exercise great care to avoid disruption of the cystic duct–common duct junction.

    iii. In general, **if the duct will not initially accept a 9-French** dilator easily, then adequate dilatation to the requisite 12-French is unlikely.

c. High-pressure, balloon-tipped catheters may be used to dilate the cystic duct.

    i. Pass a guidewire through the midclavicular port into the cystic duct and advance it into the common duct.

    ii. Advance the balloon catheter over the guidewire.

    iii. Position the balloon catheter in the cystic duct.

    iv. Inflation of the balloon distends the duct with radially directed force, which may be safer than the graduated dilators (less shear force). Still, both the pressure on the balloon and cystic duct changes must be closely observed to avoid injury. This is a more expensive way to dilate the cystic duct.

d. Insert the flexible choledochoscope through the midclavicular port and guide it into the cystic duct with atraumatic forceps inserted through the medial epigastric port. Some authors have suggested the use of a semiflexible sleeve, inserted through the midclavicular port into the cystic duct, as a guide for the choledochoscope. In the author's experience, this impedes some of the manipulations necessary for adequate choledochoscopic intervention.

e. Control the choledochoscope both at its insertion site on the abdominal wall and with the controls on the head of the choledochoscope. This allows rotational movements of the shaft of the scope and deflection movements of the scope tip.

f. Advance the choledochoscope into the common duct and visualize the stone(s). Generally a **stone basket** is the preferred tool for choledochoscopic stone extraction.

    i. Capture the stone closest to the choledochoscope first to avoid difficulty in removing the stone from the duct.

    ii. Insert the basket through the working channel of the choledochoscope and advance it to the stone under direct choledochoscopic vision.

    iii. Advance the closed basket beyond the stone. Open the basket and pull back, capturing the stone within the basket. Close the basket gently but firmly to secure the stone.

    iv. Remove the entire ensemble through the cystic duct, and deposit the stone temporarily on the omentum.

    v. Grasp the stone with forceps inserted through the medial epigastric port and remove it.

g. Stones that defy capture with a basket may be removed with a Fogarty-type balloon catheter.

    i. Pass the catheter into the ductal system alongside the scope, because the working channel of the scope is too small to admit it.

    ii. Advance the catheter beyond the stone under direct vision.

    iii. Inflate the balloon beyond the stone, and withdraw the catheter enough to impact the stone against the choledochoscope.

    iv. Remove the entire ensemble through the duct. Combined use of these techniques requires either a large-diameter cystic duct or a choledochotomy approach (see Chapter 19).

    v. In the unlikely event that stones are displaced into the common hepatic duct during balloon manipulations, flush the stones back down into the distal system by altering the position of the table, or retrieve the stones by passing the balloon catheter proximally. In the author's experience this is a rare event, and in no case have other measures been necessary to retrieve common hepatic duct stones.

5. **Lithotripsy.** Intraoperative lithotripsy is primarily indicated for impacted stones that defy less aggressive removal techniques. Both electrohydraulic (EHL) and laser lithotripters are available. The laser lithotripters are far too expensive to encourage widespread implementation, and therefore EHL devices have been used somewhat more frequently. EHL devices must be used with great caution because they may cause unwanted ductal damage if the tip of the EHL probe is not accurately applied to the stone. However, with careful, direct visualization and application of EHL energy to the stone surface, stones may be safely fragmented without undue risk.

6. **Laparoscopic antegrade sphincterotomy.** Laparoscopic antegrade sphincterotomy was first described by DePaula and coworkers in 1993.

a. In this method a sphincterotome is passed through the working channel of the choledochoscope and through the sphincter.

b. Monitor the cutting action by simultaneous side-viewing endoscopy of the duodenum.

c. Alternatively, pass the sphincterotome through the side-viewing scope, rather than through the choledochoscope.

d. While these techniques achieve excellent results as a drainage procedure, they are logistically quite difficult to accomplish.

    i. More equipment and an additional endoscopic team must be present in an already crowded operating room.

      ii. It is more difficult to pass the ERCP scope and perform sphincterotomy with the patient supine (rather than in the typical semiprone position).

      iii. Laparoscopic visualization is more difficult due to air insufflation of the duodenum and small bowel by the endoscopist.

      iv. For all these reasons, laparoscopic antegrade and retrograde sphincterotomy has not gained widespread acceptance.

    e. An alternative, when stones cannot be removed using the foregoing methods, is to pass a guide wire or cystic duct tube (C-tube) through the cystic duct and advance it into the duodenum. This assists in post procedure ERCP and sphincterotomy.

7. Biliary bypass procedures may be indicated in patients with an impacted distal stone, a stone or stones located distal to a stricture, or with dramatically dilated ducts (>2 cm) with multiple stones. Choledochoenterostomy may be accomplished laparoscopically, but this requires significant advanced laparoscopic suturing skills. These techniques are described elsewhere in this manual (see Parts IV and V).

F. Selected References

Berci G, Cuschieri A eds. Bile Ducts and Bile Duct Stones. Philadelphia: WB Saunders, 1996.

Carroll BJ, Phillips EH, Daykhovsky L, et al. Laparoscopic choledochoscopy: an effective approach to the common duct. J Laparoendosc Surg 1992;2:15–21.

DePaula AL, Hashiba K, Bafutto M. Laparoscopic management of choledocholithiasis. Surg Endosc 1994;8:1399–1403.

DePaula A, Hashiba K, Bafutto M, Zago R, Machado M. Laparoscopic antegrade sphincterotomy. Surg Laparasc Endosc 1993;3(3):157–160.

Fielding GA, O'Rourke NA. Laparoscopic common bile duct exploration. Aust N Z J Surg 1993;63:113–115.

Fletcher DR. Common bile duct calculi at laparoscopic cholecystectomy: a technique for management. Aust N Z J Surg 1993;63:710–714.

Franklin ME, Pharand D, Rosenthal D. Laparoscopic common bile duct exploration. Surg Laparosc Endosc 1994;(4)2:119–124.

Petelin J. Laparoscopic approach to common duct pathology. Surg Laparosc Endosc 1991;1:1:33–41.

Petelin JB. Laparoscopic ductal stone clearance: transcystic approach. In: Berci G, Cuschieri A, eds. Bile Ducts and Bile Duct Stones. Philadelphia: WB Saunders, 1996, 97–108.

Petelin JB. Surgical management of common bile duct stones. Gastrointest Endosc 2002;54(6):S183–S189.

Petelin JB. Laparoscopic common bile duct exploration. Surg Endosc 2003;17(11): 1705–1715.

Phillips EH, Rosenthal RJ, Carroll BJ, et al. Laparoscopic trans-cystic duct common bile duct exploration. Surg Endosc 1994;8:1389–1394.

Shapiro SJ, Gordon LA, Daykhovsky L, et al. Laparoscopic exploration of the common bile duct: experience in 16 selected patients. J Laparoendosc Surg 1991;(1)6: 333–341.

Stoker ME, Leveillee RJ, McCann JC, Maini BS. Laparoscopic common bile duct exploration. J Laparoendosc Surg 1991;1(5):287–293.

Traverso LW. A cost-effective approach to the treatment of common bile duct stones with surgical versus endoscopic techniques. In: Berci G, Cuschieri A, eds. Bile Ducts and Bile Duct Stones. Philadelphia: WB Saunders, 1996, 154–160.

Traverso LW, Roush TS, Koo K. Common bile duct stones—outcomes and costs. Surg Endosc 1995;9:1242–1244.

19. Common Bile Duct Exploration via Laparoscopic Choledochotomy

Alfred Cuschieri, M.D., Ch.M., F.R.C.S., F.R.S.E., F. Med. Sci.
Chris Kimber, M.B.B.S., F.R.A.C.S.

A. Indications and Patient Preparation

Laparoscopic common bile duct (CBD) exploration is performed when transcystic duct extraction is not appropriate or has failed. The current **indications** for laparoscopic direct CBD exploration are:

1. Failed transcystic extraction if CBD diameter exceeds 8 mm
2. Large single or multiple stones (>1.0 cm), provided the load is not excessive (see later)
3. Unsuccessful attempts at endoscopic stone extraction for large/occluding stones
4. Intrahepatic stones, which are inaccessible via a transcystic approach

Under certain circumstances, other procedures are more appropriate; these may be considered **contraindications** to laparoscopic direct simple CBD exploration, and include the following:

1. Small-caliber (<8 mm) ducts are best cleared of stone by endoscopic sphincterotomy and stone extraction. Direct exploration of the CBD is inadvisable due to the risk of stricture formation.
2. A grossly dilated duct (>2.5 cm) with multiple stones (usually brown pigment) indicates a relative obstruction at the distal CBD in the region of the ampulla of Vater. Adequate drainage must be established to prevent recurrent stone formation. Endoscopic sphincterotomy does not deal adequately with this problem, and the two options are transduodenal sphincteroplasty or choledochoduodenostomy. As these patients are elderly, the lesser of these two procedures, choledochoduodenostomy is preferred (see Section G). Often these patients are admitted on an emergency basis with jaundice and cholangitis and require endoscopic insertion of choledochoduodenal pigtail stent, intravenous fluids, and antibiotics to tide them over the acute illness before the procedure can be performed. The stent is removed at operation together with the stones.

Antibiotic prophylaxis (generally a cephalosporin) appropriate for the most likely biliary pathogens should be routine, as bile spillage is inevitable during the procedure. The remainder of the preparation is similar to that for laparoscopic cholecystectomy and should include prophylaxis against deep-vein thrombosis.

B. Patient Position and Room Setup

The basic equipment and patient positioning (head-up supine) are as for laparoscopic cholecystectomy. The following additional items are essential:

1. Modern image intensifier (fluoroscopy C-arm unit)
2. Cholangiograsper (Olsen), French (Fr) ureteric catheters 3, 4 contrast medium
3. Flexible choledochoscope (3.3 mm or Fr 10, 5.0 mm or Fr 15) with instrument channel large enough (at least 1.2 mm) to enable concomitant irrigation and instrumentation
4. Separate monitor or picture in picture setup (twin video) to enable both the laparoscopic and choledochoscopic views to be simultaneously displayed
5. Selection of retrieval baskets and balloon catheters
6. Sharp scissors
7. Semm's spoon forceps for stone removal
8. **T**-tube or Cuschieri cystic duct drainage catheter (Wilson Cook) for biliary decompression

C. Trocar Position and Choice of Laparoscope

Begin with the four standard trocars for laparoscopic cholecystectomy, with the laparoscope at the umbilicus. One further port (10.0 mm) is placed high in the right epigastrium, in line with the choledochotomy. This port is used to introduce the choledochoscope and extraction devices. A reducer sleeve is an important adjunct. This guides the choledochoscope and other flexible instruments to the choledochotomy, adds stability, and protects the choledochoscope from being damaged by the trocar valves.

The 30-degree, forward-oblique, 10-mm laparoscope provides the best visualization of the common duct and is recommended in preference to the forward-viewing (0-degree) type.

D. Performing the Choledochotomy

In the vast majority of patients, laparoscopic supraduodenal CBD exploration is performed concomitant with laparoscopic cholecystectomy, and a certain amount of dissection in Calot's triangle will precede CBD exploration.

1. Generally the operation has proceeded thus far: Calot's triangle has been dissected, the cystic artery has been divided, and a clip has been

Table 19.1. Function of preexploration cholangiogram.

1. Confirm presence, size, location, and number of stones.
2. Demonstrate anatomic relationships and diameter of the extrahepatic bile duct.
3. Exclude unsuspected pathology, such as cholangiocarcinoma, in jaundiced patients.

   placed on the distal cystic duct (at the junction with the neck of the gallbladder).

2. The cystic duct is opened and an operative cholangiogram obtained. This pre-exploration cholangiogram serves several crucial functions and should be performed even if preoperative studies of the common duct were obtained (Table 19.1). Good opacification of both the intra- and extrahepatic portions of the biliary tree must be obtained. This is particularly important in elderly patients with brown pigment stones, in whom the diagnosis of Klatskin tumor or other pathology may not have been made on preoperative ultrasound examination.

3. Maintain the **continuity of the cystic duct with the gallbladder and common bile duct**. This is essential for traction, exposure, and manipulation. Hence, defer transection of the cystic duct and removal of the gallbladder from the liver bed until the CBD exploration is completed. This differs from the usual practice during open cholecystectomy and open CBD exploration.

4. Visualize the supraduodenal CBD. The 30-degree laparoscope is essential for adequate visualization. The CBD is generally readily apparent as a large tubular blue or greenish structure. Visible pulsations in the hepatic artery are a useful landmark.

5. Use curved scissors to **divide the peritoneum** over the CBD. Displace the duodenum inferiorly. A layer of fascia surrounds the CBD. Divide this and expose the anterior wall of the CBD with gentle pledget dissection. Use electrocautery sparingly, and limit the dissection to the anterior wall of the CBD. Expose an area approximately 2 cm long and 1 cm wide.

6. Use low-voltage coagulating electrocautery to mark the line of incision on the CBD. The incision should not exceed 1 cm. The authors prefer a lengthwise incision, but some use a transverse orientation.

7. Entry into the CBD is marked by a gush of bile, gas bubbles (after failed endoscopic retrograde cholangiography [ERC]), or even a stone. Suction irrigation is often required to maintain a clear view. Make the choledochotomy with scissors, cutting electrocautery, or a sheathed knife. It is important to keep the choledochotomy **as small as possible**. Because the CBD contains a large amount of elastin, a 1.0-cm choledochotomy can be stretched to deliver a 1.5-cm stone. Avoiding a long choledochotomy reduces the amount of suturing required and minimizes the risk of stricturing due to devascularization of the CBD. There is some unresolved controversy regarding the lie of the chole-

dochotomy, with unsubstantiated statements that transverse/oblique incisions cause less devascularization of the CBD, but this has never been proven. Care must be taken, however, with vertical choledochotomies, as they are more likely to enlarge during manipulations, especially from repeated insertions of choledochoscopes, wire baskets, and balloon catheters.

E. Stone Extraction

Stone extraction is accomplished through the choledochotomy using a series of steps:

1. Apply **external compression** to the CBD from below upward, with two atraumatic forceps, gently pushing a stone toward the choledochotomy and milking the stone out through the choledochotomy. This simple maneuver is often successful for floating stones that are then grasped inside the Semm's spoon forceps and removed.

2. If step 1 fails, insert a **biliary balloon catheter** through the choledochotomy toward the distal end of the CBD. Inflate the balloon and withdraw the catheter slowly toward the choledochotomy. Ease or suction any dislodged stones out through the choledochotomy.

3. Perform visually guided extraction using the choledochoscope if the first two measures fail (as is often the case when the stones are occluding or impacted). Attach the irrigation system to the choledochoscope and insert the scope (using a reducer sleeve) through the extra trocar placed in the right subxiphoid region. (See Chapters 50 and 51 on diagnostic choledochoscopy for additional information.)

   a. Gently guide the choledochoscope into the choledochotomy. Avoid grasping the choledochoscope, as it is easy to damage the sheath or fibers.

   b. Once the scope is inside the CBD, use an atraumatic grasper to gather the choledochotomy around the endoscope, creating an adequate seal for distention and visualization of the biliary tree.

   c. Two operators working synchronously are needed for efficient visually guided stone extraction—one manipulates the scope (tip flexion and torque) to obtain the desired view of the stone, and the other is in charge of trapping the stone inside the basket (preferably four wires).

   d. Pass the closed basket and negotiate it beyond the stone. Open the wire basket and trawl it slowly backward under visual guidance.

   e. When the stone falls inside the wires, close the basket just enough to grasp the stone without crushing it.

   f. Withdraw the entire assembly (scope, basket, and stone) through the choledochotomy.

   g. Release the stone and remove it from the abdomen using a Semm's spoon forceps.

4. After all the stones have been removed, irrigate the biliary tract with warm saline to flush out any small fragments.
5. Perform a **completion check choledochoscopy** by inspecting the proximal and distal sections of the extrahepatic biliary tracts. Remove any debris, stone fragments, or residual calculi.

F. Closure of the Choledochotomy

Although some advocate primary closure without decompression of the extrahepatic biliary tract, the authors feel this is inadvisable for two reasons. First, manipulations at the lower end of the bile duct frequently cause periampullary edema, increasing the risk of bile leakage through the sutured choledochotomy. Second, primary closure precludes completion or postoperative cholangiography.

Drainage may be accomplished by placement of a T-tube or by placement of a drainage catheter through the cystic duct. Both are acceptable, but the authors prefer decompression through the cystic duct for two reasons: first, this method of drainage minimizes the postoperative hospital stay; and second, it allows primary common duct closure. Both methods will be described here.

1. Transcystic decompression requires a 1.0-m-long 8 to 10 Fr, shaped drainage cannula with a terminal S-shaped perforated segment (Cuschieri cystic duct drainage catheter set—Wilson-Cook—Fig. 19.1). The set consists of introducer needle, guidewire, dilator tube, and tear-away sheath, and allows percutaneous insertion of the drainage cannula.

    Choose an insertion site in the right flank and introduce the catheter using Seldinger technique (Fig. 19.2).

    a. Use two graspers to thread the cystic duct drainage cannula (with the guidewire projecting for a distance of 2.0 cm beyond its tip) through the cystic duct into the CBD.
    b. Advance the cannula until the perforated segment is beyond the junction of the cystic duct with the common hepatic duct.

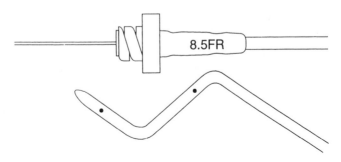

Figure 19.1. Cuschieri transcystic biliary decompression set.

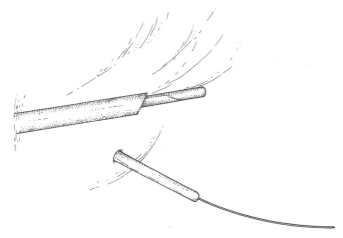

Figure 19.2. The drainage cannula is threaded over the guidewire into the peritoneal cavity.

    c.   Remove the guide wire. Confirm accurate positioning of the S-shaped segment by inspection through the choledochotomy.

    d.   Secure the catheter with two chromic catgut Roeder knots to the cystic duct.

    e.   Anchor the drainage cannula by skin sutures and attach a saline syringe (to flush the biliary tract during suture closure of the choledochotomy) (Fig. 19.3).

    f.   Maintain continuous saline irrigation through the cystic duct cannula during closure. This facilitates visualization of the edges of the wound and helps ensure a leak-proof suture line.

    g.   Closure is best performed with accurately placed interrupted sutures. Use 4/0 absorbable atraumatic sutures (Polysorb or coated Vicryl). Place the suture bites accurately, 2 mm apart.

2.   **Decompression by T-tube.** The practical considerations if this method of decompression is used include appropriate size (Fr 14) and correct exit course of the long limb of the **T**-tube.

    a.   Trim the crossbar of the **T** (the intracholedochal segment) to twice the length of the choledochotomy (generally 2 cm) and fillet this segment longitudinally.

    b.   Fold the two ends together using an atraumatic grasper and introduce the T-tube into the CBD.

    c.   Exteriorize the long limb in the right flank.

    d.   Close the choledochotomy from above downward (using interrupted 4/0 absorbable sutures, as previously discussed) so that the long limb comes to lie at the lower end of the suture line (Fig. 19.4).

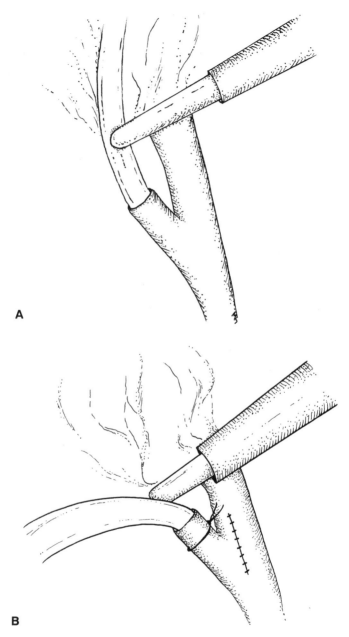

Figure 19.3. Fixation of the biliary decompression cannula to the cystic duct stump by catgut Roeder knots.

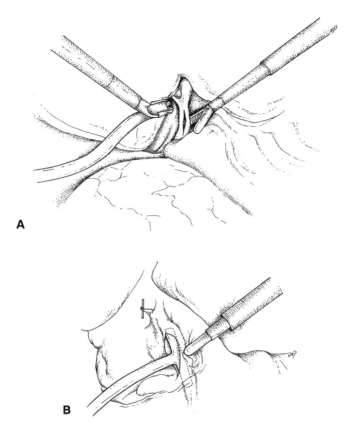

Figure 19.4. A. The folded T-tube is inserted into the choledochotomy. B. T-tube in place. The choledochotomy will be closed from above downward. The T-tube will exit from the lower end of the choledochotomy when the sutures are placed.

3. **Completion fluorocholangiogram** is advisable, even when completion choledochoscopy has been normal, as small stone fragments in the ampullary region are easily missed. Begin screening during the early filling phase with slow injection of contrast, as otherwise small calculi may be obscured by the contrast medium (see Chapter 15, Cholangiography).

4. Always **insert a subhepatic drain** via the right subcostal trocar and place the tip of the drain near the choledochotomy.

5. If exploration is unsuccessful, consider conversion to an open procedure (Table 19.2).

Decompression by internal stent. Many authors advocate insertion of a pigtail stent, which is placed across the lower choledochal sphincter before

Table 19.2. Indications for conversion to open procedure.

1. Failure to progress with the operation (beyond 2 hours); the most common problem is an impacted stone that has excavated a diverticulum; these cases frequently require open transduodenal sphincteroplasty
2. Large stone load in a grossly dilated bile duct (if the surgeon is not experienced with the performance of laparoscopic choledochoduodenostomy)
3. Difficult anatomy or unsuspected pathology of the biliopancreatic tract
4. Uncontrollable bleeding

suture closure of the CBD incision (tubeless choledochotomy). The stent is removed 4 to 6 weeks later by means of upper gastrointestinal endoscopy. This approach seems to be reasonable except that it does not allow a postoperative contrast study.

G. Laparoscopic Choledochoduodenectomy

Laparoscopic choledochoduodenectomy is indicated in patients with large stone load and a grossly dilated duct ($\geq 2.0\,cm$). It is carried out after completion of the ductal stone clearance by one of two techniques: side-to-side or end-to-side anastomosis between the CBD and the first part of the duodenum. The author's preference is for end-to-side choledochoduodenostomy, primarily because it avoids the sump syndrome. It is also technically easier to perform laparoscopically.

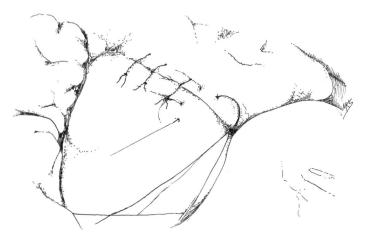

Figure 19.5. Completed sutured laparoscopic cholededochoduodenostomy.

The laparoscopic procedure entails transection of the lower end of the CBD just above its entry into the pancreatic parenchyma. The distal end is then closed with a continuous suture and the proximal end anastomosed to the first part of the duodenum using a continuous posterior layer (3/0 absorbable) and interrupted sutures for the anterior wall (Fig. 19.5). A drain is left and placed close to the completed anastomosis.

H. Postoperative Management

1. Continue perioperative antibiotics for 48 hours.
2. **Management of transcystic drainage catheter.** The average output from the 8-Fr cystic duct drainage cannula is 300 mL/day. Perform postoperative transcystic cholangiography on the second postoperative day.
   a. If the cholangiogram is normal with good entry of dye into the duodenum, clamp the drainage catheter and cover it with an occlusive dressing.
   b. Remove the subhepatic drain on the next day (if no bile drainage) and discharge the patient.
   c. Remove the transcystic drainage catheter after a minimum of 7 days (longer if the patient is elderly or diabetic) to assure that a secure tract has formed.
3. Management of T-tube:
   a. Delay performing the cholangiogram until the seventh postoperative day.
   b. If normal, clamp the tube for 6 hours.
   c. If there are no symptoms or bile drainage from the subhepatic drain (and provided the patient is not immunosuppressed, elderly, or diabetic), remove the T-tube.
   d. Remove the subhepatic drain 12 to 24 hours later.
   e. Immunosuppressed patients should be sent home with the T-tube clamped. The T-tube may be removed 2 weeks later.
4. If stones are identified on the postoperative cholangiogram, insert a guide wire into the duodenum under fluoroscopic control for use during the subsequent endoscopic retrograde cholangiopancreatography (see Chapter 61).

I. Selected References

Berci G, Cuschieri A, eds. Bile Ducts and Bile Duct Stones. Philadelphia: WB Saunders, 1997.

Crawford DL, Phillips EH. Laparoscopic common bile duct exploration. World J Surg 1999;23:343–349.

Cuschieri A, Lezoche E, Morino M, et al. EAES multicentre prospective randomized trial comparing two-stage vs single-stage management of patients with gallstones and ductal calculi. Surg Endosc 1996;13:952–957.

Dorman JP, Franklin ME Jr. Laparoscopic common bile duct exploration by choledochotomy. Semin Laparosc Surg 1997;4:34–41.

Fielding GA, O'Rourke NA. Laparoscopic common bile duct exploration. Aust N Z J Surg 1993;63:113–115.

Gersin KS, Fanelli RD. Laparoscopic endobiliary stenting as an adjunct to common bile duct exploration. Surg Endosc 1998;12:301–304.

Hensman C, Crosthwaite G, Cuschieri A. Transcystic biliary decompression after direct laparoscopic exploration of the common bile duct. Surg Endosc 1997;11:1106–1110.

Holdsworth RJ, Sadek SA, Ambikar S, Cuschieri A. Dynamics of bile flow through the choledochal sphincter following exploration of the common bile duct. World J Surg 1989;13:300–304.

Lezoche E, Paganini AM. Single-stage laparoscopic treatment of gallstones and common duct stones in 120 unselected consecutive patients. Surg Endosc 1995;9:1070–1075.

Martin IJ, Bailey IS, Rhodes M, O'Rourke N, Nathanson L, Fielding G. Towards T-tube-free laparoscopic bile duct exploration: a methodologic evolution during 300 consecutive procedures. Ann Surg 1998;228:29–34.

Millat B, Atger G, Deleuze A, et al. Laparoscopic treatment for choledocholithiasis: a prospective evaluation in 247 consecutive unselected patients. Hepatogastroenterology 1997;44:28–34.

Moroni J, Haurie JP, Judchak I, Fuster S. Single-stage laparoscopic and endoscopic treatment for choledocholithiasis: a novel approach. J Laparoendosc Adv Surg Techniques A 1999;9:69–74.

Phillips EH. Laparoscopic common bile duct exploration: long-term outcome. Arch Surg 1999;134:839–843.

20. Complications of Laparoscopic Cholecystectomy and Laparoscopic Common Duct Exploration

Mark A. Talamini, M.D., F.A.C.S.
Joseph B. Petelin, M.D., F.A.C.S.
Alfred Cuschieri, M.D., Ch.M.,
F.R.C.S., F.R.S.E., F.Med.Sci.

A. Management of Bile Duct Injury

Both the common duct and the right hepatic duct are at risk during laparoscopic biliary surgery.

1. **Cause and prevention.** The major causes are mistaken anatomy or excessive inflammation. Maintain the dissection high on the gallbladder and carefully delineate the anatomy before clipping or ligating any structures (see Chapter 15). Cholangiography (see Chapter 16) provides an invaluable roadmap. Suspect inflammation when bowel or duodenum is densely adherent to the gallbladder. Bile duct injury can also occur during common duct exploration (see Sections B and C).

2. **Recognition and management**
   a. **Intraoperative.** The danger signs listed in Table 20.1 should prompt the prudent surgeon to prove, at the very least, that a bile duct injury has not occurred. Bowel plastered to the face of the gallbladder is an early warning sign of **excessive inflammation**. Gently attempt to separate the tissues, and consider conversion to formal laparotomy, particularly if the inflammatory process precludes safe identification of structures in Calot's triangle.

   Leakage of bile after all structures have been clipped and divided (and any holes in the gallbladder repaired) should suggest a ductal injury. Cholangiography may confirm or exclude a defect in the biliary tree, but if suspicion remains, it is safest to convert to formal laparotomy. **Dissection** should normally progress several centimeters from the bifurcation of the right and left hepatic ducts. Dissection up under the liver should raise concern. In rare instances this will actually be the appropriate location for dissection. If that is the case, it probably is most safely dissected through an open incision. At the very least, when dissection is close up under the liver, one must be particularly careful about staying close to the gallbladder.

Table 20.1. Danger signs during laparoscopic biliary tract surgery.

Sign	Significance
Bile in operative field (in the absence of hole in gallbladder)	Bile duct injury
Dense adhesions to gallbladder	Excessive inflammation
Dissection progressing into hilum of liver	Mistaken anatomy
Extra or unexpected tubular structure encountered during dissection	Mistaken anatomy (aberrant right hepatic duct, or transected common duct)
Presumed cystic duct appears unusually large in diameter	Mistaken anatomy ("cystic duct" is actually common or right hepatic duct)
Extra tubular structure attached to resected gallbladder	Portion of common or right hepatic duct excised with specimen

Cholangiography is the best way to delineate anatomy. In Chapter 16, Fig. 16.14A shows the classic "cholangiogram from hell" in which the distal common duct is seen but no contrast flows proximal. This cholangiogram is a classic sign that the structure that has been identified as the "cystic duct" is actually the common duct and should prompt conversion to laparotomy. **Examination of the removed gallbladder** specimen can be a very reassuring exercise. This is particularly true after a difficult dissection. A careful dissection of the organ will quickly reveal exactly where the cystic duct was clipped and divided, and will confirm that no additional tubular structures (such as a segment of common or right hepatic duct) are attached. **Management of bile duct injury** depends on surgeon experience and comfort level with biliary tree reconstruction procedures. These are complex operations, and the best chance for a good, long-term outcome is during the first reconstruction. If the surgeon is uncomfortable or inexperienced, contact should be made with an experienced surgeon. Under some circumstances the best option may be to drain the site of injury and transfer the patient. The appropriate repair will generally be a Roux-en-Y hepaticojejunostomy to the proximal common hepatic duct or to the bifurcation of the right and left hepatic duct if necessary. The author's practice is to stent these anastomoses with Silastic stents passed through the anastomosis and brought out percutaneously. These are left in for months.

b. **Postoperative:** In the most common pattern of injury, bile leaks into the peritoneal cavity. The classic signs are pain, fever, abdominal distention, and abnormal liver function tests. Nuclear medicine scan will demonstrate leakage (Fig. 20.1).

There are three objectives when a bile duct injury is discovered postoperatively: definition and drainage of the biliary tree, control of bile peritonitis, and reconstruction of the biliary tree. **Definition and**

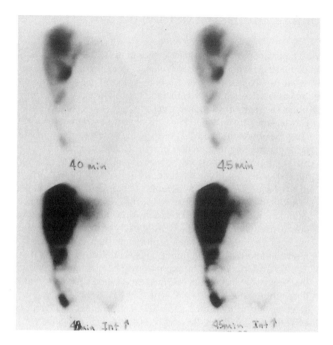

Figure 20.1. Nuclear medicine scan demonstrating free leakage of contrast. This patient had a complete transection of the common duct.

drainage of the biliary tree requires an experienced interventional radiology team that can perform complex biliary tree manipulation. Percutaneous transhepatic cholangiography and percutaneous biliary drainage are necessary to delineate biliary defect and to divert the bile away from the area by allowing it to preferentially drain into a gravity bag placed below the level of the bed. **Control of bile peritonitis** often means creating drainage for a biloma in the region of the biliary defect. If the surgeon left a percutaneous drain at the initial operation, this is usually perfectly adequate, and in fact avoids significant peritonitis. **Reconstruction of the biliary tree** usually means construction of a hepaticojejunostomy in an elective setting. Once the biliary tree has been diverted and the biloma drained, the pressure is off to move rapidly to the operating room. In fact, it is often advantageous to wait 4 to 6 weeks to allow any existent peritonitis to settle down, improving the likelihood of a good repair. Treatment of patients with laparoscopic bile duct injury requires an experienced multidisciplinary team with specialized equipment. Surgeons without such equipment and personnel at their disposal should consider transfer of the patient to another institution.

B. Complications of Transcystic Duct Exploration

Because laparoscopic common duct exploration (LCDE) is commonly performed in conjunction with laparoscopic cholecystectomy, any of the complications discussed in Chapter 16.3 (or Section A above) may occur. Additional complications associated with LCDE include the following.

1. **Failure to clear the common duct**
   a. **Cause and prevention.** There are numerous reasons for inability to clear the common duct of its obstruction. These include patient instability (prompting termination of the LCDE), intense inflammation in the porta hepatis, obese body habitus, intrahepatic stones, impacted stones, stones distal to a stricture, inadequate equipment, and surgeon inexperience. The most important of these is surgeon inexperience. While it may be difficult to gain actual experience in laparoscopic common bile duct exploration, surgeons who practice routine intraoperative cholangiography are using many of the same maneuvers that are used for transcystic ductal exploration, such as catheter and basket insertion into the ductal system. This should serve as useful preparation for LCDE. Additional training may be obtained by participation in a laparoscopic common bile duct exploration course or laparoscopic fellowship.
   b. **Recognition and management.** Completion cholangiography is essential to document the status of the ductal system after LCDE. Intraluminal opacities or failure of contrast to pass into the duodenum is usually indicative of retained intraductal material. After a thorough and careful attempt to clear the ductal system of all stones laparoscopically, decide whether to convert to open common bile duct exploration or resort to postoperative endoscopic retrograde techniques for stone removal.

2. **Bile leak**
   a. **Cause and prevention.** Bile may leak from the gallbladder bed, the cystic duct orifice used for LCDE, the cystic duct–common duct junction, or the common duct itself. This may be the result of dissection and manipulation of these structures during LCDE.
   b. Good visualization and gentle tissue-handling techniques may help reduce the incidence of this problem. The cystic duct must be secured adequately after LCDE. Consider suture ligation when the cystic duct is large, thickened, or short. Distal common duct manipulation, recent pancreatitis, or postoperative endoscopic retrograde cholangiopancreatography (ERCP) may cause temporary elevation of biliary pressure and suture ligation should be considered if any of these conditions apply.
   c. **Recognition and management.** Postoperative fever, excessive bilious drain output, ileus, and elevated liver function studies may indicate a bile leak. A radionuclide scan may confirm the presence of a leak, and the possibility of a distal obstruction in the common bile duct. Sonography or computed tomography (CT) scanning of the abdomen may help localize a bile collection if there is one.

d.   If a drain is already in place, and if there is no evidence of distal obstruction of the common bile duct, observation, intravenous fluids, and antibiotic coverage may be all that is necessary. If no drain is in place, and if a bile collection is localized, then radiographically directed placement of a drain may be adequate to allow a period of observation. The surgeon should not wait an excessively long time to intervene if there is no indication that the leak will seal itself or if generalized peritonitis is present.

e.   ERCP with or without sphincterotomy and placement of a stent is usually beneficial not only to clear any distal obstruction, but also to defeat the sphincter of Oddi in order to decrease biliary pressures and allow the leak to close.

3.   **Abscess**

a.   **Cause and prevention.** Patients requiring LCDE are often older, with more intense gallbladder inflammation than those requiring laparoscopic cholecystectomy. The bile is frequently colonized with bacteria. Hence, patients may be more prone to the development of postoperative infectious problems at the surgical site. Prophylactic antibiotics are essential here, and when acute or gangrenous cholecystitis or cholangitis is documented, therapeutic antibiotic coverage should be continued into the postoperative period.

b.   Thoroughly cleanse the perihepatic space of debris and stones before completing the case. If there has been severe inflammation or spillage of bile or stones, placement of a closed system suction drain may be prudent.

c.   **Recognition and management.** Postoperative fever, tachycardia, ileus, and abdominal pain usually signal the presence of a problem at the surgical site. Confirm the presence of an abscess by sonography or CT scanning. Management includes establishing drainage (which can often be accomplished percutaneously under ultrasound or CT guidance) and intravenous antibiotics. Surgical drainage may be needed if the symptoms do not resolve.

4.   **Common duct injury**

a.   **Cause and prevention.** Improper identification of the **anatomy** during dissection may lead to injury to the duct. This may be more likely when there is intense inflammation in the porta hepatis. A thorough knowledge of the anatomy, as seen laparoscopically, is essential. Intraoperative cholangiography via the cystic duct or the gallbladder, if necessary, may provide clues as to the location of the duct.

     During the ductal exploration itself, **aggressive manipulation of instruments** or the duct itself may lead to ductal injury. Pass all instruments gently to avoid ductal injury. Baskets are especially prone to puncture the duct, owing to the small size and configuration of the tip. Similarly, **electrohydraulic lithotripsy** must be used under direct visual control, and applied accurately and with care to avoid injury to the duct wall.

b.   **Recognition and management.** The best time to recognize this injury is at the time of surgery, when it can be either repaired primarily or bypassed if necessary. Unfortunately, most injuries are not recognized at this time and present themselves later with fever, tachycardia, abdominal pain, ileus, and jaundice. At that point, after stabilization of the patient, referral to a center specializing in reconstructive biliary tract surgery is the best option.

5. **Pancreatitis**
   a. **Cause and prevention.** Pancreatitis may be present before surgery, or exacerbated or induced postoperatively by manipulation of the distal duct. Gentle techniques are in order here to minimize the occurrence of this problem. **High-pressure balloon dilatation** of the sphincter of Oddi, advocated by some, commonly causes hyperamylasemia or frank pancreatitis and is therefore not widely recommended.

   Passage of the **choledochoscope** into the duodenum is similarly a potentially hazardous practice and should be used only when necessary to gently push debris into the duodenum, or when the orifice into the duodenum is widely patent, such as after preoperative sphincterotomy or intraoperative intravenous glucagon administration.

   b. **Recognition and management.** Pancreatitis may present postoperatively with excessive abdominal or back pain, fever, ileus, anorexia, or failure to thrive. The diagnosis may be confirmed with amylase measurement. CT scanning of the abdomen may be necessary if the patient does not improve with intravenous fluids, fasting status, and nasogastric suction. Antibiotics and/or surgical intervention may be required if pancreatic abscess is suspected or confirmed with CT scanning.

C. Complications of Laparoscopic Choledochotomy

It is conceptually useful to divide complications of laparoscopic choledochotomy into early and late complications. Many of the complications listed in Section A may also occur after laparoscopic choledochotomy.

1. **Early complications** are recognized in the first few days after laparoscopic common bile duct exploration. These include the following.
   a. **Biloma/bile leakage** through the subhepatic drain. Bile leakage is commoner after **T**-tube insertion than after transcystic drainage with primary closure. The leakage is usually from the choledochotomy site, but may be from the gallbladder bed.
      i. Excessive bile leakage indicates probable dislodgment of the **T**-tube or transcystic cannula.
      ii. The initial investigations may include ultrasound examination and radionuclide scanning of the biliary tree. The **T**-tube or transcystic duct cannula provide a convenient route for cholangiography, if needed.
      iii. Established biliary peritonitis or dislodgment of the **T**-tube are indications for reintervention laparoscopy/laparotomy.

    iv. Otherwise, percutaneous drainage under radiologic control should suffice (if adequate drainage has not been provided by the closed suction drain placed during surgery).
  b. **Missed stone**
    i. By definition, a missed stone is one that is discovered on the postoperative cholangiogram and up to 2 years after the duct exploration.
    ii. When discovered postoperatively, any missed stones should be removed either by endoscopic stone extraction or via the mature **T**-tube tract (4–6 weeks later).
    iii. Pressure-controlled flushing with heparinized saline and antispasmodic medication (glucagon, ceruletide) may be effective in some cases.
  c. **Cholangitis**
    i. Transient cholangitis is common in patients undergoing laparoscopic duct exploration after failed endoscopic sphincterotomy.
    ii. Postoperative cholangitis often indicates missed stone or other pathology.
    iii. If adequate drainage of the biliary tract is confirmed by an urgent **T**-tube/transcystic cholangiogram, the management is by antibiotic therapy. Otherwise endoscopic sphincterotomy or stenting is performed as a matter of urgency.
2. **Late complications**
  a. **Abscess formation around a spilled stone** is especially likely to occur with brown pigment stones (which usually harbor bacteria in the amorphous pits). Open drainage with removal of the stone is required.
  b. **Recurrent calculi** present beyond 2 years after surgery and are managed as new cases either laparoscopically or by endoscopic stone extraction.
  c. **Stricture** of the common duct may present several years later.

D. Selected References

Lee VS, Chari RS, Cucchiaro G, Meyers WC. Complications of laparoscopic cholecystectomy. Am J Surg 1993;165(4):527–532.

Lillemoe KD, Martin SA, Cameron JL, et al. Major bile duct injuries during laparoscopic cholecystectomy: follow-up after combined surgical and radiologic management. Ann Surg 1997;225(5):459–468.

Ponsky JL. The incidence and management of complications of laparoscopic cholecystectomy. Adv Surg 1994;27:21–41.

Sicklick JK, Camp MS, Lillemoe KD, et al. Surgical management of bile duct injuries sustained during laparoscopic cholecystectomy: perioperative results in 200 patients. Ann Surg 2005;241(5):786–792.

Talamini MA. Controversies in laparoscopic cholecystectomy: contraindications, cholangiography, pregnancy and avoidance of complications. Baillieres Clin Gastroenterol 1993;7(4):881–896.

Talamini MA. Laparoscopic cholecystectomy. In: Cameron JL, ed. Current Surgical Therapy. St. Louis: CV Mosby, 1995.

Wherry DC, Rob CG, Marohn MR, et al. An external audit of laparoscopic cholecystectomy performed in medical treatment facilities of the Department of Defense. Ann Surg 1994;220:626–634.

Laparoscopy
IV—Hiatal Hernia and Heller Myotomy

21. Laparoscopic Treatment of Gastroesophageal Reflux Disease and Hiatal Hernia

Jeffrey H. Peters, M.D., F.A.C.S.

A. Indications and Preoperative Evaluation

1. **Laparoscopic fundoplication** is indicated for the treatment of objectively documented, relatively severe gastroesophageal reflux disease (GERD). Care in patient selection and preoperative evaluation are essential for good results. Patients with gastroesophageal reflux and any of the following may be considered candidates for the procedure:
   a. Esophageal complications such as erosive esophagitis, stricture, and/or Barrett's esophagus
   b. Respiratory complications such as recurrent pneumonia or bronchiectasis
   c. Dependence upon proton pump inhibitors (PPIs) for relief of symptoms, particularly if dose escalation is required, and in the young
   d. Laryngeal and/or respiratory symptoms with a good response to PPI therapy

2. **The therapeutic approach** to patients presenting for the first time with symptoms suggestive of gastroesophageal reflux includes an initial trial of PPI therapy. Many patients will already have sought relief with readily available over-the-counter agents.
   a. **Failure of proton pump inhibitors** to control the symptoms, suggests either that the diagnosis is incorrect or that the patient has severe disease.
   b. **Endoscopic examination** at this stage of evaluation provides the opportunity for assessing the severity of mucosal damage and the presence of Barrett's esophagus (see Part II, Chapters on indications for upper gastrointestinal endoscopy). Either finding on initial endoscopy predicts a high risk for medical failure.

3. **Appropriate diagnostic evaluation** should then be undertaken. **The diagnostic approach** to patients suspected of having gastroesophageal reflux disease and being considered for antireflux surgery has three important goals (Table 21.1).

Symptoms thought to be indicative of gastroesophageal reflux disease, such as heartburn or acid regurgitation, are very common in the general population and cannot be used alone to guide therapeutic decisions, particularly when one is considering antireflux surgery. These symptoms, even when excessive, are not

Table 21.1. Goals of diagnostic evaluation for possible antireflux surgery.

- To determine that gastroesophageal reflux is the underlying cause of the patients symptoms
- To evaluate the status of esophageal body, and occasionally gastric function
- To determine the presence or absence of esophageal shortening

specific for gastroesophageal reflux and are often caused by other diseases (such as achalasia, diffuse spasm, esophageal carcinoma, pyloric stenosis, cholelithiasis, gastritis, gastric or duodenal ulcer, and coronary artery disease).

A common error is to define the presence of gastroesophageal reflux disease by the endoscopic finding of esophagitis. Limiting the diagnosis to patients with endoscopic esophagitis ignores a large population of patients without mucosal injury who may have severe symptoms of gastroesophageal reflux and could be considered for antireflux surgery. The most precise approach to define gastroesophageal reflux disease is to measure the basic pathophysiologic abnormality of the disease, that is, increased exposure of the esophagus to gastric juice. The workup consists of the following stages.

a. **24-hour pH monitoring**, to assess the degree and pattern of esophageal exposure to gastric juice. A positive 24-hour pH study is the single most important predictor of a successful outcome.

b. **Manometric examination** of the lower esophageal sphincter and motor function of the body of the esophagus. This provides insight into the reasons for reflux (i.e., sphincter incompetence) as well as the function of the esophageal body.

c. **Assessment of esophageal length to exclude esophageal shortening.** Repetitive injury causes scarring and fibrosis, and ultimately results in anatomic shortening of the esophagus. This compromises the ability to do an adequate repair without tension and leads to an increased incidence of breakdown or thoracic displacement of the repair.

    i. Esophageal length is best assessed using video roentgenographic contrast studies and endoscopic findings.

    ii. Endoscopically, hernia size is measured as the difference between the diaphragmatic crura, identified by having the patient sniff, and the gastroesophageal junction, identified as the loss of gastric rugal folds. Suspect a short esophagus if there is a large (>5 cm) hiatal hernia, particularly if it fails to reduce in the upright position on a video barium esophagram.

    iii. **Selection of a partial versus complete fundoplication**, and an open or laparoscopic approach is based upon on an assessment of esophageal contractility and length. Laparoscopic fundoplication is used in the majority of patients unless a very large (>5–6 cm) hiatal hernia or intrathoracic stomach is present, in which case it may be preferable to use an open approach. Recent data would suggest that in the absence of a named motility disorder such as achalasia or scleroderma, most patients with reflux disease will tolerate a properly constructed 360-degree Nissen fundoplication without an increased incidence of dysphagia. In addition, the failure rate of partial fundoplications has been reported to be as high as 50% after 2 to 3 years.

B. Patient Position and Room Setup

1. Position the patient supine, in a modified lithotomy position. It is important that the knees be only slightly flexed, to avoid limiting mobility of the surgeon and the instruments (Fig. 21.1).

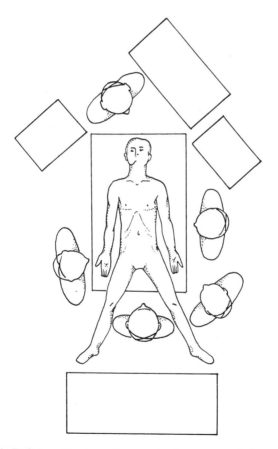

Figure 21.1. Patient positioning and room setup for laparoscopic fundoplication. The patient is placed with the head elevated 45 degrees in the modified lithotomy position. The surgeon stands between the patient's legs. One assistant, on the surgeon's right, retracts the stomach; a second assistant, on the surgeon's left, manipulates the camera.

2. The surgeon stands between the legs and works with both hands. This allows the right- and left-handed instruments to approach the hiatus from the respective upper abdominal quadrants.

3. Use 30% to 45% of reverse Trendelenburg to displace the transverse colon and small bowel inferiorly, keeping them from obstructing the view of the video camera.

C. Trocar Position and Principles of Exposure

1. Five 10-mm ports are utilized (Fig. 21.2); 5-mm ports may be substituted in the subxiphoid and right subcostal access sites.

2. **Place the camera** above the umbilicus, one third of the distance to the xiphoid process. In most patients, if the camera is placed in the umbilicus, it will be too low to allow adequate visualization of the hiatal strictures once dissected. A transrectus location is preferable to midline to minimize the prevalence of port site hernia formation.

3. **Place two lateral retracting ports** in the right and left anterior axillary lines, respectively. Position the trocar for the liver retractor in the right midabdomen (midclavicular line), at or slightly below the camera port. This allows the proper angle toward the left lateral segment of the liver and thus the ability to push the instrument toward the operating table, lifting the liver. Place the second retraction port at the level of the umbilicus, in the left anterior axillary line. Placement of these ports too far lateral or too low on the abdomen will compromise the excursion of the instruments and thus the ability to retract.

4. **The left-sided operating port (surgeon's right hand) is placed** 1 to 2 in. below the costal margin approximately at the lateral rectus border. This allows triangulation between the camera and the two instruments, and avoids the difficulty associated with the instruments being in direct line with the camera. The right-sided operating port (surgeon's left hand) is placed last, after the right lateral segment of the liver has been retracted. This prevents "swordfighting" between the liver retractor and the left-handed instrument. The falciform ligament hangs low in many patients and provides a barrier around which the left-handed instrument must be manipulated.

5. **Initial retraction** is accomplished with exposure of the esophageal hiatus. A fan retractor is placed into the right anterior axillary port and positioned to hold the left lateral segment of the liver toward the anterior abdominal wall. We prefer to utilize a table retractor to hold this instrument once properly positioned. Trauma to the liver should be meticulously avoided because subsequent bleeding will obscure the field. Mobilization of the left lateral segment by division of the triangular ligament is not necessary. Place a Babcock clamp into the left anterior axillary port and retract the stomach toward the patient's left

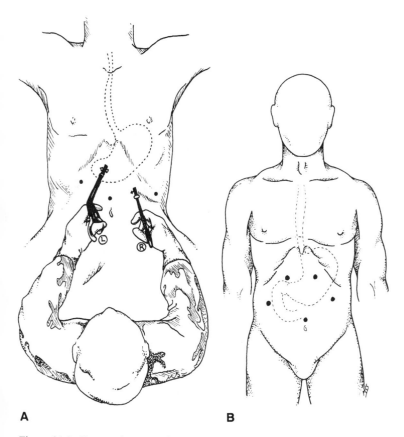

A   **B**

Figure 21.2. Trocar placement for laparoscopic antireflux surgery. Five 10-mm trocars are generally used, but the two lateral retraction ports, and occasionally others can be downsized to 5 mm with appropriate instrumentation.

foot. This maneuver exposes the esophageal hiatus (Fig. 21.3). Commonly a hiatal hernia will need to be reduced. Use an atraumatic clamp, and take care not to grasp the stomach too vigorously, as gastric perforations can occur.

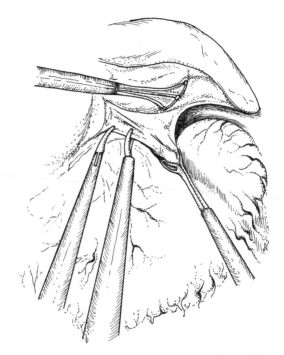

Figure 21.3. Laparoscopic exposure of the esophageal hiatus. A fan-type retractor (placed through the right subcostal port) elevates the left lateral hepatic segment anterolaterally. A Babcock clamp (placed through the left lateral port) retracts the stomach caudad. This places the phrenoesophageal membrane on traction.

D. Technique of Nissen Fundoplication

The critical elements of laparoscopic Nissen fundoplication are enumerated in Table 21.2 and will be discussed in detail.

1. **Crural dissection** begins with identification of the right crus. Metzenbaum-type scissors and fine grasping forceps are preferred for dissection. In all except the most obese patients, there is a very thin portion of the gastrohepatic omentum overlying the caudate lobe of the liver (Fig. 21.4).

    a. Begin the dissection by incising this portion of the gastrohepatic omentum above and below the hepatic branch of the anterior vagal nerve (which the author routinely spares).

    b. A large left hepatic artery arising from the left gastric artery will be present in up to 25% of patients. It should be identified and

Table 21.2. Elements of laparoscopic Nissen fundoplication.

1. Crural dissection, identification and preservation of both vagi including the hepatic branch of the anterior vagus
2. Circumferential dissection and mobilization of the esophagus
3. Crural closure
4. Fundic mobilization by division of short gastric vessels
5. Creation of a short, loose fundoplication by enveloping the anterior and posterior wall of the fundus around the lower esophagus

avoided. A right crural branch will occasionally be seen which can be divided.

c. After the gastrohepatic omentum has been incised, the outside of the right crus will become evident. Incise the peritoneum overlying the anterior aspect of the right crus with scissors and electrocautery, and dissect the right crus from anterior to posterior as far as possible.

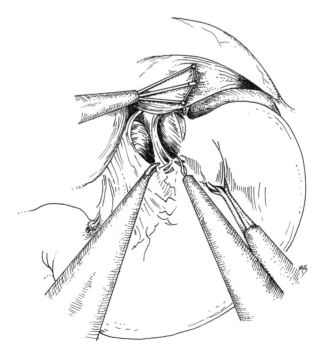

Figure 21.4. Initial dissection of the esophageal hiatus. The right crus is identified and dissected toward its posterior confluence with the left crus.

d. The medial portion of the right crus leads into the mediastinum and is entered by blunt dissection with both instruments.

e. At this juncture the esophagus usually becomes evident. Retract the right crus laterally and perform a modest dissection of the tissues posterior to the esophagus. Do not attempt to dissect behind the gastroesophageal junction at this time.

f. Meticulous hemostasis is critical. Blood and fluids tend to pool in the hiatus and are difficult to remove. Irrigation should be avoided. Take care not to injure the phrenic artery and vein as they course above the hiatus. A large hiatal hernia often makes this portion of the procedure easier because it accentuates the diaphragmatic crura. On the other hand, dissection of a large mediastinal hernia sac can be difficult.

g. Following dissection of the right crus, attention is turned toward the anterior crural confluence. Use the left-handed grasper to hold up the tissues anterior to the esophagus, and sweep the esophagus downward and to the right, separating it from the left crus.

h. Divide the anterior crural tissues and identify the left crus. The anterior vagus nerve often "hugs" the left crus and can be injured in this portion of the dissection if not carefully searched for and protected (Fig. 21.5).

i. Dissect the left crus as completely as possible, including taking down the angle of His and the attachments of the fundus to the left diaphragm (Fig. 21.6). A complete dissection of the lateral and inferior aspect of the left crus and fundus of the stomach is

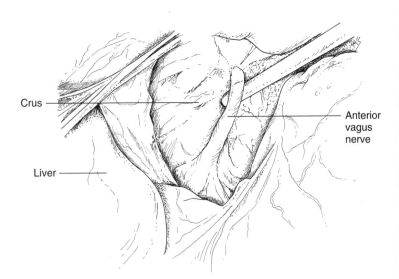

Figure 21.5. Anterior dissection of the esophageal hiatus. The anterior (left) vagus nerve often "hugs" the inside of the left crus and can be injured if not dissected off before crural dissection.

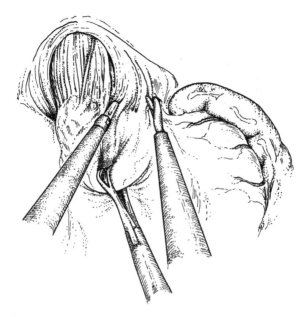

Figure 21.6. Dissection of the left crus. The left crus is dissected as completely as possible, and the attachments of the fundus of the stomach to the diaphragm are taken down.

the key maneuver allowing circumferential mobilization of the esophagus. Failure to make a complete dissection will result in difficulty in encircling the esophagus, particularly if approached from the right. Repositioning of the Babcock retractor toward the fundic side of the stomach facilitates retraction for this portion of the procedure. The posterior vagus nerve may be encountered in the low left crural dissection. It should be looked for and protected.

2. **Circumferential dissection of the esophagus** is achieved by careful dissection of the anterior and posterior soft tissues within the hiatus. If the crura have been completely dissected, then dissection posterior to the esophagus to create a window will not be difficult.

   a. From the patient's right side, use the left-handed instrument to retract the esophagus anteriorly. This allows the right hand to perform the dissection behind the esophagus. Reverse this maneuver for the left-sided dissection.

   b. Leave the posterior vagus nerve on the esophagus.

   c. Identify the left crus and keep the dissection caudad to it. There is a tendency to dissect into the mediastinum and left pleura.

   d. In the presence of severe esophagitis, transmural inflammation, esophageal shortening, and/or a large posterior fat pad, this dissection may be particularly difficult. If unduly difficult, abandon this route of dissection and approach the hiatus from the left side by dividing the short gastric vessels (see later) at this point in the procedure rather than later.

e. After completing the posterior dissection, pass a grasper (via the surgeon's left-handed port) behind the esophagus and over the left crus. Pass a Penrose drain around the esophagus and use this as an esophageal retractor for the remainder of the procedure.

3. **Fundic mobilization.** Complete fundic mobilization allows construction of a tension-free fundoplication.

a. Suspend the gastrosplenic omentum anteroposteriorly, in a clothesline fashion via two Babcock forceps, and enter the lesser sac approximately one third the distance down the greater curvature of the stomach (Fig. 21.7). Sequentially dissect and divide the short gastric vessels with the aid of ultrasonic shears (Ethicon Endo-Surgery, Cincinnati, OH). An anterior–posterior rather than medial-to-lateral orientation of the vessels is preferred, with the exception of those close to the spleen. The dissection includes pancreaticogastric branches posterior to the upper stomach and continues until the right crus and caudate lobe can be seen from the left side (Fig. 21.8). With caution and meticulous dissection, the fundus can be completely mobilized in virtually all patients. Although generally possible via the right- and left-handed

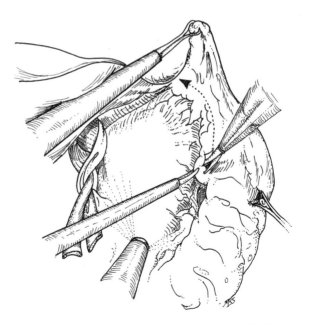

Figure 21.7. Proper retraction of the gastrosplenic omentum facilitates the initial steps of short gastric division.

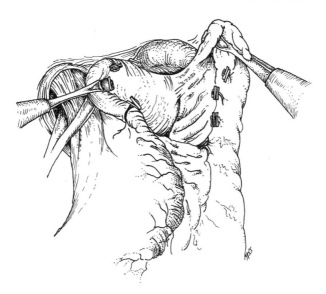

Figure 21.8. Retract the stomach rightward and the spleen and omentum left and downward to complete mobilization of the fundus. These maneuvers open the lesser sac and facilitate division of the high short gastric vessels.

surgeon's access ports, occasionally this dissection will require removal of the liver retractor and placement of a second Babcock forceps through the right anterior axillary port to facilitate retraction during division of the short gastric vessels.

4. **Esophageal mobilization.** The esophagus is mobilized into the posterior mediastinum for several centimeters to provide maximal intraabdominal esophageal length. Posterior and right lateral mobilization is readily accomplished. Take care during the anterior and left lateral mobilization not to injure the anterior vagus nerve. Gentle traction on the penrose drain around the gastroesophageal junction facilitates exposure. The right and left pleural reflections often come into view and should be avoided.

5. **Crural closure.** Continue the crural dissection to enlarge the space behind the gastroesophageal junction as much as possible.

   a. Holding the esophagus anterior and to the left, approximate the crura with two to four interrupted figure-of-eight 0-gauge Ethibond sutures, starting just above the aortic decussation and working anterior (Fig. 21.9).

   b. The author prefers a large needle (CT1) passed down the left upper 10-mm port to facilitate a durable crural closure.

   c. Because space is limited, it is often necessary to use the surgeon's left-handed (nondominant) instrument as a retractor, facilitating placement of single bites through each crus with the surgeon's

218   J.H. Peters

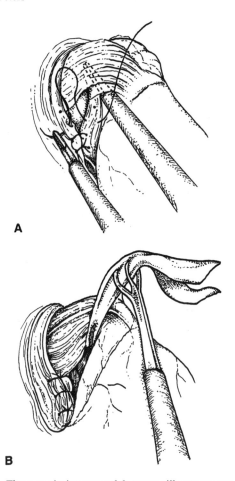

Figure 21.9. A. Three to six interrupted 0-gauge silk sutures are used to close the crura. B. Exposure of the crura and posterior aspect of the esophagus is facilitated by traction on a Penrose drain encircling the gastroesophageal junction.

right hand. The aorta might be punctured while suturing the left crus. Identification of its anterior surface and often retracting the left crus away from the aorta via the left handed grasper will help avoid inadvertent aortic puncture (Fig. 21.10).

d. The author prefers extracorporeal knot tying using a standard knot pusher or a "tie knot" device, although tying within the abdomen is perfectly appropriate.

6. **Create a short, loose fundoplication** with particular attention to the geometry of the wrap.

a. Grasp the posterior fundus and pass it left to right rather than pulling right to left. This assures that the posterior fundus is used for the posterior aspect of the fundoplication. This is accomplished by placing a Babcock clamp through the left lower port, and grasping the midportion of the posterior fundus (Fig. 21.11). Gently bring the posterior fundus behind the esophagus to the right side with an upward, rightward, and clockwise twisting motion. This maneuver can be difficult particularly for the novice. If so, placement of a 0 silk suture in the midposterior fundus and grasping it from the right side facilitates brining the posterior fundus around to create the fundoplication.

b. Bring the anterior wall of the fundus anterior to the esophagus above the supporting Penrose drain.

c. Manipulate both the posterior and anterior fundic lips to allow the fundus to envelope the esophagus without twisting (Fig. 21.12). Laparoscopic visualization has a tendency to exaggerate the size of the posterior opening that has been dissected. Consequently, the space for the passage of the fundus behind the esophagus may be tighter than thought and the fundus relatively ischemic when brought around. If the right lip of the fundoplication has a bluish discoloration, the stomach should be returned to its original position and the posterior dissection enlarged.

d. Pass a 60-French bougie to properly size the fundoplication, and suture it utilizing a single U-stitch of 2–0 Prolene buttressed

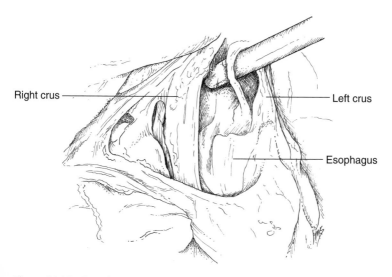

Figure 21.10. Crural closure. The left crus sits in close approximation to the aorta, which is at risk of being punctured during crural closure. Retraction of the left crus away from the aorta during suture placement will prevent injury.

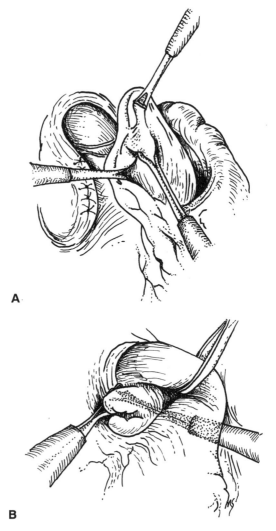

Figure 21.11. A. Placement of Babcock clamp on the posterior fundus in preparation for passing it behind the esophagus to create the posterior or right lip of
the fundoplication. To achieve the proper angle for passage, place the Babcock
through the left lower trocar. B. Pass the posterior fundus from left to right and
grasp it from the right with a Babcock clamp (passed through the right upper
trocar).

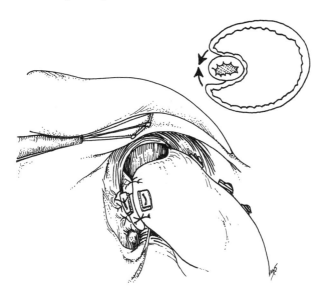

Figure 21.12. The fundoplication is sutured in place with a single **U**-stitch of 2–0 Prolene pledgeted on the outside. A 60-French mercury-weighted bougie is passed through the gastroesophageal junction prior to fixation of the wrap to assure a floppy fundoplication. Inset illustrates the proper orientation of the fundic wrap.

with felt pledgets. The most common error is an attempt to grasp the anterior portion of the stomach to construct the right lip of the fundoplication rather than the posterior fundus. The esophagus should comfortably lie in the untwisted fundus prior to suturing.

e. Place two anchoring sutures of 2–0 silk above and below the U-stitch to complete the fundoplication. When finished, the suture line of the fundoplication should be facing in a right anterior direction.

f. Irrigate the abdomen, assure hemostasis, and remove the bougie and Penrose drain.

E. Laparoscopic Partial Fundoplication

Although the orientation of partial fundoplication may be either anterior, posterior, or lateral, the most commonly performed laparoscopic partial fundoplication is the modified Toupet procedure, a 270-degree posterior hemifundoplication.

1. **Patient positioning**, trocar placement, hiatal dissection, crural closure, and fundic mobilization are performed exactly as for laparoscopic Nissen fundoplication.

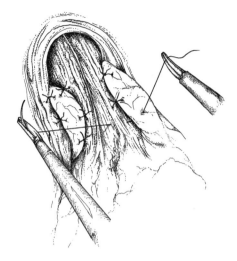

Figure 21.13. Completed 270-degree posterior hemifundoplication (Toupet fundoplication).

2. **Fixation of the fundoplication** is the only portion of the procedure that differs from that of Nissen fundoplication. The posterior lip of the fundoplication is created as described for Nissen fundoplication.
3. With adequate fundic mobilization the posterior fundus should lie comfortably on the right side of the esophagus prior to suturing it in place.
4. Place a Babcock clamp on the superior aspect of the right lip and suture the posterior fundus to the crural closure with three interrupted sutures of 2–0 silk.
5. Rather than bringing the lips together (as in a Nissen fundoplication), suture the right limb of the fundoplication to the esophageal musculature at the 11 o'clock position and the left at the 1 o'clock position on the esophagus (Fig. 21.13). Three interrupted sutures of 2–0 silk are placed along the lower esophagus just above the gastroesophageal fat pad to fix each limb. (see also Chapter 23, in which Toupet and Dor fundoplications are discussed in the context of laparoscopic cardiomyotomy).

F. Postoperative Considerations

Recovery is more rapid than usual after the corresponding open procedure, and several aspects of postoperative management are correspondingly different.

1. **A nasogastric tube** is not necessary.
2. **Pain** is managed with parenteral narcotics or ketorolac for the first 24 hours and oral hydrocodone thereafter as necessary.

3. **A Foley** catheter is placed following induction of anesthesia and left in place until the morning after surgery. The incidence of urinary retention is approximately 10% to 25% if bladder decompression is not used.

4. **A diet** of clear liquids ad libitum is allowed the morning following surgery. Soft solids are begun on the second postoperative day and continued for 2 weeks. The patient should be instructed to eat slowly, chew carefully, and avoid bread and meats for a minimum of 2 weeks.

G. Complications

The safety of laparoscopic fundoplication has now been established. **Mortality** is rare following an elective antireflux procedure, whether open or closed. The complication rate is similar to that of open fundoplication, averaging 10% to 15%, but the spectrum of the morbidity has changed. Complications associated with surgical access and postoperative recovery have improved. With the exception of a reduction in the number of splenic injuries and splenectomies performed during laparoscopic fundoplication, intraoperative complications such as gastric or esophageal perforation are slightly higher. Initial concern of the possibility of an increased incidence of pulmonary embolism has not proven true. Cumulative results suggest an incidence of pulmonary embolism of 0.49%, similar to that of open fundoplication.

Several excellent series of laparoscopic fundoplication have been published. Three of the best come from Atlanta, Omaha, and Adelaide. These reports document the ability of laparoscopic fundoplication to relieve typical symptoms of gastroesophageal reflux, that is, heartburn, regurgitation, and dysphagia, in over 90% of patients. Atypical respiratory and laryngeal symptoms are relieved less reliably improving on average in 65% to 80% of patients.

Long-term outcome studies (5 years and beyond) have also been published. These studies show a small but definite incidence of recurrent reflux, with 80 to 85% of patients free of reflux symptoms at 5 years. Patients with long-segment Barrett's esophagus and those with hiatal hernias larger than 5 cm may be at higher risk of recurrence, although even in this population most will enjoy long-lasting reflux control.

A few complications are particularly noteworthy and are described briefly here.

1. **Pneumothorax and surgical emphysema** have occurred in 1% to 2% of patients. This is most likely related to excessive hiatal dissection and should decrease with increasing experience of the surgical team.

2. **Unrecognized perforations of esophagus or stomach** are the most life-threatening problems. Perforations of the esophagus and stomach occur during hiatal dissection and are related to operative experience. Intraoperative recognition and repair is the key to preventing life-threatening problems.

3. Although uncommon, **acute paraesophageal herniation** has been noted by a number of authors and usually results in early reoperation.

H. Selected References

Bammer T, Hinder RA, Klaus A, Klinger PJ. Five to eight year outcome of the first laparoscopic fundoplications. J Gastrointest Surg 2001;5:42–48.

Campos GMR, Peters JH, DeMeester TR, et al. Multivariate analysis of the factors predicting outcome after laparoscopic Nissen fundoplication. J Gastrointest Surg 1999;3:292–300.

Carlson MA, Frantzides CT. Complications and results of primary minimally invasive antireflux procedures; a review of 10,735 reported cases. J Am Coll Surg 2001; 193:428–439.

DeMeester TR, Bonavina L, Albertucci M. Nissen fundoplication for gastroesophageal reflux disease—evaluation of primary repair in 100 consecutive patients. Ann Surg 1986;204:9.

Hinder RA, Filipi CJ, Wetscher G, Neary P, DeMeester TR, Perdikis G. Laparoscopic Nissen fundoplication is an effective treatment for gastroesophageal reflux disease. Ann Surg 1994;220(4):472–483.

Horgan S, Pohl D, Bogetti D, Eubanks T, Pellegrini C. Failed antireflux surgery; what have we learned from reoperations? Arch Surg 1999;134:809–817.

Horvath KD, Swanstrom LL, Jobe BA. The short esophagus; pathophysiology, presentation and treatment in the era of laparoscopic antireflux surgery. Ann Surg 2000;282:630–640.

Hunter JG, Trus TL, Branum GD, Waring JP, Wood WC. A physiologic approach to laparoscopic fundoplication for gastroesophageal reflux disease. Ann Surg 1996;223: 673–687.

Jamieson GG, Watson DI, Britten-Jones R, Mitchell PC, Anvari M. Laparoscopic Nissen fundoplication. Ann Surg 1994;220:137–145.

Peters JH, Heimbucher J, Kauer WKH, Incarbone R, Bremner CG, DeMeester TR. Clinical and physiologic comparison of laparoscopic and open Nissen. J Am Coll Surg 1995;180:385–393.

Reardon PR, Matthews BD, Scarborough TK, Preciado A, Marti JL, Kamelgard JI. Geometry and reproducibility in 360° fundoplication. Surg Endosc 2000;14:750–754.

Schauer PR, Meyers WC, Eubanks S, Norem RF, Franklin M, Pappas TN. Mechanisms of gastric and esophageal perforations during laparoscopic fundoplication. Ann Surg 1996;223:43–52.

Waring JP, Hunter JG, Oddsdottir M, Wo J, Katz E. The preoperative evaluation of patients considered for laparoscopic antireflux surgery. Am J Gastroenterol 1995;90:35–38.

Watson D, Balgrie RJ, Jamieson GG. A learning curve for laparoscopic fundoplication; definable, avoidable or a waste of time? Ann Surg 1996;224:198–203.

Watson DI, de Beaux AC. Complications of laparoscopic antireflux surgery. Surg Endosc 2001;15:344–352.

22. Laparoscopic Paraesophageal Hernia Repair

Ketan M. Desai, M.D.
Nathaniel J. Soper, M.D.

A. Introduction

Laparoscopy is accepted as the standard operative approach for the surgical treatment of gastroesophageal reflux disease (GERD), and it is widely used for the repair of paraesophageal hernia (PEH). Although technically challenging, this approach provides excellent exposure of the surgical field and adds the known general advantages of laparoscopy in terms of reduced morbidity, more rapid recovery, short hospital stay, and decreased pain medication requirements compared with laparotomy or thoracotomy. These advantages are especially valuable in this patient population, since most PEH patients are elderly and have multiple comorbidities.

The technical difficulty of laparoscopic repair of PEH is greater than that for laparoscopic antireflux surgery (LARS). The inherent difficulties of this operation include a compromised gastric wall (which has been incarcerated chronically in a mediastinal hernia sac), the necessity of excising the hernia sac without damaging critical structures, the difficulty of gaining exposure in a closed abdomen where there is a great laxity of the tissues, and the problem of closing the enlarged hiatus adequately. It is unwise for a laparoscopic surgeon to attempt repair of a PEH before performing 20 to 50 laparoscopic antireflux operations, the typical "learning curve" for LARS.

A classification system for hiatal hernias is given in Table 22.1.

B. Indications for Surgery

Paraesophageal hernias account for only 5% of all hiatal hernias. In both types of PEH (II and III), the herniated stomach lies besides the thoracic esophagus. When left untreated, PEH may lead to life-threatening complications, which include hemorrhage, strangulation, and volvulus (Table 22.2). If the blood supply is compromised, necrosis and perforation may occur, with mortality rate at his stage of disease approaching 50%. Traditionally, most surgeons believed that all paraesophageal hernias should be corrected electively on diagnosis, irrespective of symptoms, to prevent the development of complications and to avoid the risk of emergency surgery. However, recent evidence suggests that

Table 22.1. Types of hiatal hernia.

I.   Sliding hiatal hernia; migration of the gastroesophageal junction (GEJ) into the thorax
II. Isolated paraesophageal hernia with the GEJ in its normal anatomic location below the diaphragm; however, the proximal stomach protrudes through the hiatus, "rolling" alongside the distal esophagus
III. Upward displacement of the GEJ above the diaphragm, with the stomach protruding cephalad adjacent to the esophagus
IV. Herniation of other viscera through the esophageal hiatus, usually in association with types I to III

Table 22.2. Complications of paraesophageal hernia.

---

1. Bleeding from associated esophagitis, erosions (Cameron ulcers), or a discrete esophageal ulcer resulting in anemia.
2. Gastric volvulus with strangulation is a surgical emergency if the stomach cannot be decompressed. The stomach becomes angulated in its midportion just proximal to the antrum (Fig. 22.1). (**Borchardt's triad:** chest pain, retching but no vomiting, and inability to pass a nasogastric tube.)
3. Incarceration of a paraesophageal hernia. Patients present with abrupt onset of vomiting and pain; may require immediate operative intervention.
4. Torsion, obstruction, gangrene, perforation.

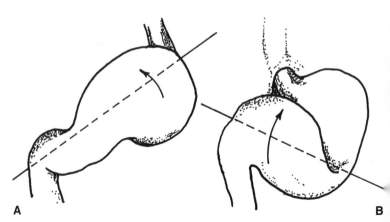

A   **B**

Figure 22.1. A. Organoaxial rotation. B. Mesentericoaxial rotation.

nonoperative management of asymptomatic patients is a reasonable alternative. Surgical repair of PEH is generally recommended for symptomatic patients. However, the operative strategy remains a matter of debate, and there is not a single technique guaranteeing uniform long-term success.

There are several controversies regarding laparoscopic repair of paraesophageal hiatal hernias. These include the necessity of excising the hernia sac, the best technique for closing the diaphragm, the requirement of an antireflux procedure, and the need to perform a gastropexy. The reported recurrence rate for laparoscopic PEH repair has varied widely. If patients are followed closely, the reported recurrence rates range from 10% to 42%, especially when routine postoperative x-ray contrast studies are performed.

C. Preoperative Evaluation

1. **Clinical presentation.**
   Most patients are symptomatic, but there is no clear correlation between the size of the hiatal hernia and severity of the symptoms.
   a. **Symptoms**
      i. Asymptomatic in a minority of patients
      ii. Vague epigastric or substernal discomfort
      iii. Postprandial fullness, nausea, dysphagia
      iv. Pulmonary complications are common: recurrent pneumonia; chronic atelectasis; dyspnea (pleural space compression by the huge hernia sac)
      v. GERD symptoms (heartburn, regurgitation)
   b. **Diagnostic Evaluation**
      i. **Chest radiograph** often demonstrates a retrocardiac air–fluid level.
      ii. **Barium upper-gastrointestinal series** establishes the diagnosis with greater accuracy and helps distinguish a sliding from a paraesophageal hernia.
      iii. **Upper endoscopy** is used to diagnose complications such as erosive esophagitis, ulcers, Barrett esophagus, and/or tumor. A hiatal hernia is confirmed by endoscopy on retroflexed views once inside the stomach.
      iv. **Esophageal manometry** for evaluation of esophageal motility disorders: Measurement of esophageal body peristalsis and lower esophageal sphincter position/length/pressure.
      v. **Optional: 24-hour pH test** to document GERD.
   c. **Medical therapy.** Management of PEH includes the reduction of gastroesophageal reflux, improving esophageal clearance, and reducing acid production. This is achieved in the majority of patients by modifying lifestyle factors, use of acid-reduction medication, and enhancing esophageal and gastric motility.

    d. **Surgical therapy**
        i. A PEH in a symptomatic patient of suitable anesthetic risk is an indication for repair.
       ii. Complications of GERD (strictures, ulcers, and bleeding) despite medical treatment (proton pump inhibitors) may also prompt repair. In addition, young patients with PEH and severe or recurrent complications of GERD may prefer to avoid long-term medication use.
      iii. Patients with PEH and pulmonary complications (asthma, recurrent aspiration pneumonia, chronic cough, or hoarseness) are also potential surgical candidates.

D. Patient Position and Room Setup

1. Prepare and position the patient as for laparoscopic antireflux surgery (see Chapter 21). The operating room personnel and equipment are arranged with the surgeon between the patient's legs, the assistant surgeon on the patient's right, and the camera holder to the left.
2. Place video monitors at either side of the head of the table. These should be viewed easily by all members of the operating team.
3. Irrigation, suction, and electrocautery connections come off the head of the table on the patient's right side. Special instruments include endoscopic Babcock graspers, cautery scissors, curved dissectors, clip applier, atraumatic liver retractor, 5-mm needle holders, and ultrasonic coagulating shears.
4. Port arrangement should allow easy access to the hiatus and permit comfortable suturing by placing the optics between the surgeon's hands. Access to the abdominal cavity is achieved by either a closed or open technique superior to the umbilicus. The initial laparoscopic camera port should be placed higher on the abdominal wall than for Nissen fundoplications, because the dissection often needs to be performed well up into the mediastinum, and a low port placement renders adequate visualization difficult.
5. The initial port is placed 12 to 15 cm below the xiphoid. Four additional ports are placed under direct vision of the laparoscope. Ports are typically placed in the following locations to optimize visualization, tissue manipulation, and facilitate suturing (Fig. 22.2). A port is placed 3 to 4 cm inferior and to the right of the xiphoid process. Subcostal ports are placed in the midclavicular line on the right and left sides. The fifth port is placed in the far right lateral subcostal position.
6. With current 5-mm equipment and optics, we generally use only one 10- to 12-mm port, for the surgeon's right hand, to allow insertion of an SH needle through the valve mechanism.

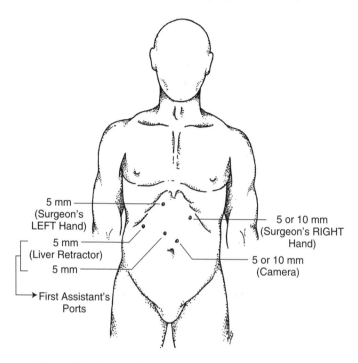

Figure 22.2. Trocar placement for laparoscopic PEH repair.

E. Hernia Reduction

1. The surgeon and assistant first reduce as much of the intrathoracic con-
    tents of the hiatal hernia sac as much as possible, using atraumatic
    graspers and careful hand-over-hand technique.
2. Divide the gastrohepatic ligament, beginning just superior to the
    hepatic branch of the vagus nerve; this dissection is carried orad up to
    the medial border of the right crus of the diaphragm (Fig. 22.3).
3. To gain the appropriate plane for dissecting the hernia sac out of the
    mediastinum, aggressively divide the tissues that form the border
    between the sac and crural margin. Use the ultrasonic shears to target
    the medial border of the right crus of the diaphragm, and divide
    the endoabdominal and endothoracic fascia layers to create a plane
    between the right crus and the hernia sac in the supradiaphragmatic
    mediastinum.

4. Spreading motions of the surgeon's instruments then open this plane further and allow the insufflated carbon dioxide to dissect some of the tissues away. Blunt dissection is continued up into the mediastinum while the sac is swept back toward the abdominal cavity. This combination of sharp and blunt dissection is continued until the entire anterior circumference of the crural arch has been freed from the hernia sac (Fig. 22.4). Long blunt motions are used to sweep the sac inferiorly, exposing the right lateral border of the esophagus and posterior vagus nerve, as well as the anterior and left side of the esophagus and anterior vagus nerve. In a patient with no previous operations, the tissues usually separate readily.

5. There are usually adhesions of variable density between the sac and the pleura and other mediastinal structures that must be divided with the harmonic shears. Small blood vessels connect the aorta directly to the esophagus posteriorly, which also must be divided.

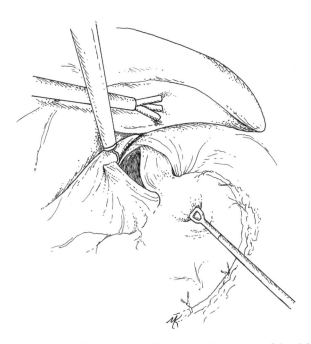

Figure 22.3. Division of gastrohepatic ligament and exposure of the right crus of the diaphragm.

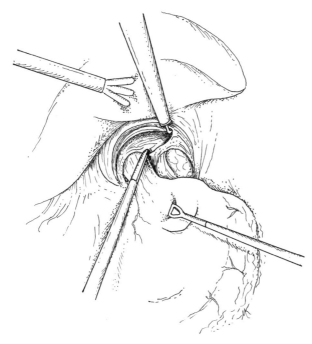

Figure 22.4. Dissection of the hernia sac away from the right crus.

F. Excision of the Hernia Sac

1. After the dissection of as much of the plane anterior to the esophagus as possible, divide the short gastric vessels. Enter the lesser sac to the left of the stomach, and divide the perifundic tissues up to the base of the left crus of the diaphragm.
2. Divide the endoabdominal and endothoracic fascia posterior to the esophagus at the medial border of the crura until a circumferential dissection has been undertaken and all of the sac has been pulled down beyond the lower esophagus and over the proximal stomach (Figs. 22.5 and 22.6).
3. The sac itself may be allowed to remain attached to the proximal stomach if small, unobtrusive, and well vascularized; otherwise it can be excised with impunity, while taking care to preserve the vagus nerves and avoid injury to the gastric and esophageal wall.

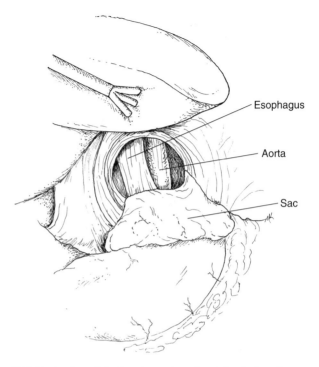

Figure 22.5. Reduction of the hernia sac into the abdominal cavity away from mediastinal structures.

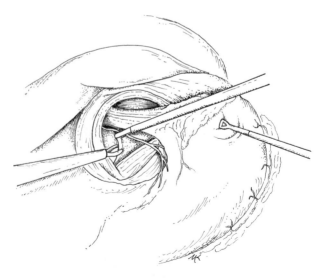

Figure 22.6. Dissection posterior to the esophagus within the mediastinum.

G. Closure of the Hiatal Defect

1. After the hernia sac has been dissected completely from the mediastinum, there is a space of variable size separating the crura. Because this space is shaped like an inverted teardrop, there is less distance between the right and left crura posterior to the esophagus (near the origin of the crural leaves) than anterior to it.

2. Approximate the right and left crura, beginning posteriorly and working anteriorly. In closing the crura from their posterior aspect, the esophagus is transposed anteriorly toward the dome of the diaphragm, thereby effectively lengthening it, because the distance between the dome of the diaphragm and the oropharynx is less than that from the oropharynx to the posterior aspect of the diaphragm.

3. We currently use pledgeted 0-gauge Ethibond sutures for the closure and try to incorporate endoabdominal fascia on the abdominal surface of the crura to minimize tearing of the crural muscle (Fig. 22.7).

4. Place sutures until either the hiatal hernia is completely closed posterior to the esophagus or the esophagus has been moved anteriorly to the point that it appears to be angulated. The crura can almost always be closed primarily.

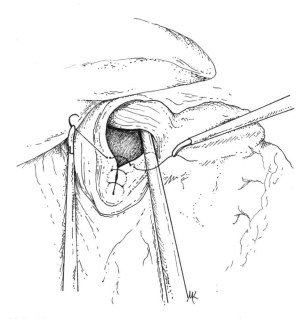

Figure 22.7. The crural opening is closed with simple, interrupted nonabsorbable suture (0 Ethibond). For large defects, pledgets and/or bioprosthetic mesh may be used.

5. If the hiatal defect is too large to be closed primarily without tension, a bioprosthetic patch may be used.
6. If a space remains between the crura anterior to the esophagus, additional anterior sutures may be placed after the fundoplication has been performed.

H. Fundoplication

1. After the hiatal hernia has been repaired, we advocate performing a fundoplication (Fig. 22.8; see also Chapter 21) to prevent postoperative GERD.
2. In patients with normal preoperative esophageal motor function, a complete fundoplication is performed, whereas a partial fundoplication is used in patients with poor esophageal motility.

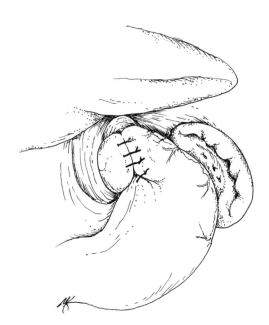

Figure 22.8. A 2-cm, 360 degree wrap is created using three interrupted, nonabsorbable sutures with care to avoid the anterior vagus.

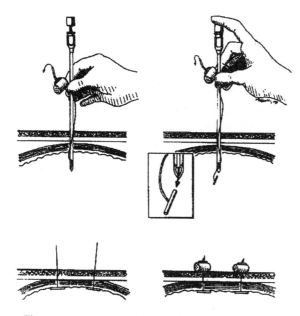

Figure 22.9. Use of **T**-fasteners for anterior gastropexy.

I. Gastropexy

1. After the completion of the fundoplication, an anterior gastropexy may be performed. We reserve gastropexies for patients in whom most of the stomach is in the chest and those with organoaxial volvulus of the stomach. In these situations, anterior gastropexy can either be performed by placing a gastrostomy tube, or the anterior gastric wall can simply be sutured to the posterior abdominal wall.

2. Brown-Mueller **T**-fasteners (Ross Laboratories, Columbus, OH). are ideally suited to performing a simple, fast, and effective anterior gastropexy (Fig. 22.9). Grasp the anterior gastric wall with Babcock forceps at the greater curvature of the antrum of the stomach. Gently pull this portion of the stomach anteriorly to assess whether it reaches the posterior abdominal wall without tension, remembering that the pneumoperitoneum increases this distance.

3. If necessary, reduce the pneumoperitoneum pressure.

4. Lightly score the gastric wall with monopolar electrocautery to stimulate subsequent adhesion formation.

5. Place a **T**-fastener within the slotted needle and pass it percutaneously through the skin of the epigastrium several centimeters inferior to the costal margin. Pass the needle tip into the gastric lumen while elevating the stomach slightly.

6. Next, use the stylet to dislodge the metal bar of the **T**-fastener from the needle, causing the bar to turn sideways and reside within the lumen of the stomach.

7. Place two additional **T**-fasteners in a triangulated configuration with a distance of approximately 2 cm around each **T**-fastener.

8. After these three **T**-fasteners have been placed, slowly exsufflate the abdominal cavity, allowing the carbon dioxide to escape while gently retracting all three **T**-fasteners. In this manner, the stomach is pulled to the anterior abdominal wall under direct vision, preventing interposition of colon or other intra-abdominal viscera between the stomach and anterior abdominal wall.

9. The **T**-fasteners are allowed to remain for 2 to 4 weeks, at which time the nylon suture is cut at the level of the skin, and the metal bar is allowed to pass through the intestinal tract.

J. Postoperative Care

1. A nasogastric tube is not used unless the patient requires gastric decompression for relief of nausea or abdominal distention. Intravenous antiemetics are administered prophylactically.

2. The patients are more frail and elderly and often do not take a full diet as quickly.

3. Clear liquids are given the morning of the first postoperative day and advanced to a soft diet as tolerated.

4. Patients are usually discharged on the first or second postoperative day.

K. Complications

1. Pleural injury/pneumothorax is the result of inadvertent entry into the pleura during the mediastinal dissection. Clinically significant pleural injuries rarely occur. The balance between positive airway pressure and pneumoperitoneum pressure may be adjusted if necessary. Dissection close to the esophagus may prevent pleural injury. At the conclusion of the procedure, suction is applied transhiatally to the mediastinum while administering vital capacity breaths to allow venting of the pneumoperitoneum through the trocar sites. A postoperative chest radiograph is obtained only if the patient experiences respiratory distress.

2. Bleeding from the short gastric vessels is an uncommon complication, which can be managed with the ultrasonic scalpel or a clip.

3. Splenic injury/liver injury during retraction and dissection can occur. An atraumatic liver retractor and gentle, meticulous technique will in general prevent severe hemorrhage. Most bleeding can be stopped by direct pressure or with topical hemostatic agents.

4. Esophageal perforation occurs in less than 1% of cases. Patients with
    severe periesophageal inflammation are at greater risk for injury given
    that tissue planes are less clear. Prevention of injury includes circum-
    ferentially dissecting the esophagus under direct vision with an angled
    laparoscope, and not directly grasping the esophagus for retraction.
    Repair of simple perforations can involve laparoscopic placement of
    interrupted sutures with coverage by the fundoplication.

Acknowledgment.

The authors gratefully acknowledge support from: Washington University Institute for Minimally Invasive Surgery (WUIMIS).

L. Selected References

Diaz S, Brunt LM, Klingensmith ME, Frisella P, Soper NJ. Laparoscopic paraesophageal
    hernia repair, a challenging operation. Medium-term outcome of 116 patients. J
    Gastrointest Surg 2003;7(1):59–67.

Gantert WA, Patti MG, Arcerito M, et al. Laparoscopic repair of paraesophageal hiatal
    hernias. J Am Coll Surg 1998;186:428–432.

Hashemi M, Peters JH, DeMeester TR, et al. Laparoscopic repair of large type III hiatal
    hernia: objective follow-up reveals high recurrence rate. J Am Coll Surg 2000;
    190:553–560.

Mattar SG, Bowers SP, Galloway KD, Hunter JG, Smith CD. Long-term outcome of laparo-
    scopic repair of paraesophageal hernia. Surg Endosc 2002;16:745–749.

Oddsdottir M. Paraesophageal hernia. Surg Clin North Am 2000;80:1243–1252.

Stylopulos N, Gazzele MS, Rattner DW. Paraesophageal hernias: operation or observation.
    Ann Surg 2002;236(4):492–500.

Trus TL, Bax T, Richardson WS, et al. Complications of laparoscopic paraesophageal
    hernia repair. J Gastrointest Surg 1997;1221–1228.

Willekes CL, Edoga JK, Frezza EE. Laparoscopic repair of paraesophageal hernia. Ann
    Surg 1997;225:31–38.

Wu JS, Dunnegan DL, Soper NJ. Clinical and radiologic assessment of laparoscopic para-
    esophageal hernia repair. Surg Endosc 1998;13:497–502.

23.1 Laparoscopic Cardiomyotomy (Heller Myotomy)

Margret Oddsdottir, M.D.

A. Indications and Patient Preparation

Laparoscopic cardiomyotomy (Heller myotomy) is performed for achalasia. The **diagnostic workup** must exclude several diseases that can mimic achalasia (malignant obstruction, gastroesophageal reflux with stricture formation, diffuse esophageal spasm, and nutcracker esophagus), as treatment of these is quite different. A complete diagnostic workup is outlined in Table 23.1.1.

Patients who can tolerate general anesthesia are candidates for laparoscopic cardiomyotomy. Pneumatic balloon dilation is an alternative treatment. Botulinum toxin (Botox) injection is an alternative that should be reserved for patients who are not candidates for operation or dilatation. Who should be referred for laparoscopic cardiomyotomy?

1. **Young patients**—patients under the age of 40 do not respond well to pneumatic dilation
2. Patients who **fail pneumatic dilations**
3. Patients who are fit for surgery and choose to have surgery

Because patients with achalasia frequently retain food and secretions within the esophagus, preoperative fasting for at least 8 hours is recommended. Some surgeons evacuate the dilated esophagus with an Ewald tube or esophagoscope. *Candida albicans* frequently colonizes this dilated esophagus, and oral antifungal therapy may be warranted. These measures decrease the likelihood of aspiration upon induction of anesthesia, and minimize the consequences of inadvertent mucosal perforation during myotomy.

B. Patient Positioning and Room Setup

1. Position the patient supine on the operating table, with the legs spread apart on leg boards (Fig. 23.1.1). If possible, tuck both arms at the patient's side. Once the first trocar has been introduced, the patient is placed in a steep reverse Trendelenburg position.
2. Place an orogastric tube and Foley catheter (optional). Most surgeons use sequential pneumatic compression devices (or perioperative low-molecular-weight heparin injections) as prophylaxis for deep venous thrombosis.

Table 23.1.1 Diagnostic workup for laparoscopic cardiomyotomy.

Test	Results consistent with
Barium swallow	Dilated esophagus, tapering distally, with a so-called bird's beak deformity
Upper gastrointestinal endoscopy (EGD) with biopsy if necessary	Smooth mucosa and a tight distal esophageal sphincter, which the endoscopist is able to traverse
Esophageal manometry	Loss of peristalsis in the esophageal body and a normal or hypertensive lower esophageal sphincter that fails to relax upon swallowing
24-hour pH study*	No evidence of gastroesophageal reflux
Computed tomography (CT) scan*	No evidence of malignancy

* Optional tests, depending upon clinical presentation.

3. Stand between the patient's legs facing the monitors, maintaining coaxial alignment with the gastroesophageal junction and the laparoscope. The camera operator stands on the patient's right side. Alternatively the camera can be held by a robotic arm. The first assistant and scrub nurse stand on the patient's left.

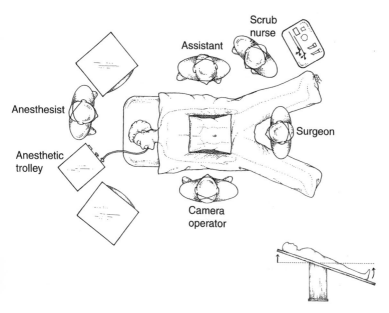

Figure 23.1.1. The operating room setup.

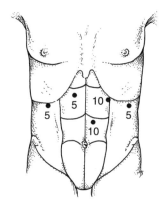

Figure 23.1.2. Trocar placement. The supraumbilical trocar and the right sub-costal trocar are placed 15 cm from the xiphoid, the left subcostal trocar about 10 cm from the xiphoid. The epigastric trocar is placed as high as the liver edge allows and as lateral as the falciform ligament allows. The left flank port is about 7 cm lateral to the left subcostal trocar.

C. Trocar Position and Choice of Laparoscope

1. Place the first trocar through the left rectus sheath, medial to the epi-gastric vessels. This trocar will be used for the laparoscope. It is imper-ative to use an angled (30- or 45-degree) laparoscope for adequate visualization of the hiatus.
2. Insert the remaining four trocars under direct vision (Fig. 23.1.2).
3. Pass a liver retractor through the right subcostal trocar and place it under the left liver lobe to expose the hiatus. Several types of self-holding devices are available to hold the liver retractor in place.
4. Place an atraumatic grasper through the 5-mm left flank port. The assistant should use this grasper to retract the epiphrenic fat pad.
5. The left subcostal port and the right epigastric port are the working trocars for the surgeon.

D. Performing the Cardiomyotomy

It is convenient to conceptualize the dissection in three phases: the hiatal dissection, the myotomy, and the antireflux procedure (if desired).
1. **The hiatal dissection**
    a. Take scissors or a hook electrocautery in the right hand and an atraumatic grasper in the left hand.
    b. Begin by incising the avascular area of the gastrohepatic omentum above the hepatic branch of the vagus. This exposes the caudate lobe of the liver and the right crus.

c. Continue the dissection across the hiatus, dividing the phreno-esophageal ligament above the epiphrenic fat pad with electrocautery and sharp dissection. The assistant should retract the epiphrenic fat pad down and to the left.

d. Identify the right and left crura of the diaphragm and dissect these from the esophagus with blunt dissection.

e. Divide the posterior esophageal attachments under direct vision with blunt and sharp dissection. Retain the posterior vagus with the posterior esophageal wall.

f. Pass the left-hand grasper behind the esophagus under direct vision, and place the grasper in front of the left crus. Pull an 8-cm long segment of 0.25-in. Penrose drain around the esophagus. Clip the two ends of the drain together and use this sling to retract the esophagus. Special angled or reticulating graspers are available for this purpose.

g. Complete the periesophageal dissection by dissecting both crura free of all epiphrenic tissue, mobilizing an adequate length of the esophagus and developing a posterior window large enough for a loose partial (270-degree) fundoplication.

h. Divide the short gastric vessels, beginning about one third of the way down the greater curvature using the ultrasonically activated shears or a dissector and clips. Continue the dissection of the gastric fundus, finally taking down the attachments to the diaphragm and left crus. A redundant fundus is thus prepared and will be used for partial fundoplication at the conclusion of the myotomy. Thus far, the dissection is essentially the same as that performed for hiatal hernia repair (see Chapter 21).

i. Dissect the epiphrenic fat pad from the anterior surface of the gastroesophageal junction and the cardia.

2. **The myotomy**

a. Begin the myotomy on the anterior surface of the esophagus, to the left of the anterior vagus nerve, just proximal to the gastroesophageal junction.

b. Use dissecting scissors or a dissector to separate the outer longitudinal fibers, using the twin action of the scissors.

c. Separate the inner circular fibers from the underlying mucosa with blunt dissection, using the scissors or the dissector, then divide these circular fibers with scissors or hook cautery. Tent the fibers away from the mucosa before applying electrocautery if a monopolar electrocautery is being used. When the submucosal plane is reached, the mucosa bulges up. This is clearly seen in the magnified laparoscopic view.

d. Carry the myotomy proximally for about 5 to 6 cm from the gastroesophageal junction (Fig. 23.1.3).

e. Distally, carry the myotomy across the gastroesophageal junction and onto the stomach for about 1 cm. On the stomach site, the separation of the muscle layers from the mucosa is more difficult to achieve, the mucosa becomes thinner, and there are more bridging vessels than on the esophagus. This results in more

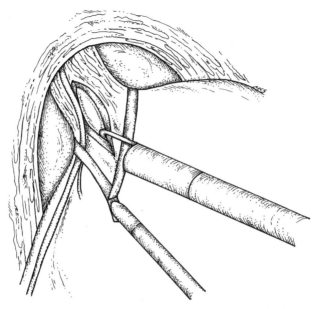

Figure 23.1.3. The myotomy being carried distally, using hook electrocautery. Care must be taken to elevate the muscle fibers away from the mucosa before the electrocautery is applied. The myotomy extends about 5 to 6 cm proximal to the gastroesophageal junction and about 1 cm onto the stomach. (Reprinted with permission from Oddsdottir M. Laparoscopic management of achalasia. Surg Clin North Am 1996;76:451–457.)

> bleeding than is encountered during the esophageal myotomy and increased risk of perforation.
>
> f. When the myotomy is completed, separate the muscle edges from the underlying mucosa for approximately 40% of the esophageal circumference.
>
> g. Some surgeons place a flexible upper gastrointestinal (UGI) endoscope in the esophagus and visualize the distal esophagus to confirm adequacy of myotomy.
>
> h. Pull the orogastric tube back into the distal esophagus and instill about 100 mL of methylene blue solution (one ampule diluted in 250 mL NaCl) down the tube. This will clearly demonstrate any mucosal perforation. If any perforation is encountered, close it with a stitch (4-0 absorbable suture).

3. **Antireflux procedures.** Either a Toupet (a posterior fundoplication) or a Dor (an anterior fundoplication) is recommended in conjunction with the myotomy. The partial fundoplication holds the raw edges of the myotomy open and provides some protection against gastro-esophageal reflux, while being sufficiently loose that passage of food

and liquids is not obstructed (recall that the esophagus lacks normal peristalsis in this disorder). If the hiatus is patulous, the crura are approximated with one or two sutures posteriorly.

a. **Toupet procedure.** The first fundoplication sutures anchor the fundic wrap posteriorly to the crura or the crural closure using two or three interrupted, nonabsorbable, 2-0 sutures. Suture the right side of the wrap to the right edge of the myotomy with three interrupted sutures. Similarly, suture the fundus on the left to the left edge of the myotomy (Fig. 23.1.4).

b. **Dor procedure.** In this partial fundoplication, the redundant fundus is rolled over the exposed mucosa. This may be used to buttress a mucosal repair. Place two or three interrupted sutures between the fundus of the stomach and the left edge of the myotomy. Then place another two or three sutures between the

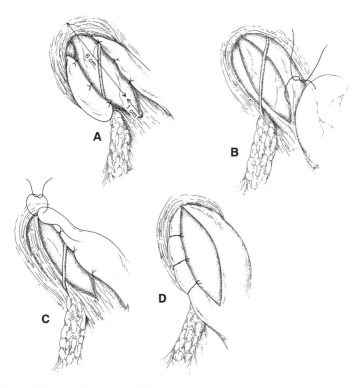

Figure 23.1.4. A. Completed abdominal myotomy with Toupet posterior fundoplication. B–D. Completed abdominal myotomy with Dor anterior fundoplication. (Reprinted with permission from Hunter et al, Laparoscopic Heller myotomy and fundoplication for achalasia. Ann Surg 1997;225:655–664.)

fundus and the anterior crural arch. Finally, suture the fundus to the right edge of the myotomy.

E. Complications

1. **Mucosal perforation**
   a. **Cause and prevention.** This is the most common complication, and the most frequent cause is probably electrosurgical injury. As previously noted, on the gastric side, separation of the muscle layers from the mucosa is more difficult to achieve and the mucosa becomes thinner than on the esophagus. This results in increased risk of perforation. Late perforations are rare, and are probably due to sloughing of a burned mucosa. When performing the myotomy it is very important to tent up the mucosa before applying the electrocautery. The cut edge of the muscularis may bleed, but care should be taken not to apply electrocautery close to the mucosa. Bleeding there usually stops spontaneously.
   b. **Recognition and management.** Mucosal perforations are easily recognized, if not immediately then during the installation of methylene blue dye into the esophagus. These lacerations are clean and are easily repaired with a stitch. As of today, there are no reports of an infection from a small, recognized mucosal laceration during laparoscopic cardiomyotomy. Late perforations are very rare.

2. **Pneumothorax**
   a. **Cause and prevention.** Pneumothorax is not uncommon during laparoscopic hiatal dissection and esophageal mobilization (5%–10%). One can frequently see the pleural edges during these procedures.
   b. **Recognition and management.** These pneumothoraces are usually small and self-limited. They are best recognized on a postoperative chest film. Intervention is rarely needed, as the lung reexpands rapidly as carbon dioxide is absorbed.

3. **Dysphagia**
   a. **Cause and prevention.** Heller myotomy offers relief of dysphagia in 90% to 97% of patients. Postoperative dysphagia may be due to either incomplete myotomy or a megaesophagus in "end-stage" achalasia. Incomplete myotomy occurs more commonly at the distal end of the myotomy, the stomach side. It is important to carry the myotomy across the gastroesophageal junction and onto the stomach for about 1 cm.
   b. **Recognition and management.** The magnification during laparoscopic surgery offers excellent views of the myotomy and of uncut muscle fibers. If incomplete myotomy is not recognized intraoperatively, postoperative dilation can help. If esophageal manometry shows clearly an uncut, high-pressure zone at the gastroesophageal junction, reoperation should be considered.

Patients with extremely dilated aperistaltic esophagus generally require esophageal replacement. Workup of postoperative dysphagia requires careful assessment with esophageal manometry and should prompt reconsideration of the underlying diagnosis.

F. Selected References

Abid S, Champion G, Richter JE, et al. Treatment of achalasia: the best of both worlds. Am J Gastroenterol 1994;89:979–985.

Ackroyd R, Watson DI, Dewitt PG, Jamieson GG. Laparoscopic cardiomyotomy for achalasia. Surg Endosc 2001;15:683–686.

Andreollo NA, Earlam RJ. Heller's myotomy for achalasia: is an added anti-reflux procedure necessary? Br J Surg 1987;74:765–769.

Anselmino M, Zaninotto G, Costantini M, et al. One-year follow-up after laparoscopic Heller-Dor operation for esophageal achalasia. Surg Endosc 1997;11:3–7.

Crookes PF, Wilkinson AJ, Johnston GW. Heller's myotomy with partial fundoplication. Br J Surg 1989;76:98.

Csendes A, Braghetto I, Henriquez A, et al. Late results of a prospective randomised study comparing forceful dilatation and oephagomyotomy in patients with achalasia. Gut 1989;30:299–304.

Ellis FH. Functional disorders of the esophagus. In Zuidema GD, Orringer MB, eds. Shackelford's Surgery of the Alimentary Tract. 3d ed. Philadelphia: WB Saunders, 1991;150–156.

Hunter JG, Trus TL, Branum GD, et al. Laparoscopic Heller myotomy and fundoplication for achalasia. Ann Surg 1997;225:655–664.

Oddsdottir M. Laparoscopic management of achalasia. Surg Clin North Am 1996;76:451–457.

Patti MG, Tamburini A, Pellegrini CA. Cardiomyotomy. Semin Laparosc Surg 1999; 6:186–193.

Pechlivandes G, Chrysos E, Athanasakis E, et al. Laparoscopic Heller cardiomyotomy and Dor fundoplication for esophageal achalasia: possible factors predictiong outcome. Arch Surg 2001;136:1240–1243.

Raiser F, Perdikis G, Hinder RA, et al. Heller myotomy via minimal-access surgery: an evaluation of antireflux procedures. Arch Surg 1996;131:593–597.

Swanstrom LL, Pennings J. Laparoscopic esophagomyotomy for achalasia. Surg Endosc 1995;9:286–292.

23.2 Operations for Esophageal Diverticula

D. Mario del Pino, M.D.
Hiran Fernando, M.D.

A. Indications

Esophageal diverticula can be classified according to their location into cervical (Zenker's diverticulum), midesophageal, and epiphrenic. The approach and operation performed for esophageal diverticula (ED) is tailored to the location of the diverticulum and the underlying esophageal functional abnormality.

Midesophageal diverticula are rarely seen. These are usually traction diverticula that are often associated with inflammatory diseases such as histoplasmosis or tuberculosis. Because of the degree of adhesions seen and the proximity of these diverticula to the airway, they are usually approached with open techniques. In the rare cases that can be approached with minimal invasiveness, an appropriate video-assisted thoracic surgery (VATS) approach similar to that used for mobilization of the esophagus during esophagectomy is used (see Chapter 75).

This chapter will focus on the use of minimally invasive operations for cervical diverticulum (Zenker's diverticulum) and epiphrenic diverticulum, both of which are more commonly seen.

1. Zenker's Diverticulum (ZD)

Zenker's diverticula are thought to be a form of pulsion diverticula that occurs in an area of muscular weakness (Killian dehiscence) located between the inferior constrictor and cricopharyngeus (CP) muscles. Typically elderly people, especially males, are affected. Symptoms include dysphagia, regurgitation of undigested food, globus sensation, halitosis, and aspiration pneumonia. Operation is the only effective treatment and has been shown to result in improvement of symptoms and quality of life despite the advanced age of many affected patients. The goals of surgical treatment for ZD are (1) release of the upper esophageal sphincter by division or myotomy of the cricopharyngeus muscle and (2) elimination of the reservoir (the diverticulum) trapping food particles and secretions. The most important aspect of operation is division or myotomy of the cricopharyngeus. Approaches to the diverticulum include diverticulectomy, diverticulopexy (by suspending the diverticulum sac to the prevertebral fascia), and imbrication of the diverticulum (by dissecting the diverticulum and inverting it into the lumen of the esophagus with a "purse-string" suture). Endoscopic approaches have recently gained popularity for ZD, particularly with the use of the linear stapler for division of the cricopharyngeus muscle. Since many ZD patients are elderly, often with significant comorbid disease, an endoscopic approach, avoiding the need for a neck incision, offers potential advantages for this patient population. A key factor when using this approach is to select patients with a diverticulum at least 3 cm in diameter. This operation is unlikely to succeed with smaller diverticula, since there will be inadequate division of the cricopharyngeus muscle, and there may be difficulties in placement of the stapler. Other factors that make endoscopic stapling technically difficult include the presence of prominent upper incisors, limited mouth opening, and inability to adequately extend the neck.

2. Epiphrenic Diverticulm

Epiphrenic diverticula are generally regarded as pulsion diverticula that develop secondary to increased intraesophageal pressure usually associated with motility disorders. Controversy exists regarding the management of these patients primarily owing to our incomplete understanding of the pathophysiology and the risks associated with operation. In the past, operative treatment was favored for symptomatic patients only, although some authors have advocated operative intervention on all patients with epiphrenic diverticula regardless of symptoms. The extent of the esophageal myotomy and the need for an antireflux procedure are also issues of contention. At our institution operative management is reserved for patients with major symptoms. The mortality rates for open surgery for ED are not insignificant, and range from 0% to 11%. Our treatment of choice for epiphrenic diverticula associated with achalasia, hypertensive lower esophageal sphincter, or other motility disorders with abnormal manometry isolated to the distal esophagus is a laparoscopic diverticulectomy, gastroesophageal myotomy, and partial fundoplication. This approach is described next.

B. Zenker's Diverticulum

1. Patient position and room setup for Zenker's Diverticulum
    a. General anesthesia is used.
    b. Place the patient in the supine position, with the neck carefully extended.
    c. The surgeon stands behind the head of the patient.
    d. Place monitors at the foot of the bed and behind the surgeon.
2. Endoscopic transoral stapling of a Zenker's diverticulum
    a. First perform flexible esophagoscopy to make a final assessment of the diverticulum and its suitability for endoscopic stapling.
    b. Suction out any retained material found in the diverticulum.
    c. We then perform rigid esophagoscopy using the Weerdascope (Karl Storz, Tuttlingen, Germany). This scope has two jaws (Fig. 23.2.1).

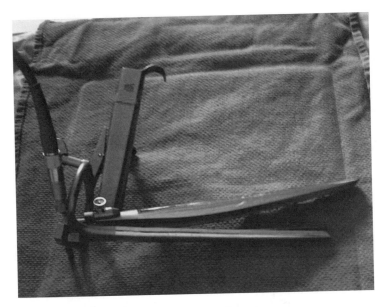

Figure 23.2.1. Weerdascope.

d. Place one jaw in the esophagus and the second in the diverticulum.
Next, expand the jaws to clearly visualize the diverticulum and
the common septum formed by the cricopharyngeal muscle.

e. Place a traction suture in the common septum (Fig. 23.2.2). We
use the Endo-Stitch (U.S. Surgical, Norwalk, CT), as this simpli-
fies manipulation of the suture within the Weerdascope.

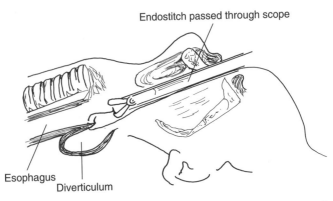

Figure 23.2.2. Placement of stay suture on common wall between esophagus
and diverticulum.

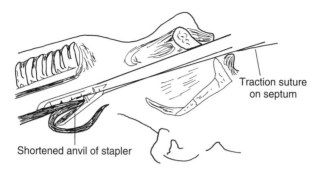

Traction suture
on septum

Shortened anvil of stapler

Figure 23.2.3. Stapling of diverticulum using modified Endo-GIA 30.

f. Using the suture to provide traction on the common septum, a
    stapler for endoscopic gastrointestinal anastomosis (Endo-GIA
    30, U.S. Surgical, Norwalk, CT), modified as shown shortly, is
    placed across the septum and fired (Fig. 23.2.3). Further firings
    of the stapler are performed as needed to ensure that the common
    septum is divided to the base of the diverticulum.

g. The stapler is modified by shortening the tip of the anvil (Fig.
    23.2.4). This is necessary so that the stapler will both cut and
    staple to the end of the stapler tip. The modified anvil is placed

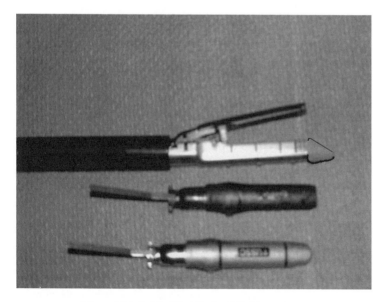

Figure 23.2.4. Modified Endo-GIA 30 stapler.

within the diverticulum and the disposable cartridge within the esophageal lumen (Fig. 23.2.3).

h.   We do not place a nasogastric tube.

i.   Obtain a barium swallow on the first postoperative day and start the patient on liquids if the results are satisfactory.

C. Epiphrenic Diverticulum

1.   Patient positioning and room setup

a.   General anesthesia is used.

b.   Position the patient supine on the operating table, slightly to the right side of the table to facilitate placement of a lateral port for a liver retractor.

c.   Use a foot board, so that the patient can be placed in reverse Trendelenburg position during the operation without sliding down the table.

d.   The surgeon stands on the patient's right, and one assistant stands on the patient's left.

e.   Use two monitors, one on either side of the head of the table.

2.   Performing the laparoscopic diverticulectomy, gastroesophageal myotomy, and Toupet fundoplication

a.   First perform flexible esophagoscopy.

b.   Leave the endoscope in the esophagus during the procedure.

c.   Five laparoscopic ports are used: one 10-mm port and four 5-mm ports.

d.   Place a liver retractor to elevate the left lobe of the liver and expose the hiatus.

e.   Open the gastrohepatic ligament. We prefer to use the ultrasonic shears for most of this dissection.

f.   Identify the right crus and dissect the esophagus away from this, taking care to preserve the peritoneal lining over the crus.

g.   Perform a limited division of the short gastric vessels using the ultrasonic shears, with hemoclips for the larger vessels. This allows exposure and facilitates dissection of the left crus and also mobilizes the gastric fundus to allow creation of a tension-free wrap.

h.   Dissect the anterior fat pad from the gastroesophageal junction. This is performed in a left-to-right direction, taking care to protect and mobilize the vagus nerves with the fat pad. This dissection allows the surgeon to clearly identify the gastro-esophageal junction and facilitates determination of the optimal length and location of the myotomy.

i.   Dissect the distal esophagus at the hiatus into the mediastinum and identify the diverticulum. Sometimes endoscopy will facilitate identification of the diverticulum.

j.   Dissect the ED dissected with careful exposure of the entire neck.

k. Resect the ED with an Endo-GIA 30 stapler (U.S. Surgical, Norwalk, CT). To prevent narrowing of the esophagus during the stapling, we usually remove the endoscope and place a bougie in the esophagus under direct vision with the laparoscope.

l. The ED is a mucosal outpouching without a muscular covering. Following resection of the ED, the overlying esophageal muscle layer is closed using the Endo-Stitch (U.S. Surgical, Norwalk, CT) with intracorporeal knot tying.

m. Epinephrine (1 mL, 1 : 1000, in 20 mL of normal saline) is injected into the muscular layers of the anterior esophagus and stomach on the opposite side of the stapled diverticulum. This improves hemostasis and facilitates the myotomy.

n. Perform a myotomy on the opposite side of the diverticulum (see also Chapter 23.1).
    i. This myotomy should extend from the level of the myotomy down onto the first centimeter or two of the stomach.
    ii. We use a combination of sharp dissection with ultrasonic shears and blunt dissection with an Endo-Peanut dissector (U.S. Surgical, Norwalk, CT).

o. The endoscope is used to assess the completeness of the myotomy and also to check for mucosal perforations.

p. We routinely include a posterior partial fundoplication (Toupet) with the laparoscopic approach. Sutures are placed between the fundus and the myotomized esophageal muscle to help keep the myotomy open (see Fig. 23.1.4A).

D. Complications

1. **Endoscopic transoral stapling of cervical (Zenker's) diverticulum**
    a. **Failure or recurrence of ZD**
        i. Division of the common wall or cricopharyngeal muscle is the key part of this operation. Inadequate division of the cricopharyngeal muscle will lead to persistent symptoms or future recurrence. If the diverticulum is too small, this will lead to an inadequate division of the cricopharyngeus. For this reason we recommend that ES be reserved for diverticula at least 3 cm or more in size. The inclusion of the traction suture helps to bring the common wall into the jaws of the stapler.
        ii. If a small diverticulum is identified, then the endoscopic technique should be abandoned and an open approach used.
    b. **Perforation of the cervical esophagus**
        i. Previous endoscopic approaches utilized a laser to divide the common wall. The introduction of the mechanical stapler has minimized the incidence of perforation.

        ii. Difficulty in placement of the stapler can lead to perforation. In addition to the inappropriate use of this technique with small diverticula, other factors may contribute. These include the presence of prominent upper incisors, limited mouth opening, and inability to adequately extend the neck. Again a low threshold for a standard open approach should be present when this situation arises.

2. **Laparoscopic diverticulectomy, gastroesophageal myotomy, and Toupet fundoplication**

    a. **Intraoperative perforation.** Small mucosal perforations recognized in traoperatively are usually repaired with interrupted sutures. We use the Endo-Stitch (U.S. Surgical, Norwalk, CT) with intracorporeal tying for this. Additionally, an anterior partial wrap may be performed to place the mobilized fundus over this mucosal repair.

    b. **Postoperative leak.** Operations for ED are among the most complex and challenging of esophageal problems. Even with open techniques, leak rates as high as 18% can occur. We routinely obtain a barium swallow in the early postoperative period. If a leak is identified, the patient is taken back to the operating room. Repair is performed when possible. If repair is not feasible, drains and occasionally an esophageal T-tube are placed around the leak site to create a controlled fistula.

    c. **Pneumothorax.** Occasionally a pneumothorax may occur intraoperatively during the dissection of the ED in the mediastinum. This may result in difficulty with ventilation and/or hypotension. Usually a pigtail catheter or chest tube will resolve the situation. This may require conversion to open operation because of difficulties in maintaining pneumoperitoneum after placement of the chest tube.

E. Selected References

Benacci JC, Deschamps C, Trastek VF, et al. Epiphrenic diverticulum: results of surgical treatment. Ann Thorac Surg 1993;55:1109–1114.

Collard JM, Otte JB, Kestens PJ. Endoscopic stapling technique of esophagodiverticulostomy for Zenker's diverticulum. Ann Thorac Surg 1993;56:573–576.

Crescenzo DG, Trastek VF, Allen MS, Deschamps C, Pairolero PC. Zenker's diverticulum in the elderly: is operation justified? Ann Thorac Surg 1998;66:347–350.

Luketich JD, Alvelo-Rivera M, Buenaventura PO, et al. Minimally invasive esophagectomy: outcomes in 222 patients. Ann Surg 2003;238(4):486–494.

Luketich JD, Fernando HC, Christie, et al. Outcomes after minimally invasive esophagomyotomy. Ann Thorac Surg 2001;72:1909–1913.

Patti MG, Pellegrini CA, Horgan S, et al. Minimally invasive surgery for achalasia: an 8-year experience with 168 patients. Ann Surg 1999;230:587–593.

Rosati R, Fumagalli U, Bona S, et al. Diverticulectomy, myotomy, and fundoplication through laparoscopy. A new option to treat epiphrenic diverticula? Ann Surg 1998;227(2):174–178.

Laparoscopy
V—Laparoscopic Gastric Surgery

24. Laparoscopic Gastrostomy

John D. Mellinger, M.D.
Thomas R. Gadacz, M.D.

A. Indications

The indications for gastrostomy include access to the stomach for feeding or prolonged gastric decompression. Laparoscopic gastrostomy is indicated when a percutaneous endoscopic gastrostomy (PEG) cannot be performed or is contraindicated (see Chapter 57, Percutaneous Endoscopic Feeding Tube Placement). Specific situations in which this is likely to occur include:

1. an obstructing oropharyngeal lesion
2. a lesion in the esophagus when the stomach is not to be used for reconstruction
3. concern that the colon, omentum, or liver is overlying the stomach, precluding adequate access via a percutaneous blind approach

Other methods of achieving enteral nutrition (such as Dobhoff tube placement) should be considered, and pyloric obstruction and gastroesophageal reflux should be ruled out. If recurrent aspiration is a problem, a jejunal feeding tube may be more appropriate (but aspiration, including from oropharyngeal sources, may still occur).

B. Patient Position and Room Setup

1. Position the patient supine on the operating room table with the arms tucked.
2. As with most upper abdominal procedures, some surgeons prefer a modified lithotomy position and operate from between the legs of the patient.
3. The surgeon generally stands on the left side of the patient, and the first assistant and scrub nurse on the right side.
4. The monitors are placed at the head of the bed and as close to the operating room table as the anesthesiologist permits.
5. The general setup is very similar to laparoscopic cholecystectomy in most respects, but less equipment is required.

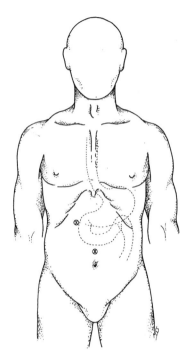

Figure 24.1. Cannula placement for laparoscopic gastrostomy. Consider adequate working distance from anticipated site of gastrostomy placement.

C. Cannula Position and Choice of Laparoscope

Generally only two cannulas are needed for a laparoscopic gastrostomy (Fig. 24.1).

1. Place the cannula for the 30-degree laparoscope below the umbilicus in short patients and at the umbilicus in tall patients. Estimate the working distance to the probable site of gastrostomy placement. Do not place the laparoscope too close, as a short working distance makes it difficult to proceed.
2. Place a second 5-mm cannula in the right subcostal region at the midclavicular line.

D. Performing the Gastrostomy

Two methods of laparoscopic gastrostomy have been described. The first method constructs a simple gastrostomy without a mucosa-lined tube. This is appropriate for most indications. The tract will generally seal without surgical closure when the tube is removed.

An alternative method utilizes the endoscopic stapler to construct a mucosa-lined tube in a fashion analogous to the open Janeway gastrostomy. This provides a permanent stoma that is easily recannulated. Both methods will be described here.

1. **Simple gastrostomy**
    a. Identify the anterior wall of the body of the stomach. Avoid the classic error of mistaking colon for stomach by confirming the absence of taeniae.
    b. Select a location in the left subcostal area for gastrostomy construction.
    c. Pass an atraumatic grasper from the second cannula and grasp the midportion of the selected region. Lift the gastric wall and simultaneously indent the selected region of the abdominal wall with one finger.
    d. Confirm that the area of the stomach selected for the gastrostomy comfortably reaches the corresponding area selected in the left upper abdominal wall. Reassess and choose different sites if necessary.
    e. Reduce the pneumoperitoneal pressure to 6 to 8 mmHg to avoid tension on the stomach.
    f. Pass the T-fasteners though the skin and abdominal wall, and then through the anterior wall of the stomach (Fig. 24.2).
        i. There is a slight give in resistance as the needle passes thought the gastric wall.

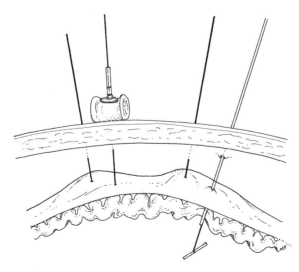

Figure 24.2. T-fasteners through the abdominal wall and anterior gastric wall.

      ii.   Elevate the anterior gastric wall with a grasper to prevent passing the T-fastener through both walls of the stomach.

      iii.   Insert the most proximal T-fasteners and pull up slightly to expose the distal sites of the T-fasteners. By pulling on the T-fasteners, the correct placement can usually be determined.

      iv.   Place a total of four T-fasteners outlining a 2- to 3-cm square on the abdominal and gastric walls.

  g.   Make a 5- to 8-mm stab incision in the skin to adequately accommodate the diameter of the gastrostomy tube.

  h.   Pass a 14-gauge needle through the center of the square of the T-fasteners in the abdominal wall and stomach.

  i.   Pass a 0.35-mm guidewire through the lumen of the needle and thread at least 25 cm into the stomach.

  j.   Enlarge the tract with dilators and pass an 18-French gastrostomy tube using Seldinger technique.

  k.   Release the pneumoperitoneum and pull up the T-fasteners. Tie these to secure the gastric wall to the abdominal wall.

  l.   Pull up the gastrostomy tube to approximate the gastric and abdominal walls. Secure the gastrostomy tube to the skin with sutures or with a Silastic plate.

2. **Construction of gastrostomy with mucosa-lined tube**

  a.   Place three cannulas, in addition to the umbilical port for the laparoscope:

      i.   Left upper quadrant (10 mm)—preferably placed at the approximate site of entry of the gastrostomy

      ii.   Right upper quadrant (10 mm)

      iii.   Right midabdomen (to right of umbilicus) (12 mm)

  b.   Place two endoscopic Babcock clamps through the left and right upper quadrant cannulas and elevate a fold of gastric wall on the anterior surface of the stomach.

  c.   Pass the endoscopic linear stapling device through the 12-mm cannula and use it to create a gastric tube. Generally a single application of the stapler will produce a tube of adequate length (Fig. 24.3). Take care to construct a tube with adequate lumen; this is accomplished by placing the stapler 1 cm from the edge of the gastric fold.

  d.   Evacuate the pneumoperitoneum.

  e.   Pull the cannula, Babcock clamp, and finally the end of the gastric tube out through the left upper quadrant trocar site.

  f.   Open the gastric tube and mature the end to the skin with several interrupted absorbable sutures.

  g.   Cannulate the gastrostomy with a small-diameter Foley catheter. Test the gastrostomy by instilling saline or methylene blue.

  h.   Reestablish a limited (6–8 mmHg) pneumoperitoneum sufficient to visualize the gastric wall with the laparoscope and confirm that the stomach lies comfortably against the anterior abdominal wall and that there is no leakage.

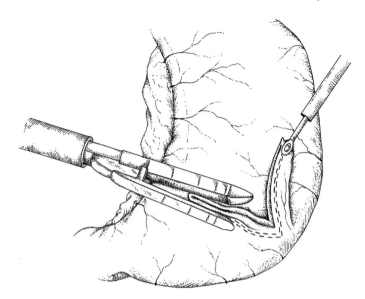

Figure 24.3. Construction of mucosa-lined tube (Janeway-style gastrostomy). A fold of stomach is elevated and the endoscopic stapler applied. Approximately 1 cm of stomach must be included in the staple line to assure an adequate lumen. The tube is grasped and elevated and will be pulled out through the left upper quadrant cannula site.

E. Complications

1. **Leakage of the gastrostomy**
    a. **Cause and prevention.** The gastrostomy can leak if the gastrostomy tube and T-fasteners are not approximated to the abdominal wall. Prevent this by directly observing the T-fasteners being pulled up and ensuring that the gastric wall is adherent to the abdominal wall. The balloon of the gastrostomy tube should be inflated and pulled with gentle traction to approximate the anterior gastric wall to the abdominal wall. This is confirmed by visualization though the laparoscope. If a stapled tube is constructed, an incomplete staple line may result in leakage.
    b. **Recognition and management.** If visualization of the stomach to the abdominal wall is unsatisfactory at the time of operation, inject methylene blue through the gastrostomy tube while visualizing the gastric wall. If any dye is seen in the abdominal cavity, assume inadequate approximation between the stomach and abdominal wall. Fix this either by loosening the gastrostomy tube and inserting more T-fasteners around the gastrostomy site, or by

using a gastrostomy tube with a larger balloon and applying sufficient retraction to provide a better seal between the stomach and abdominal wall.

2. **Gastric perforation**

   a. **Cause and prevention.** Gastric perforation may occur during laparoscopic gastrostomy if there is too much tension on the T-fasteners, or if the selected sites cannot be approximated without tension. Prevent this by careful site selection and by reducing the pressure of the pneumoperitoneum to 6 to 8 mmHg. Excessive use of electrocautery may produce a delayed perforation, and the patient may present with intra-abdominal sepsis 2 to 5 days after operation.

   b. **Recognition and management.** Confirm a suspected perforation by injecting water-soluble contrast through the gastrostomy tube under fluoroscopic observation. If no leak is seen and the patient is stable or improving, nasogastric decompression may be sufficient. Free leakage of contrast, clinical evidence of peritonitis, or clinical deterioration mandates exploratory laparotomy. Oversew the perforation or convert to a formal gastrostomy.

F. Selected References

Arnaud J-P, Casa C, Manunta A. Laparoscopic continent gastrostomy. Am J Surg 1995; 169:629–630.

Duh Q-Y, Way LW. Laparoscopic gastrostomy using T-fasteners as retractors and anchors. Surg Endosc 1993;7:60–63.

Edelman DS, Unger SW. Laparoscopic gastrostomy. Surg Gynecol Obstet 1991;173:401.

Duh QY, Senokozlieff-Englehart AL, Choe YS, Siperstein AE, Rowland K, Way LW. Laparoscopic gastrostomy and jejunostomy: safety and cost with local vs. general anesthesia. Arch Surg 1999;134:151–156.

Peitgen K, von Ostau C, Walz MK. Laparoscopic gastrostomy: result of 121 patients over 7 years. Surg Laparosc Endosc Percut Techniques 2001;11:76–82.

25. Laparoscopic Plication of Perforated Ulcer

John D. Mellinger, M.D.
Thomas R. Gadacz, M.D.

A. Indications

Laparoscopic plication of perforated ulcer is indicated in patients with a suspected or confirmed duodenal ulcer when laparoscopic access to the perforation is possible. It is an alternative to the standard open Graham patch plication and is appropriate whenever this procedure would be considered.

B. Patient Position and Room Setup

Laparoscopic exposure for treatment of a perforated duodenal ulcer is analogous to that used for laparoscopic cholecystectomy. Some surgeons prefer to stand between the legs of the patient for all upper abdominal laparoscopic procedures. (See Chapters 21–23 for additional positioning information.)

C. Cannula Position and Choice of Laparoscope

The cannula position and laparoscope are shown in Figure 25.1. The use of an angled (30- or 45-degree) laparoscope is preferred to facilitate visualization.

D. Performing the Laparoscopic Plication

1. Perform a careful, thorough exploration and lavage the abdominal cavity. If the liver has sealed the perforation, leave this seal undisturbed until the remainder of the abdomen has been explored and lavaged. This minimizes contamination.
2. Pass an irrigating cannula into the right cannula and a Babcock or other atraumatic grasping instrument in the left cannula and irrigate any fibrin away to expose the site of perforation.

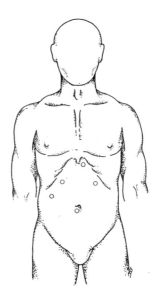

Figure 25.1. Cannula placement for laparoscopic placation of perforated ulcer.

3. If the liver is adherent to the site of perforation, a fan, balloon, or noodle retractor passed through an additional trocar may be necessary.
4. Assess the size, location, and probable cause of perforation. Large perforations, particularly those for which all borders cannot be clearly identified (e.g., large duodenal perforations that extend onto the back wall of the duodenum) are difficult to plicate. Always consider the possibility of gastric malignancy or gastric lymphoma if the perforation is on the stomach. Exercise good judgment and convert to an open surgical procedure if the situation is not conducive to simple Graham patch closure (Fig. 25.2). As a general rule, perforated gastric ulcers should be excised and not simply plicated because of the risk of malignancy.
5. Close the perforation with three or four sutures placed 8 to 10 mm from the edge of the perforation.
6. Tie these sutures as they are placed.
7. Place omentum over the plication, if possible. The authors prefer to close the perforation first and then overlay omentum, rather than placing omentum in the perforation, depending on the size of the defect, tissue intergrity, and caliber of the adjacent duodenal lumen (Fig. 25.3). The sutures are retied over the omentum to secure it to the plication site.
8. If the omentum is surgically absent or insufficient, the ligamentum teres and adjacent falciform ligament may be mobilized and used for

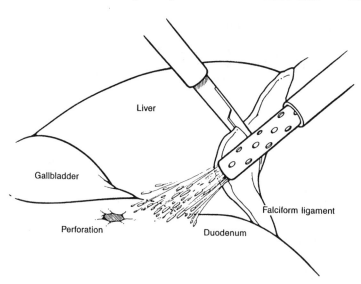

Figure 25.2. Exposure of a typical perforated duodenal ulcer using the suction irrigator to wash away fibrin.

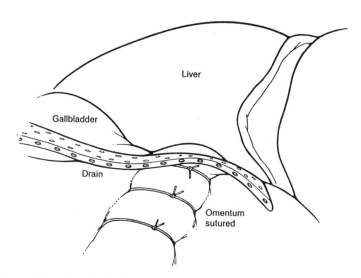

Figure 25.3. Completed plication buttressed with omentum. A drain may be placed if desired.

the tissue patch. Irrigate the area with saline to dilute and remove as much of the gastric contents as possible.

9. Air insufflation via a nasogastric tube with gentle manual compression of the duodenum distal to the plication site may be used to test the integrity of the closure.

E. Complications

1. In general, the complications of laparoscopic plication are similar to those previously described for laparoscopic gastrostomy (Chapter 24) and recognition, prevention, and management are similar.

2. Additional problems with this procedure are incorrect diagnosis (which can be avoided if the laparoscopist is scrupulously careful to visualize the site of perforation), recurrent ulcer (which is likely to occur in 30% of cases if treatment of the underlying ulcer diathesis is not followed), and inadvertent plication of a malignancy or lymphoma. These complications can be avoided by exercising good surgical judgment and converting to formal laparotomy if the diagnosis is unclear or plication does not appear feasible.

3. Gastric outlet obstruction may result if the plicating sutures are placed too deep or if the ulcer has produced significant pyloric stenosis.

F. Selected Reference

Lorand I, Molinier N, Sales JP, Douchez F, Gayral F. Results of laparoscopic treatment of perforated ulcers. Chirurgie 1999;124:149–153.

Mouret P, François Y, Vignal J, Barth X, Lombard-Platet R. Laparoscopic treatment of perforated peptic ulcer. Br J Surg 1990;77:1006.

Munro WS, Bajwa F, Menzies D. Laparoscopic repair of perforated duodenal ulcers with a falciform ligament patch. Ann R Coll Surg Engl 1997;79:156–157.

26. Gastric Resections

Alfred Cuschieri, M.D., Ch.M., F.R.C.S.
F.R.S.E, F. Med. Sci.

A. Indications for Laparoscopic Gastric Surgery

The indications for laparoscopic gastrectomy (in the author's practice) are as follows.

1. **Intractable peptic ulceration** that fails to heal on medical treatment. Successful medical management (including treatment for *Helicobacter pylori*) has made this a rare indication. In the author's experience, the peptic ulcers that require resection are prepyloric ulcers (antectomy and truncal vagotomy) and gastric ulcers.

2. **Gastrointestinal stromal tumors of the stomach** (previously known as leiomyomas and leimyosarcomas). These usually present with bleeding, less often perforation. The distinction between benign and malignant is size dependent and can be difficult even on pathologic examination.

3. **Some gastric cancers.** Case selection is important here, and the indications are still evolving. Early gastric cancers not involving the submucosa are suitable for laparoscopic or endoluminal local resection. Early gastric cancer involving the submucosa requires gastrectomy with removal of greater omentum and level 1 lymph nodes (D_1 gastrectomy). This can be performed safely laparoscopically. Advanced gastric cancer (involving the muscularis propria but not the serosa, T_2 tumor) requires a more extensive regional lymphadenectomy (D_2) with the gastrectomy. Although not in established practice, D_2 resection for T_2 gastric tumors can be performed safely without jeopardizing outcome and is facilitated by use of the hand-assisted laparoscopic surgical (HALS) technique. Operable bulky tumors involving the serosa (T_3), are still considered unsuitable for the laparoscopic approach. **Incurable (distant metastasis, peritoneal deposits) but resectable disease** is a good indication for laparoscopic palliative resection.

4. **Gastric lymphoma** (from gut-associated lymphoid tissue [GALT lymphoma]) is suitable for laparoscopic gastric resection.

5. **Polyps and other benign lesions** are suitable for a laparoendogastric approach.

B. Approaches

The techniques of minimal access gastric resection may be categorized as follows.

1. **Interventional flexible endoscopy** is suitable for superficial gastric cancer not involving the submucosa on endoluminal ultrasound scanning (even if caught early, tumors with significant involvement of the submucosa have a 15%–20% incidence of regional node spread). These approaches include submucosal resection after adrenaline/saline instillation in the submucosal layer, and laser ablation (see Chapter 50).

2. **Laparoendoluminal resection** is an alternative to the interventional flexible endoscopic approach and is suitable for small superficial lesions.

3. **Laparoscopic partial or total gastrectomy** with internal reconstruction of the upper gastrointestinal tract.

4. **Laparoscopic assisted partial or total gastrectomy** with reconstruction through a midline 5.0-cm minilaparotomy, used for both specimen extraction and reconstruction.

5. **Hand-assisted laparoscopic gastric resections.** In the HALS technique, a hand access device is used to enable the insertion of the assisting hand of the surgeon (or of the assistant) in the peritoneal cavity for exposure and retraction of tissue planes, for palpation of diseased areas, and for immediate control of bleeding. The second-generation devices are easy to insert through a mini-incision (Omniport, Lapdisk, Gelport) and protect the wound edges; some enable withdrawal/insertion of the hand without loss of pneumoperitoneum (Omniport, Gelport).

C. Patient Position and Setup

Two options are available for laparoendoluminal gastric resection, laparoscopic gastrectomy, and HALS gastrectomy:

1. Patient in the supine head-up tilt position with the surgeon operating from the right side of the operating table and the main video monitor facing the surgeon.

2. Patient in the supine position with head-up tilt and abduction of the lower limbs with the surgeon operating between the legs of the patient. The main monitor should go at the head of the table. This is easier and more comfortable for the surgeon but may increase calf vein compression trauma and the risk of deep venous thrombosis (DVT), especially if leg stirrups are used.

Irrespective of position, DVT prophylaxis with subcutaneous heparin and graduated compression stockings is recommended, as is antibiotic prophylaxis.

D. Endoluminal Gastric Surgery

The technique described here works well for lesions on the posterior wall, fundus, and esophagogastric junction. An experienced laparoscopic surgeon and a skilled endoscopist (stationed at the head of the table, outside the sterile field) work together.

1. Place a laparoscope through an **umbilical port** and perform a thorough laparoscopic inspection of the peritoneal cavity and stomach.
2. The assistant then passes a flexible upper gastrointestinal endoscope with a large (3.4-mm) instrument channel and inflates the stomach. An instrument passed through this endoscope will provide additional manipulation and assistance during the surgery.
3. Choose the appropriate point for intragastric entry, usually halfway between the greater and lesser curvature in the proximal half of the stomach (Fig. 26.1). The exact site is dictated by the topography of the intragastric lesion. After evaluating various types of trocar/cannula

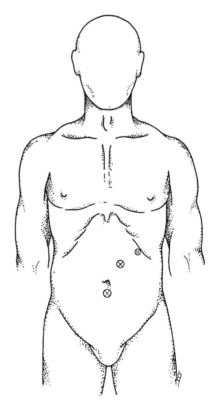

Figure 26.1. Trocar sites for endoluminal gastric surgery. The laparoscope is first placed through an umbilical port and initial inspection of the peritoneal cavity performed. The two additional left upper quadrant trocars are placed under direct vision and an operating laparoscope passed into the stomach via the 11-mm port. The 5-mm port is an additional intragastric operating port.

system, the author's preference is for the Innerdyne (Innerdyne, Inc., Sunnyvale, CA) system. This is ideal for endoluminal work.

    a.   Make a small gastric perforation with a straight electrosurgical needle in the cutting mode.

    b.   Place a Veress needle through the abdominal wall of the left upper quadrant and into the stomach via the small perforation.

    c.   Insert the nonexpanded polymer sheath over the Veress needle (Fig. 26.2).

4.   Place a second 5.0-mm cannula, more lateral and cephalad than the operating laparoscope port.

5.   The "second" assisting instrument is provided by the instruments passed through the channel of the flexible endoscope, operated by a trained flexible endoscopist. The completed setup is shown in Figure 26.3.

6.   Surgery is then performed within the lumen of the stomach. Instruments passed through the operating channel of the laparoscope and the second port are used to elevate, resect, and suture as needed. At the conclusion of the case, instruments are withdrawn and the two holes in the stomach are closed.

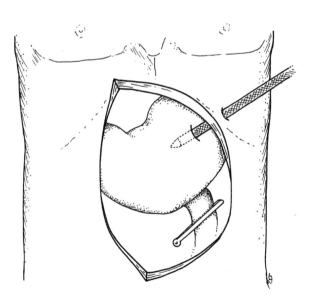

Figure 26.2. Insertion of the Innerdyne gastric cannula into inflated stomach. Thereafter, the radially expandable polymer sheath is stretched by an 11.0-mm port for intragastric insertion of the operating laparoscope.

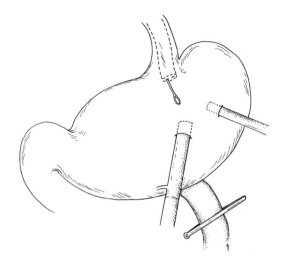

Figure 26.3. Access for endoluminal gastric surgery.

E. Laparoscopic Gastric Resection

1. Place the laparoscope through an umbilical trocar. The author favors a 30-degree forward-oblique viewing laparoscope; others prefer a 0-degree laparoscope.
2. Place three additional ports as shown in Figure 26.4.
3. If the resection is planned for gastric cancer, first **assess resectability**. Fixation of the tumor to the pancreas and celiac axis indicates inoperability. Hepatic metastases or peritoneal deposits confirm incurability but do not preclude palliative resection unless there is extensive involvement.
4. **Laparoscopic distal partial gastrectomy** is performed for intractable ulcer disease and for early distal gastric cancer. In the latter instance the duodenal bulb, greater omentum, and level-1 lymph nodes (lesser and greater curvature, infra- and suprapyloric nodes) are included in the resection.
   a. Begin **mobilizing the greater curvature** by proximal stapler transection of the gastroepiploic vessels. Continue the mobilization toward the duodenum.
   b. Divide adhesions between stomach and lesser sac with scissors.
   c. The author prefers to **ligate the right gastroepiploic** artery as it comes off the gastroduodenal, but some double-clip this vessel before division.

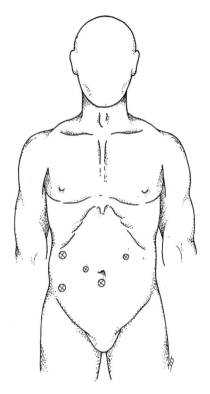

Figure 26.4. Port sites for laparoscopic gastric resections.

d. In cancer cases, the mobilization is different and consists of detachment of the greater omentum from the transverse colon and mesocolon until the greater curvature of the stomach is reached. This detachment requires traction of the transverse colon by an atraumatic grasper by the assistant and is performed either with electrocautery scissors or with the harmonic scalpel. The right gastroepiploic artery is secured as outlined previously.

e. Next pass a **vascular sling** along the posterior aspect of the stomach and then through an avascular window in the lesser omentum. Use this sling to pull the stomach up and away from the lesser sac and pancreas (Fig. 26.5).

f. Dissect and expose the **right gastric artery** from behind the stomach and secure it high up at the origin from the hepatic artery (especially in cancer cases, to ensure removal of the suprapyloric nodes). The author prefers ligature with an external slipknot but others clip the artery before division.

g. Mobilization of the **duodenal bulb** is needed in cancer cases. Secure the paraduodenal veins and divide fibrous attachments between the first part of the duodenum and the head of the pancreas.

    i. **Billroth II.** Divide the duodenum with an endoscopic linear stapler well beyond the pylorus. Carefully inspect the staple line and reinforce it with interrupted sutures when necessary.

    ii. **Billroth I.** Maintain duodenal continuity until the stomach is ready for resection.

h. **Ligation of the left gastric vessels in continuity.** The easiest and safest technique is to visualize the fold of the left gastric vessels as the stomach is pulled away from the retroperitoneum, then to underrun this fold containing the vessels with a 0-gauge suture, which is then tied intracorporeally in continuity. This completes the devascularization of the stomach.

i. **Gastric resection.** Select the proximal transection site. Clear the appropriate sites on the greater and lesser curves of fat and blood vessels.

    i. **Billroth II.** Transect the stomach vertically from the greater to the lesser curvature, using the endoscopic linear stapler. Usually, three applications of the 3.0-cm endoscopic linear

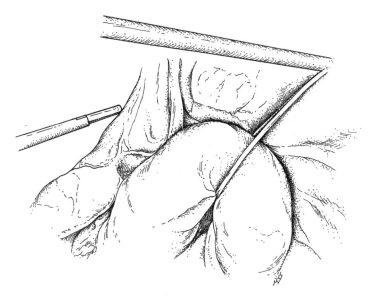

Figure 26.5. Sling retraction of the stomach.

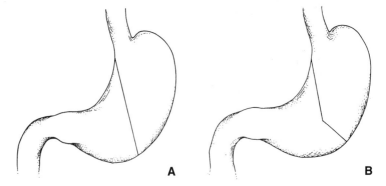

Figure 26.6. Stapler transection of proximal stomach for (A) Billroth II and (B) Billroth I gastrectomy.

      stapler (blue cartridge) are necessary. Remove the specimen through a protected upper midline minilaparotomy.

    ii. **Billroth I.** Make the first application of the endoscopic stapler vertically from the lesser curvature. The second and third applications are at an angle to the first application so that the transection line reaches the lesser curvature more proximally (Fig. 26.6). Divide the duodenum just beyond the pylorus with cutting electrocautery. Remove the specimen through a small midline laparotomy.

5. **Laparoscopic total gastrectomy** (total R1 gastrectomy) is usually performed for early cancers in the middle and upper third of the stomach and for gastric lymphomas. The technique is similar to that for laparoscopic distal gastrectomy with these important differences:

    a. **Mobilization of the greater curvature.** This involves detachment of the entire greater omentum from the transverse colon/mesocolon and is the most laborious part of the procedure.

        i. Apply downward traction on the transverse colon with a large atraumatic forceps. This is crucial.

       ii. Separate the greater omentum along a line extending from the right side (duodenum and hepatic flexure) to the inferior pole of the spleen and adjacent left paracolic gutter.

     iii. Transect the short gastric vessels using an endoscopic linear stapler (vascular cartridges) with preservation of the spleen.

     iv. On the right side, the right gastroepiploic vessels and the right gastric artery are ligated or clipped as described in connection with distal gastric resection (item 4.2).

b. **Division of lesser omentum** should be as cephalad as possible, extending from the divided right gastric vessels up to the left gastric vessels. Some small vessels in the lesser omentum may need to be coagulated.

c. **Elevate the stomach with a vascular sling** as previously described.

d. **Hiatal dissection with mobilization of the abdominal esophagus and bilateral truncal vagotomy**
    i.   Begin this dissection on the left with division of the gastrophrenic peritoneal reflection and blunt separation of the posterior aspect of the esophagogastric junction from the left crus until the hiatal canal is entered from the left side.
    ii. Then move to the right side, medial to the left gastric vessels with separation of the right crus from the esophagus to access the hiatal canal and mediastinum from the right side.
    iii. Identify the plane between the posterior wall of the esophagus and the preaortic fascia and dissect bluntly behind the esophagus until the left crus is reached.
    iv. Pass a sling around the mobilized esophagus and pull the esophagus away from the mediastinum. Complete the posterior separation of the esophagogastric junction.
    v.   Identify and divide the posterior vagus between the lower end of the right crus and the right edge of the esophagus. Similarly, identify and divide the anterior vagal trunk. Vagal division allows the surgeon to pull more of the mediastinal esophagus into the peritoneal cavity.

e. **Dissection of the celiac axis with division of the left gastric artery at its origin and division of the left gastric (coronary) vein**
    i.   Use the sling to retract the esophagogastric junction downward and to the left, and gently depress the superior margin of the pancreas.
    ii. Dissect carefully with scissors until the origin of the left gastric artery is identified without any doubt. The safest method of securing the left gastric artery is double ligation with external slip knots (using braided 1/0 ligatures) in continuity before the artery is divided (proximal to any lymph node mass). Other surgeons clip the artery but the author does not consider this to be safe. Often, there is insufficient space behind the artery to introduce the limb of the endoscopic linear stapler.

f. **Ligature (or clipping) of the right gastric artery.** This step is identical to that used in distal gastric resections.

g. **Duodenal mobilization and transection.** This step is identical to that used in distal gastric resections. At this stage the completely mobilized stomach (with greater omentum) is only attached to the esophagus.

h. **Proximal transection, removal of specimen, and reconstruction through upper midline minilaparotomy.** After the creation of the minilaparotomy, a noncrushing clamp is placed over the esophagus, some 2.5 cm proximal to the transection site, the esophagus is divided, and the specimen removed through the protected wound.

i. **Reconstruction** after laparoscopic gastrectomy can be performed intracorporeally (by staplers, suturing, or both) or through an upper midline minilaparotomy following the completed mobilization (open). In the latter instance, the protected minilaparotomy serves as the route for extraction of the resected specimen. The author rarely performs intracorporeal reconstruction except in palliative distal gastrectomy for incurable cancer with closure of duodenal stump and an antecolic stapled gastrojejunostomy. The reason for this change in practice is the poor functional results after intracorporeal reconstruction of the upper gastrointestinal tract, with open revision for postgastric symptoms being required in 5 out of 19 patients. Open reconstruction saves time and permits a more functional anastomosis.

6. **Reconstruction after distal gastrectomy for cancer (Billroth II)** is best performed with an open Roux-en-Y anastomosis through the minilaparotomy.

7. **Reconstruction after distal gastrectomy for benign disease (Billroth I).** The author's preference is for a sutured gastroduodenostomy through a minilaparotomy.

8. **Reconstruction after total gastrectomy for cancer.** Place a purse-string suture (2–0 Prolene) at the cut end of the esophagus. Introduce the anvil of the circular stapler into the lumen of the esophagus and tie the purse string over the stem. A classical Hunt-Lawrence Roux-en-Y is created from the upper jejunum using established open surgical technique for this procedure. The pouch is then stapled to the esophagus in standard fashion.

F. HALS D_1 and D_2 Gastrectomy

A. Access Devices

The second-generation hand access devices (Omniport, Lapdisk, Gelport) are now generally used. The author's experience and preference is for the Omniport (Fig. 26.7). The Omniport has a number of advantages for this procedure:

- Easy to insert (Fig. 26.8A)
- Consists of one component
- Provides comfortable hand seal and maintains the capnoperitoneum
- Provides full protection of the abdominal parieties
- Enables withdrawal, reinsertion of hand(s) and instruments, sponges, and staplers without loss of capnoperitoneum
- Enables good hand reach (Fig. 26.8B)

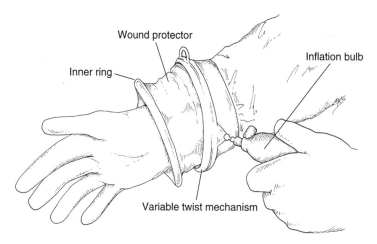

Figure 26.7. The Omniport: its two flexible rubber rings that straddle the abdominal wall after insertion are connected to a double-layer spiral cuff that closes on the surgeon's wrist and expands over the wound edges when inflated.

B. Procedure

1. The port locations for HALS D_1 and D_2 gastrectomies are shown in Figure 26.9.
2. It is preferable for the access port to be inserted before the creation of the pneumoperitoneum. Make a small (6.0-cm) vertical incision (for surgeons who wear $7–7\frac{1}{2}$ gloves) in the lower epigastric region. Alternatively the wound is transverse, starting at the junction of the upper with lower two thirds of the epigastric midline and extending to the right hypochondrium. This gives slightly more working space and is preferable in patients with a narrow subcostal angle.
3. Then, stretch the wound manually and insert both rings of the Omniport device through the wound inside the peritoneal cavity, with the external ring (has attachment to the insufflating bulb) uppermost.
4. Exteriorize this superficial ring in a circular fashion to lie externally on the anterior abdominal wall (Fig. 26.8). When proper placement of the two rings has been checked, the assisting hand of the surgeon is inserted into the peritoneal cavity, the insufflating bulb attached, and the cuff inflated around the wrist and over the external ring. The site of the optical port is then selected and the port introduced through a small skin incision with the "internal hand" cupped beneath the site to protect the intestines.

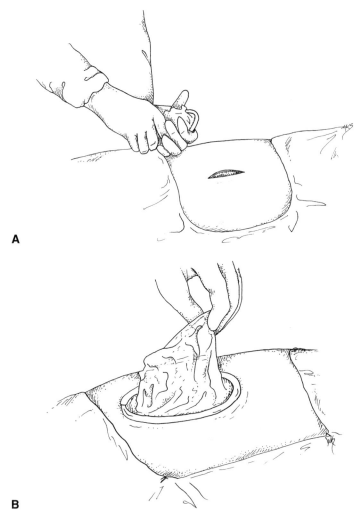

A

B

Figure 26.8. A. Insertion of Omniport. B. Omniport in place.

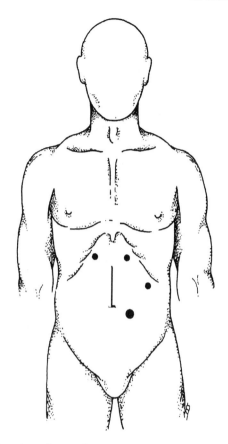

Figure 26.9. Location of ports for HALS D_1 and D_2 gastrectomy: Omniport; optical port; instrument ports.

5. The technique of gastric resection (partial, distal, D_1, D_2) is essentially the same as that used in the laparoscopically assisted approach. Nowadays, newer forms of hemostatic dissection (ultrasonic and Liga-Sure cutting devices) are increasingly used for the gastric mobilization as they are probably safer and certainly reduce instrument traffic.

6. The Omniport is opened but left in place as a wound protector at the end of the operation to extract the specimen and for the reconstruction of the upper gastrointestinal tract after both partial and total gastrectomy.

G. Complications

1. **Laparoendoluminal resections**
   a. **Bleeding** requiring transfusion occurred in one case (out of 10) in the author's experience.
   b. Other possible complications include unrecognized or delayed gastric perforation (excessive electrocutting/coagulation with collateral damage) at the site of local submucosal excision. In full-thickness local resections, suture line leakage is also possible.

2. **Laparoscopic partial or total gastrectomy**
   a. **Pneumothorax** can occur if the pleura is damaged during mobilization of the mediastinal esophagus. Carbon dioxide then insufflates into the pleural space and tension pneumothorax results. Placement of a chest tube corrects the cardiopulmonary compromise but may cause desufflation of the pneumoperitoneum through the chest drain. If this happens, intermittent occlusion of the chest drain allows completion of the operation.
   b. **Bleeding from suture line.** In our experience postoperative oozing from intracorporeally stapled gastrojejunal anastomosis is not uncommon (18%), may require transfusion, and generally stops. It is less frequent (5%) after hand-sutured anastomosis.
   c. **Anastomotic leak** results in a localized collection in the supracolic compartment with fever and leukocytosis. Drainage is required (open or percutaneous) and is often followed by an external fistula. Intravenous hyperalimentation is needed until closure of the fistula.
   d. **Pancreatic injury:** this usually declares itself in the postoperative period with ileus, pain, and hyperamylasemia. The pancreatitis may be severe and necrotizing.
   e. **Poor functional result** is common (25%) after intracorporeal reconstruction. The most common problems are vomiting and bile reflux.

G. Selected References

Cuschieri A. Gastric resections. In: Cuschieri A, Buess G, Perissat J, eds. Operative Manual of Endoscopic Surgery. New York: Springer-Verlag, 1993.

Goh P. Laparoscopic Billroth II gastrectomy. Semin Laparosc Surg 1994;1:171–181.

Goh PMY, Alpont A, Mak K, Kum CK. Early international results of laparoscopic gastrectomy. Surg Endosc 1997;11:650–652.

Hyung WJ, Cheong JH, Kim J, Chen J, Choi SH, Noh SH. Application of minimally invasive treatment for early gastric cancer. J Surg Oncol 2004;85:181–185.

Kitano S, Shiraishi N. Current status of laparoscopic gastrectomy for cancer in Japan. Surg Endosc 2004;18:182–185.

Kitano S, Iso Y, Moriyama M, Sugimacki K. Laparoscopic assisted Billroth I gastrectomy. Surg Laparosc Endosc 1994;4:146–148.

Lorente J. Laparoscopic gastric resection for gastric leiomyoma. Surg Endosc 1994;8: 887–889.

Uyama I, Ogiwara H, Takahara T, Kato Y, Kikuchi K, Iida S. Laparoscopic and minila-parotomy Billroth I gastrectomy for gastric ulcer using an abdominal wall-lifting method. J Laparoendosc Surg 1994;4:441–445.

27.1 Laparoscopic Bariatric Surgery: Principles of Patient Selection and Choice of Operation

Daniel R. Cottam, M.D.
Giselle G. Hamad, M.D.
Philip R. Schauer, M.D.

A. Indications

Morbid obesity, a serious health problem that causes substantial morbidity and mortality, is reaching epidemic proportions in the United States. More than 58 million adult Americans (one third of the adult population) are overweight, and there are approximately 260,000 to 380,000 deaths a year from factors related to obesity. This exceeds the aggregate U.S. totals of lung (154,000), colon (48,000), breast (4,000), and prostate (30,200) cancer combined.

Obesity is defined as a body weight that exceeds ideal body weight by 20%, or a body mass index of 30 to 35 kg/m². Morbidly obese persons generally exceed ideal body weight by 100 pounds or more or are 100% over ideal body weight. In 1991, the National Institutes of Health defined *morbid obesity* as a body mass index of 35 kg/m² or greater with severe obesity-related comorbid illness or a body mass index of 40 kg/m² or greater without comorbid illness. Approximately 4 million Americans have a body mass index between 35 and 40 kg/m², and an additional 4 million have a body mass index exceeding 40 kg/m².

Patients with a body mass index greater than 40 kg/m² without comorbid illness and patients with a body mass index of 35 to 40 kg/m² with comorbid illness are candidates for bariatric surgery. The patient must have previously attempted weight loss by diet, exercise, behavior modification, or medication. He or she must understand and accept the risks of surgery and the commitments required in terms of lifestyle and diet. Furthermore, the patient must be motivated to comply with lifelong vitamin supplementation and follow-up.

The goal of bariatric surgery is to improve the health of morbidly obese patients by achieving long-term, durable weight loss. It reduces caloric intake or absorption of calories from food and may modify eating behavior by promoting slow ingestion of small boluses of food.

B. Preoperative and Postoperative Care

Preoperatively all patients must undergo a thorough history and physical examination, during which medical comorbid illnesses are identified. Preoperative testing should be performed, and additional studies should be considered depending on the patient's burden of comorbid illness.

Morbidly obese persons are at an increased risk for postoperative cardiovascular events. This results from the higher rates of hypertension, coronary artery disease, left ventricular hypertrophy, congestive heart failure, and pulmonary hypertension among the morbidly obese. Preoperative electrocardiography should be done in all patients. Patients with cardiovascular disease should undergo preoperative evaluation by a cardiologist. Echocardiography, stress testing, and cardiac catheterization may be indicated in some patients.

Loud snoring or daytime hypersomnolence in a morbidly obese patient should prompt a workup for respiratory insufficiency. Patients with significant sleep apnea should be treated with nasal continuous positive airway pressure. These patients are at high risk for acute upper airway obstruction in the postoperative period. The obesity hypoventilation syndrome is characterized by hypoxemia (partial pressure of arterial oxygen <55 mm Hg) and hypercarbia (partial pressure of arterial carbon dioxide >47 torr) with severe pulmonary hypertension and polycythemia. Patients with obstructive sleep apnea, the obesity hypoventilation syndrome, or severe asthma should undergo preoperative evaluation by a pulmonologist.

Patients with gastroesophageal reflux should undergo upper endoscopy with possible biopsy to rule out esophagitis or Barrett's esophagus.

Nutritional evaluation and education is invaluable in the preoperative period. The dietician may help determine whether the patient understands the necessary changes in postoperative eating habits and food choices.

Additionally some patients may require endocrine, gastroenterology, nephrology, or gynecology consults, depending on individual circumstances.

The operations currently used to manage morbid obesity involve gastric restriction with or without intestinal malabsorption. The only widespread purely gastric restrictive procedure practiced in the United States today is adjustable Silatic gastric banding. Purely malabsorptive procedures include biliopancreatic diversion, and biliopancreatic diversion with duodenal switch. The Roux-en-Y gastric bypass offers both restriction and malabsorption.

Postoperative care and follow-up is critical to promptly diagnose and manage postoperative complications. Routine thromboprophylaxis with sequential compression devices, subcutaneous heparin, or low-molecular-weight heparin is important to prevent thromboembolic events. Oral liquid diet is initiated generally after a water-soluble contrast swallow examination has confirmed the absence of an anastomotic leak. After a variable interval, the patient is advanced to a pureed diet and gradually to soft and then solid food.

Patients must comply with lifelong follow-up, exercise, and vitamin supplementation after undergoing bariatric surgery. They must significantly alter their eating behavior for life because of their revised gastrointestinal anatomy. Follow-up includes assessment of weight loss trends; compliance with diet, exercise, and vitamin supplementation; and regular monitoring of metabolic and nutritional status.

Overall, surgery is the most effective method of achieving durable, medically significant weight loss in morbidly obese persons. In 1991, the National Institutes of Health Consensus Development Conference stated that surgical therapy should be offered to morbidly obese patients unresponsive to nonsurgical programs for weight loss. The operations advocated at that time were gastric bypass and vertical banded gastroplasty. In an update in 1996, the panel reaffirmed that "surgery remains the only effective treatment for patients with morbid obesity." It stated that its previous endorsement of vertical banded gastroplasty may have been "premature" and that laparoscopic gastric banding and biliopancreatic diversion merit consideration.

C. Laparotomy Versus Laparoscopy

Compared with access by laparotomy, laparoscopic approaches to major abdominal operations have been shown to reduce organ-system impairment, resulting in significantly reduced perioperative morbidity and recovery time. Physiologically these advantages include less inflammatory insult, less immune suppression, and better pulmonary function. Clinically these advantages are fewer ventral hernias formed, fewer hospital days required, fewer wound infections, fewer adhesive related complications, and better cosmesis.

D. Laparoscopic Adjustable Gastric Banding

1. Mechanism of Action

Laparoscopic adjustable gastric banding (LAGB) involves the placement of a silicone band around the proximal stomach to restrict the amount of solid food that can be ingested at one time (see Chapter 27.3). Because the band is adjustable, the amount of restriction can be increased or decreased depending on the patient's weight loss or the onset of side effects (e.g., vomiting).

2. Efficacy

Mean excess weight loss at one year is between 45% and 55% at 1 year and 50% and 56% at 2 years. These weights can be maintained with proper follow-up. Initial reports indicate that a body mass index of 31 to $34\,kg/m^2$ at 6 years can be expected. Furthermore, there is complete resolution or improvement of diabetes, hypertension, asthma, dyslipidemia, reflux esophagitis, and sleep apnea. Quality-of-life measurements improve substantially after laparoscopic adjustable gastric banding.

The impressive weight loss results after laparoscopic adjustable gastric banding reported in Australia and Europe have not been reproduced in the United States. Intermediate results show a maximum weight loss of 34% to 42% in the United States, which is lower than that observed in Australia and Europe. Excess weight loss at one of the original U.S. centers performing laparoscopic adjustable gastric banding was 18% (range, 5–38%).

There is also concern whether LAGB should be performedin the super morbidly obese (body mass index >50) as these patients tend to be refractory to restrictive procedures.

3. Complications

The mortality (0.0–0.5%) and conversion rates are low (0–4%). Intraoperative complications include splenic injury, esophageal or gastric injury (0–1% of patients), and bleeding (0–1%). Early postoperative complications include bleeding (0.0–0.5%), wound infection (0–1%), and food intolerance (0–11%). Late complications include slippage of the band (7.3–21%), band erosion (1.9–7.5%), tubing-related problems (4.2%), leakage of the reservoir, persistent vomiting (13%), pouch dilatation (5.2%), and poor weight loss. Fixation of the band to the stomach has reduced the incidence of postoperative gastric prolapse to less than 5% in most series with the use of the pars flaccida technique.

E. Laparoscopic Biliopancreatic Diversion

1. Mechanism of Action

Laparoscopic biliopancreatic diversion (LBPD) and laparoscopic biliopancreatic diversion with duodenal switch (LBPDS) are minimally invasive bariatric surgical procedures that provide modest gastric restriction but significant intestinal malabsorption (see Chapter 27.5). A 50- to 100-cm common absorptive alimentary channel is created proximal to the ileocecal valve; digestion and absorption are limited to this segment of bowel.

2. Efficacy

Weight loss after laparoscopic biliopancreatic diversion is similar to open procedures with 45% to 52% excess weight loss at 6 months and 68% to 90% at one year. Median operative time ranges from 195 to 210 minutes. Operative times, in general, increase with rising body mass index.

3. Complications

Mortality is 0% to 2.5%, major morbidity varies from 12.5% to 15%, including venous thrombosis (0–2.5%), pulmonary embolism (0–5%), staple-line hemorrhage (0–10%), and subphrenic abscess (0–2.5%) and anastomotic leak (0–2.5%) in reported series. Long-term morbidity includes anemia, fat-soluble vitamin deficiencies, and protein calorie malnutrition However, experience with this laparoscopic procedure is limited to four small series; thus the true rate of complications may be hard to ascertain.

F. Laparoscopic Roux-en-Y Gastric Bypass

1. Mechanism of Action

Laparoscopic Roux-en-Y gastric bypass (see Chapter 27.4) creates a small gastric pouch to restrict food intake, while the Roux-en-Y configuration provides modest malabsorption of calories and nutrients.

2. Efficacy

In the literature, the mean excess weight loss after laparoscopic Roux-en-Y gastric bypass ranges from 69% to 82%, in the first 24 months or less. A mean excess weight loss of 73% can be maintained of up to 5 years following laparoscopic gastric bypass. Most comorbid conditions were improved or eradicated, including diabetes mellitus, hypertension, sleep apnea, and reflux. Quality of life was improved significantly.

3. Complications

Postoperative complications include pulmonary embolism (0–1.5%), anastomotic leak (1.5–5.8%), bleeding (0–3.3%), and pulmonary complications (0–5.8%). Stenosis of the gastrojejunostomy is observed in 1.6% to 6.3% of patients. Other complications include internal hernia (2.5%), gallstones (1.4%), marginal ulcer (1.4%), and staple-line failure (1%). Late complications include anemia and vitamin deficiencies.

G. Summary

Curently there is no universal standard defining the most appropriate weight loss procedure to perform. What is certain, however, is that the laparoscopic approach can safely be applied to all types of bariatric operation. All laparoscopic bariatric procedures significantly reduce perioperative morbidity and mortality, thereby justifying the acquisition of skills needed to perform these complex procedures.

H. Selected References

Allison DB, Fontaine KR, Manson JE, et al. Annual deaths attributable to obesity in the United States. JAMA 1999;282:1530–1538.

Angrisani L, Alkilani M, Basso N, et al. Italian Collaborative Study Group for the Lap-Band System. Laparoscopic Italian experience with the Lap-Band. Obes Surg 2001;11(3):307–310.

Brolin, R. Update: NIH Consensus Conference Gastrointestinal Surgery for Severe Obesity. Nutrition 1996;12:403–404.

Chevallier JM, Zinzindohoué F, Elian N, et al. Adjustable gastric banding in a public university hospital: prospective analysis of 400 patients. Obes Surg 2002;12:93–99.

DeMaria EJ, SH, Kellum JM, Meador JG, Wolfe LG. Results of 281 consecutive total laparoscopic Roux-en-Y gastric bypasses to treat morbid obesity. Ann Surg 2002;235(5):640–645.

Favretti F, Cadiere GM, Segato G. Laparoscopic banding: selection and technique in 830 patients. Obes Surg 2002;12:385–390.

Gastrointestinal Surgery for Severe Obesity; Consensus Development Conference Panel. Ann Intern Med 1991;115:956–961.

Higa KD, HT, Boone KB. Laparoscopic Roux-en-Y gastric bypass: technique and 3-year follow-up. J Laparoendosc Adv Surg Techniques A 2001;11(6):377–382.

Nguyen NT, Wolfe BM. Laparoscopic versus open gastric bypass. Semin Laparosc Surg 2002;9(2):86–93.

O'Brien PE, Dixon J, Brown W, et al. The laparoscopic adjustable gastric band (Lap-Band): a prospective study of medium-term effects on weight, health and quality of life. Obes Surg 2002;12(5):652–660.

Ren CJ, Patterson E, Gagner M. Early results of laparoscopic biliopancreatic diversion with duodenal switch: a case series of 40 consecutive patients. Obes Surg 2000;10:514–523.

Schauer PR, Ikramuddin S. Outcomes after laparoscopic Roux-en-Y gastric bypass for morbid obesity. Ann Surg 2000;232:515–529.

Schauer PR, Ikramuddin S. Laparoscopic surgery for morbid obesity. Surg Clin North Am 2001;81:1145–1179.

Schauer P, Ikramuddin S, Hamad G, Gourash W. The learning curve for laparoscopic Roux-en-Y gastric bypass is 100 cases. Surg Endosc 2003;17:212–215.

Scopinaro N, Marinari G, Camerini G. Laparoscopic standard biliopancreatic diversion: technique and preliminary results. Obes Surg 2001;12:362–365.

Wittgrove AC, Clark G. Laparoscopic gastric bypass: a five year prospective study of 500 patients followed from 3 to 60 months. Obes Surg 1999;9:123–143.

27.2 Instrumentation, Room Setup, and Adjuncts for Laparoscopy in the Morbidly Obese

Ninh T. Nguyen, M.D., F.A.C.S.

A. Instrumentation

The two most commonly performed bariatric surgical procedures are the laparoscopic Roux-en-Y gastric bypass and laparoscopic adjustable gastric banding. These procedures are technically challenging operations and require certain specialized instrumentation. The following instruments are considered an integral part of these bariatric procedures.

1. **The Veress insufflation needle** is often used for initial introduction of pneumoperitoneum and is the preferred method of access.

    a. The initial intra-abdominal pressure in the morbidly obese tends to be high, in the range of 9 to 10 mm Hg. Intra-abdominal pressure of the nonobese is normally less than 4 mm Hg.

    b. An alternative method of access is the Hasson open cannula technique. The Hasson technique is not commonly performed in the morbidly obese because the thick layer of subcutaneous tissue makes it difficult to provide exposure of the fascial layer through a small skin incision.

2. **Trocars** with normal length are sufficient in most cases; however, in the super-superobese (body mass index >60 kg/m²), longer trocars can be helpful.

    a. Normally five or six trocars are used for laparoscopic bariatric surgery. Five abdominal trocars should be sufficient in most cases, but in difficult cases affording poor exposure, a sixth trocar is placed.

    b. The trocars range in size from 5 to 15 mm in diameter. Normally, three 5-mm trocars are placed to introduce grasping instruments, an 11-mm trocar is placed for the laparoscope, and a 12-mm trocar is placed for the mechanical stapling instruments. For laparoscopic adjustable gastric banding, a 15-mm trocar is required for insertion of the band.

    c. The initial trocar position can be either at the umbilicus or at the left midclavicular line. Technique for introduction of the trocar is very important in the morbidly obese. All trocars should be placed through the surgical incision and perpendicular to the abdominal cavity. If a trocar is placed tangentially, so that the

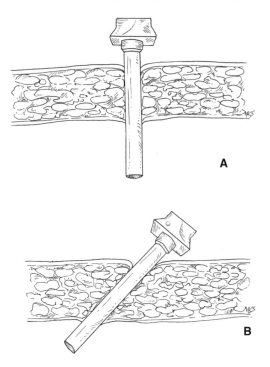

Figure 27.2.1. A. Correct placement of trocar in morbidly obese patients.
B. Incorrect placement of trocar.

surgical incision and the fascial entrance are in different planes,
its movement will be severely limited (Fig. 27.2.1).
3. **The liver retractor** is used to retract the left lobe of the liver for expo-
    sure of the gastroesophageal junction and the gastric cardia. There are
    two different types of liver retractor. The Nathanson liver retractor
    (Cook Surgical, Bloomington, IN) is placed in the subxiphoid posi-
    tion, and the Snowden Pencer retractor (Snowden Pencer, Tucker, GA)
    is placed through a 5-mm trocar positioned at the right anterior axil-
    lary line in the subcostal region. Once positioned, these devices are
    attached to a self-retaining mechanical arm.
4. **The ultrasonic devices** (Harmonic Scalpel, Ethicon Endo-Surgery,
    Cincinnati, OH; AutoSonix Ultrashears, US Surgical, Norwalk, CT)
    are instruments that utilize ultrasonic vibration to achieve hemostasis
    and tissue cutting.
5. **Laparoscopic mechanical staplers** are used for division and recon-
    struction of intestinal continuity. Mechanical staplers consist of either
    the linear or circular stapler.

       a.   Linear staplers can be used for creation of the gastric pouch, the jejunojejunostomy, and the gastrojejunostomy in laparoscopic gastric bypass.

       b.   Some surgeons use the circular stapler for creation of the gastro-jejunostomy anastomosis. In this procedure, the anvil of the circular stapler is placed into the gastric pouch. The original description for placement of the anvil into the gastric pouch is the transoral technique, similar to the technique for percutaneous gastrostomy tube (PEG) placement. The size of the circular stapler used for construction of the gastrojejunostomy is 21 or 25 mm.

   6.   **Laparoscopic instruments** consist of the following: scissors, atraumatic graspers, needle drivers, suturing instruments, and clip appliers. Suturing instruments consist of either a conventional needle driver or specialized instruments to facilitate intracorporeal suturing.

B. Room and Equipment Setup

   1.   **Room layout** for laparoscopic bariatric surgical procedures is very similar to that for other laparoscopic operations. General considerations include the size of the operating room and the location of the doors, as the fiberoptic gastroscope is commonly brought in for evaluation of the gastrojejunostomy anastomosis. Figure 27.2.2 shows a typical setup for a laparoscopic bariatric surgical procedure.

   2.   **Video equipment** should include a three-chip camera, a 10-mm laparoscope with 45-degree angle, a light source, an insufflator, and two monitors. A monitor is placed on the right and left sides of the patient at the head of the operating table.

   3.   **The operating room table** should have the capacity to bear heavy patients and to move them in Trendelenburg and reverse Trendelenburg positions.

C. Patient Preparation and Adjuncts

   1.   A bowel preparation is performed the day before the surgery.

   2.   The patient is positioned supine with both arms extended on the arm board. An egg-crate mattress is placed underneath both arms to avoid pressure injury. The surgeon stands on the patient's right side and the assistant stands on the patient's left side. A foot board is used to securely position the patient's feet on a flat platform in preparation for placement into reverse Trendelenburg position. The patient's legs are taped securely to the bed and a safety strap is placed around the patient's thighs.

   3.   **Sequential compression device** and graduated compression stockings are applied to the lower extremities as prophylaxis for deep venous thrombosis.

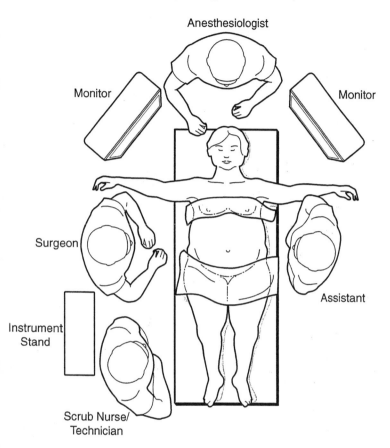

Figure 27.2.2. Room setup and patient position for laparoscopic bariatric surgery.

4. A Foley catheter and an orogastric tube are inserted to evacuate the bladder and stomach before insertion of the Veress needle.
5. Prophylactic antibiotics are used prior to making the initial surgical incision.

D. Selected References

Ammori BJ, Vezakis A, Davides D, Martin G, Larvin M, McMahon MJ. Laparoscopic cholecystectomy in morbidly obese patients. Surg Endosc 2001;15:S91.

Higa KD, Boone KB, Ho T. Complications of the laparoscopic Roux-en-Y gastric bypass: 1,040 patients—what have we learned? Obes Surg 2000;10:509–513.

Miles RH, Carballo RE, Prinz RA, et al. Laparoscopy: the preferred method of cholecystectomy in the morbidly obese. Surgery 1992;112:818–823.

Nguyen NT, Goldman C, Rosenquist CJ, et al. Laparoscopic versus open gastric bypass: a randomized study of outcomes, quality of life, and costs. Ann Surg 2001; 234:279–289.

Schauer PR, Ikramuddin S. Laparoscopic surgery for morbid obesity. Surg Clin North Am 2001;81:1145–1179.

Schauer PR, Ikramuddin S, Gourash W, et al. Outcomes after laparoscopic Roux-en-Y gastric bypass for morbid obesity. Ann Surg 2000;232:515–529.

Wittgrove AC, Clark GW. Laparoscopic gastric bypass, Roux-en-Y 500 patients: technique and results, with 3–60 month follow-up. Obes Surg 2000;10:233–239.

27.3 Laparoscopic Gastric Banding

Todd A. Kellogg, M.D.
Sayeed Ikramuddin, M.D.

A. Introduction

The history of gastric banding can be traced back to Edward Mason at the University of Iowa. Having been exposed to the jejunoileal bypass operations of the 1950s, he set forth to describe procedures that were safer, with a more predictable outcome. He described the first purely restrictive gastric operation in 1971. By the 1980s the technique had evolved to a vertically stapled gastric pouch with an outlet reinforced by a Silastic ring. One of the main drawbacks of the operation was the limiting nature of the stoma, resulting in intolerance of certain foods in particular breads and meat. A few years before this final technique was published, surgeons began to experiment with true gastric banding. Wilkinson reported the use of a fixed band rather than a reinforced pouch in 1978. In 1986 Kuzmak introduced the Silastic adjustable gastric band. It is important to note that this operation was true gastric banding with lateral imbrication of the band with the body and fundus of the stomach.

The emergence of laparoscopic surgery was extended to laparoscopic gastric and later esophagogastric banding, with Mitiku Belachew of Belgium being instrumental in the development of this field. There are at least four types of band available today. The only adjustable gastric band that is approved for use in the Unites States by the Food and Drug Administration is the LapBand™ (INAMED Corporation, Santa Barbara, CA). Three sizes are available: 9.75, 10.0, and 11.0 cm. The Swedish Adjustable Gastric Band is undergoing clinical trials in the United States.

B. The Adjustable Gastric Band

The laparoscopic adjustable gastric band (LAGB) is composed of three main parts: a Silastic inflatable circular 5-mL balloon, 30 cm of Silastic tubing, and an access port (Fig. 27.3.1). The ends of the balloon are connected by means of a self-locking mechanism around the cardia of the stomach. The tubing is exteriorized on the abdominal wall and attached to the access port, which is then secured to the anterior fascia, typically over the left rectus muscle.

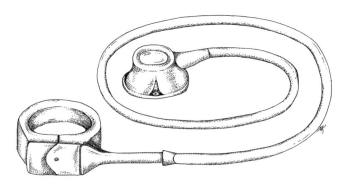

Figure 27.3.1. The LapBand system consists of a Silastic, inflatable, circular 5-mL balloon, 30 cm of Silastic tubing, and an access port.

C. Patient Preparation

1. As is the case for all bariatric surgery patients, preoperative multi-disciplinary evaluation is mandatory for patients being considered for LAGB placement. Medical evaluation allows preoperative optimization of comorbid conditions such as hypertension, diabetes, and sleep apnea. The role of the psychologist has been growing in most bariatric practices. Although postoperative success is not possible to accurately predict with such an evaluation, it is possible to identify preclusive conditions such as borderline personality disorder and severe depression.
2. A careful history and physical examination must be performed. It is especially important to preoperatively determine a history of dysphagia or gastroesophageal reflux disease. If there is any question of dysmotility, manometry and an upper gastrointestinal series should be performed preoperatively. In the setting of prolonged gastroesophageal reflux disease, an upper endoscopy should be performed to rule out the presence of Barrett's metaplasia.
3. Patients are asked to take a bottle of magnesium citrate the day prior to surgery. Bowel preparation instructions are given to the patient one-week prior to surgery. Postoperative dietary instructions are emphasized during the preoperative period. No routine preoperative ultrasound examination of the gallbladder is performed unless the patient is symptomatic.
4. Heparin and prophylactic antibiotics are administered to all patients 30 minutes prior to incision.

D. Techniques of Placement

1. Patient positioning
    a. The patient is placed supine on the operating room table with a foot board and two security belts to prevent slippage on the table. The arms are positioned out at 90 degrees.
    b. Pneumatic compression devices are placed on the lower extremities and activated prior to induction of general anesthesia.
    c. A pillow is placed under the legs of patients with severe degenerative joint disease.
2. Port placement
    a. We use a five- to six-port technique for placement of the lap band. There are many acceptable arrangements for port placement. The objective is to have the midline camera port near the hiatus to facilitate optimal exposure.
    b. Initial access is achieved in the left upper quadrant in the midclavicular line by using a Veress needle. This is a safe and reproducible technique in the vast majority of patients. Use of the Veress needle is dependent on the comfort level of the surgeon. Care should be taken in patients with extreme central obesity, who may be more prone to hepatic steatosis and subsequent liver enlargement. Once ports have been placed, initial inspection of the abdomen is carried out to rule out the presence of occult malignancy, gynecologic pathology, or other conditions that may change the operative plan.
3. Initial dissection. Two dissection techniques are described for placement of the band around the gastric cardia: the perigastric, and pars flaccida techniques.
    a. **Perigastric.** This was the original technique for band placement. It involves dissection at the lesser curvature, into the lesser sac, and toward the angle of His. It is now universally recognized that this technique increases the incidence of posterior gastric herniation (15–20%). This has resulted in a shift toward use of the pars flaccida technique whenever possible.
    b. **Pars flaccida** (Fig. 27.3.2): This is the most common approach used today. It begins in the very proximal lesser curve fatty tissue and extends retrogastrically beneath the gastroesophageal junction just in front of (inferior to) the confluence of the right and left crura, toward the angle of His. Care must be taken to avoid injury to the esophagus. It is important not enter the lesser sac. The dissection is made in the posterior gastric fatty tissue, which is adherent to the posterior stomach. When the dissection is completed, a grasper is placed within this retrogastric tunnel, exiting at the angle of His.
4. Band placement and positioning
    a. With tubing attached, the band is introduced into the abdomen through the 15-mm port, handed to the retrogastric grasper,

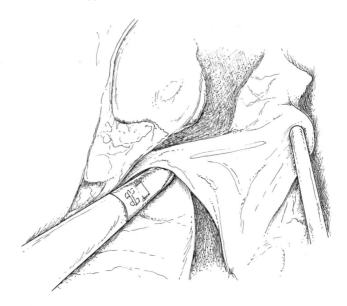

Figure 27.3.2. The pars flaccida technique. A tunnel is made in the posterior gastric fatty tissue at the level of the gastroesophageal junction and just inferior to the crural confluence. This technique decreases the incidence of posterior gastric herniation.

and pulled behind the stomach through the tunnel and into place. Once appropriately positioned, the band is closed by pulling the band tail through the buckle until the locking mechanism engages.

b.   A balloon catheter is available to assist in determining the site of dissection (INAMED Corporation, Santa Barbara, CA). The balloon is introduced transorally until its tip is in the stomach. It is then inflated with 25 mL of saline and withdrawn until it lodges in the gastroesophageal junction. The equator of the balloon represents the appropriate site of dissection for formation of a 15-mL pouch.

5.   Securing the band. Once the band has been appropriately positioned and locked, three to four anterior gastrogastric fixation sutures are placed, effectively imbricating gastric tissue around the band to prevent herniation anteriorly.

6.   Access port placement

a.   The band tubing is brought out through the 15-mm port. The ports are removed under direct laparoscopic visualization to

ensure hemostasis. A suprafascial subcutaneous pocket is developed.
b. The access port is attached to the tubing and secured to the fascia by using four interrupted 2–0 nonabsorbable sutures. Redundant tubing is replaced into the abdomen.
c. The fascial defect is closed with interrupted absorbable suture. The wound is irrigated with normal saline and all loose debris removed from the wound. The subcutaneous tissue is reapproximated with absorbable suture to cover the access port. The skin is reapproximated with a continuous suture.

D. LAGB Adjustment

1. The key to a successful weight loss after LAGB placement is to make periodic adjustments that allow control over the degree of restriction. This intervention is unique to the adjustable band and may hold an advantage over vertical banded gastroplasty. Various algorithms for adjustment have been suggested. In general, we wait at least 6 weeks after LAGB placement before performing the first adjustment. The patient's weight loss and food volume tolerance are followed closely, and further adjustments are performed when there is a plateau in further weight loss. There are two general methods for performing LAGB adjustments.
   a. **Office-based adjustments** are performed by accessing the subcutaneous port under sterile conditions and injecting saline (typically 0.25–0.5 mL), while the ability of the patient to ingest water is assessed. The adjustment is complete when the patient experiences a renewed sense of fullness without regurgitation of water.
   b. **Fluoroscopically guided adjustments** are performed in the radiology department. The procedure is similar to office-based adjustments except that the result is objectively assessed fluoroscopically while the patient ingests thin barium. Fine adjustments in band restriction can then be made based on a combination of patient feedback and fluoroscopic appearance. A general algorithm for fluoroscopic band adjustment is depicted in Figure 27.3.3.
2. As is the case after all bariatric procedures, success is contingent upon comprehensive nutritional follow-up and a consistent exercise regimen. The primary cause of weight loss failure after band placement is noncompliance with the recommended postprocedure diet. High-carbohydrate and high-fat liquid foodstuffs should be avoided under all circumstances.

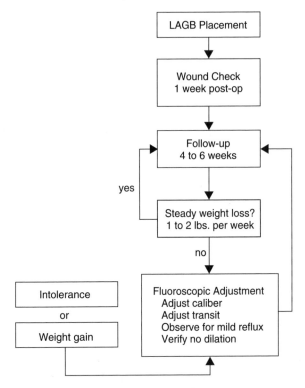

Figure 27.3.3. A suggested algorithm for LapBand adjustment under fluoroscopic guidance. The volume injected varies depending on the appearance under fluoroscopy and patient feedback. Intolerance generally manifests as persistent vomiting or regurgitation of ingested liquids.

E. Complications

1. Port-related complications
    a. **Access port dysfunction, flipping or angulation** (0.5–7.3%) occurs occasionally in our practice despite four-corner anchoring to the fascia. This situation makes port access very difficult or impossible. Fluoroscopic guidance is necessary to access the port. If the port has flipped radically, it is best to relocate the port under anesthesia.
    b. **Tubing breakage** (0.5–2%) can more readily occur if there is angulation of the tubing at any point in its course. We have seen this happen near the port twice. In both cases the patients complained of right lower quadrant pain. Imaging studies demonstrated the tubing extending to the right lower quadrant, with the

fractured end irritating the peritoneum of the anterior abdominal wall of the right lower quadrant. In such a case, laparoscopic exploration with retrieval and inspection of the fractured tubing is performed. Reattachment to a new port relocated to a different subcutaneous site is preferred. Careful attention to technique to avoid potential angulation or kinking of the tubing will help prevent this complication.

   c. **Port site infection** occurs uncommonly (0.4–4%). A superficial cellulitis, which can be treated with antibiotics initially in an attempt to salvage the port, can be difficult to distinguish from an immune-mediated foreign body reaction seen in some patients. Removal of the port is necessary to resolve any draining wound. In cases of extensive infection, the entire LAGB should be removed and antibiotic therapy initiated. Replacement with a new LAGB can be performed when the infection has completely resolved.

2. Band slippage

   a. **Anterior band slippage** (1.5–2.2%) with consequent **gastric herniation** can occur if anterior fixation of the band was inadequate or as a result of early severe vomiting. Immediate band deflation followed by laparoscopic exploration should be performed, with reduction of the herniated stomach, band repositioning, and anterior fixation of the band.

   b. **Posterior band slippage** occurred with much higher frequency (15–20%) prior to development of the pars flaccida technique (see Section D.3.6). Management of posterior gastric herniation should be approached in a manner similar to that of the anterior variant. If the perigastric technique was used initially, a pars flaccida technique should be used subsequently.

3. Band erosion

   a. Band erosion occurs in 1.5% of patients by most reports. Patients can be asymptomatic, or they may present with a latent port site infection or an acute abdomen.

   b. Diagnosis is made by contrast radiograph or by upper endoscopy. Contrast radiographic studies can often be negative and should always be followed by upper endoscopy if there is clinical suspicion.

   c. Laparoscopic or open removal of the band and its components with gastrotomy repair should be performed as soon as the diagnosis is made. In the case of an acute perforation with associated abscess, laparotomy, closure of the perforation, and wide drainage should be performed.

   d. Some have advocated endoscopic removal, though this practice cannot be recommended at this time.

E. Outcomes

Outcomes reported in the literature are summarized in Table 27.3.1 and discussed briefly here.

Table 27.3.1. Reported outcomes after laparoscopic adjustable band placement.

Author	n	Percent Female	BMI (kg/m²)	OR time (min)	Conversions (%)	Complications (%)	Mean LOS (days)	Percent Reop	Follow-up (months)	Percent EWL
Zimmermann	894	85	42.0	35	1 (0.11%)	3 (0.33)	3.0	2	12	40
Belachew	763	78	42.0	62	0 (1.3)	92 (12.1)	NR	11.1	60	50
Dargent	500	80	43.0	NR	NR	40 (8)	NR	3.6	21	64
Fielding	335	82	46.7	71	3 (0.9)	26 (7.8)	1.4	3.6	18	62
Ren	115	85	47.5	NR	NR	25 (22)	NR	13	12	41.6*
O'Brien	277	88	44.5	57	5 (1.8)	12 (4.3)	3.9	4	48	70
Favretti	830	72	45.5	90	22 (2.7)	125 (15.2)	2.0	15	NR	NR
Zinzindohoué	500	88	44.3	105	12 (2.4)	52 (10.4)	4.5	10.4	36	55
Greenstein	250	NR	48.0	NR	NR	14 (5.6)	NR	5.2	72	42

BMI, body mass index; EWL, excess weight loss; LOS, length of stay; OR, operating room; Reop, reoperations; NR, not reported.
*% EWL of 43 patients followed for 12 months.

1. Weight loss
   a. Weight loss generally occurs in a slow steady and steady manner. Percent excess weight loss (EWL) is 40% to 70% at up to 6 years follow-up.
   b. Overall (early and late) complication rates vary from 0.33% to 22% as reported in the literature. However, most reports suggest overall complication rates in the 10% to 20% range.
   c. Mortality is generally reported to be less than 1%.
   d. Success or failure is highly dependent on postoperative follow-up. Band adjustments need to be performed in a timely fashion.
   e. Dietary counseling is extremely important for LAGB success. The majority of failures are due to noncompliance with diet.
2. Resolution of comorbidities. Most studies demonstrate a 60% to 72% improvement or complete resolution in comorbid conditions.

F. Conclusions

To this point, it has been demonstrated that the LAGB is safe and effective. However, excellent results require meticulous operative technique, vigilant systematic follow-up and adjustments, and close adherence by the patient to diet and exercise recommendations. As more data become available, firmer conclusions can be made regarding the long-term efficacy of the procedure.

G. Selected References

Belachew M, Belva PH, Desaive C. Long-term results of laparoscopic adjustable gastric banding for the treatment of morbid obesity. Obes Surg 2002;12(4):564–568.

Dargent J. Laparoscopic gastric banding: lessons from the first 500 patients in a single institution. Obes Surg 1999;9(5)446–452.

Favretti F, Cadiere GB, Segato G, et al. Laparoscopic banding: selection and technique in 830 patients. Obes Surg 2002;12(3):385–390.

Fielding GA, Rhodes M, Nathanson LK. Laparoscopic gastric banding for morbid obesity surgical outcome in 335 cases. Surg Endosc 1999;13:550–554.

Greenstein RJ, Martin L, MacDonald K, et al. The Lap-Band® system as surgical therapy for morbid obesity: intermediate results of the USA, multicenter, prospective study. Surg Endosc 1999;13:S1–S18.

O'Brien PE, Brown A, Smith PJ, et al. Prospective study of a laparoscopically placed, adjustable gastric band in the treatment of morbid obesity. Br J Surg 1999;85:113–118.

Ren CJ, Fielding GA. Laparoscopic adjustable gastric banding: surgical technique. J Laparoendosc Adv Surg Techniques A 2003;13(4):257–263.

Ren CJ, Horgan S, Ponce J. US experience with the Lap-Band system. Am J Surg 2002;184:46S–50S.

Zimmermann JM, Mashoyan PH, Michel G, et al. Laparoscopic adjustable silicon gastric banding: une étude préliminaire personnelle concernant 900 cas operés entre Juillet 1995 et Decembre 1998. J Coelio-Chirugie 1999;29:77.

Zinzindohoué F, Chevallier JM, Douard R, et al. Laparoscopic gastric banding: a minimally invasive surgical treatment for morbid obesity: prospective study of 500 consecutive patients. Ann Surg 2003;237(1):1–9.

27.4 Roux-en-Y Gastric Bypass

Daniel R. Cottam, M.D.
Giselle G. Hamad, M.D.
Philip R. Schauer, M.D.

A. Introduction

Gastric bypass introduces the variable of malabsorption to the concept of solid food restriction utilized by the open vertical-banded gastroplasty and the laparoscopic adjustable band techniques. The advantages of this procedure over a gastric restrictive operation include a 10% to 15% greater sustained weight loss and less difficulty in eating solid food. The disadvantages include a higher mortality rate, interference with absorption of iron, calcium, and vitamin B_{12} (imposing a lifelong requirement that these essential nutrients be supplemented), difficult accessibility for radiographic and endoscopic examination of the excluded segment, and an increased lifelong risk of peptic ulceration and closed-segment bowel obstruction.

B. Patient Position and Room Setup

Use an operating table capable of accommodating a morbidly obese patient. Position the patient supine, with legs spread as shown in Figure 27.4.1. The surgeon stands between the patient's legs, with an assistant and camera operator on the sides.

C. Technique:

1. Establish pneumoperitoneum and insert five or six access ports (Fig. 27.4.2).
2. Obtain access to the proximal stomach as described in Chapter 27.3. A balloon catheter may be placed to calibrate the size of the pouch (Fig. 27.4.3).
3. Divide the stomach by sequential application of a linear endoscopic stapler to produce a vertically oriented proximal gastric pouch measuring 15 to 30 mL (Fig. 27.4.4).
4. Identify the ligament of Treitz, and divide the jejunum 30 to 50 cm distally with a linear stapler (Fig. 27.4.5).

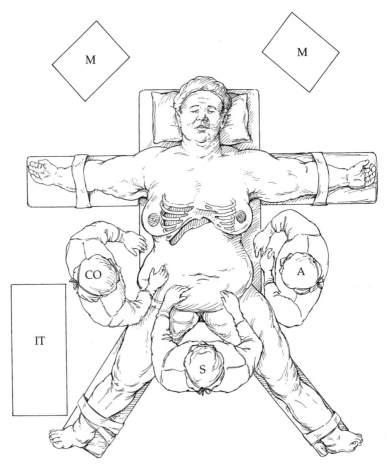

Figure 27.4.1. Patient position and room setup for laparoscopic gastric bypass: S, surgeon; A, assistant; CO, camera operator; M, monitor; IT, instrument table. (Soper NJ, Swanstrom LL, Eubanks WS, eds. Mastery of Endoscopic and Laparoscopic Surgery. 2d ed. Philadelphia: Lippincott Williams & Wilkins, 2005. Used by permission.)

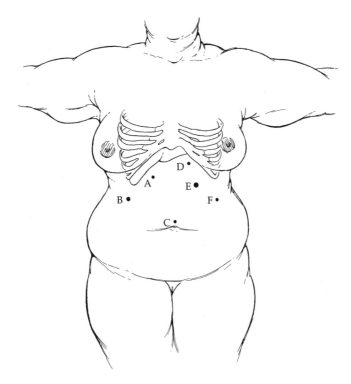

Figure 27.4.2. Port placement for laparoscopic gastric bypass. Ports B and E should be 12-mm ports. The remaining ports may be 5- or 11-mm ports, depending upon instrumentation; C is the camera port. (Soper NJ, Swanstrom LL, Eubanks WS, eds. Mastery of Endoscopic and Laparoscopic Surgery. 2d ed. Philadelphia: Lippincott Williams & Wilkins, 2005. Used by permission.)

5. Fashion a 75- to 150-cm Roux limb and create a side-to-side jejunostomy with linear endoscopic staplers (Fig. 27.4.6). A sutured technique is, of course, also applicable for this anastomosis.
6. In superobese patients, some surgeons use an elongated Roux limb of 150 to 250 cm, which has been shown to achieve greater weight loss in this population.
7. Pass the end of the Roux limb into proximity to the gastric pouch, taking care to avoid twisting. This may be done in either an antecolic or retrocolic fashion. Many surgeons prefer the retrocolic route, which takes a direct route, passing the limb behind the fat-laden mesentery and colon. Create an opening in the transverse mesocolon and pass the Roux limb cephalad behind the stomach (retrogastric) so that it reaches the gastric pouch without tension. This is the most common approach.

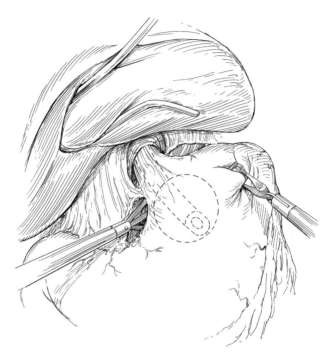

Figure 27.4.3. The stomach is exposed and mobilized. A gastric balloon catheter may be used to define the pouch and facilitate pouch creation. (Soper NJ, Swanstrom LL, Eubanks WS, eds. Mastery of Endoscopic and Laparoscopic Surgery. 2d ed. Philadelphia: Lippincott Williams & Kilkins, 2005. Used by permission.)

Take care to close the mesenteric defect to prevent internal herniation. Several other variations exist, including retrocolic antegastric and antecolic retrogastric.

8. The gastrojejunal anastomosis may be stapled or hand sewn. Several stapling techniques have been described.

    a. For a circular stapled anastomosis with transoral passage of the anvil, upper endoscopy is then performed.

    b. A percutaneous intravenous cannula is placed by the surgeon and is used to introduce a loop of wire into the lumen of the gastric pouch.

    c. The endoscopist grasps this and attaches it to the anvil of a 21- or 25-mm circular stapler.

    d. The anvil is then passed through the oropharynx and esophagus and into the gastric pouch.

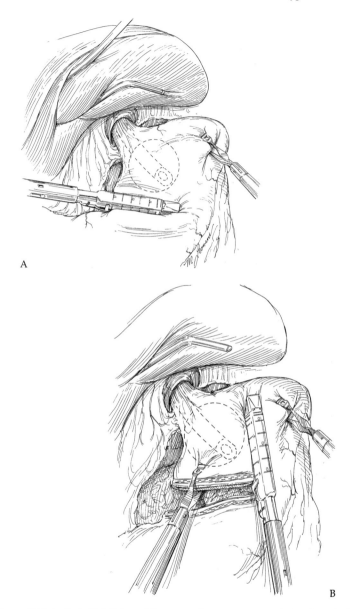

Figure 27.4.4. A. Initial firing of linear stapler to create pouch. B. Completion of pouch. (Soper NJ, Swanstrom LL, Eubanks WS, eds. Mastery of Endoscopic and Laparoscopic Surgery. 2d ed. Philadelphia: Lippincott Williams & Wilkins, 2005. Used by permission.)

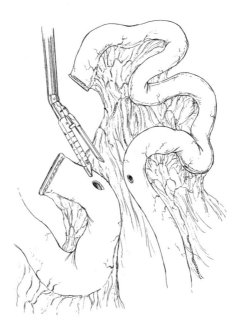

Figure 27.4.5. The Roux limb is created using a linear stapler. A hand-sewn technique may also be employed. (Soper NJ, Swanstrom LL, Eubanks WS, eds. Mastery of Endoscopic and Laparoscopic Surgery. 2d ed. Philadelphia: Lippincott Williams & Wilkins, 2005. Used by permission.)

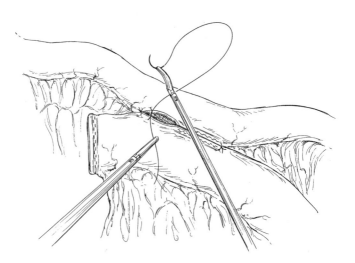

Figure 27.4.6 The jejunostomy is completed by closing the enterotomies (stapled technique, with sewn closure of enterotomies). (Soper NJ, Swanstrom LL, Eubanks WS, eds. Mastery of Endoscopic and Laparoscopic Surgery. 2d ed. Philadelphia: Lippincott Williams & Wilkins, 2005. Used by permission.)

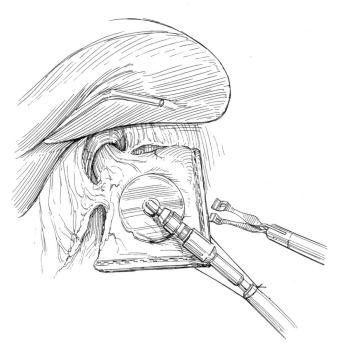

Figure 27.4.7. The anvil is pulled through the gastric wall after transoral delivery. (Soper NJ, Swanstrom LL, Eubanks WS, eds. Mastery of Endoscopic and Laparoscopic Surgery. 2d ed. Philadelphia: Lippincott Williams & Wilkins, 2005. Used by permission.)

   e. Electrocautery is applied over the stem of the anvil to bring it through the gastric wall (Fig. 27.4.7).

   f. A left-sided port is enlarged to allow a circular stapler to be passed.

   g. An incision is made in the Roux limb 8 to 10 cm from the stapled end to admit the circular stapler, which is mated with the anvil to create the stapled anastomosis (Fig. 27.4.8).

   h. The enterotomy is closed with a linear stapler (Fig. 27.4.9).

9. Alternative techniques for the gastrojejunostomy include variations in how the circular stapler is introduced, and a hand-sewn and linear-stapled anastomosis. For this combination anastomosis, a posterior layer of continuous nonabsorbable sutures is placed to approximate the Roux limb to the pouch. The ultrasonic dissector is used to create gastrotomies and enterotomies through which the 45-mm linear stapler is passed and fired to create the anastomosis. The remaining openings are then closed with two layers of running nonabsorbable sutures.

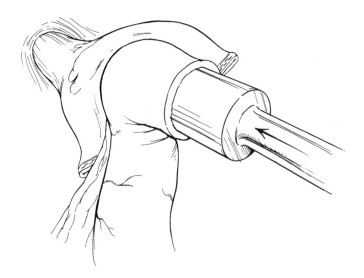

Figure 27.4.8. The gastrojejunostomy is created by connecting the anvil and shaft of the circular stapler and firing it. (Soper NJ, Swanstrom LL, Eubanks WS, eds. Mastery of Endoscopic and Laparoscopic Surgery. 2d ed. Philadelphia: Lippincott Williams & Wilkins, 2005. Used by permission.)

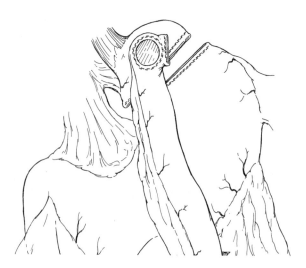

Figure 27.4.9. Completed bypass. The bypass is tested by insufflation of air under saline, or by instillation of methylene blue. (Soper NJ, Swanstrom LL, Eubanks WS, eds. Mastery of Endoscopic and Laparoscopic Surgery. 2d ed. Philadelphia: Lippincott Williams & Wilkins, 2005. Used by permission.)

10. Insufflate the gastric pouch with air by endoscopy or through a naso-gastric (NG) tube to test the integrity of the anastomosis, which is submerged in irrigation fluid. Alternately, a methylene blue solution may be flushed through the NG tube to identify extravasation
11. Close port sites larger than 5 mm at the fascial level.

C. Selected References

Schauer PR, Ikramuddin S. Outcomes after laparoscopic Roux-en-Y gastric bypass for morbid obesity. Ann Surg 2000;232:515–529.

Schauer PR, Ikramuddin S, Hamad G, Gourash W. The learning curve for laparoscopic Roux-en-Y gastric bypass is 100 cases. Surg Endosc 2003;17:202–205.

27.5 Other Laparoscopic Procedures for Obesity

Emma Patterson, M.D., F.R.C.S.C., F.A.C.S.

As mentioned in Chapter 27.1, only small series with limited follow-up exist for biliopancreatic diversion and duodenal switch. Major complications include the sequelae of malabsorption and may be significant. These procedures are included for completeness.

A. Biliopancreatic Diversion

Biliopancreatic diversion consists of a significant antrectomy, leaving an approximately 200- to 300-mL gastric pouch. The duodenum is transected. Continuity is restored with a long alimentary limb (which drains the gastric pouch) and a relatively short "common channel" through which bile and pancreatic secretions admix with the intestinal contents (Fig. 27.5.1).

1. Patient Position

a. Position the patient supine on the operating room table with the arms abducted and the legs split.
b. The surgeon operates from the patient's left side to perform the common channel and between the legs to do the antrectomy and gastrojejunostomy.
c. Place a Foley catheter.
d. Use sequential compression devices for prophylaxis for deep venous thrombosis (perioperative low-molecular-weight heparin could also be used).
e. Administer preoperative prophylactic antibiotics.

2. Trocar Placement

a. Place a 10-mm trocar at the umbilicus. This will be used as the viewing port for a 30-degree laparoscope.
b. Place a 12-mm trocar in the midepigastrium.
c. Place a second 12-mm trocar in the right upper quadrant.

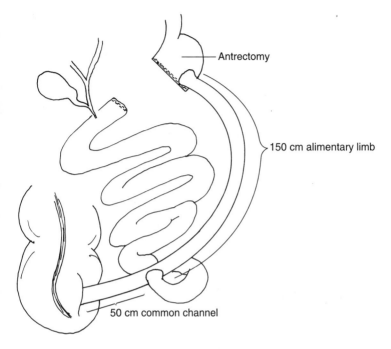

Figure 27.5.1. Laparoscopic biliopancreatic diversion.

d. Place two additional 5-mm trocars. Position one in the left upper quadrant and the second to the left of the xiphoid. Remove the second trocar and place a Nathanson liver retractor through the tract to retract the left lobe of the liver.

3. Performing the Biliopancreatic Diversion

a. Creating the common channel
    i.   Place the patient in Trendelenburg position with the right side up.
    ii. Identify the terminal ileum. Using an umbilical tape, measure 50 cm proximally and mark this point with a silk suture.
    iii. From this point, measure another 150 cm proximally using the umbilical tape and transect the bowel at this point with an endoscopic cutting linear stapler, 45 mm × 2.5 mm (this is the 200-cm mark).
    iv. Divide 2 cm of mesentery using a harmonic scalpel.

      v. Anastomose the proximal end (the biliopancreatic limb) of the transection point to the 50-cm mark of the terminal ileum to create a 50-cm common channel.

          (1) Create enterotomies on the antimesenteric side of both pieces of bowel using the harmonic scalpel.

          (2) Apply a reticulating 60-mm × 2.5-mm laparoscopic stapler to the approximated loops of bowel.

          (3) Close the remaining common enterotomy with a running 2-0 silk suture.

      vi. The distal end of the transected bowel will form the 150-cm alimentary limb.

b. Performing the antrectomy

      i. Place the patient in reverse Trendelenburg position.

      ii. Mark a transection point across the stomach using cautery, starting at the incisura and proceeding horizontally.

      iii. Retract the stomach superiorly and devascularize the greater curve by using the harmonic scalpel. Continue devascularization until just past the pylorus.

      iv. Create a window in the gastrohepatic ligament next to the pylorus. Divide the duodenum just past the pylorus with a reticulating 60-mm × 3.5-mm stapler for endoscopic gastrointestinal anastomosis (V.S. Surgical, Norwalk, CT, Endo-GIA).

      v. Devascularize the lesser curve of the stomach using the harmonic scalpel to the previously marked transection point.

      vi. Divide the stomach using serial firings of a 60-mm × 3.5-mm Endo-GIA stapler.

      vii. Remove the specimen in a retrieval bag via the right upper quadrant 12-mm trocar site. This will have to be dilated to permit removal.

c. Creating the gastrojejunostomy

      i. Divide the omentum with the harmonic scalpel down to the transverse colon to create an omental pathway.

      ii. Place a 2-0 silk tacking suture from the alimentary limb to the greater curve of the stomach to facilitate stapling of the gastrojejunostomy.

      iii. Using the harmonic scalpel, create a gastrotomy posterior to the staple line on the stomach.

      iv. Similarly create an enterotomy on the antimesenteric border of the alimentary limb.

      v. Create the anastomosis with an articulating 45-mm × 3.5-mm Endo-GIA stapler.

      vi. Close the common enterotomy with a running 2-0 silk suture.

d. Test the anastomosis

      i. The anesthesiologist places an orogastric tube into the stomach, just proximal to the gastrojejunostomy.

      ii. Clamp the Roux limb with a noncrushing bowel clamp to occlude the lumen.

iii. The anesthesiologist instills 100 to 150-mL of diluted methylene
      blue dye through the orogastric tube to distend the stomach and
      test the anastomosis.
iv.   Placing a drain near the duodenal stump is optional.

B. Duodenal Switch

The duodenal switch procedure consists of a sleeve resection of the stomach,
with preservation of the pylorus (Fig. 27.5.2).

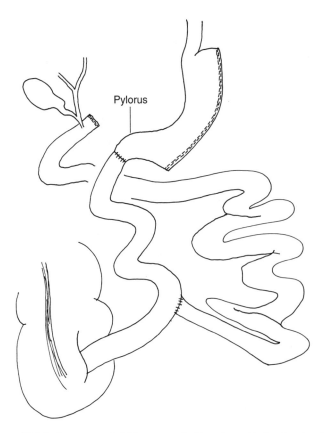

Figure 27.5.2. Laparoscopic biliopancreatic diversion with duodenal switch.

1. Patient Position

a.   Position the patient in the supine, split-leg position with the arms abducted.

b.   The surgeon operates from between the patient's legs to do the sleeve gastrectomy, prepare the stomach, and create the duodenojejunostomy. The surgeon stands on the patient's left side when preparing the limbs and creating the common channel.

c.   Insert a Foley catheter.

d.   Use sequential compression devices for prophylaxis for deep venous thrombosis (perioperatively, low-molecular-weight heparin could be used).

e.   Administer prophylactic antibiotics.

2. Trocar Position

a.   Place a 5-mm trocar in the left upper quadrant.

b.   Place a 12-mm trocar in the right upper quadrant.

c.   Place a 12-mm trocar at the umbilicus.

d.   Place a 5-mm trocar in the suprapubic region.

e.   Place a 5-mm trocar to the left of the xiphoid; then remove the trocar and insert a Nathanson liver retractor through the tract.

3. Create the Common Channel

The common channel is created as described for the biliopancreatic diversion.

4. Prepare the Stomach

a.   Devascularize the greater curve of the stomach with the ultrasonic shears by dividing the gastroepiploic vessels.

b.   Leave the omental attachments to the antrum.

c.   Use blunt dissection to create a window 3 to 5 cm distal to the pylorus.

d.   Transect the duodenum 3 to 5 cm distal to the pylorus using a laparoscopic linear cutting stapler 60 mm × 2.5 mm.

e.   Create a gastrostomy on the greater curve of the stomach, just superior to the antrum (in the portion of stomach to be resected as part of the sleeve gastrectomy).

   f.   Suture the anvil of a 25-mm circular stapler with the cap in the flipped position. Leave the suture ends long.

   g.   Grasp the suture with a Maryland dissector, and feed it through the gastrostomy, toward the duodenum.

   h.   Make a duodenotomy just at the staple line using the harmonic scalpel.

   i.   Feed the suture through this duodenotomy, and pull the suture through until the anvil sits in the duodenum.

5. Performing the Sleeve Gastrectomy

   a.   The anesthesiologist passes a 56-French bougie into the stomach.

   b.   Resect two thirds of the stomach using multiple firings of a 60-mm $\times$ 3.5-mm laparoscopic linear cutting stapler. Use the bougie as a guide to ensure that the stomach is not too narrow.

   c.   Divide any remaining short gastric vessels with the ultrasonic shears.

   d.   Place the stomach in an endoscopic specimen retrieval bag and extract it via the right upper quadrant port.

6. Create the Duodenojejunostomy

   a.   Using the ultrasonic shears, open the staple line of the alimentary limb.

   b.   Dilate the right upper quadrant incision.

   c.   Attach a camera drape to a 25-mm circular stapler using a rubber band; this will serve as a wound protector.

   d.   Insert the 25-mm circular stapler into the abdominal wall through the dilated right upper quadrant incision, and intubate the opened small bowel of the alimentary limb.

   e.   Rotate the stapler up toward the anvil in clockwise fashion to create the anastomosis.

   f.   Pull the camera drape off the stapler, and remove the stapler and donuts from the abdominal cavity.

   g.   Using a 45-mm $\times$ 2.5-mm linear cutting stapler trim off the open end of the bowel. Remove in an endoscopic retrieval bag.

7. Test the Anastomosis

Testing is done as previously described for the biliopancreatic diversion.

318   E. Patterson

C. Selected References

Ren CJ, Patterson E, Gagner M. Early results of laparoscopic biliopancreatic diversion
with duodenal switch: a case series of 40 consecutive patients. Obes Surg 2000;
10:514–523.
Scopinaro N, Marinari G, Camerini G. Laparoscopic standard biliopancreatic diversion:
technique and preliminary results. Obes Surg 2001;12:362–365.

27.6 Complications of Laparoscopic Bariatric Surgery

Adolfo Z. Fernandez, Jr., M.D.
David S. Tichansky, M.D.
Eric J. DeMaria, M.D., F.A.C.S.

A. Complications of the Laparoscopic Gastric Bypass

1. Intestinal Leak

a. **An intestinal leak is** defined as any anastomotic leak, staple line disruption, or intestinal perforation. It can occur at the gastrojejunostomy, jejunojejunostomy, the bypassed stomach staple line, the gastric pouch staple line, or anywhere along the intestinal tract. Leak rates as high as 6.9% have been reported.

b. **Diagnosis** can be made clinically or by upper gastrointestinal (UGI) series. Greater than 50% of leaks can be missed by the UGI series. Symptoms of a leak include feeling of "impending doom," left shoulder pain, back pain, pelvic pressure or pain, tenesmus, or worsening abdominal pain. Signs include fever, tachypnea, oliguria, fluid sequestration, hypotension, hypoxia, or shock. Abdominal pain and peritonitis are not reliably found in this group of patients. Most of the findings are nonspecific and can be confused with an acute myocardial infarction or pulmonary embolus. It is imperative that the appropriate tests be expeditiously performed to guide the therapy. Empiric abdominal exploration may be the only appropriate diagnostic test. Failure to act quickly can result in the patient's demise.

c. Leak **treatment** depends on the clinical situation. If the leak is well contained and the patient is hemodynamically stable, the patient can be treated conservatively with fasting, intravenous antibiotics, and intravenous nutrition. If the leak is not contained or the patient is hemodynamically unstable, laparoscopic or open exploration is indicated. Exploration for a leak entails three basic principles: (1) large-bore drainage, (2) repair of the leak if possible, and (3) gastrostomy tube placement in the bypassed stomach.

2. *Pulmonary Embolus*

a. Obesity is a risk factor for the development of deep venous thrombosis (DVT). The combination of increased intra-abdominal pressure and a baseline hypercoagulable state found in obesity puts this patient population at high risk for DVT. The rates of DVT and pulmonary embolus (PE) are about or less than 1% in multiple series of laparoscopic gastric bypass procedures (L-GBP).

b. **Prevention** of DVT includes the use of perioperative heparin or low-molecular-weight heparin (LMWH) and sequential compression devices. Placement of inferior vena caval filters is recommended in patients with a history of prior DVT or PE, venous stasis disease, or pulmonary hypertension and obesity hypoventilation syndrome. The main benefit is prevention of a fatal PE.

3. *Acute Gastric Dilatation*

a. **Dilatation of the bypassed stomach** most commonly occurs as a result of obstruction at the jejunojejunostomy but can also occur spontaneously. Interruption of the nerves of Laterjet resulting in loss of vagal innervations may be a contributing factor. This complication can still be seen in patients despite the preservation of these nerves.

b. **Diagnosis** is made either clinically or radiographically. Signs and symptoms include hiccoughs, bloating, tympani, tachycardia, and ultimately cardiopulmonary compromise. A plain abdominal radiograph may show a large gastric bubble or air fluid level. If the stomach is fluid filled without air, the radiograph may not be helpful.

c. **Treatment** involves urgent needle decompression of the excluded stomach under fluoroscopy or surgical gastrostomy. If the patient becomes hemodynamically unstable, laparotomy may reveal gastric blowout with a high risk for mortality.

4. *Stomal Stenosis*

a. Occurrence of stricture at the gastrojejunostomy site has been reported to be as high as 6.6%. The reason for which stomal stenosis occurs is not well understood. **Symptoms** include dysphagia, nausea/vomiting, or odynophagia.

b. **Diagnosis** and **treatment** are achieved by upper endoscopy. Balloon dilatation is usually successful after the first attempt, though multiple dilatations may be necessary.

5. Internal Hernia

a. The L-GBP has three potential sites of internal herniation, which must be repaired at surgery: the mesocolic, Petersen's, and the **jejunojejunostomy** defects. The **mesocolic** defect is created only if the Roux limb is brought retrocolic. **Petersen's** defect is the space between the cut edge of the Roux limb mesentery and the mesocolon. The reported risk of herniation is less than 2%.

b. **Diagnosis** can be problematic. The symptoms associated with an internal hernia are vague and most commonly include intermittent periumbilical or left-sided crampy abdominal pain. Multiple episodes may occur with only transient symptoms. Patients may also present with a small bowel obstruction. The diagnostic tests of choice include a UGI series or a computed tomography (CT) of the abdomen with oral and intravenous contrast. Unfortunately results of these tests will likely be normal if performed after symptoms have subsided.

c. Optimal **treatment** is laparoscopic reduction and closure of the hernia defect. Rarely is open exploration needed, unless there is necrotic bowel, confused anatomy, or poor visualization due to dilated small bowel.

6. Marginal Ulcer

a. Marginal ulcers can occur early or late and are usually located on the jejunal side of the anastomosis. The rate of ulceration is 5% or less.

b. **Diagnosis** is based on strong clinical suspicion and an upper endoscopy.

c. **Treatment** is acid suppression using proton pump inhibitors. If these should fail, a UGI series should be performed to rule out a gastrogastric fistula with regurgitation of acid from the excluded stomach. In this case treatment requires surgical ablation of the gastrogastric fistula.

7. Wound Complications

a. One of the advantages of the laparoscopic approach to GBP is the significant decrease in wound complications including hernias and infections. The rate of trocar site hernia is less than 1%, and wound infection rates are less than 8%.

b. **Treatment** for simple wound infections or cellulitis includes antibiotic therapy and incision and drainage of any fluid collections. Asymptomatic hernias may be postponed till the patient's weight has stabilized to increase the success of the repair. If the hernia is incarcerated, strangulated, or symptomatic, prompt repair is necessary.

8. Cholelithiasis

a.   Rapid weight loss is associated with the formation of gallstones as a result of the increased concentration of cholesterol in the bile. This likely leads to the formation of sludge with cholesterol crystals that serve as the nidus for gallstone formation.

b.   The best treatment is **prevention**. Sugerman et al. showed that in patients without gallstones, 32% would form gallstones after the GBP. The addition of prophylactic ursodiol for the first 6 months postoperatively reduces the risk to 2%.

9. Nutritional Deficiencies

Nutritional deficiencies are common in noncompliant patients but quite rare when patients maintain good follow-up and take prescribed supplements including multivitamins, calcium, and vitamin B_{12} daily. Menstruating females require iron supplementation.

10. Inadequate Weight Loss

a.   Wittgrove and Clark reported that 15% of their patients failed to lose more than 50% of their excess weight after the L-GBP. This correlates well with what is known from the open literature. The solution to this problem is not easy, and a revisional procedure is more risky for the patient.

b.   Two mechanical causes of inadequate weight loss are gastrogastric fistula and dilated stoma. **Diagnosis** of these is made simply with a UGI series. Another cause of inadequate weight loss is noncompliance. Patients can eat through a GBP if they have a large daily intake of high-fat foods or drinks. Some will overcome the dumping syndrome and not adhere to dietary recommendations.

c.   **Treatment** for a gastrogastric fistula is surgical. In selected cases the reexploration can be performed laparoscopically because of the minimal adhesions produced by the initial L-GBP. Surgical treatment for a dilated stoma has been met with a high failure rate and a higher risk of leak for the patient. The noncompliant patient with inadequate weight loss should be treated with dietetic interventions to help the patient attain more weight loss. The added risk of a second procedure in these patients is not justified if the patient's compliance is the issue.

For compliant patients who are not satisfied with their weight loss, conversion to a malabsorptive procedure should be done only if serious comorbidities remain. The risk of malnutrition is too high if the only reason for conversion to a malabsorptive procedure is aesthetics.

11. Death

The risk of death in the L-GBP is reported in most series to be less than 1%. The two most significant postoperative events that cause mortality are intestinal leak and PE. Early aggressive diagnosis and treatment are necessary to prevent mortality.

B. Complications of the Laparoscopic Adjustable Gastric Band

Gastric perforation and death are rare complications of the laparoscopic adjustable gastric band (LAGB). Both have been reported in various series with incidences less than 1%. The LAGB has been shown to have an overall reoperative rate as high as 50%, which decreases with the surgeon's experience. The more common complications of the LAGB are listed in the subsections that follow.

1. Band Slippage

a. Band slippage can occur early or late (>30 days after the procedure). Its reported incidence in larger series is a high as 13.9%. Signs or symptoms include gastric prolapse, pouch dilatation, reflux, vomiting, dysphagia, epigastric pain, or acute obstruction. The incidence of this complication has been reduced with the use of the pars flaccida approach.

b. **Diagnosis** is made either clinically or through UGI series.

c. **Treatment** involves surgical repositioning or replacement of the LAGB.

2. Band Erosion

a. Band erosion is a late complication occurring in 1 to 3% of patients. Patients may present with symptoms of weight gain as their restriction to food is alleviated, as well as pain between the shoulder blades or signs of tubing or port infection.

b. The **diagnosis** can be made with upper endoscopy or UGI series.

c. **Treatment** requires removal of the band and repair of the gastric perforation. Reports of immediate and delayed replacement of the LAGB have provided good results, though long-term follow-up is lacking.

3. Esophageal Dilatation

a. Dilatation of the esophagus is a worrisome complication. Its incidence is variable in the literature and is usually not identified for at least 3 years following the procedure. The incidence in the literature probably underestimates the prevalence of this complication because it can be asymptomatic and therefore undiagnosed unless a contrast study is done. Its significance long term is unknown, but concerns of esophageal dysmotility and emptying problems have been raised. Pulsion diverticulum, pseudoachalasia syndrome, or sigmoid esophagus may result.

b. **Diagnosis** can be made clinically with symptoms of dysphagia or reflux or radiographically via a UGI series.

c. **Treatment** involves deflation of the band. If symptoms or dilatation persist or if the patient has coexistent poor weight loss, band removal is indicated.

4. Port Infections/Malfunction

The band is susceptible to reservoir leaks, tubing breaks, tubing disconnections, balloon leaks, or infection. The incidence of these complications ranges from 2% to 5%. Treatment requires LAGB revision, removal, or replacement.

5. Inadequate Weight Loss

Many of the Australian and European studies have defined inadequate weight loss as less than 20% or 25% of excess weight. By this measure the failure rate have been as high as 30% at 3 years follow-up. Most of these data are with follow-up of less than 3 years. In the United States, the weight loss failures may be greater, requiring removal of the bands in as many as half the patients. The long-term outcomes are still lacking.

C. Selected References

DeMaria EJ, Sugerman HJ, Kellum JK, et al. High failure rate following laparoscopic adjustable silicone gastric banding for treatment of morbid obesity. Ann Surg 2001;223:809–818.

DeMaria EJ, Sugerman HJ, Kellum JK, et al. Results of 281 consecutive total laparoscopic Roux-en-Y gastric bypasses to treat morbid obesity. Ann Surg 2002;235:640–647.

Doherty C, Maher JW, Heitshusen DS. Long-term data indicate a progressive loss in efficacy of adjustable silicone gastric banding for the surgical treatment of morbid obesity. Surgery 2002;132:724–728.

Favretti F, Cadiere GB, Segato G, et al. Laparoscopic banding: selection and technique in 830 patients. Obes Surg 2002;12:385–390.

Hauri P, Steffen R, Ricklin T, et al. Treatment of morbid obesity with the Swedish adjustable gastric band (SAGB): complication rate during a 12-month follow-up period. Surgery 2000;127:484–488.

Higa KD, Boone KB, Ho T. Complications of the laparoscopic Roux-en-Y gastric bypass: 1,040 patients—what have we learned? Obes Surg 2000;10:509–513.

Lonroth H, Dalenback J. Other laparoscopic bariatric procedures. World J Surg 1998;22:964–968.

O'Brien PE, Dixon JB. Weight loss and early and late complications—the international experience. Am J Surg 2002;184:42S–45S.

Schauer PR, Ikramuddin S. Laparoscopic surgery for morbid obesity. Surg Clin North Am 2001;81:1145–1179.

Schauer PR, Ikramuddin S, Gourash W, et al. Outcomes after laparoscopic Roux-en-Y gastric bypass for morbid obesity. Ann Surg 2000;232:515–529.

Sugerman HJ, Brewer WH, Shiffman ML, et al. A multicenter, placebo-controlled, randomized, double-blind, prospective trial of prophylactic ursodiol for the prevention of gallstone formation following gastric-bypass-induced rapid weight loss. Am J Surg 1995;169:91–97.

Sugerman HJ, Sugerman EL, Wolfe L, et al. Risks/benefits of gastric bypass in morbidly obese patients with severe venous stasis disease. Gastroenterology 2000;118:A1051.

Wittgrove AC, Clark GW. Laparoscopic gastric bypass, Roux-en-Y—500 patients: technique and results, with 3–60 month follow-up. Obes Surg 2000;10:233–239.

Laparoscopy
VI—Laparoscopic Procedures
on the Small Intestine,
Appendix, and Colon

28. Small Bowel Resection, Enterolysis, and Enteroenterostomy

Bruce David Schirmer, M.D., F.A.C.S.

A. Indications

Laparoscopic small bowel resection has been used for essentially all situations for which a small bowel resection might otherwise be done via celiotomy, where circumstances allow the favorable technical performance of the procedure using a laparoscopic approach. Specific indications include the following:

1. Inflammatory bowel disease (Crohn's disease)
2. Diverticula
3. Ischemia or gangrenous segment of bowel
4. Obstructing lesions
5. Stricture (postradiation, postischemic, etc.)
6. Neoplasms (some controversy exists owing to concern about the appropriateness of laparoscopy for maximizing oncologic principles of resection of potentially curable malignant neoplasms, as with current concerns for colon carcinoma; these concerns stem from reports of port site tumor recurrences when this approach has been used)

Nonresectional laparoscopic small bowel procedures and their indications include **laparoscopic enterolysis** for acute small bowel obstruction, **"second-look" diagnostic laparoscopy** for possible ischemic bowel, and **laparoscopic palliative enteroenterostomy** for bypassing obstructing nonresectable tumors.

B. Patient Positioning and Room Setup

1. Position the patient supine. Tuck the arms, if possible, to create more space for surgeon and the camera operator.
2. The surgeon should stand facing the lesion:
   a. on the patient's right for lesions in the patient's left abdominal cavity or those involving the proximal bowel
   b. on the patient's left for lesions in the patient's right abdominal cavity, or those involving the terminal ileum.
3. The camera operator stands on the same side as the surgeon.
4. The assistant stands on the opposite side.

5.   Two monitors should be set up if lesion location is in doubt or if it is likely that the lesion may be manipulated from side to side within the peritoneal cavity. Monitors should be near the left shoulder and near either the right shoulder or right hip. Under some circumstances a single monitor, placed opposite the surgeon, will suffice.

6.   Follow the basic principles of laparoscopic surgery setup: the surgeon should stand in line with the view of the laparoscope, having within comfortable reach a port for each hand. The monitor should be directly opposite the surgeon and facing the line of view of the telescope.

7.   An ultrasound machine with laparoscopic probe should be available for use if a condition such as intestinal ischemia or neoplasm (requiring hepatic assessment) is encountered.

C. Trocar Position and Instrumentation

1.   Place the initial trocar in the umbilical region and insert the laparoscope. (See Chapter 2, Access to Abdomen, and 10.2, Previous Abdominal Surgery, for tips on gaining access in the previously operated or difficult abdomen). Look at the intestine and determine whether the lesion is proximal or distal in the small bowel, and which is the best position from which to perform the resection.

2.   **For distal intestinal lesions**
   a.   Place the monitor by the patient's right hip.
   b.   Place additional trocars in the right upper quadrant and lower midline (10–12 mm) and in the left abdomen just below the level of the umbilicus and near the cecum (5 mm or larger, depending upon instruments) (Fig. 28.1).

3.   **For proximal intestinal lesions**
   a.   Place the monitor near the left shoulder.
   b.   The surgeon stands near the right hip.
   c.   Place large (10–12 mm) trocars in the right upper and left lower quadrants. Additional trocars are placed in the left upper quadrant and right midabdomen, slightly above the level of the umbilicus, as needed.

4.   An angled (30- or 45-degree) laparoscope gives the best view of the small bowel mesentery and is much preferred over a 0-degree scope.

5.   Other essential equipment includes atraumatic graspers for safely handling the bowel. Laparoscopic intestinal staplers, both linear dividing (gastrointestinal anastomosis [GIA]-type) and linear closing (TA-type) greatly facilitate anastomosis. Mesenteric division may be accomplished by using a combination of vascular endoscopic staplers, clips, and Roeder loops, or by using the ultrasonic scalpel. The latter is also quite helpful for initial dissection of the mesentery and division of the nonmajor mesenteric vessels. Laparoscopic scissors with attachment to monopolar cautery are also useful in performing enterolysis when that is required.

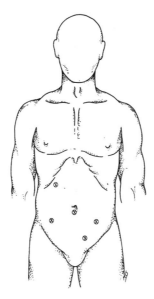

Figure 28.1. Suggested trocar placement for resection of distal small bowel lesions. For a more proximal lesion, move the left lower quadrant trocar to the left upper quadrant. Trocars 4 and 5 are per the surgeon's preference.

D. Technique of Small Bowel Resection

Because of the potential for multifocal lesions or unsuspected disease in other segments, small bowel resection should be preceded by a thorough exploration and visualization of the entire small bowel, where this is feasible. If preoperative studies localize a lesion well, and there are extensive adhesions that preclude "running" the entire small bowel, then this rule may not apply.

1. **Laparoscopic assisted small bowel resection**
   a. Let gravity assist in visualizing the bowel.
       i.   Use initial Trendelenburg position. Locate and grasp the transverse colon and maintain upward traction.
       ii. While maintaining upward traction, change the position to reverse Trendelenburg. The small intestine will slip down, away from the transverse colon, allowing identification of the ligament of Treitz.
   b. Run the small intestine between a pair of atraumatic bowel clamps or endoscopic Babcock clamps. Identify the segment to be resected. Lyse adhesions to surrounding loops of bowel (see Chapter 10.2, Previous Abdominal Surgery).

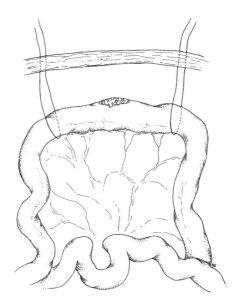

Figure 28.2. The small bowel segment chosen for resection has been suspended by traction sutures passed through the anterior abdominal wall. This facilitates subsequent dissection of mesenteric vessels and provides retraction without additional graspers or trocars.

    c.   Mark and suspend the section of bowel by placing traction sutures through the mesentery just below the mesenteric side of the bowel at the proximal and distal points of intended resection.

        i.   These sutures are most easily placed by using large straight needles passed through the abdominal wall, through the mesentery, and back through the same area of abdominal wall, thereby suspending the bowel near the anterior abdominal wall.

        ii.   This suspends the segment of small bowel like a curtain (Fig. 28.2).

        iii.   Silastic vessel loops may be used if preferred, but they must be passed through trocars.

        iv.   Choose the site for suspension near one of the large trocars, which will be enlarged for extracorporeal anastomosis.

    d.   With scissors or ultrasonic scalpel, score the peritoneum overlying the mesentery, on the side facing the surgeon, along the line of intended resection. This outlines the V-shaped part of small bowel and mesentery that will be resected. Make the V just deep enough for the intended purpose: for example, wide mesenteric excision is appropriate when operating for cancer but unnecessary when a resection is performed for a benign stricture.

e. Next, divide the mesentery along one vertical limb using the ultrasonic scalpel, placing additional clips or ligatures if needed to control bleeding, or for added security for large transverse crossing vessels.

f. Divide the vascular pedicle between ligatures, using the endoscopic linear stapler, or with the ultrasonic scalpel (for vessels <4 mm in size).

g. Divide the bowel at the site of mesenteric division using the endoscopic stapler with the intestinal size (usually 3.5 mm) staples. The end of the bowel is now free for removal through the abdominal wall.

h. Grasp the divided bowel end just proximal to the stapled division with an atraumatic grasper, for easy subsequent identification. Do the same with the distal end.

i. Enlarge the adjacent trocar site (usually to around 4 cm) to allow removal of both ends of bowel. Eliminate the pneumoperitoneum and pull the end of the segment to resected (and associated mesentery) out through the incision. Use wound protection if neoplasm is suspected (Fig. 28.3).

j. Divide the remaining portion of scored mesentery extracorporeally using a standard technique. Divide the bowel extracorporeally using an intestinal stapler.

k. Remove the other end of the bowel through the incision and perform an extracorporeal anastomosis with a stapler (functional end to end, Fig. 28.4) or by hand suturing.

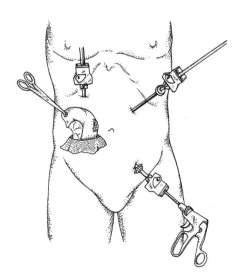

Figure 28.3. External view of exteriorized segment of small intestine prior to resection. Note wound protector.

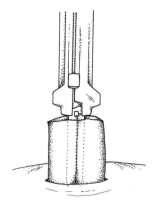

Figure 28.4. Construction of an extracorporeal stapled anastomosis using a linear endoscopic stapler. The jaws of the stapler are being advanced into small enterotomies. Traction sutures help steady the bowel in position.

      l.   Close the mesenteric defect extracorporeally (if possible) or intracorporeally after reestablishment of pneumoperitoneum (see later).

      m. Return the reanastomosed bowel to the peritoneal cavity. Close the small incision in layers, and then reestablish the pneumoperitoneum, confirm hemostasis, and inspect the bowel anastomosis. Perform any additional mesenteric suturing needed at this time.

2. **Laparoscopic small bowel resection.** The totally laparoscopic technique uses an intracorporeal anastomosis. Begin as outlined in steps 1.a through 1.d.

      a.   Divide the remaining mesentery to completely devascularize the segment to be resected.

      b.   Use a laparoscopic stapler loaded with the 3.5-mm staples to divide the bowel at the proximal and distal points of resection.

      c.   Enlarge a trocar site, using wound protection as needed, and remove the specimen. Close the trocar site and reestablish pneumoperitoneum.

      d.   Align the divided bowel ends with stay sutures placed through the antimesenteric surface of the bowel just proximal and distal to the intended anastomosis.

      e.   Cut off a corner from the staple line of each segment, then pass one limb of the endoscopic gastrointestinal stapler into each enterotomy, approximating the segments. Close the stapler and verify correct alignment.

      f.   Fire the stapler and remove it.

    g.   Use the traction sutures to inspect the anastomotic staple line for bleeding. Control any bleeding sites with intracorporeally placed figure-of-eight sutures of absorbable suture material along the staple line.

    h.   Close the enterotomies with an endoscopic linear stapler.

        i.   Place three traction sutures (one at each end and one in the middle) to approximate the enterotomy and elevate the edges.

        ii.   Place the endoscopic TA stapler just beneath the cut edges. Be careful to ensure that both edges are completely enclosed within the stapler, but avoid including excessive amounts of the bowel (which can narrow the enteroenterostomy).

        iii.   Fire the stapler and use scissors to remove excess tissue from the staple line.

        iv.   Alternatively, the defect from the stapler may be closed by using one or two layers of interrupted sutures. These sutures are best placed and tied in an intracorporeal fashion, since extracorporeal tying may place excessive tension on the suture as the knot pusher is being advanced.

        v.   A running suture line may be used as an alternative, but the surgeon must take great care to maintain the appropriate degree of tension on the suture line as subsequent sutures are placed. This also requires an intracorporeal technique.

    i.   Close the mesenteric defect with interrupted sutures, carefully placed in a superficial fashion (to avoid injuring the blood supply).

E. Technique of Enterolysis

    Enterolysis is performed for acute small bowel obstruction or as an initial step in performing any intra-abdominal laparoscopic procedure where previous adhesions preclude adequate visualization or access to abdominal organs. Each procedure is different, but here are some general rules, followed by details of the technique for enterolysis in the presence of small bowel obstruction. Additional information is given in Chapter 10.2, Previous Abdominal Surgery.

    1.   Use laparoscopic scissors to sharply lyse adhesions between the intestine, omentum, other viscera, and abdominal wall.

    2.   Use atraumatic graspers to carefully grasp the viscera or omentum, providing traction and assisting in division. Do not rely simply on traction to tear adhesions, as damage to viscera or bleeding may result.

    3.   The main precaution to take against visceral damage is adequate visualization of all surfaces to be cut before actual division with the scissors.

    4.   It may be necessary to reposition the laparoscope to begin work in an area of limited adhesions; then move into others areas as exposure is obtained.

5. **Enterolysis for acute small bowel obstruction**
    a. The usual limiting factor is bowel distention. A laparoscopic approach is feasible only if distention is not excessive.
    b. Use the Hasson technique to place the first trocar.
    c. Trace the bowel from the area of proximal distention to the transition point, identifying the site of obstruction and the distal decompressed bowel.
    d. Sometimes it is easier to work retrograde from the decompressed area. In any case, a clear transition point should be identified and freed, if possible.
    e. Finally, perform full examination of the entire small intestine if at all possible.

F. Technique of Enteroenterostomy

The performance of an enteroenterostomy essentially mimics the anastomotic portion of small bowel resection. In most cases, the anastomosis will need to be performed intracorporeally, since mobilization of both bowel segments proximal and distal to the obstructing point will usually be technically difficult. In addition, the proximal bowel is often dilated and not amenable to exteriorization through an incision that is limited in size. The anastomosis may be performed using a stapled or a sutured technique.

1. **Stapled enteroenterostomy**
    a. Define the segments of bowel proximal and distal to the obstruction point and mobilize these sufficiently to approximate without tension.
    b. Place traction sutures to maintain alignment. Do not tie these, as bowel mobility facilitates insertion of the endoscopic linear stapler.
    c. Make an enterotomy in each segment of bowel. Suction enteric contents and contain spillage as much as possible.
    d. Insert one limb of the endoscopic linear stapler into each enterotomy. Close the stapler and verify good alignment. Fire the stapler to create the anastomosis. Inspect the inside of the staple line for hemostasis, and close the enterotomies as previously outlined.
    e. Reinforce the corners of the staple line for the gastrointestinal anastomosis, if necessary, with seromuscular interrupted sutures placed and tied intracorporeally.

2. **Hand-sewn enteroenterostomy**
    a. Approximate the bowel as described earlier for stapled anastomosis.
    b. Perform a one- or two-layer anastomosis according to the surgeon's preference. A standard two-layer closure is feasible. All sutures should be placed and tied intracorporeally. (See Chapter 7.)

G. Complications

1. **Anastomotic leak**
   a. **Cause and prevention.** Anastomotic leak most frequently results from technical error, excess tension on the anastomosis, or poor blood supply to the anastomosis. A number of technical errors can occur:
      i. Incomplete closure of the enterostomies with the linear stapler. This is particularly likely if the two ends of the staple lines are apposed in the center rather than at the end points (resulting in poor tissue approximation at the double staple site). Prevent this by always placing these two staple lines at the two ends of the stapled enterotomy closure.
      ii. Similar technical problems can occur if the enterostomy is hand sewn and the sutures are not placed carefully.
      iii. Take care that the anastomosed ends have adequate blood supply and are not under tension. Evidence of ischemia mandates further resection back to clearly well-vascularized intestine. Excessive tension requires mobilization of additional length of bowel.
      iv. Edematous bowel is best approximated by a hand-sewn, rather than a stapled, anastomosis. This may require an extracorporeal technique.
   b. **Recognition and management.** Maintain a high index of suspicion. A small leak may seal and present with minimal symptoms. The more classic presentation includes postoperative fever, abdominal tenderness, and leukocytosis. Treatment is based on the clinical condition of the patient. Small leaks occasionally seal, or manifest as low volume enterocutaneous fistulas through an abdominal wound. Favorable conditions (absence of distal obstruction, intravenous antibiotics, limiting oral intake) may allow the situation to resolve without surgery.

      Clinical deterioration, sepsis, persistence of the fistula, high-volume or proximal location of the fistula, or the presence of conditions likely to prevent fistula closure (such as distal obstruction, foreign body, or neoplasm) are all indications for reoperation as treatment for anastomotic leak.

      In general, suture closure of the leak will not work because the tissues are too edematous and friable to hold suture, and there is an intense local inflammatory reaction. Recurrence of the fistula is the norm when this is the treatment. Give strong consideration to proximal diversion of the enteric stream (through creation of an ileostomy or jejunostomy), or repair plus drainage of the fistula to control any likely postoperative leak. The former is more definitive and hence greatly preferred unless precluded by the condition of the intestinal tissue itself (e.g., intestinal loops virtually "frozen" by severe intra-abdominal adhesions). Proximal diversion may require placement of a feeding tube for administration of an elemental formula or even total parenteral nutrition. Occasionally bypass of the leaking anastomosis may be feasible; adequate diversion of the enteric stream should be assured by this technique to prevent likely releakage. Do not attempt to restore intestinal continuity for at least 3 months. It is prudent to wait longer if severe inflammation and adhesions were encountered at the second operation. These management principles are no different from those followed when an open small bowel resection results in leak.

2. **Anastomotic stricture**

   a. **Cause and prevention.** Anastomotic stricture is usually caused by one of three factors—technical error, ischemia, or tension on the anastomosis—probably in that order of frequency.

      i. The technical errors that most frequently result in anastomotic stricture include creation of an inadequate size opening, including the opposite side of the bowel wall in a suture (thereby effectively closing the opening at that point), turning in too much bowel wall, incorporating excess bowel wall in a staple enterotomy closure (hence narrowing the outflow), and creation of a hematoma at the anastomotic site (which may produce transient stenosis).

      ii. Prevent these errors through diligence and careful visualization of tissues as sutures are placed.

      iii. In some situations it is possible to pass a dilator through the anastomosis to prevent inadvertent inclusion of the back wall in a suture when the front walls are being approximated to complete the anastomosis.

      iv. Remember, during intracorporeal anastomosis it is not possible to palpate the anastomosis to confirm patency. Exercise vigilance and inspect the anastomosis carefully.

      v. Ischemia results from resecting excess mesentery relative to the length of bowel wall resected, or from sutures placed in the mesentery to reapproximate it or control hemorrhage.

      vi. In situations where low flow states or thromboembolic events have resulted in bowel ischemia requiring resection, the potential for anastomotic ischemia postoperatively remains high owing to persistence of the conditions causing thromboembolic events or low flow status. Prevention of this low flow state is often impossible inasmuch as it usually results from intrinsic cardiovascular disease and its complications.

      vii. Tension on the anastomosis will often result in leakage or complete disruption. When it does not, it may result in excessive scarring and narrowing of the anastomotic lumen.

   b. **Recognition and management.** Recognize intraoperative technical errors by vigilance and by testing the anastomosis for patency afterward (milk succus or intestinal gas across the anastomosis and observe the result). If an error is recognized, redo the anastomosis.

      i. When anastomotic strictures are recognized during the postoperative period, the severity of obstructive symptoms dictates whether reoperation and revision of the anastomosis is indicated.

      ii. Usually in this situation, a picture of mechanical postoperative bowel obstruction arises. Confirm the site with contrast studies such as barium small bowel follow-through, but take care to avoid vomiting and aspiration. Confirmation of postoperative obstruction at the anastomotic site demands reoperation and anastomotic revision.

c. **Summary considerations.** Intestinal ischemia, if recognized at the time of the original procedure, must be addressed by further resection of ischemic intestine and performance of an anastomosis only in well-vascularized bowel if the ischemia resulted from a technical error. Ischemia from low flow mandates careful correction of the underlying hemodynamic abnormality with optimization of cardiopulmonary status to prevent recurrence. A second-look procedure should be performed 24 hours later. Depending on the severity of the condition and the potential for rethrombosis, primary anastomosis may be contraindicated and the patient better served by anastomosis at the time of second look. Alternatively, if a primary anastomosis was performed, the integrity can be assessed at the second look.

Anastomotic tension is often appreciated at the time of anastomotic construction. If present, the anastomosis should be abandoned until adequate mobilization has been performed to allow construction without tension. If tension is unrecognized and anastomotic stricture results, reoperation is indicated if obstructive symptoms of significant severity arise, since such symptoms almost always will persist or worsen.

3. **Small bowel obstruction**
a. **Cause and prevention.** The majority of small bowel obstructions occur as a result of postoperative adhesions. There is no certain way to avoid this problem, but limiting the amount of dissection and hemorrhage intraoperatively will usually limit the extent of postoperative adhesions. On occasion, a technical error will result in obstruction, such as failure to close a mesenteric defect with resultant internal herniation of bowel and obstruction.
b. **Recognition and management.** Bowel obstruction presents with the typical picture of nausea, vomiting, distention, and cramping abdominal pain. Radiographic confirmation is helpful. Partial small bowel obstruction, particularly in the early postoperative period, is usually successfully managed with bowel rest, decompression, and intravenous fluid support until spontaneous resolution. In cases of significant mechanical small bowel obstruction, surgical intervention is indicated. Reoperation should be done emergently if there is any concern that tissue compromise (strangulation obstruction) exists.

4. **Prolonged postoperative ileus**
a. **Cause and prevention.** Postoperative ileus is a normal response after abdominal surgery. While its severity is often lessened by using a laparoscopic approach, it nevertheless does occur, even if subtle enough to have few clinical manifestations. The etiology of postoperative ileus is unknown, as are factors that govern its usual spontaneous reversal. Postoperative ileus is particularly likely in settings of ongoing intra-abdominal sepsis and inflammation, and should raise the suspicion of a postoperative infection, particularly an anastomotic leak.
b. **Recognition and management.** The signs and symptoms of postoperative ileus typically include lack of signs of intestinal peristalsis,

abdominal bloating and distention, nausea, and vomiting. The condition must be differentiated from mechanical obstruction. Treatment for ileus is nonoperative and consists of intravenous fluids and bowel rest until peristalsis begins. Prokinetic agents may, on occasion, be of some help in treatment.

5. **Hemorrhage**

   a. **Cause and prevention.** Intra-abdominal hemorrhage almost always arises as a result of technical error from inadequately securing vascular structures as they are divided. Less frequently it may arise as a result of delayed trocar-site bleeding. On occasion, it results from postoperative anticoagulation. Prevention of this problem relies on careful assessment of vascular structures for hemostasis intraoperatively, and use of appropriate ligature or hemostatic measures for vascular structures. Cautery is an inadequate means of dividing significant-sized vessels. Instead, vascular staples, clips, or ligatures are required. The ultrasonically activated scissors may be used to safely divide vessels up to 3 mm in diameter; larger ones require the foregoing measures. Trocar sites should be checked for hemostasis as the pneumoperitoneum is being decompressed and the trocars are being removed. Postoperative anticoagulation medication is rarely indicated for the first few days. If it is, care should be taken to administer heparin or Coumadin in conservative doses with careful monitoring of clotting parameters.

   b. **Recognition and management.** A drop in hematocrit, abdominal distention, and hemodynamic instability with hypotension and tachycardia are the symptoms, either singly or in combination, that suggest postoperative hemorrhage. An abdominal wall hematoma may also be detected for trocar-site bleeding. Management is based on the severity of the problem: hemorrhage of a quantity sufficient to cause hemodynamic instability requires reoperation, while a simple drop in hematocrit of 5 points may be best treated conservatively with fluids and, if necessary, transfusions. The time course is also important: the earlier the problem arises after surgery, the more likely significant-sized vessels are involved and the more urgent the need for reoperation.

Bleeding arising as a result of excessive anticoagulation should be treated by correcting the clotting factors, transfusion, and then determination if hemorrhage is ongoing. If it is not, nonoperative treatment is indicated.

6. **Inadvertent enterotomy (during enterolysis)**

   a. **Cause and prevention.** Most enterotomies result from technical errors and are more likely in the previously operated abdomen or when extensive tumor is present (e.g., carcinomatosis). Prevention involves careful sharp dissection in the proper plane. When extremely difficult dissection is encountered, consider converting to open laparotomy.

   b. **Recognition and management.** Usually a full-thickness enterotomy is recognized at the time of surgery. Sutured repair is immediately indicated. When tissue quality precludes adequate repair and closure, a diverting ostomy or tube drainage via the site to create a controlled fistula may be the only options. When partial-thickness violation of the bowel wall has occurred but an enterotomy has not been done, attempt to ascertain the likelihood that the injured area will convert to a full-thickness injury in the postoperative period. Many partial-thickness injuries require suture reinforcement. Small deserosalized segments usually do not require such repair, and overzealous reinforcement of such areas may do more harm than good. This is no different from the open situation, but the laparoscopic surgeon may have greater difficulty judging the degree of injury. Delayed recognition of an enterotomy (in the postoperative period) is treated in the same manner as an anastomotic leak.

H. Selected References

Adams S, Wilson T, Brown AR. Laparoscopic management of acute small bowel obstruction. Aust N Z J Surg 1993;63:39–41.

Chopra R, McVay C, Phillips E, Khalili TM. Laparoscopic lysis of adhesions. Am Surg 2003;69:966–968.

Duh QY. Laparoscopic procedures for small bowel disease, Baillieres Clin Gastroenterol 1993;7:833–850.

Ibrahim IM, Wolodiger F, Sussman B, et al. Laparoscopic management of acute small-bowel obstruction. Surg Endosc 1996;10:1012–1015.

Lange V, Meyer G, Schardey HM, et al. Different techniques of laparoscopic end-to-end small-bowel anastomoses. Surg Endosc 1995;9:82–87.

Schlinkert RT, Sarr MG, Donohue JH, Thompson GB. General surgical laparoscopic procedures for the "nonlaparologist." Mayo Clin Proc 1995;70:1142–1147.

Scoggin SD, Frazee RC, Snyder SK, et al. Laparoscopic-assisted bowel surgery. Dis Colon Rectum 1993;36:747–750.

Soper NJ, Brunt LM, Fleshman J Jr, et al. Laparoscopic small bowel resection and anastomosis. Surg Laparosc Endosc 1993;3:6–12.

Waninger J, Salm R, Imdahl A, et al. Comparison of laparoscopic handsewn suture techniques for experimental small-bowel anastomoses. Surg Laparosc Endosc 1996; 6:282–289.

29. Placement of Jejunostomy Tube

Bruce David Schirmer, M.D., F.A.C.S.

A. Indications

Placement of a jejunostomy tube is indicated when the proximal gastrointestinal system is unable to be used safely as a route for delivery of enteral nutrition, but intestinal function is otherwise unimpaired. Tube placement may be the sole indication for the operation, or it may accompany another procedure. Where tube placement is the sole procedure, the indications include the following:

1. Documented gastroparesis with nutritional compromise
2. Proximal gastrointestinal obstruction precluding percutaneous gastrostomy placement
3. Specific requirements for a jejunostomy rather than a gastrostomy, such as for the delivery of L-DOPA to treat Parkinson's disease (where the medication is less effective if exposed to an acid environment).

Jejunostomy tube placement may also be incorporated as part of a larger operation. Common indications for its placement regardless of using celiotomy or laparoscopic approaches include the following:

1. Major upper gastrointestinal reconstruction where postoperative anastomotic problem, if present, will preclude enteral feeding. Examples include esophagogastrostomy, total gastrectomy, and pancreaticoduodenectomy.
2. Operations to treat pancreatic or duodenal trauma, and severe pancreatitis.

B. Patient Positioning and Room Setup

1. Position the patient supine. Place a monitor near the patient's left shoulder.
2. The surgeon stands by the patient's right hip, with the camera operator on the same side. The assistant may stand on the opposite side.

C. Trocar Position and Instrumentation

1. Place the initial trocar in the infraumbilical region. Where jejunostomy accompanies another procedure, this may already have occurred.

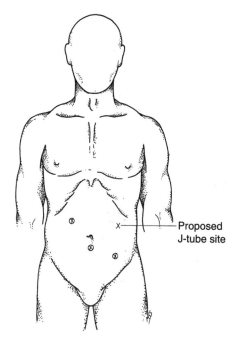

Figure 29.1. Trocar placement for laparoscopic jejunostomy.

2. Place a second trocar in the left lower quadrant. This must be of suf-
    ficient size to allow intracorporeal suturing (10–12 mm, or smaller
    depending upon instrumentation and needle size.
3. Place the final trocar in the right upper quadrant, not far from the
    midline, in a comfortable position for use by the surgeon's left hand
    (Fig. 29.1).
4. In addition to standard laparoscopic instruments, a 30-degree laparo-
    scope, two needle holders, and a pair of atraumatic bowel graspers are
    needed.
5. A commercially available gastrostomy or jejunostomy kit is helpful:
    a Silastic catheter with an inflatable balloon, separate channels for
    decompression and feeding, and an outer bolster to secure the catheter
    to the skin. Serial dilators and a percutaneous needle and guidewire
    for tube insertion via a Seldinger technique are also required for the
    technique described here.

D. Technique of Jejunostomy Tube Placement

1. As described in Chapter 28, initial Trendelenburg positioning with retraction of the transverse colon helps visualize the ligament of Treitz. It is essential that the proximal jejunum be clearly identified.
2. Once the ligament of Treitz is seen, place the patient in slight reverse Trendelenburg to allow easier tracing of the bowel and to permit the remainder of the distal intestine to fall away. Trace the proximal jejunum to a convenient point, usually 1 to 2 feet beyond the ligament, where the bowel can be elevated to touch the left upper quadrant abdominal wall.
3. Determine the location for the tube site in the left upper quadrant (See Chapter 24 for more information about tube siting.)
4. Place four anchoring sutures in a diamond configuration around this site. The author uses 3-0 nylon suture on a straight needle to pierce the abdominal wall, and a laparoscopic needle holder to then pull the needle into the abdominal cavity.
5. Take a seromuscular bite of the antimesenteric border of the intestine, in a position corresponding to the diamond configuration proposed for the suture placement (Fig. 29.2).

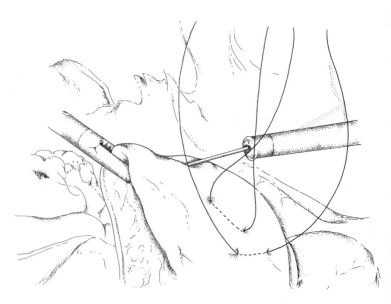

Figure 29.2. The anchoring sutures are being placed. The suture is passed through the abdominal wall, a seromuscular bite of intestine is taken, and the suture is then passed out of the abdomen. Four sutures are placed in a diamond-shaped configuration, providing both retraction and anchoring.

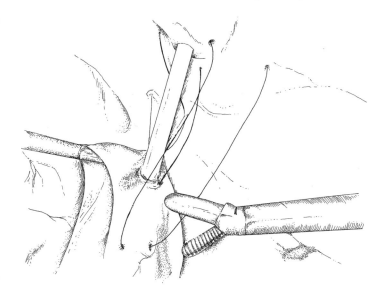

Figure 29.3. Passing one of the dilators through the abdominal wall and into the lumen of the jejunum. Care is taken to pass the dilator just into the lumen of the bowel (under visual laparoscopic control), not far enough to risk posterior intestinal wall perforation.

6. Pass the needle out through the abdominal wall adjacent to its entry site. Do not tie these sutures at this point.
7. If desired, additional absorbable 3-0 braided sutures may be placed (and subsequently tied intracorporeally) to anchor the bowel wall to the underside of the abdominal wall and safeguard against leakage.
8. Insert the jejunostomy tube via a Seldinger technique.
   a. Pass the percutaneous needle through the abdominal wall in the center of the diamond configuration of anchoring sutures.
   b. Take care to position the bowel and advance the needle only far enough to penetrate into the lumen. Do not allow the needle to pierce the back wall.
   c. Pass the guidewire through the needle, into the lumen of the jejunum. Laparoscopic visualization of intestinal movement from wire manipulation is used to confirm the wire's position within the lumen of the bowel. Turn the bowel and inspect it to confirm that penetration or injury to the back wall has not occurred. Repositioning the laparoscope to the left lower quadrant trocar facilitates this maneuver.
   d. With the guidewire in place, enlarge the skin site with a knife and pass serial dilators percutaneously to dilate the track for the tube (Fig. 29.3). Take care to avoid excessive passage of the stiff

dilators into the jejunum; posterior bowel wall perforation may result.

9. Once the largest of the dilators has been passed and withdrawn, pass the tube into the jejunum under laparoscopic vision, using the stent available in the kit (Fig. 29.4). Remove the stent.

10. Tie the anchoring sutures. If additional intracorporeal sutures are needed, these may be placed and tied at this point rather than earlier.

11. Inflate the balloon with 3 mL of saline. Overdistention of the balloon may cause intestinal obstruction. Position the catheter so that the balloon is snug against the abdominal wall within the lumen of the jejunum.

12. Adjust the outer bolster to the skin level and secure it with nylon skin sutures.

13. Test the catheter for ease of gravitational flow of saline into the jejunum, and observe the resulting flow into the bowel with the laparoscope. Methylene blue may be used if there is concern about leakage.

14. Secure the four anchoring sutures without excessive skin trauma by passing the needle through a small cotton dissector roll, both before entering and after exiting the abdominal wall. This roll serves as a bolster to prevent skin damage from the suture (Fig. 29.5).

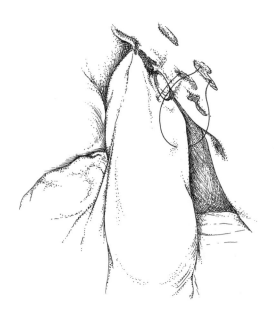

Figure 29.4. Passing the Silastic feeding jejunostomy tube into the lumen of the jejunum and tying the sutures.

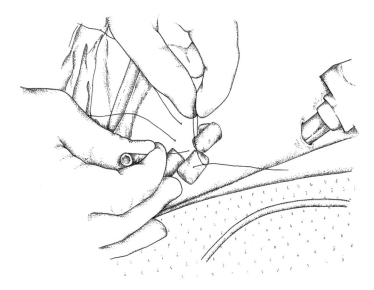

Figure 29.5. The abdominal wall upon completion of the procedure. The external and anchoring sutures are secured to the skin.

E. Complications

1. **Intestinal perforation**
   a. **Cause and prevention.** Intestinal perforation may result if the guidewire or dilator is passed too far, injuring the back wall. Careful attention to technique as described should prevent this complication.
   b. **Recognition and management.** Intraoperative recognition is the goal; this requires careful intraoperative inspection of the posterior intestinal wall. Any injuries that are recognized need immediate suture repair and confirmation that the repair is watertight. Absence of leakage of methylene blue from the repaired site provides good reassurance that the repair is sound.
2. **Intestinal obstruction**
   a. **Cause and prevention.** The most common cause of postoperative intestinal obstruction is overinflation of the intraluminal balloon. To prevent this problem, do not use more than 3 (or at most 4) mL of saline.
   b. **Recognition and management.** Maintain a high index of suspicion for this problem. Balloon deflation is both diagnostic and therapeutic.

348   B.D. Schirmer

3. **Leakage from balloon site**
   a. **Cause and prevention.** The most likely causes are inadequate fixation of the bowel to the abdominal wall or an unrecognized perforation. Prevention is through careful technique.
   b. **Recognition and management.** Index of suspicion for this problem should be high when signs and symptoms of peritonitis result postoperatively. A water-soluble contrast study through the tube is indicated to help determine whether a leak is present. If the study is negative and strong suspicion still exists that the tube is the source of the peritonitis, reexploration is indicated.

      If a tube site leak is identified, it must be repaired operatively with sutures or even reconstruction if needed. On occasion, the leak may result from balloon deflation, and balloon reinflation to the appropriate size should be performed and the contrast study repeated to determine whether the leak has been corrected.

4. **Dislodgment of catheter**
   a. **Cause and prevention.** Most often a catheter is dislodged when a disoriented patient pulls on the tube. When the patient's condition predisposes to such action, protect all but the very end of the tube under an occlusive dressing or abdominal binder. Make connections to external feeding or drainage tubes **loose** so that a pull on the tube results in disruption of the external connection rather than tube dislodgment. Careful intraoperative securing of the tube and postoperative protective dressing should prevent this problem.
   b. **Recognition and management.** Recognition is usually obvious clinically. Management depends on the time course after surgery and after tube dislodgment. In all cases, an attempt to replace the tube into the intestinal lumen should be made immediately. If this is felt to be successful, radiographic confirmation of correct tube positioning and absence of tube site leak is mandatory in the first 10 days after surgery or if questions about tube position remain at any time thereafter. If the tube cannot be replaced, and the patient is less than 10 days from tube placement, emergent reoperation for tube replacement and to prevent potential intraperitoneal contamination is indicated. If the tube has been in place for more than 10 days, elective reoperation to replace it may be performed.

F. Selected References

Duh QY, Senokozlieff-Englehart AL, Siperstein AE, et al. Prospective evaluation of the safety and efficacy of laparoscopic jejunostomy. West J Med 1995;162:117–122.

Edelman DS. Laparoendoscopic approaches to enteral access. Semin Laparosc Surg 2001;8:195–201.

Edelman DS, Unger SW. Laparoscopic gastrostomy and jejunostomy: review of 22 cases. Surg Laparosc Endosc 1994;4:297–300.

Fan AC, Baron TH, Rumalla A, Harewood GC. Comparison of direct percutaneous endoscopic jejunostomy and PEG with jejunal extension. Gastrointest Endosc 2002; 56:890–894.

Hotokezaka M, Adams RB, Miller AD, et al. Laparoscopic percutaneous jejunostomy for long term enteral access. Surg Endosc 1996;10:1008–1011.

Murayama KM, Johnson TJ, Thompson JS. Laparoscopic gastrostomy and jejunostomy are safe and effective for obtaining enteral access. Am J Surg 1996;172:591–594.

Nagle AP, Murayama KM. Laparoscopic gastrostomy and jejunostomy. J Long Term Eff Med Implants 2004;14:1–11.

Rosser JC Jr, Rodas EB, Blancaflor J, Prosst RL, Rosser LE, Salem RR. A simplified technique for laparoscopic jejunostomy and gastrostomy tube placement. Am J Surg 1999;177:61–65.

Saiz AA, Willis IH, Alvarado A, Sivina M. Laparoscopic feeding jejunostomy: a new technique. J Laparoendosc Surg 1995;5:241–244.

Sangster W, Swanstrom L. Laparoscopic-guided feeding jejunostomy. Surg Endosc 1993;7:308–310.

30. Laparoscopic Appendectomy

Keith N. Apelgren, M.D.

A. Indications

1. Laparoscopic appendectomy is indicated when acute appendicitis is suspected or confirmed by computed tomographic (CT) scan. It is especially helpful in the obese patient, in young women, or when the diagnosis is in doubt.
2. Laparoscopic removal of the normal appendix is indicated if the indication for the procedure was right lower quadrant pain.
3. Incidental laparoscopic appendectomy (i.e., as part of laparoscopic cholecystectomy) is not generally indicated.

B. Patient Position and Room Setup

1. Position the patient supine.
2. Some surgeons prefer to use the lithotomy position in women. This allows access to the perineum so that a cervical manipulator may be used to elevate and provide better visualization of the pelvic organs.
3. Tuck the patient's arms at the sides. This is **extremely important** to allow sufficient room for the assistant and camera operator to move cephalad as required.
4. The surgeon stands on the patient's left side.
5. Place the monitor at the patient's hip on the right or directly below the feet.
6. Place a Foley catheter to decompress the bladder.

C. Trocar Position and Choice of Laparoscope

1. Place the initial 10-mm trocar at the umbilicus. Use a 0-degree telescope for visualization.
2. Place the second 5-mm trocar in suprapubic midline to accommodate a grasping instrument. A 10-mm trocar may be needed to accommodate an endoscopic Babcock clamp. This trocar must be placed far

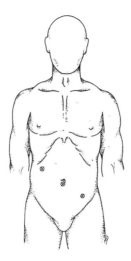

Figure 30.1. Trocar placement for laparoscopic appendectomy. The laparoscope is inserted through an umbilical port. A second trocar (5 or 10 mm) is placed in the suprapubic region and used to elevate the appendix. The third trocar is the working port and should be placed above trocar #2 or on the left side, beyond the border of the rectus muscle. Placement through the rectus muscle should be avoided because it risks injury to the inferior epigastric vessels with subsequent bleeding.

      enough from the appendix to allow sufficient working distance. Occasionally it will need to be placed in the right upper abdomen or even right lower quadrant.

3. The third trocar is usually a 12-mm trocar inserted in the hypogastrium, if the endoscopic linear stapler is to be used, or a 5- or 10-mm trocar if clips or ultrasonic scalpel will be employed. Place this trocar in the midline or lateral to the rectus muscle to avoid injury to the inferior epigastric vessels.

4. A fourth trocar may be necessary to assist in grasping or dissecting the appendix (Fig. 30.1).

D. Performing the Appendectomy

1. Place the patient in steep Trendelenburg position to allow the intestines to slide out of the pelvis, and perform a thorough exploration to confirm the diagnosis.

2. If the appendix is normal, seek other sources for abdominal pain. If no other source is found, it is reasonable to proceed with appendec-

tomy. In many cases a fecalith or other evidence of pathology will be found.

3. Identify the appendix by blunt dissection at the base of the cecum. Elevate the cecum or terminal ileum with an endoscopic Babcock clamp, placed through the right upper quadrant trocar. Generally the base of the appendix will come into view first.

4. Grasp the appendix with an atraumatic grasper or Babcock clamp placed through the suprapubic trocar. An extremely inflamed appendix may be lassoed with a pretied suture ligature, which provides a handy way to elevate it with minimal trauma (Fig. 30.2).

5. Depending upon how the appendix presents, it may be simplest to divide the base before the mesentery. In general, dividing the mesentery first provides the greatest assurance that the dissection of the appendix is carried all the way to the base.

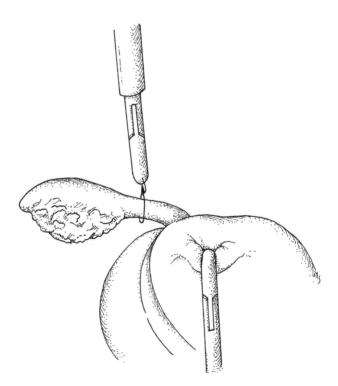

Figure 30.2. A pretied ligature may be used to elevate a grossly inflamed appendix with minimal trauma.

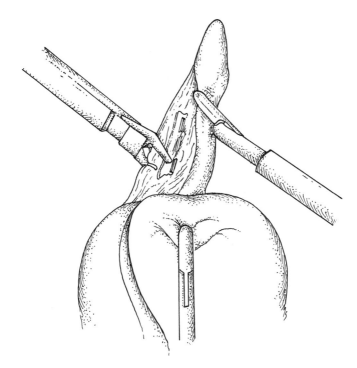

Figure 30.3. The mesoappendix is divided serially with clips, ligatures, or other hemostatic devices. Both the endoscopic stapler and the ultrasonic scalpel may also be used for this purpose.

6. Divide the mesoappendix serially with clips, cautery, ultrasonic scalpel, or endoscopic stapler (Fig. 30.3).
7. Divide the base of the appendix (Fig. 30.4). Ligatures or the endoscopic stapling device may be used. The endoscopic stapling device saves time but is more costly than using two pretied sutures. If the appendix is normal, the appendiceal base and mesoappendix may be divided by a single application of the stapler.
8. Remove the appendix by pulling it into the 12-mm trocar and removing trocar and appendix together, thus protecting the abdominal wall from contamination. An extremely bulky or contaminated appendix may be placed in a specimen bag to facilitate removal (see Chapter 8).

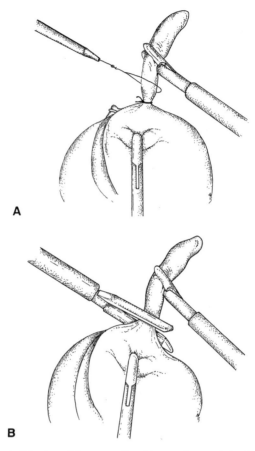

Figure 30.4. A. Division of the appendiceal base using pretied sutures. B. Division of the base using the endoscopic stapling device.

E. Complications

1. **Bleeding**
   a. **Cause and prevention.** Aggressive dissection of the meso-appendix may lead to troublesome bleeding. Likewise, bleeding from omental vessels or the retroperitoneum may occur as the inflamed appendix is dissected out. Careful dissection with early control of the mesoappendix with minimal dissection should prevent this complication.

b. **Recognition and management.** Bleeding is not difficult to recognize. Suction, adequate lighting, and pressure will aid in identifying the bleeding site. An additional trocar may be needed to allow retraction around the field or grasping of the vessel. Control with an endoloop or clip seems more certain than the application of cautery.

2. **Leakage of appendiceal pus or fecalith**

   a. **Cause and prevention.** This problem may be seen when the appendix is tensely distended and inflamed but not yet perforated. Careful dissection with the use of a sterile specimen bag for extraction may prevent leakage.

   b. **Recognition and management.** This complication is easy to recognize and quite distressing. Irrigate the field and suction carefully after removal of the specimen. Retrieve any dropped fecaliths immediately, while still visible. It is easy for a small object like a fecalith to become lost in the pelvis or between loops of bowel. Continue antibiotic coverage for several days after surgery, at least until the patient is afebrile with a normal white blood cell count.

3. **Incomplete appendectomy**

   a. **Cause and prevention.** This problem, although rare, may lead to recurrent appendicitis. It is caused by ligation of the appendix too far from the cecum. It may be prevented by carefully identifying the junction of the base of the appendix with the cecum before ligating and dividing the appendix.

   b. **Recognition and management.** See item 2.b. The surgeon must be aware that a patient who has had a laparoscopic or open appendectomy may later present with signs and symptoms of appendicitis owing to this complication.

F. Selected References

Apelgren KN, Cowan BD, Metcalf AM, Scott-Conner CEH. Laparoscopic appendectomy and the management of gynecologic pathologic conditions found at laparoscopy for presumed appendicitis. Surg Clin North Am 1996;76:469–482.

Cosgrove JM, Gallos G. Laparoscopic appendectomy. In: Brooks DC, ed. Current Review of Minimally Invasive Surgery. New York, Springer-Verlag, 1998, ch. 5.

Guller U, Hervey S, Purves H, et al. Laparoscopic versus open appendectomy: outcomes comparison based on a large administrative database. Ann Surg 2004;239: 43–52.

Macarulla E, Vallet J, Abad JM, et al. Laparoscopic versus open appendectomy: a prospective randomized trial. Surg Laparosc Endosc 1997;7:335–339.

Milne AA, Bradbury AW. Residual appendicitis following laparoscopic appendectomy. Br J Surg 1996;83:217.

Scott-Conner CEH, Hall TJ, Anglin BL, et al. Laparoscopic appendectomy. Am Surg 1992;215:660–667.

Troidl H, Gaitzsch A, Winkler-Wilforth A, et al. Fehler und Gafähren bei der laparoskopis-chen Appendektomie. Chirurg 1993,64:212–220.

31. Laparoscopic Colostomy

Anne T. Mancino, M.D., F.A.C.S.

A. Indications

1. Laparoscopic colostomy is an effective tool for management of un-resectable cancer and severe perianal disease, whenever proximal fecal diversion is required. The ability to perform a thorough exploration of the rest of the abdomen, with biopsy of any suspicious areas (staging), to mobilize a loop, and to create a stoma with minimal adhesion formation, makes it an attractive option for obstructing anorectal cancers (prior to neoadjuvant therapy). Laparoscopic colostomy formation is indicated in the following circumstances:
   a. Unresectable pelvic cancer
   b. Rectovaginal fistula
   c. Complex fistula-in-ano
   d. Perianal sepsis
   e. Fecal incontinence
   f. Obstructing cancers of the anus or rectum, prior to neoadjuvant therapy
   g. Extraperitoneal rectal injuries or severe perineal trauma.
2. In cases of a proximal obstruction or an immobile colon from carcinomatosis, a **laparoscopic loop ileostomy** or transverse colostomy can be formed in a similar manner, with similar advantages.

B. Patient Position and Room Setup

1. Position the patient supine on the operating table with the right arm tucked to the side. The modified lithotomy position (low stirrups) may also be used.
2. Place the patient in the Trendelenburg position and rotate the table to left side up, to move the small intestine out of the pelvis and expose the desired segment of colon.
3. The surgeon stands on the patient's right with the first assistant on the left.
4. Monitors are positioned toward the foot of the bed or toward upper right if transverse colostomy is planned.
5. If an ileostomy or transverse colostomy is planned, the left arm is tucked and the surgeon stands on the patient's left.

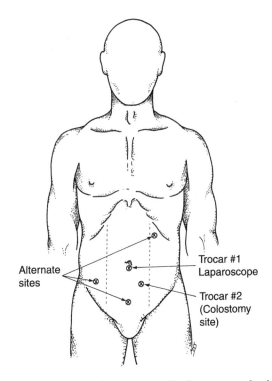

Figure 31.1. Trocar placement for colostomy. The laparoscope should be placed through trocar #1 and the site for trocar #2 inspected for suitability prior to port insertion. The other trocar sites should be used as needed to facilitate exposure and mobilization. If a loop ileostomy is planned, the port sites will be reversed (mirror image).

C. Trocar Placement and Choice of a Laparoscope

1. The first trocar is placed at or just inferior to the umbilicus (Fig. 31.1). A 0-degree (straight-viewing) laparoscope is used to explore the abdomen and verify that the planned ostomy site is free of adhesions.

2. The second trocar is a 10- to 12-mm port placed at the planned ostomy site. This site should be identified and marked by an enterostomal therapist or surgeon prior to the procedure.

3. Further trocars can be positioned in the opposite iliac fossa lateral to the rectus muscle, in the midline suprapubic area, or in the ipsilateral upper quadrant to allow for better mobilization of the bowel. If an end stoma is planned, one of these ports should be 12 mm to accommodate an endoscopic stapler. Otherwise 5-mm ports are in order.

D. Technique of Colostomy

1. Insert the laparoscope through the umbilical port and perform a thorough inspection of the abdominal contents and perform any needed biopsies (see Chapter 13).
2. Assess the suitability of the predetermined stoma site and ascertain that a proximal loop of sigmoid colon or transverse colon will reach without tension.
3. If the site is acceptable, excise a disk of skin and subcutaneous tissue down to the anterior fascia and insert a 10- to 12-mm port through the center of the incision.
4. Pass an atraumatic clamp such as a Babcock into the port, grasp the colon, and pull it toward the abdominal wall to assess mobility.
5. If there are adhesions or mesenteric attachments to the paracolic gutters, a third trocar is inserted to allow countertraction. The lateral attachments or greater omentum can be dissected through the left lower quadrant port using coagulating scissors.
6. Once mobilized, the colon is again grasped with the Babcock clamp (Fig. 31.2A).
7. Back the trocar out over the clamp, withdraw the laparoscope into its trocar, and remove other instruments (except for the Babcock) from the abdomen.
8. Enlarge the fascial defect to allow the colon to be exteriorized. At this point, pneumoperitoneum will be lost.
9. Construct an end colostomy by dividing the colon with a linear stapler, either extracorporeally, which is the simplest method, or under laparoscopic vision using a linear stapling device.
10. Place the distal colon back into the peritoneal cavity and fashion an end stoma in the usual manner (Fig. 31.2B).
11. If an end stoma is not desired, the loop of colon may be matured as a loop colostomy.
12. Do not fully mature the stoma at this point.
13. Reestablish pneumoperitoneum and inspect the intestine to verify:
    a. Absence of any tension or twist
    b. Adequacy of hemostasis
    c. Correct identification of proximal and distal segments
14. Remove the trocars, close the fascial defects, and mature the ostomy.

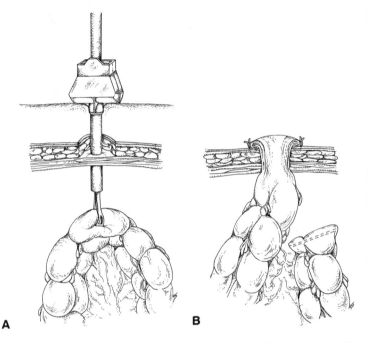

Figure 31.2. Laparoscopic colostomy. A. The preselected colostomy site has been prepared by excising a disk of skin and subcutaneous tissue down to fascia. Fascia is left intact to prevent loss of pneumoperitoneum. A trocar is placed through the center of the ostomy site and a loop of sigmoid colon is grasped. The fascial defect is enlarged and the colon exteriorized. B. The loop has been divided extracorporeally with a linear stapler and the distal segment dropped back into the abdomen. An end stoma has been fashioned in the usual manner. Alternatively, a loop colostomy could be constructed.

E. Complications

1. **Stricture of the stoma**
   a. **Cause and prevention.** A narrowed stoma results from inadequate incision of the fascia. This is more likely to occur in patients with excessive adipose tissue or when the surgeon is trying to prevent the loss of pneumoperitoneum. Excision of the skin and subcutaneous tissue prior to cannula insertion will allow for better visualization. The fascia should then be incised to allow two fingers to pass easily.
   b. **Recognition and management.** The patient will exhibit signs of bowel obstruction with minimal output. Digital examination will usually identify a stricture at the fascial level. Self-intubation of

the stoma serves to dilate the stoma adequately in the majority of cases. If stenosis persists, then surgical revision is necessary.

2. **Malrotation of intestinal loop**
   a. **Cause and prevention.** On occasion the intestinal loop becomes twisted as it is pulled through the abdominal wall. This malrotation can usually be identified intraoperatively by reinsufflating the abdomen and evaluating the position of the loop by direct visualization. The proximal and distal limbs can be marked prior to exteriorization using sutures, staples, or methylene blue injected through a long spinal needle.
   b. **Recognition and management.** The patient will exhibit signs of bowel obstruction with minimal output. If the obstruction appears to be proximal to the stoma on digital exam, then evaluation with endoscopy or water-soluble contrast through the stoma is indicated. If a malrotation of the intestine is identified, it should be repaired operatively.

F. Selected References

Almquist PM, Bohe M, Montgomery A. Laparoscopic creation of loop ileostomy and sigmoid colostomy. Eur J Surg 1995;161:907–909.

Bogen GL, Mancino AT, Scott-Conner CEH. Laparoscopy for staging and palliation of gastrointestinal malignancy. Surg Clin North Am 1996;76:557–569.

Hallfeldt K, Schmidbauer S, Trupka A. Laparoscopic loop colostomy for advanced ovarian cancer, rectal cancer and rectovaginal fistulas. Gyn Oncol 2000;76:380–382.

Khoo REH, Montrey J, Cohen MM. Laproscopic loop ileostomy for temporary fecal diversion. Dis Colon Rectum 1993;36:966–968.

Kini SU, Perston Y, Radcliffe AG. Laparoscopically assisted trephine stoma formation. Surg Laparosc Endosc 1996;6:371–374.

Lange V, Meyer G, Schardey HM, Schildberg FW. Laparoscopic creation of a loop colostomy. J Laparoendosc Surg 1991;1:307–312.

Ludwig KA, Milsom JW, Garcia-Ruiz A, Fazio VW. Laparoscopic techniques for fecal diversion. Dis Colon Rectum 1996;59:285–288.

Lyerly HK, Mault JR. Laparoscopic ileostomy and colostomy. Ann Surg 1994;219:317–322.

Navsaria PH, Graham R, Nicol A. A new approach to extraperitoneal rectal injuries: laparoscopy and diverting loop colostomy. J Trauma-Injury Inf Crit Care 2001;51:532–535.

Oliviera L, Reissman P, Nogueras J, Wexner SD. Laparoscopic creation of stomas. Surg Endosc 1997;11:19–23.

Roe AM, Barlow AP, Durdey P, Eltringham WK, Espiner HJ. Indications for laparoscopic formation of intestinal stomas. Surg Laparosc Endosc 1994;4:345–347.

Sakai T, Yamashita Y, Maekawa T, Shirakusa T. Techniques for determining the ideal stoma site in laparoscopic sigmoid colostomy. Intern Surg 1999;84:239–240.

32. Laparoscopic Segmental Colectomies, Anterior Resection, and Abdominoperineal Resection

Eric G. Weiss, M.D.
Steven D. Wexner, M.D.
Mirza K. Baig, M.D.

A. Indications

1. **Laparoscopic colon resection** may be considered whenever resection of a segment of colon is required. Large masses such as a phlegmon in Crohn's disease or a large bulky tumor may not be amenable to the laparoscopic technique. Laparoscopic colectomy is most commonly performed for one of the following indications:
   a. Endoscopically unresectable benign colon polyps
   b. Crohn's disease
   c. Volvulus
   d. Diverticulitis
   e. Colon carcinoma
2. **Laparoscopic anterior resection** is primarily indicated for neoplasms of the colon, sigmoid, and upper rectum, for which surgical removal is the treatment of choice. This includes the following:
   a. Endoscopically unresectable benign polyps
   b. Rectosigmoid or upper-third rectal cancers
3. **Laparoscopic abdominoperineal resection** is indicated whenever surgical extirpation of the entire rectum and anus is required, and is almost always reserved for cure or palliation of low colorectal malignancies. Indications for this procedure include the following:
   a. Rectal cancer
   b. Squamous cell carcinoma of the anus
   c. Anal or rectal melanoma
   d. Anal or rectal sarcomas
   e. Crohn's disease of the rectum

B. Patient Position and Room Setup

1. Position the patient supine on the operating table with both arms tucked, padded, and protected at the sides.

2. Place the patient in a modified lithotomy position using Allen stirrups (Lloyd-Davies or other designs may be used). It is imperative that the thighs be at or lower than the level of the abdominal wall to obviate difficulty in maneuvering the lower abdominal instruments. This position enables intraoperative colonoscopy, if needed, as well as the introduction of a circular stapler through the anus for construction of a low anastomosis.

3. In general, the surgeon stands on the side of the patient opposite the pathology and site of dissection, with the first assistant standing across the table.

   a. Thus, for **right hemicolectomy or ileocolic resection**, the surgeon typically stands on the patient's left side. At times it may be beneficial to stand between the patient's legs. Two monitors are placed at the head of the table.

   b. For **left colon resections (including abdominoperineal resection)**, the surgeon usually stands on the patient's right side. During mobilization of the splenic flexure it is often easier to stand between the patient's legs. Two monitors are placed at the foot of the table.

4. **Trocar position and choice of laparoscope** will be discussed with each individual procedure.

C. Performing the Laparoscopic Assisted Ileocolic Resection or Right Hemicolectomy

1. Place the **first (10–12 mm) trocar** in the supraumbilical region at the site of the planned incision for specimen extraction. In certain instances where an infraumbilical extraction may be possible (based on pathology and patient's body habitus), this site may be used. Threaded trocars are sometimes helpful in heavy patients with thick abdominal walls.

2. Pass a **0-degree laparoscope** through this trocar.

3. Place **two 10- to 12-mm trocars** in the left upper and left lower quadrants, lateral to the rectus muscles.

4. **Additional trocars** may be needed for retractors (Fig. 32.1). These are generally placed in the right upper or right lower quadrants (again lateral to the rectus muscles). Occasionally, a third additional trocar may be placed very high in the left upper quadrant.

5. Position the patient in steep Trendelenburg position with the left side of the table down.

6. Identify the terminal ileum and base of cecum. Grasp the cecum with an endoscopic Babcock-type clamp.

7. Incise along the white line of Toldt with ultrasonic scissors or electrocautery scissors, and mobilize the right colon superiorly to the level of the liver.

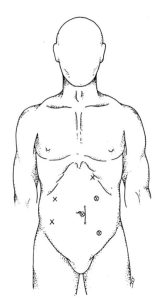

Figure 32.1. Positions of the 10- to 12-mm trocars for ileocolic resection and right hemicolectomy. The small midline incision is made as an extension of a trocar site and is used for exteriorization of the specimen and extracorporeal resection and anastomosis: ⊗, typical trocars; ×, optional trocars.

8. Continually regrasp and manipulate the right colon as needed for further medial dissection to expose the ureter, Gerota's fascia, and the duodenum (see Figs. 32.2 and 32.3).
9. Grasp the hepatic flexure and divide the hepaticocolic ligament with ultrasonic or electrocautery scissors. When using electrocautery scissors, it is necessary to have ligaclips or endoclips available as bleeding may occur.
10. Finally, grasp the transverse colon and divide the greater omentum distal to the gastroepiploic vessels to the level of the middle colic artery. The ultrasonic scissors work better than other modalities for this dissection.
11. Once the right colon has been completely mobilized as described, grasp the cecum with an endoscopic Babcock clamp passed through the selected site of specimen removal. Place the laparoscope in one of the other trocar sites if necessary.
    a. In patients with Crohn's disease, it is imperative to "run" the small bowel.
    b. Accomplish this maneuver by a "hand-over-hand" technique using two Babcock clamps under direct vision.

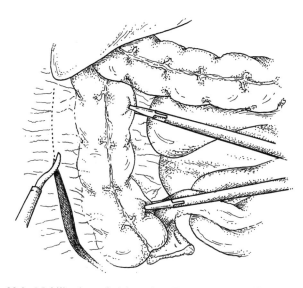

Figure 32.2. Mobilization of right colon. Two graspers pull the right colon medially as the white line of Toldt is incised.

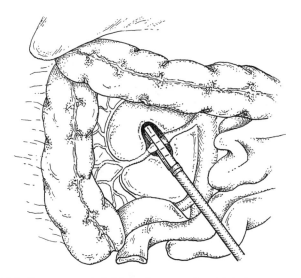

Figure 32.3. Intracorporeal division of mesenteric pedicle is an alternative to totally extracorporeal resection.

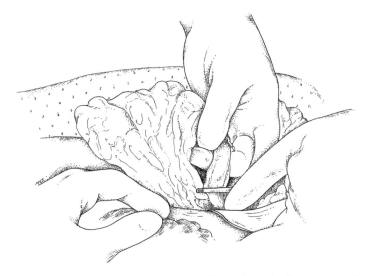

Figure 32.4. Terminal ileum, cecum, ascending and proximal transverse colon eviscerated through the small midline incision. Resection and anastomosis will be performed in an extracorporeal manner. The anastomosis is then returned to the abdominal cavity.

12. At the site of the initial trocar placement, usually in the supraumbilical position, make a 2- to 5-cm vertical incision in the skin.

13. Make the fascial incision along the insulated sheath of the forceps (which is attached to the cecum). Allow the pneumoperitoneum to collapse.

14. Deliver the cecum to the midline wound, and eviscerate the terminal ileum, cecum, and ascending and proximal transverse colon onto the abdominal wall (see Fig. 32.4).

   a. The vascular ligation, bowel division, anastomosis, and closure of the mesenteric defect are performed as they would be during a laparotomy.

   b. Typically, a stapled functional end-to-end anastomosis is performed. The mesenteric defect is closed in the usual fashion.

   c. When the anastomosis is complete, return it to the abdominal cavity, taking great care not to damage or tear the bowel or mesentery during this manipulation.

   d. Close the incision using interrupted absorbable sutures.

15. Reestablish pneumoperitoneum through one of the other trocar sites, and insert the laparoscope.

16. Inspect the bowel, anastomosis, and abdomen; irrigate and assure hemostasis. Close trocar sites in the usual fashion.

D. Laparoscopic Assisted Sigmoid Colon Resection or Left Hemicolectomy

1. Place the patient in **steep Trendelenburg position** with the right side of the table down.
2. Introduce the first trocar in the supraumbilical region and insert a **0-degree laparoscope**. Next, place two 10- to 12-mm trocars in the right upper and lower quadrants, lateral to the rectus muscle. Place a third 10- to 12-mm trocar in the left upper quadrant. This trocar will be exchanged for a 33-mm port using the Seldinger technique.
3. Rarely, a fourth 10- to 12-mm trocar placed in the left upper quadrant lateral to the rectus muscle is used for additional retraction. This site also provides an excellent vantage point for laparoscopic visualization of the anastomosis. A fifth trocar is sometimes high in the right upper quadrant if needed (Fig. 32.5).
4. Grasp the sigmoid colon with an endoscopic Babcock clamp and retract it medially to expose the white line of Toldt.
5. Using either a ultrasonically activated scissors or a cautery scissors, incise the peritoneum to mobilize the sigmoid and left colon to the level of the splenic flexure (Fig. 32.6).

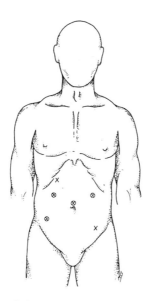

Figure 32.5. Placement of 10- to 12-mm trocars for laparoscopic assisted left colon resection. Two optional trocar sites (right upper quadrant and left lower quadrant) are occasionally helpful: ⊗, typical trocars; ×, optional trocars.

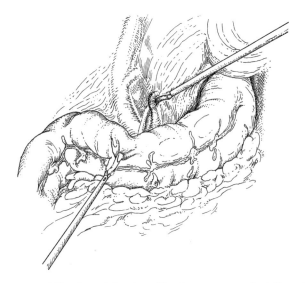

Figure 32.6. Mobilization of the sigmoid colon to expose the left ureter as it crosses the pelvic brim. The iliac vessels are seen to the left of the ureter.

6. Continually regrasp and manipulate the colon as the dissection progresses medially to expose Gerota's fascia, the ureter, and the sacral promontory.
7. Next, mobilize the splenic flexure and distal transverse colon. The dissection may be easier if the surgeon stands between the patient's legs and uses a left lower quadrant port site.
8. Divide the gastrocolic omentum with an ultrasonic scalpel or cautery scissors to the level of the middle colic artery.
9. Grasp the transverse colon with an endoscopic Babcock clamp and dissect transverse colon and splenic flexure free of the retroperitoneum inferior to the spleen.
10. After complete mobilization, ligate the vascular pedicle intracorporeally.
    a. Medially isolate either the superior hemorrhoidal and the left colic arteries or the inferior mesenteric artery.
    b. Anterolateral retraction of the left colon facilitates this identification.
    c. **Isolate the vessels** by scoring the mesentery and creating windows in the mesentery on each side.
    d. These vessels are typically divided by using an endoscopic stapler with a (white) **vascular cartridge** introduced via the right lower quadrant port site.
    e. Visualize the blades on the lateral side of the mesentery. **This is crucial** to ensure that nothing else is incorporated into them.

    f.   After confirming satisfactory positioning, fire the stapler.

    g.   Typically, only the above-named vessels and possibly the inferior mesenteric vein are divided in this manner.

    h.   After isolating the smaller vessels in the sigmoid mesentery, control them with clips, ligatures, or the ultrasonic scalpel.

11. Identify the distal extent of resection and circumferentially expose the colonic or rectal wall.

12. Exchange the right lower quadrant 10- to 12-mm trocar for an 18-mm trocar over an exchange rod under direct vision.

13. Insert a 45- to 60-mm linear cutting stapler, encompass the bowel wall between the blades (making sure that laterally nothing else is incorporated into the blades), and fire the stapler (Fig. 32.7).

14. In the left upper quadrant, enlarge the skin incision and exchange the previously placed 10- to 12-mm port over a rod for a 33-mm port.

15. Place a Babcock clamp through this trocar and grasp the proximal staple line.

16. Extrude the specimen through the port or in continuity with the port. If the specimen is too large, remove the port and deliver the bowel through an enlarged incision protected by a plastic wound drape.

17. Perform the proximal resection extracorporeally in the conventional fashion. Place a pursestring suture and insert the circular stapling anvil into the proximal end of bowel. Secure the pursestring suture and replace the bowel into the abdominal cavity (Fig. 32.8).

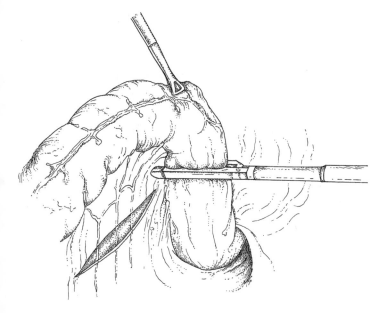

Figure 32.7. The endoscopic linear stapler is used to divide the bowel at the distal resection margin.

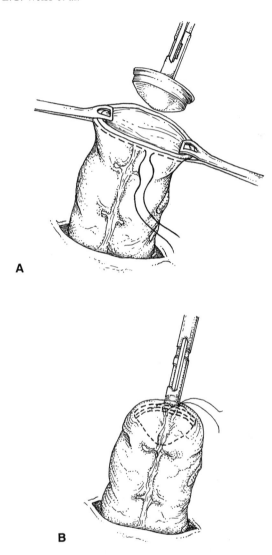

Figure 32.8. A. The anvil of the circular stapler is inserted in the proximal end of the bowel (which has been drawn out of the abdomen through an enlarged trocar site). B. The pursestring suture is tied. The bowel is then returned to the abdomen.

18. Replace the 33-mm trocar (if it was removed) and reestablish pneumoperitoneum.
19. Grasp the anvil with an anvil-grasping clamp, usually passed through the right upper or lower quadrant trocar sites. Assess the ability of the anvil to reach the planned anastomotic site. Further mobilization and/or vascular division may be needed, and should be performed if necessary. Verify the correct orientation (i.e., no twist) for the proximal bowel.
20. Insert a circular stapler transanally and advance it to the distal staple line. Under direct laparoscopic visual control, extend the spike of the stapler through the distal staple line. Attach the anvil (Fig. 32.9).

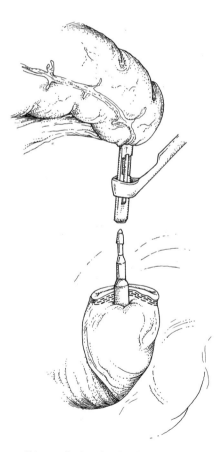

Figure 32.9. The anvil is attached to the circular stapler (which has been passed transanally); the stapler will be closed and fired in the usual fashion.

21. Move the laparoscope to the right or left lower quadrant port to best visualize the anvil and stapler head coming together. Once satisfied, close, fire, and remove the stapler. Inspect the two donuts for completeness.
22. Test the anastomosis by placing an atraumatic Dennis-type clamp across the bowel proximal to the anastomosis. Use the suction-irrigator to fill the pelvis with saline and immerse the anastomosis. Insufflate the rectum with air, using a bulb syringe, proctoscope, or flexible sigmoidoscope, and observe for air bubbles.
23. Irrigate the abdomen, obtain hemostasis, and close the trocar sites. Close the 33-mm port site with interrupted absorbable sutures.

E. Performing the Laparoscopic Anterior Resection

1. Patient position is similar to that described in Section D.
2. A thorough inspection is required for patients with cancer to exclude any metastatic disease.
3. Place the first three (10–12 mm) trocars in the supraumbilical region (laparoscope) and right upper and right lower quadrants, lateral to the rectus muscle.
4. Place a fourth (10–12 mm) trocar in the left upper quadrant lateral to the rectus muscle. This will be exchanged for a 33-mm trocar later. Additional (10–12 mm) trocars may be needed for retraction.
5. After mobilizing the left colon (see Section D), grasp the rectosigmoid junction using an endoscopic Babcock clamp and retract it anteriorly toward the abdominal wall.
6. Enter the presacral plane posteriorly with ultrasonic or cautery scissors. Dissect posteriorly to well below the level of the pathology, using sharp dissection.
7. Intraoperative rigid proctoscopy is often helpful to confirm the exact level of the lesion. Mark the site with clips.
8. Continue the dissection laterally and finally anteriorly to circumferentially free the mesorectum at least 5 cm distal to the distal edge of the tumor.
9. Serially divide and ligate the mesorectum (at right angles to the rectum) with a series of clips, vascular stapler, or ultrasonically activated scissors. Bare rectum should be demonstrated circumferentially. Perform a total mesorectum excision for tumors in the lower two thirds of the rectum, to obtain adequate tumor control.
10. The remainder of the procedure is analagous to that described above for a sigmoid or left colectomy (Section D).

F. Performing a Laparoscopic Abdominoperineal Resection

1. The patient position and trocar sites are as previously described, except that the third 10- to 12-mm trocar should be placed at the site of the proposed colostomy (which will have been marked by the enterostomal therapist prior to surgery). This mark will typically overlie the rectus muscle. Insert this trocar with great care to avoid laceration of the inferior epigastric vessels.
2. The initial mobilization is similar to that already described for a sigmoid colectomy, left colectomy, or anterior resection.
   a. Depending on the length and mobility of the sigmoid colon, it may not be necessary to mobilize the splenic flexure.
   b. The level of vascular ligation may vary based on the same considerations.
3. Choose a point at which to divide the bowel. Serially divide the mesentery at this level using ultrasonically activated scissors, ligatures, clips, or vascular stapler. At this site, the mesentery is serially divided to this level using either the ultrasonically activated scissors, vessel loops, ligaclips, or vascular stapler.
4. Transect the bowel as previously described for sigmoid and left colectomy.
5. Grasp the distal colonic staple line and retract it anteriorly or inferiorly to expose the presacral space. The presacral space is entered posteriorly using either cautery scissors or an ultrasonic scalpel.
6. Dissect the presacral space posteriorly to the level of Waldeyer's fascia. Open this fascia to expose the levator muscles.
7. Continue this dissection laterally on both sides.
8. Perform the anterior dissection last.
   a. Retract the rectum superiorly and posteriorly. In the female, retract the uterus (if present) anteriorly and inferiorly.
   b. Dissect the rectum from vagina (in females) or seminal vesicles and prostate (in males).
9. At this point, with the rectum fully mobilized intracorporeally, the perineal dissection is made.
   a. Make an elliptical incision around the external sphincter.
   b. Deepen this incision into the ischiorectal fat to expose the levator muscles. Posteriorly, place the levator plate at the level of the tip of the coccyx. Introduce a finger into the pelvis posteriorly and visualize it with the laparoscope.
   c. Divide the levators laterally and posteriorly.
   d. Insert a ring forceps into the pelvis from below. Under laparoscopic control, the tip of the rectum/sigmoid colon is handed to the perineal operator via the ring forceps. The rectosigmoid colon is then extracted from below.
   e. Complete the remaining dissection from the perineal aspect in the usual fashion.

10. Pass an endoscopic Babcock clamp via the trocar at the stoma site, and grasp the remaining end of sigmoid colon. Excise a 2-cm disk of skin around the trocar site and enlarge the trocar site. Bring out the end of the colon as a colostomy. Mature this in the usual fashion.

11. From the perineal wound, pass an endoscopic Babcock clamp into the abdomen and guide it up retrograde through the right lower quadrant trocar site. Grasp and pull an irrigation sump catheter through the trocar site and position it just above the levators. Close the levators and perineum, and complete the operation in the usual fashion.

G. Complications

1. **Anastomotic leak**
   a. **Cause and prevention.** A well-vascularized, tension-free, circumferentially intact anastomosis is necessary to prevent anastamotic leakage. If any of the foregoing requirements are not present during a laparoscopic assisted colectomy, then the anastomosis must be revised. It is often prudent, if not mandatory, to convert to a laparotomy at this point. Identification of ischemia may be difficult and the aid of intravenous fluorescein should be used. One ampule of fluorescein given intravenously followed by inspection with a Wood's lamp allows for identification of ischemic bowel. Resection proximally to viable colon will alleviate this problem. Intraoperative testing of the anastomosis is mandatory as described earlier. Any leak requires, at minimum, reinforcement if not complete revision. The use of only a diverting stoma to protect such an anastomosis is inadequate.
   b. **Recognition and management.** Postoperative fevers, prolonged ileus, elevated leukocyte counts, and abdominal pain are all hallmarks of postoperative anastomotic leak. Aggressive detection and delineation will often allow conservative therapy to be employed. Perform prompt radiologic evaluation of the anastomosis using a water-soluble contrast enema (perhaps in concert with a computed tomography [CT] scan of the abdomen and pelvis). If a small leak or a leak associated with a localized abscess is identified, percutaneous drainage, antibiotics, bowel rest, and total parenteral nutrition often allow for spontaneous closure. If a large, free leak is identified, prompt laparotomy with stoma creation is necessary.

2. **Postoperative small bowel obstruction**
   a. **Cause and prevention.** Postoperative small bowel obstruction is almost universally caused by adhesion formation. Postoperative adhesions may be less common with the laparoscopic approach. However, internal hernias or port site hernias may still occur. Closing mesenteric defects and closing all port sites of 10 mm or greater should help minimize this problem.

b. **Recognition and management.** Abdominal distention, cessation or no passage of flatus, and the inability to tolerate oral intake associated with nausea or vomiting are all common signs and symptoms of small bowel obstruction. When these symptoms occur early in the postoperative course (3–10 days), it is often difficult to distinguish a bowel obstruction from a normal postoperative ileus. Initial management is similar in both cases with nasogastric tube decompression, intravenous fluids, and possibly nutritional support. This conservative management may continue in the absence of fevers, rising white blood counts, or peritonitis (which would indicate leak, see above). Consider evaluation of the port sites via CT scan or ultrasound in any patient who develops a bowel obstruction after a laparoscopic procedure. Failure to resolve mandates reexploration (usually via laparotomy) for lysis of adhesions and possible bowel resection. If possible, the addition of an antiadhesion product should be employed to prevent further postoperative adhesions.

H. Selected References

Bernstein MA, Dawson JW, Reissman PR, et al. Is complete laparoscopic colectomy superior to laparoscopic assisted colectomy? Am Surg 1996;62:507–511.

Braga M, Vignalli A, Gianotti L, et al. Laparoscopic versus open colorectal surgery: a randomized trial on short term outcome. Ann Surg 2002;236:759–767.

Cohen SM, Wexner SD. Laparoscopic right hemicolectomy. In: Lezoche E, Paganini AM, Cuschieri A, eds. Minimally Invasive Surgery. Milan, Italy: Documento Editoriale, 1994:23–26.

Darzi A, Lewis C, Menzies-Gow, et al. Laparoscopic abdominoperineal excision of the rectum. Surg Endosc 1995;9:414–417.

Duepree HJ, Senagore AJ, Delaney CP, Brady KM, Fazio VW. Advantages of laparoscopic resection for ileocecal Crohn's disease. Dis Colon Rectum 2002;45:605–610.

Fine AP, Lanasa S, Gannon MP, et al. Laparoscopic colon surgery: report of a series. Am Surg 1995;61:412–416.

Franklin ME. Laparoscopic low anterior resection and abdominoperineal resections. Semi Colon Rectal Surg 1994;5:258–266.

Hamel CT, Hildebrandt U, Weiss EG, Feifelz G, Wexner SD. Laparoscopic surgery for inflammatory bowel disease. Surg Endosc 2001;15:642–645.

Hong D, Lewis M, Tabet J, Anvari M. Prospective comparison of laparoscopic versus open resection for benign colorectal disease. Surg Laparosc Endosc Percutan Techniques 2002;12:238–242.

Jacobs M, Verdeja JC, Goldstein MD. Minimally invasive colon resection (laparoscopic colectomy). Surg Laparosc Endosc 1991;1:144–150.

Kockerling F, Scheidbach H, Schneider C, et al. Laparoscopic abdominoperineal resection: early postoperative results of a prospective study involving 116 patients. The

Laparoscopic Colorectal Surgery Study Group. Dis Colon Rectum 2000;43: 1503–1511.

Lacy AM, Garcia-Valdercasas JC, Delgado S, Grande L, et al. Postoperative complications of laparoscopic assisted colectomy. Surg Endosc 1997;11:119–122.

Lacy AM, Garcia-Valdecassas JC, Delgado S, et al. Laparoscopy-assisted colectomy versus open colectomy for treatment of nonmetastatic colon cancer: a randomized trial. Lancet 2002;359:2224–2229.

Larach SW, Salomon MC, Williamson PR, Goldstein E. Laparoscopic assisted abdominoperineal resection. Surg Laparosc Endosc 1993;3:115–118.

Ludwig KA, Milsom JW, Church JM, Fazio VW. Preliminary experience with laparoscopic intestinal surgery for Crohn's disease. Am J Surg 1996;171:52–56.

Marcello PW, Milsom JW, Wong SK, et al. Laparoscopic restorative proctocolectomy: case matched comparative study with open restorative proctocolectomy. Dis Colon Rectum 2000;43:604–608.

Milsom JW, Hammerhofer KA, Bohm B, Marcello P, Elson P, Fazio VW. Prospective randomized trial comparing laparoscopic versus open conventional surgery for refractory ileocolic Crohn's disease. Dis Colon Rectum 2001;44:1–8.

Phillips EH, Franklin M, Carroll BJ, et al. Advances in surgical technique: laparoscopic colectomy. Ann Surg 1992;216:703–707.

Pietrabissa A, Moretto C, Carobbi A, Boggi U, Ghilli M, Mosca F. Hand assisted laparoscopic low anterior resection: initial experience with a new procedure. Surg Endosc 2002;16:431–435.

Pikarsky AJ, Rosenthal R, Weiss EG, Wexner SD. Laparoscopic total mesorectal excision. Surg Endosc 2002;16:558–562.

Poulin EC, Schlachta CM, Seshardi PA, Cadeddu MO, Gregoire R, Mamazza J. Septic complications of elective laparoscopic colorectal resection. Surg Endosc 2001; 15:203–208.

Quattlebaum JK, Flanders D, Usher CH. Laparoscopically assisted colectomy. Surg Laparosc Endosc 1993;3:81–86.

Reissman P, Salky BA, Pfeifer J, et al. Laparoscopic surgery in the management of inflammatory bowel disease. Am J Surg 1996;171:47–51.

Sackier JM, Berci G, Hiatt JR, Hartunian S. Laparoscopic abdominoperineal resection of the rectum. Br J Surg 1992;1207–1208.

Schiedbach H, Schneider C, Konradt J, et al. Laparoscopic abdominoperineal resection and anterior resection with curative intent for carcinoma of the rectum. Surg Endosc 2002;16:7–13.

Tate JJT, Kwok S, Dawson JW, et al. Prospective comparison of laparoscopic and conventional anterior resections. Br J Surg 1993;80:1396–1398.

Trebuchet G, Lechaux D, Lecalve JL. Laparoscopic left colon resection for diverticular disease. Surg Endosc 2002;16:18–21.

Young-Fadok TM, Nelson H. Laparoscopic right colectomy: five step procedure. Dis Colon Rectum 2000;43:267–271.

Zucker KA, Pitcher DE, Martin DT, Ford RS. Laparoscopic assisted colon resection. Surg Endosc 1994;8:12–18.

33. Laparoscopic-Assisted Proctocolectomy with Ileal-Pouch-Anal Anastomosis

Amanda Metcalf, M.D., F.A.C.S.

A. Indications

Laparoscopic assisted proctocolectomy with ileal-pouch anal anastomosis is indicated for young patients with ulcerative colitis or familial polyposis.

1. In patients with **ulcerative colitis**, the most common indication is intractible disease or carcinoma prophylaxis in patients who wish a continence-preserving procedure. It is **not indicated** in the surgical management of toxic megacolon.
2. The procedure is indicated for patients with **familial polyposis**, when multiple adenomatous colonic polyps are detected on surveillance endoscopy.

B. Patient Position and Room Setup

1. Place the patient in the dorsolithotomy position, with arms extended, and legs in Allen stirrups (Allen Medical Co., Bedford Heights, OH), with minimal hip flexion, (i.e., with the upper legs almost parallel to the floor). The arms should be abducted less than 90 degrees to minimize the possibility of brachial plexopathy. This position allows the surgeon and assistants to manipulate instruments from between the legs with full mobility.
2. Prepare and drape both the abdominal wall and perineum to allow full access to both areas.
3. The surgeon usually stands on the side opposite to the site of dissection: on the left side during mobilization of the right colon, between the legs for the transverse colon, and on the right side for the left colon.
4. The camera operator should stand adjacent to the surgeon, ensuring that the camera view of the operative field is parallel to the surgeon's view.
5. Other assistants usually stand on the opposite side of the table.
6. Place the monitors on each side, toward the head of the patient for the abdominal portions of the procedure, and then toward the feet if the pelvic dissection is performed laparoscopically.

C. Trocar Position and Choice of Laparoscope

1. Place the first trocar just inferior to the umbilicus.
2. A 30-degree angled laparoscope is useful during the majority of the procedure.
3. In general, four additional port sites will be placed, one in each quadrant of the abdomen (Fig. 33.1). The exact number and location depends upon the habitus of the patient and the location and mobility of the colon.
4. All trocar sites should be at least 10 mm in size, and those in the lower abdomen optimally should be 12 mm in size, to allow use of the Multifire Endo-GIA stapler (US Surgical, Norwalk, CT).
5. Use of a 12-mm site in all quadrants will add versatility in the application of the endostapler on all the major mesenteric pedicles.
6. Port sites are ideally placed lateral to the rectus sheath, but modification of placement locations can allow one to "hide" a site in, for example, the proposed right lower quadrant ostomy site, or to the left of the midline in the anticipated site of a Pfannenstiel incision. This incision is usually made after full laparoscopic mobilization of the colon, for specimen delivery and construction of the ileal pouch. Threaded cannula oversleeves are useful in each port site to prevent accidental dislodgment of cannulas during manipulation.

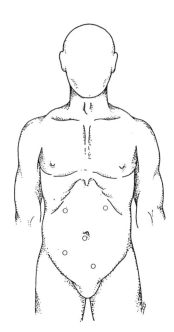

Figure 33.1. Suggested port sites for laparoscopic proctocolectomy.

7. An alternative technique is to use the Pfannenstiel incision for place-
    ment of a hand-access port (HandPort: Smith and Nephew, Andover,
    MA). This is usually made after the placement of the port site in the
    subumbilical location. The size of the incision is the same size as the
    surgeon's glove. The fascial incision is made in the linea alba, and
    the lower ring of the donut device is inserted into the peritoneal cavity.
    The device is then insufflated. The surgeon then uses his or her non-
    dominant hand through this device for retraction and palpation. Addi-
    tional port sites are placed as needed in the positions illustrated.

D. Performing the Abdominal Colectomy

1. The dissection **begins in the right lower quadrant** and follows the
    colon around to the sigmoid.
2. **Mobilization of the right colon**
    a. Rotate the operating table to the left, and place the patient in the
        Trendelenburg position to facilitate displacement of small bowel
        loops from the right lower quadrant. Place the laparoscope
        through the infraumbilical or the left upper quadrant port.
    b. The assistant retracts the ascending colon medially using an
        atraumatic bowel grasper. Babcock forceps may be used instead,
        but this tends to cause serosal tears that can convert to inadver-
        tent enterotomies. In patients with friable bowel, the mesentery
        or epiploical appendices of the colon can be grasped instead to
        minimize trauma to the bowel wall.
    c. The surgeon will generally work through the lower abdominal
        cannula sites, using a bowel-grasping instrument through one
        cannula and the dissecting instrument through the other site
        (Fig. 33.2).
    d. If a hand port device is utilized, the surgeon retracts the colon
        medially through the hand port site and uses the upper abdomi-
        nal cannula sites for the dissecting instruments.
    e. Incise the peritoneum along the white line of Toldt using
        Endoshears with electrocautery or the harmonic scalpel (Ethicon
        Endosurgery, Cincinnati, OH) to minimize bleeding, which can
        quickly obscure the operative field.
    f. As dissection is performed in this areolar plane, apply increasing
        traction to the right colon to facilitate complete dissection of even
        flimsy attachments.
    g. Recognize complete dissection of all attachments by clear iden-
        tification of Gerota's fascia overlying the right kidney and the
        duodenal sweep.
    h. Incomplete dissection will make intracorporeal ligation of the
        vascular pedicles extremely difficult.
3. **Mobilization of transverse colon**
    a. Place the patient in reverse Trendelenburg position during this
        portion of the procedure, with traction applied in a caudad direc-

tion to either the omentum overlying the transverse colon or the transverse colon itself.

b. Stand between the patient's legs or on either side of the patient as preferred.

c. As the dissection progresses around the hepatic flexure, divide the greater omentum and expose the lesser sac with the harmonic scalpel (The omental vessels are too larger to be reliably controlled with cautery, and endoclips are tedious to apply to each omental vessel).

d. Retract the stomach cephalad by grasping it opposite the colonic retractor (Fig. 33.3).

e. After division of several omental vessels, the defect in the omentum will allow the use of a fan-shaped retractor on either the colon or the stomach.

f. As in all portions of this procedure, application of the appropriate amount of traction and countertraction greatly facilitates the dissection.

g. In the region of the splenic flexure, it may be easier to divide the omentum in a caudad direction to enter the avascular plane between the colon and the omentum.

4. **Mobilization of the left colon**

a. Position the patient in reverse Trendelenburg position and rotate the table to the right.

b. Stand on the patient's right side, or between the legs.

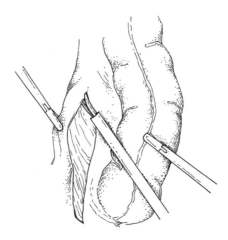

Figure 33.2. With the patient rotated to the left in steep Trendelenburg position, the surgeon retracts the peritoneum laterally while the assistant retracts the right colon medially.

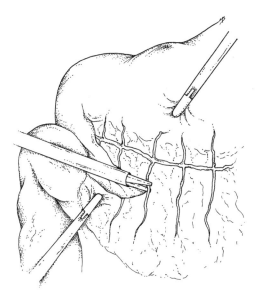

Figure 33.3. The stomach is retracted cephalad as the transverse colon is retracted caudad while the omentum is divided with the harmonic scalpel.

    c. Retract the left colon with atraumatic bowel graspers, a fan-shaped retractor, or by hand if using the hand port device.

    d. Dissect in the areolar plane all the way from the splenic flexure to the left pelvic brim, taking care to identify both the gonadal vessels and the left ureter. Gentle blunt dissection is sufficient to sweep these structures laterally and posteriorly from the mesocolon.

5. **Transection of the mesenteric vessels** is most rapidly accomplished by using the endostapler with vascular staples.

    a. The assistant (or the surgeon if using the hand port device) grasps either the colon itself or the mesentery adjacent to the colon, and retracts the mesentery toward the anterior abdominal wall.

    b. With sufficient traction, the position of vessels can be determined by identifying the lines of traction they produce on the stretched mesentery.

    c. Make openings on each side of the vessels close to the base of the mesentary using either the endoshears or the harmonic scalpel.

    d. Transect the vascular pedicles with the vascular endostapler (Fig. 33.4).

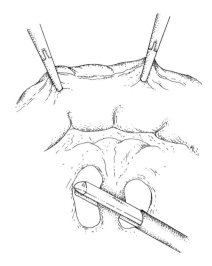

Figure 33.4. The colon is retracted toward the anterior abdominal wall as the vascular pedicle is divided with the linear cutting stapler.

E. Completion of the Operation

1. Remove the cannulas, and make a Pfannenstiel incision.
2. Mobilization of the rectum from the presacral space is performed through this incision.
3. Transect the ileum and rectum with an endoscopic linear stapler and remove the specimen.
4. Construct the pouch in the usual fashion and create the ileoanal anastomosis.
5. Choose a suitable portion of the ileum for construction of the diverting loop ileostomy, if desired, and draw this loop through the right lower quadrant trocar site.
6. Place a pelvic drain.
7. Close all trocar sites.
8. Finally, close the Pfannenstiel incision and then mature the loop ileostomy.

F. Complications

1. **Bowel trauma.** Inadvertent enterotomy is usually due to excessive trauma to the bowel during retraction. Avoid this problem by using atraumatic bowel graspers when feasible and retracting the colon by

the taenia. Sometimes the colon is excessively fragile, secondary to fulminant colitis; inability to retract without tearing the colon may preclude a laparoscopic assisted approach in this situation. As mentioned in earlier sections, damage to the bowel can result from electrocautery or the ultrasonic scalpel and can present as a bowel perforation several days postoperatively.

2. **Bleeding.** This complication can occur during a variety of maneuvers. A few situations in which it may occur, and their management or prevention, are the following.

   a. Bleeding frequently occurs during division of the omentum as a result of shearing of the omentum, especially in the region of the splenic flexure.

   b. If the omentum is thickened and foreshortened in the region of the splenic flexure, it may be wise to use the linear cutting stapler with vascular staples to transect the omentum.

   c. There will often be slight oozing from a mesenteric or omental pedicle if smaller vessels are divided with the stapler. This can usually be managed with the application of either a large endoclip or an endoloop.

3. **Ureteral injury.** Ureteral injury can be caused by inadvertent energy transfer from the electrocautery unit or the harmonic scalpel, or from inclusion in the stapling device during transection of the mesenteric pedicle. This complication can be manifest by postoperative fever, ileus, or excessive drainage from pelvic drains that is high in creatinine. Minimize the risk of this complication by clearly identifying the ureter during dissection, and convert to an open procedure if this is not possible. Recognition of a ureteral injury usually mandates conversion to an open procedure for repair.

4. **Pressure injuries.** The length of the procedure, with frequent operating table position changes, increases the risk of pressure injuries to the ulnar, peroneal, and brachial plexus nerves. Careful patient positioning with padding of pressure points is imperative, as is securing the patient to the table. Use sequential compression devices to minimize the incidence of deep venous thrombosis.

G. Selected References

Bruce CJ, Coller MA, Murray JJ, Schoetz DJ, Roberts PL, Rusin LC. Laparoscopic resection for diverticular disease. Dis Colon Rectum 1996;39(10 Suppl):S1–S10.

Darzi A. Hand-assisted laparoscopic colorectal surgery. Surg Endosc 2000;14:999–1004.

Franklin ME Jr, Rosenthal D, Abrego-Medina D, et al. Prospective comparison of open vs. laparoscopic colon surgery for carcinoma. Five year results. Dis Colon Rectum 1996;39(10 Suppl):S35–S46.

Jacobs M, Plasencia G. Laparoscopic colon surgery: some helpful hints. Intern Surg 1994;79:233–234.

Jager RM, Wexner SD. Laparoscopic Colorectal Surgery. New York: Churchill-Livingstone, 1996.

Liu MD, Rolandelli R, Ashley SW, Evans B, Shin M, McFadden DW. Laparoscopic surgery for inflammatory bowel disease. Am Surg 1995;61:1054–1056.

Lointier PH, Lautard M, Massoni C, Ferrier C, Dapoigny M. Laparoscopically assisted subtotal colectomy. J Laparoendosc Surg 1993;3:439–453.

Marcello PW, Milsom JW, Wong SK, et al. Laparoscopic restorative proctocolectomy: a case-matched comparative study with open restorative proctocolectomy. Dis Colon Rectum 2000;43:604–608.

Mathis CR, MacFayden BV Jr. Laparoscopic colorectal resection: a review of the current experience. Intern Surg 1994;79:221–225.

O'Reilly MJ, Saye WB, Mullins SG, Pinto SE, Falkner PT. Technique of hand-assisted laparoscopic surgery. J Laparoendosc Surg 1996;6:239–244.

Schirmer BD. Laparoscopic colon resection. Surg Clin North Am 1996;76:571–583.

34. Laparoscopy in Inflammatory Bowel Disease

Carol E.H. Scott-Conner, M.D. Ph.D.

A. Introduction

The term "inflammatory bowel disease" refers to a family of disorders characterized by chronic inflammation. The precise pathogenesis of these disorders remains to be elucidated. The two disorders most commonly requiring surgical intervention are chronic ulcerative colitis (UC) and Crohn's disease (CD). For the surgeon, UC and CD differ in anatomic extent of disease within the tubular gastrointestinal tract, depth of involvement, continuity of disease, risk for subsequent of development of carcinoma, and predilection for recurrence (Table 34.1). Both disorders have extraintestinal manifestations, but the current laparoscopic management of these diseases targets only the intestinal manifestations. Section E lists references that deal with these issues in greater detail.

B. Indications for Surgery

As medical management has improved, surgery is less frequently required. The most common indications for surgery reflect the clinicopathologic differences (Table 34.2) and are discussed in greater detail here.

1. Ulcerative Colitis

a. **Cancer prophylaxis.** Carcinoma is estimated to develop in 7 to 14% of patients who have had ulcerative colitis for 25 years. The rate may reach 30% in patients who have had disease for more than 35 years. The risk is increased in patients with
   i. Young age at onset
   ii. Long duration of active disease
   iii. Dysplasia at surveillance colonoscopy
   iv. Pancolitis rather than isolated left colon involvement
   v. Associated diagnosis of primary sclerosing cholangitis (one of the extraintestinal manifestations)
   The operation that is performed is total proctocolectomy, generally with some sort of sphincter preservation (reservoir formation),

Table 34.1. Anatomic extent of disease in chronic ulcerative colitis (UC) and Crohn's disease (CD) within the tubular gastrointestinal tract.

	UC	CD
Anatomic extent of disease	Colon and rectum	Entire gastrointestinal tract
Depth of involvement	Mucosal	Transmural
Continuity of disease	Continuous (no skip lesions)	Skip lesions are common
Risk of cancer in diseased bowel	High	Slightly increased
Recurs after surgical resection of involved bowel	No	Yes

discussed in detail in Chapter 33. By removing all diseased mucosa, this operation cures the colorectal disease but does not eliminate the extraintestinal manifestations.

b. **Emergency resection** for bleeding, toxic megacolon, or perforation. Because these patients are often in very poor condition, the operation is chosen to minimize operative time and trauma. Diseased bowel is removed and if possible, a remnant of the anorectum is preserved to allow subsequent reconstruction. The operation that is generally performed is total abdominal proctocolectomy with ileostomy (see Chapters 32 and 33).

2. Crohn's Disease

Crohn's disease cannot be cured by surgery, even when all diseased bowel is resected. The risk of subsequent development of carcinoma is slight, and hence surgery is reserved for symptoms. Because the small intestine is so commonly

Table 34.2. Indications for surgery in chronic ulcerative colitis (UC) and Crohn's disease (CD).

	UC	CD
Cancer prophylaxis	++++	−
Toxic megacolon	+	+
Bleeding	++	+
Free perforation	++	+
Refractory symptoms	++++	++++
Obstruction	−	++++
Fistula formation	−	++

Ranked from − (very uncommon) through ++++ (very common indication).

involved, surgery for CD emphasizes conservation of bowel length by stricture-plasty where possible. When resection is needed, it should be limited to the minimum possible length of bowel.

a. **Acute Ileocolic Crohn's Disease.** Acute ileocolic Crohn's disease may simulate acute appendicitis. It is occasionally encountered during laparoscopic or open exploration for appendicitis. Clues that assist in the correct preoperative diagnosis include anemia and history of previous gastrointestinal symptoms in CD, as well as the characteristic appearance on computed tomographic scan.

  When acute CD is encountered during laparoscopy for presumed appendicitis, perform appendectomy if the base of the cecum appears normal. Do not resect diseased bowel; rather refer the patient for medical management. Other inflammation conditions such as presence of *Yersinia* and mesenteric adenitis can produce a similar appearance.

  In a patient with known ileocolonic CD in whom medical management has failed, resection may be required and can be accomplished laparoscopically. This procedure is analogous to laparoscopic right colon resection (see Chapter 32) but is somewhat more difficult because the mesentery is typically thicker and shorter than normal. Because wide resection does not prevent recurrence, margins should be selected to obtain soft pliable bowel suitable for anastomosis. The general rule is to excise visible mucosal disease. Typically the bowel is exteriorized through a small incision and an extracorporeal anastomosis is performed.

b. **Obstruction.** Obstruction may be limited to a single area, or it may involve discontinuous segments. Careful delineation of anatomic extent of disease is particularly important when laparoscopic surgery is performed. Strictured bowel may be resected or, alternatively, relief of obstruction may be achieved by strictureplasty (see later: Section C).

  In the past, obstructed segments were bypassed in the hope of preserving bowel length by allowing the intestine to heal. This is no longer recommended because the bypassed bowel rarely heals, intestinal continuity is not restored, and carcinoma developing in a forgotten bypassed segment is particularly difficult to diagnose.

c. **Refractory Disease.** Disease localized to a limited segment may be resected to improve quality of life, especially when refractory to medical management. A standard small bowel or colon resection with anastomosis is performed.

d. **Crohn's Proctocolitis.** Rarely, Crohn's disease is limited to the colon and rectum, and proctocolectomy may be required. Pouch formation for restoration is generally not advocated because of concerns about recurrence and desire to preserve length of small intestine. Crohn's disease is occasionally diagnosed as an unexpected finding after pathologic examination of the resected proctocolectomy specimen, and a small number of cases will fall into a pathologically indeterminate category. Generally resection and pouch formation will have been performed at the time of initial surgery; no further intervention is recommended unless symptoms occur.

e. **Bleeding, Perforation.** Emergency resections are usually limited to the involved segment. Intestinal continuity is restored.

f. **Fistula.** Patients with CD are prone to form fistulas to adjacent loops of bowel, other hollow viscera, or to the skin. Many of these fistulas close with current aggressive medical management. Rarely, a chronic fistula necessitates resection. Isolated reports of laparoscopic enterocutaneous fistula closure (by firing a laparoscopic stapler across the fistula) lack numbers or long-term follow-up.

C. Technical Considerations

For small bowel or colon resections, see Chapters 28 and 32. Total proctocolectomy with and without ileostomy is discussed in Chapter 33.

Strictureplasty requires that narrowed segments be identified, opened longitudinally, and then closed either in a simple transverse fashion or as a side-to-side Finney-type closure (Figs. 34.1 and 34.2). This procedure is most commonly done for chronic "burned-out" strictures. Multiple segments of bowel may be involved, and it is important to identify and fix all areas of stricture. Careful preoperative evaluation with small bowel radiography, and intraoperative evaluation by passage of a calibrated marble or intestinal tube with the balloon blown up are helpful adjuncts. While these strictureplasties could be performed intracorporeally, most surgeons exteriorize the bowel through a small incision and perform the anastomosis in a standard hand-sewn extracorporeal fashion.

D. Complications

In addition to the complications listed for each procedure, in the respective chapters, there are some unique aspects to operating upon this patient population. First, resection of active disease does not appear to alter incidence of extraintestinal manifestations. Second, patients with UC are more likely to develop pouchitis than patients with polyposis syndromes after restorative proctocolectomy. Finally, patients with CD are particularly prone to develop recurrence and fistulas. These complications are briefly discussed here.

1. **Recurrence.** There are no currently accepted effective strategies to avoid recurrence. Neither wide surgical excision nor postoperative adjunctive medical management has proven effective.

2. **Fistula.** Recurrent disease often develops just proximal to an anastomosis and may manifest by fistula to the abdominal wall. Late presentation of a wound abscess (months or even years after surgery) is often the initial sign, and it is important to warn the patient that a fistula may result when such an abscess is drained. Management is by drainage of any associated abscess and then medical therapy. Occasionally, resection of involved bowel may be required.

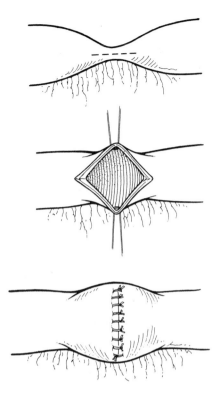

Figure 34.1. For a short stricture, open the bowel longitudinally and close it transversely as shown.

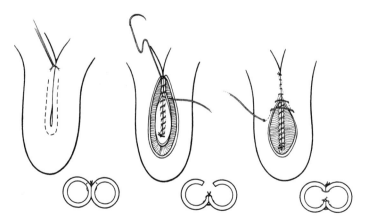

Figure 34.2. Longer strictures may be managed by a Finney-type plastic closure, essentially a side-to-side anastomosis.

3. **Postoperative small bowel obstruction.** Recurrent disease or adhesions may cause this condition. Adhesions may be less common with a laparoscopic approach.

E. Selected References

Bemelman WA, Slors JP, Dunker MS, et al. Laparoscopic-assisted versus open ileocolic resection for Crohn's disease. A comparative study. Surg Endosc 2000;14:721–725.

Bergamaschi R, Pessaux P, Arnaud JP. Comparison of conventional and laparoscopic ileocolic resection for Crohn's disease. Dis Colon Rectum 2003;46:1129–1133.

Duepree JH, Senagore AJ, Delaney CP, Brady KM, Fazio VW. Advantages of laparoscopic resection for ileocecal Crohn's disease. Dis Colon Rectum 2002;45:605–610.

Milsom JW, Hamonerhofer KA, Bohm B, Marcello P, Elson P, Fazio VW. Prospective randomized trial comparing laparoscopic versus conventional surgery for refractory ileocolic Crohn's disease. Dis Colon Rectum 2001;44:1–8.

Tabet J, Hong D, Kim CW, Wong J, Goodacre R, Anvari M. Laparoscopic versus open bowel resection for Crohn's disease. Can J Gastroenterol 2001;15:237–242.

Watanabe M, Hasegawa H, Yamamoto S, Hibi T, Kitajima M. Crohn's disease with fistulas. Dis Colon Rectum 2002;45:1057–1061.

Wu JS, Burnbaum EH, Kodner IJ, Fry RD, Read TE, Fleshman JW. Laparoscopic-assisted ileocolic resections in patients with Crohn's disease: are abscesses, phlegmons, or recurrent disease contraindications? Surgery 1997;122:682–688.

Laparoscopy

VII—Laparoscopic Approaches to the Pancreas, Spleen, and Retroperitoneum

35. Distal Pancreatectomy

Barry Salky, M.D., F.A.C.S.

A. Indications

1. Laparoscopic **distal pancreatectomy with splenectomy** is indicated for tumors of the tail and distal body of the pancreas. The procedure is most commonly applied to benign tumors in which the splenic vein or artery cannot be separated from the pancreatic lesion. It can also be used in palliative resection of the distal pancreas for malignant disease. Conditions in which this may be appropriate include:
   a. Cystadenoma
   b. Neuroendocrine tumors
   c. Cysts
   d. Carcinoma of the pancreatic tail
2. When the splenic vein and artery are uninvolved by the disease process, laparoscopic distal pancreatectomy **with splenic salvage** may be considered. This is more common with cysts and small cystadenomas. The incidence of splenic salvage has increased with the added experience of this type of surgery.

B. Patient Position and Room Setup

1. Position the patient in the modified lithotomy position with both arms tucked to the side. As with other advanced upper abdominal procedures, this enhances access and facilitates a two-handed suturing and knot-tying technique.
2. The thighs must be parallel to the floor (rather than flexed at hip and knee) so that movements of the instruments are not impeded.
3. If an arm needs to be out for anesthesia access, it should be the left one.
4. Place a bolster beneath the left thoracic cage to elevate the left side 15 to 20 degrees.
5. Place the camera operator to the left and the first assistant to the patient's right.
6. Place the video monitor above the head of the patient in the midline. A suitable alternative position is to place the monitor opposite the patient's left shoulder.
7. A Foley catheter is optional.

C. Trocar Position and Choice of Laparoscope

1. Place the first trocar just above and to the left of the umbilicus. This should be a 10/11-mm trocar. Use an angled laparoscope (30- to 45-degree) to facilitate visualization of the left upper quadrant structures.
2. Place a 5-mm trocar in the epigastric midline just below the xiphoid.
3. Place another trocar (10–12 mm) in the left midclavicular line. This will be used for dissection and placement of an endoscopic linear stapler for pancreatic transection. This trocar must be low enough in the abdomen to allow the jaws of the stapler to open completely. Usually, placement at the level of the umbilicus, or just below it, is sufficient.
4. Place the fourth trocar in the anterior axillary line. This site will be used for retraction and suction and irrigation. Although the size of this trocar (5 vs 10/11 mm) depends upon the instrumentation, use of the

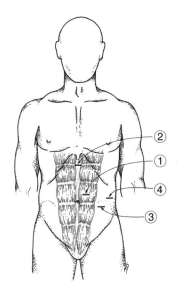

Figure 35.1. Trocar placements for distal pancreatectomy. These sites are proper for both splenic salvage and with splenectomy. There should be at least a hand's breadth distance between trocars 1, 3, and 4. The trocar for the laparoscope should be above the umbilicus; otherwise, visualization of the upper short gastric vessels and splenic attachments will be difficult. The third trocar must be of sufficient size for placement of the gastrointestinal anastomosis (GIA) stapler (12 mm). On occasion, replacement of the laparoscope into the third or fourth trocar will be helpful in delineating the anatomy. Suturing and knot tying are prerequisites for advanced laparoscopic surgery. The angle of attack should be at about 90 degrees, which explains the placement of trocars 2 and 3.

larger trocar allows the laparoscope to be repositioned if needed to enhance visualization (Fig. 35.1).

D. Initial Dissection and Mobilization of Pancreas

1. First explore the abdomen for other pathology before commencing the pancreatic dissection.
2. Position the angled laparoscope to look down on the abdominal structures.
3. **Enter the lesser sac** by dividing the gastrocolic omentum.
   a. This is facilitated by superior retraction of the stomach (trocar 2) and lateral traction of the ligament (trocar 4).
   b. The operating port is trocar 3.
   c. The dissection can be accomplished with the harmonic scalpel (Ultracision, Ethicon Endo-Surgery, Cincinnati, OH) scissors, monopolar electrocautery, and titanium clips. Liga-Sure (U.S. Surgical, Norwalk, CT) uses bipolar electric energy and is a relatively new addition to the instruments in laparoscopic surgery. In some cases, the mobilization can be facilitated with this instrument.
   d. It is easier to stay outside the gastroepiploic vessels.
   e. Wide mobilization of the gastrocolic omentum is required to fully visualize the pancreas.
4. Incise the posterior peritoneum at the inferior border of the pancreas. Identify the inferior mesenteric vein and avoid it. With that exception, the plane is fairly avascular.
5. Mobilize medial to lateral. Divide the splenocolic ligament and visualize the splenorenal attachments.
6. Dissect the posterior aspect of the pancreas to ascertain involvement of the splenic vein and/or artery. **The decision to remove or salvage the spleen is made now.** Each procedure will be described separately in the sections that follow.

E. Distal Pancreatectomy with Splenectomy

1. Identify the splenic artery beneath the posterior peritoneum at the superior border of the pancreas.
2. It may be advantageous to divide the short gastric vessels at this stage (Fig. 35.2). Clips or the laparoscopic coagulating shear (LCS) work well here, as does the Liga-Sure device. (See Chapter 37, Laparoscopic Splenectomy.)
3. Dissect the splenic artery by staying in the adventitial plane next to it. The site of division should be at the planned line of pancreatic transection. Doubly clip the and divide the artery. The author places a

pretied suture ligature on the artery for extra security. The Liga-Sure device can also be used for splenic artery division.

4. Bluntly dissect the posterior pancreas from the retroperitoneal tissues at the site of the previously divided splenic artery. Elevate the gland medially (trocar 2) and laterally (trocar 4) with graspers to expose the area. The splenic vein should be on the posterior aspect of the gland. This is a delicate part of the operation and hemorrhage here must be avoided.

5. Once the posterior gland is fully mobilized, the dissector should be visible at the superior border of the pancreas at the previously divided splenic artery.

6. Pass the vascular endoscopic GIA stapler through trocar 3, and divide the gland and splenic vein as a unit (Fig. 35.3). Two applications of the stapler are usually necessary to completely transect the pancreas. The remainder of the dissection of the pancreatic tail, splenorenal ligament, and splenodiaphragmatic attachments is facilitated by the pancreatic division.

7. After the remaining attachments have been divided, remove trocar 3 and roll up a sturdy retrieval bag and insert it into the abdomen. The 5-cm × 7-cm Cook urological bag has worked well for the author.

8. Reinsert trocar 3 and regain pneumoperitoneum. The author prefers to insert another 5-mm trocar to hold the bag open with three-point traction (graspers in trocars 2, 4, and 5).

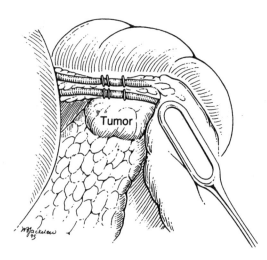

Figure 35.2. Once the lesser sac has been entered, lateral traction on the splenogastric attachments will allow exposure of the short gastric vessels. These can be clipped (as shown) or divided with the LCS. (Reprinted with permission from Salky BA, Edye M. Laparoscopic pancreatectomy. Surg Clin North Am 1996;76(3):539–545.)

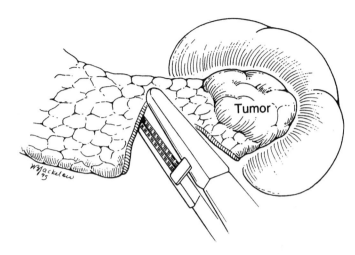

Figure 35.3. Distal pancreatectomy with splenectomy. The figure demonstrates the proper angle of approach when transecting the pancreatic body with the 30-mm GIA stapler. The posterior aspect of the pancreas must be dissected completely to allow free passage of the stapler. Include the splenic vein in the staple line, and transect pancreas and splenic vein at the site of the previously divided splenic artery. (Reprinted with permission from Salky BA, Edye M. Laparoscopic pancreatectomy. Surg Clin North Am 1996;76(3):539–545.)

9. Manipulate the specimen with a grasper inserted through trocar 3. Tilt the table to take advantage of gravity as the specimen is brought into the bag (see Chapter 8).
10. Thoroughly check hemostasis, irrigate, and place a closed suction drain via trocar 4. The operation is concluded in the usual fashion.

F. Pancreatectomy with Splenic Salvage

Performing pancreatectomy with splenic salvage implies that the benign pathology is not adherent to the splenic artery or vein. Size and location of the pathologic process to the vessels determine the best approach. In general, there are multiple small vascular branches that have to be dissected. Traction and countertraction, meticulous avascular dissection, and fine working instruments are key here. Both sharp and blunt dissection techniques are employed, but sharp dissection tends to be more avascular. On occasion, laparoscopic ultrasound can be helpful in delineating the relationship of the pathologic process to the pancreatic duct. This can decrease the incidence of ductal injury and, therefore, potentially decrease the incidence of post-operative pancreatic fistula.

1. As the blood vessels are small, the LCS or 5-mm titanium clips are better choices for hemostasis. At present, the Ligasure device is too large (1 cm) to use in this setting. It is a good idea to limit the amount of electrocautery energy applied to the pancreatic tissue.
2. Clip any identifiable pancreatic ductal branches to the main duct.
3. As in pancreatectomy with splenectomy, trocars 2 and 3 are the operating ports with trocar 4 utilized for countertraction and suction.
4. Hemostasis, irrigation, aspiration, and placement of a closed system suction drain via trocar 4 complete the procedure.

G. Complications

1. **Hemorrhage**
    a. **Cause and prevention.** The most common event leading to conversion to open procedure is inability to control hemorrhage. Both the splenic artery and vein are the main sources. Dissection in the proper adventitial plane and gentle laparoscopic techniques will limit this complication.
    b. **Recognition and management.** Rapid hemorrhage which cannot be controlled promptly requires laparotomy to treat. Temporary control may be obtained by exerting pressure with 10-mm instruments. This allows time to ascertain what exactly is the problem. Laparoscopic hemostatic techniques include vascular staples, titanium clips, electrocautery, LCS, and suturing, and knot tying capability (Chapter 6).
2. **Pancreatic leak**
    a. **Cause and prevention.** Disruption of the pancreatic duct closure can lead to leakage of pancreatic juice. The enzymes in pancreatic fluid are caustic to surrounding tissue. Inspect the stump of the pancreatic remnant before closure. If necessary, suture-ligate the duct with a nonabsorbable suture. Fibrin glue placed on the proximal cut end of the pancreas can possibly decrease the incidence of fistula.
    b. **Recognition and management.** A closed suction drain is routinely placed at the cut end of the pancreas. Check the drainage fluid for amylase on the second postoperative day, and remove the drain if the amylase level is normal. Elevation of amylase is consistent with a pancreatic leak. Management is dependent on amount of leakage and the clinical status of the patient. Barring a proximal obstruction of the pancreatic duct or a foreign body, the pancreatic leak should close. Adjunctive measures such as somatostatin analogues, total parenteral nutrition (TPN), and antibiotics may be required, depending upon the patient's clinical status.
3. **Infection**
    a. **Cause and prevention.** Pancreatic leak and hematoma formation at the surgical site in the left upper quadrant can lead to abscess

formation. The incidence is around 5%. Meticulous hemostasis, closure of the pancreatic duct, gentle handling of the pancreatic gland, and minimal electrocautery usage will decrease, but not eliminate infection. There is no evidence that prophylactic antibiotics prevent infection in this setting. Most surgeons will place a closed-system suction drain at the time of surgery.

b. **Recognition and management.** Respiratory difficulty, sepsis, pleural effusion, and left upper quadrant pain are all signs of a left subphrenic abscess, which is best confirmed by computed tomography (CT) scan. Antibiotics and percutaneous or operative drainage may be required. (See Chapter 37 for additional discussion of complications).

H. Suggested References

Fernandez-Cruz L, Saenz A, Astudillo E, et al. Outcome of laparoscopic pancreatic surgery: endocrine and nonendocrine tumors. World J Surg 2002;26(8):1057–1065.

Gagner M, Ponp A. Laparoscopic pylorus-preserving pancreatoduodenectomy. Surg Endosc 1994;8:408–410.

Patterson EJ, Gagner M, Salky B, et al. Laparoscopic pancreatic resection: single institution experience of 19 patients. J Am Coll Surg 2001;193(3):281–287.

Salky BA, Edye M. Laparoscopic pancreatectomy. Surg Clin North Am 1996;76(3): 539–545.

36. Laparoscopic Cholecystojejunostomy and Gastrojejunostomy

Carol E.H. Scott-Conner, M.D., Ph.D.

A. Indications

1. **Laparoscopic cholecystojejunostomy** is indicated when bypass of the biliary tract is needed and the cystic duct is known to be patent. The procedure is most commonly used to palliate unresectable malignancies of the region of the ampulla of Vater. It may also be used in chronic pancreatitis. Internal stenting is an alternative procedure. Conditions in which this procedure is used include the following:
   a. Carcinoma of the head of the pancreas
   b. Chronic pancreatitis
   c. Other obstructive processes of the ampullary region for which no alternative treatment exists
2. **Laparoscopic gastrojejunostomy** is used alone or in conjunction with laparoscopic cholecystojejunostomy. Used alone, the procedure is indicated for bypass of distal gastric, pyloric, or duodenal obstruction, generally when the patient is not considered to be a candidate for a more definitive procedure. Such conditions include the following:
   a. Gastric carcinoma
   b. Severe peptic ulcer disease (often in conjunction with vagotomy)
   c. Carcinoma of the pancreas in the absence of jaundice
3. **Laparoscopic cholecystojejunostomy and gastrojejunostomy** are occasionally performed as a double-bypass procedure when both biliary and gastric diversion are indicated. This is occasionally needed in carcinoma of the ampullary region, particularly carcinoma of the pancreas.
4. These bypass procedures may be done at the time of laparoscopic exploration for resectability when unresectable gastric or pancreatic cancer is confirmed.

B. Patient Position and Room Setup

1. Position the patient supine on the operating table with arms extended.
2. The surgeon stands at the right side of the patient. Some surgeons prefer to stand between the patient's legs, particularly if a sutured anastomosis is planned. This is a matter of individual preference.
3. Place the monitors at the head, in positions similar to those used for laparoscopic cholecystectomy.

C. Trocar Position and Choice of Laparoscope (Fig. 36.1)

1. Place the first trocar at or just below the umbilicus. Use an angled laparoscope (30 degree) to facilitate visualization of the anastomosis.
2. Place a 5-mm trocar to the left of the midline, lateral to the rectus, at approximately the level of the umbilicus. Place a 10- or 12-mm trocar (use a 12-mm trocar if a gastrojejunostomy is planned in addition to the cholecystojejunostomy) to the right of the midline, in the subcostal region but lateral to the gallbladder. The trocar on the right should be large enough (generally 10 mm, unless a smaller laparoscope is available) to permit passage of the laparoscope through this port if needed. Use a long needle passed through the abdominal wall to test trocar locations and angles. These two trocars will be used for manipulation and suturing.
3. The fourth trocar will be used for the endoscopic stapling device. It must be placed low on the right side (just above the iliac fossa). Placement of this trocar must be low enough to allow sufficient working space within the abdomen. If the trocar is placed too close to the gallbladder, it will be difficult to manipulate the stapling device (remember that to properly open the device, the jaws must be completely out of the trocar). Take care to ensure that you are satisfied with the alignment and spatial relationships before you place this trocar. To accommodate the stapler, use a 12-mm trocar here.

D. Performing the Cholecystojejunostomy

1. The simplest method is an **antecolic loop cholecystojejunostomy**, performed with the endoscopic linear stapling device. To perform this anastomosis,
   a. Identify the ligament of Treitz and run the bowel to a point at least 50 cm distal to the ligament of Treitz. The loop selected

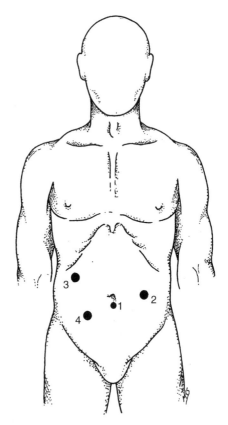

Figure 36.1. Trocar placement for cholecystojejunostomy. If you plan to do a gastrojejunostomy as well, modify the trocar placement as shown later (Fig. 36.4). In each case, trocar placement must be individualized. A standard umbilical or subumbilical location for trocar 1 will place the laparoscope in a good position. Trocars 2 and 3 will be used to manipulate the bowel and gallbladder, and to place sutures. If you plan to use the endoscopic stapler to close the enterotomies, then trocar 2 must be large enough (generally 12 mm) to accommodate this device. Otherwise a 5-mm trocar will suffice. Trocar 3 should be large enough to accept passage of the laparoscope, should it become necessary to inspect the inside of the anastomosis. Trocar 4 will be used to pass the endoscopic stapling device. It must be placed low enough to allow sufficient working distance to open the jaws and should also allow the stapler to line up with the long axis of the gallbladder, if possible. As with all advanced laparoscopic procedures, trocar placement is crucial, and you should take time and explore your planned placement with a long needle, if necessary, to assure good alignment and positioning.

should reach comfortably to the gallbladder without tension, when passed in an antecolic fashion. Verify that the loop passes comfortably up into the right upper quadrant; if the loop does not pass easily, try selecting a more distal small bowel site (and hence farther from the ligament of Treitz).

b. Place a stay suture on the loop of jejunum. With the same suture, take a bite of the fundus of the gallbladder. Use this stay suture to approximate the two hollow viscera in apposition. Tie the suture loosely and pass it out trocar 3. Place a second stay suture about 1 cm from the first, tie it loosely, and pass it out through trocar 2. The stab wounds will be placed between these two sutures. An alternative technique, without the use of stay sutures, may be used and is described shortly (see Section D.2).

c. Use electrocautery or endoscopic scissors to make two stab wounds, each large enough to accommodate one jaw of the endoscopic linear stapling device (approximately 8 mm long). Suction the bile from the gallbladder, note its color, and send a sample for culture. The gallbladder bile should be golden. If the gallbladder bile is white (hydrops) the cystic duct is not patent, and the procedure should not be performed (see Complications, Section F).

d. Pass the endoscopic linear stapling device, with a 3.5-mm cartridge, from trocar 4. Place one jaw within each stab wound (Fig. 36.2). Take care to ensure that the jaws pass into the lumen of the two viscera rather than into a submucosal plane. When you are satisfied, close the stapler and fire it. Open the stapler and remove it from the region of the anastomosis. Some advocate keeping the stapler closed for 1 to 1.5 minutes, feeling that this period of gentle compression facilitates hemostasis.

e. Inspect the staple line for bleeding. Irrigate the staple line and check the color of the effluent (see Complications, Section F).

f. Close the stab wounds by simple running suture (Fig. 36.3). An alternative method is to pass the endoscopic linear stapling device through the left lateral port and staple the closure.

g. Inspect the completed anastomosis and place a closed suction drain in proximity. If there is omentum, place it in the right upper quadrant as well. Irrigate the abdomen and close in the usual fashion.

2. **Alternate technique (no stay sutures).** Make the enterotomy in the jejunal loop first. Insert the narrow end of the linear stapler and gently close, but do not fire, the linear stapler. This will serve to hold the jejunal loop in position. Next, make an enterotomy on the gallbladder. Bring the stapler, carrying the jejunal loop, up into the right upper quadrant and open the jaws, taking care not to drop the jejunal loop. Pass the wide end of the stapler into the gallbladder. Use atraumatic graspers to position the bowel and gallbladder in the proper alignment. Close and fire the stapler.

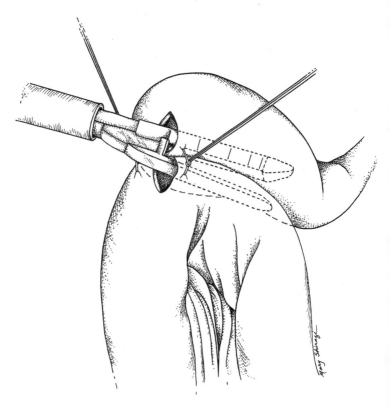

Figure 36.2. Stay sutures have been placed and tied. Two enterotomies have been made and the stapler is inserted into the two enterotomies. The bowel and gall-bladder must be carefully positioned to fully utilize the entire length of the sta-pling device (by pulling the two viscera up into the "crotch" of the device) and to avoid catching other structures in the staple line. In this illustration the stapler is being passed through a trocar relatively high on the right side. This can be done only when the patient is large and the abdominal wall anatomy allows suf-ficient working distance. In smaller patients, the stapler will be passed from a trocar low in the right lower quadrant. (Reprinted with permission from Bogen GL, Mancino AT, Scott-Conner CE. Laparoscopy for staging and palliation of gastrointestinal malignancy. Surg Clin North Am 1996;76:557–569.)

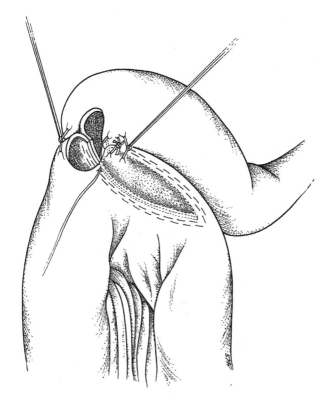

Figure 36.3. After the staple line has been inspected for hemostasis, the enterotomies are closed with a running suture. (Reprinted with permission from Bogen
GL, Mancino AT, Scott-Conner CE. Laparoscopy for staging and palliation of
gastrointestinal malignancy. Surg Clin North Am 1996;76:557–569.)

E. Gastrojejunostomy

1. Trocar placements are similar (Fig. 36.4) except that trocar 2 may be
   placed lower on the left side (to create sufficient working distance from
   the stomach).
2. Identify a loop of jejunum as previously described.
3. Choose a site low on the greater curvature of the stomach, but away
   from the tumor (if the bypass is performed for malignancy). Instillation of some air into the nasogastric (NG) tube will elevate the
   stomach, making it easier to identify the proper site.
4. Place two stay sutures to approximate the stomach and the jejunum.
   Pass these sutures out through trocars 2 and 3.

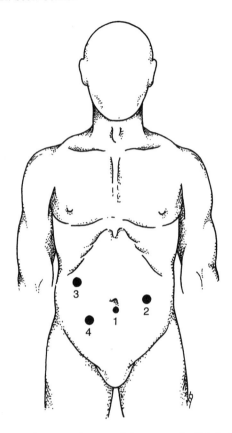

Figure 36.4. Trocar placement for gastrojejunostomy is slightly different, in that trocar 2 is placed lower, to allow adequate working distance from the stomach. If you plan to do both procedures, use this trocar arrangement (rather than that in Fig. 36.1).

5. Make two enterotomies; pass and fire the stapling device with a 3.5-mm cartridge (Fig. 36.5). The 60-mm stapler provides an adequate lumen. If this is not available, perform a second firing of the 30-mm device, taking care to extend the stapling line directly back from the apex.

6. Inspect the staple line for hemostasis. Close the enterotomies with a running suture or with the endoscopic stapler, passed through trocar 2 (Fig. 36.6). Check the anastomosis with air under saline, or by instillation of methylene blue into the NG tube.

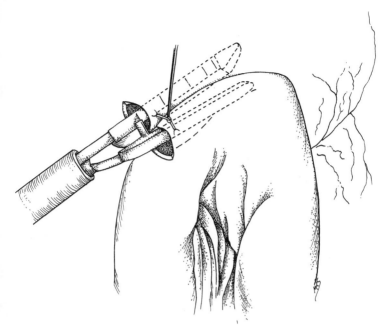

Figure 36.5. A loop of jejunum has been selected and affixed to the greater curvature of the stomach, above the gastroepiploic vessels, with two stay sutures. Two enterotomies have been made and the stapling device inserted.

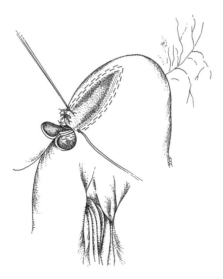

Figure 36.6. The stapler has been fired and removed. The staple line has been inspected for hemostasis and is being closed with a simple running suture.

F. Complications

1. **Leakage of the cholecystojejunostomy**
   a. **Cause and prevention.** Bile is a detergent and will go through a pinhole; hence, small leaks at biliary-enteric anastomotic sites are common. Many surgeons routinely place a closed suction drain in close proximity to a biliary-enteric anastomosis, so that any such leakage is easily recognized and controlled. The resulting bile leak usually subsides spontaneously in the absence of distal obstruction.
   b. **Recognition and management.** Bilious output from the closed suction drain should be monitored and outputs recorded. Excessive (more than 100–200 mL/day) or prolonged (>1 week) output may be a sign of distal obstruction. A radionuclide biliary scan is an easy, noninvasive way to confirm that the jejunal loop is patent. The scan will show passage of radionuclide into the distal small intestine if the loop is patent. Sequential scans over time will confirm rapid transit of bile through the gut. If the loop is obstructed or the leak is very large, the radionuclide will pass out through the drain or puddle in the right gutter, and little or no activity will be seen to go into the gut. Distal obstruction is generally mechanical in nature and requires operative correction.

If no drain has been placed, a subphrenic collection or generalized peritonitis may result. Generally this is signaled by fever or ileus, and diagnosed by computed tomography or ultrasound. A localized collection may be amenable to percutaneous drainage. Generalized peritonitis will usually require exploration, with repair of the leak and establishment of adequate external drainage. Similar concerns about distal obstruction of the jejunal loop exist and should be kept in mind.

2. **Leakage of the gastrojejunostomy**
   a. **Cause and prevention.** To minimize the possibility of leakage, test the gastrojejunostomy by air under water, or by instillation of dilute methylene blue through the NG tube. Reinforce any areas that appear weak or are leaking.
   b. **Recognition and management.** A localized collection or generalized peritonitis may result. Fever, ileus, abdominal tenderness, and distention are symptoms. A Gastrografin upper gastrointestinal series may demonstrate the site of leakage. Revision of the anastomosis will generally be required.

3. **Bleeding from the staple line**
   a. **Cause and prevention.** All gastrointestinal stapling devices are designed to approximate tissues without strangulating or devascularizing them. The potential for bleeding always exists. The rich submucosal blood supply of the stomach makes it particularly prone to staple line bleeding. To avoid this complication, inspect the staple line carefully before closing the stab wounds. Use the suction irrigator to irrigate the staple line, and carefully inspect the color and quantity of the effluent. The effluent should be clear or bilious.
   b. **Recognition and management.** If the effluent is persistently bloody, suspect a staple line bleeder and place the laparoscope into the lateral

port. You can then advance the laparoscope through the stab wounds to look inside. Cauterize or suture-ligate any bleeding points under direct vision. Use cautery with caution to avoid thermal damage and delayed perforation.

4. **Failure of the cholecystojejunostomy to produce biliary diversion**
   a. **Cause and prevention.** Obstruction of the anastomosis by blood clot can cause recurrent jaundice. This can be avoided if hemostasis is carefully checked as noted earlier. An unrecognized blocked cystic duct will cause the anastomosis to fail. Avoid this complication by careful patient selection and knowledge of individual anatomy. The cystic duct enters the common duct at a variable distance from the duodenum. A cholecystojejunostomy uses the cystic duct as a conduit for bile from the common hepatic duct. If the cystic duct is not patent, or is blocked by tumor, the conduit will not function. At laparoscopy, the gallbladder should appear grossly distended (Courvoisier's sign). The cystic duct should be dilated and the gallbladder should contain bilious material. White bile (hydrops) indicates the presence of cystic duct obstruction and is a contraindication to performing a biliary-enteric bypass.

Cholangiography is the best way to delineate biliary anatomy. If you are uncertain about the anatomy, perform a transcystic cholangiogram by placing a needle in the gallbladder and injecting contrast. The cholangiogram should visualize the common duct.

   b. **Recognition and management.** If cholecystojejunostomy does not produce biliary diversion, or if the conduit fails as the tumor grows, stenting, transhepatic drainage, or conversion to choledochojejunostomy should be considered. Decision to employ one of these procedures should be based upon careful consideration of the anatomy and the patient's overall medical condition.

5. **Obstruction of the jejunum at the anastomotic site**
   a. **Cause and prevention.** Problems during the construction of the anastomosis, particularly during closure of the enterotomies, can narrow the lumen of the jejunal loop or even totally obstruct it. This causes a high small bowel obstruction. Avoid this complication by taking care not to narrow the jejunal lumen, particularly if you use the stapler to close the enterotomies. Visually inspect the anastomosis after you construct it, and if it does not look right, consider revising it.
   b. **Recognition and management.** Signs of high small bowel obstruction (vomiting, inability to tolerate feeds) suggest the diagnosis, which may be confirmed by Gastrografin upper gastrointestinal series. The anastomosis must be revised or a jejunojejunostomy (to bypass the obstruction) constructed.

6. **Distal mechanical obstruction of the jejunal loop**
   a. **Cause and prevention.** Avoid kinking by visually verifying that the chosen site allows the jejunum to lie in a comfortable and loose position as it passes over the transverse colon. Rarely, a trocar site hernia may present as small bowel obstruction.
   b. **Recognition and management.** Distal obstruction may cause the anastomosis to leak. If the anastomosis does not leak, obstructive symptoms of distention, inability to tolerate feedings, and vomiting

suggest the diagnosis. The diagnosis may be confirmed by flat and upright abdominal films, hepatoiminodiacetic acid scan (cholecysto-jejunostomy), or Gastrografin upper gastrointestinal series (gastroje-junostomy). Generally, revision of the anastomosis will be required.

G. Selected References

Bogen GL, Mancino AT, Scott-Conner CEH. Laparoscopy for staging and palliation of gastrointestinal malignancy. Surg Clin North Am 1996;76:557–569.

Casaccia M, Diviacco P, Molinello P, Danavaro L, Casaccia M. Laparoscopic palliation of unresectable pancreatic cancers: preliminary results. Eur J Surg 1999;165:556–569.

Chekan EG, Clark L, Wu J, Pappas TN, Eubanks S. Laparoscopic biliary and enteric bypass. Semin Surg Oncol 1999;16:313–320.

Cogliandolo A, Scarmozzino G, Pidoto RR, Pollicino A, Florio MA. Laparoscopic pallia-tive gastrojejunostomy for advanced recurrent gastric cancer after Billroth I resec-tion. J Laparoendosc Adv Surg Techniques A 2004;14:43–46.

Cuschieri A. Laparoscopy for pancreatic cancer: Does it benefit the patient? Eur J Surg Oncol 1988;14:41–44.

Fletcher DR, Jones RM. Laparoscopic cholecystojejunostomy as palliation for obstructive jaundice in inoperable carcinoma of pancreas. Surg Endosc 1992;6:147–149.

Hawasli A. Laparoscopic cholecysto-jejunostomy for obstructive pancreatic cancer: tech-nique and report of two cases. J Laparoendosc Surg 1992;2:351–355.

Mittal A, Windsor J, Woodfield J, Casey P, Lane M. Matched study of three methods for palliation of malignant pyloroduodenal obstruction. Br J Surg 2004;91:205–209.

Nagy A, Brosseuk D, Hemming A, Scudamore C, Mamazza J. Laparoscopic gastroen-terostomy for duodenal obstruction. Am J Surg 1995;169:539–542.

Nathanson K. Laparoscopy and pancreatic cancer; biopsy, staging, and bypass. Baillieres Clin Gastroenterol 1993;7:941–960.

Rangraj MS, Mehta M, Zale G, Maffucci L, Herz B. Laparoscopic gastrojejunostomy; a case presentation. J Laparoendosc Surg 1994;4:81–87.

Shimi S, Banting S, Cuschieri A. Laparoscopy in the management of pancreatic cancer: endoscopic cholecystojejunostomy for advanced disease. Br J Surg 1992;79:317–319.

Sosa JL, Zalewski M, Puente I. Laparoscopic gastrojejunostomy technique: case report. J Laparoendosc Surg 1994;4:215–220.

Targarona EM, Pera M, Martinez J, Balague C, Trias M. Laparoscopic treatment of pan-creatic disorders: diagnosis and staging, palliation of cancer and treatment of pan-creatic pseudocysts. Intern Surg 1996;81:1–5.

Wyman A, Stuart RC, Ng EK, Chung SC, Li AK. Laparoscopic truncal vagotomy and gas-troenterostomy for pyloric stenosis. Am J Surg 1996;171:600–603.

37. Laparoscopic Splenectomy

Robert V. Rege, M.D.

A. Indications

Laparoscopic splenectomy is indicated in patients with hematological disorders not responding to medical therapy if removal of the spleen is expected to improve the patient's condition. Indications for laparoscopic splenectomy are essentially the same as for open splenectomy (Table 37.1).

Although laparoscopic splenectomy has been successfully performed for splenic artery aneurysm, ruptured spleen, tumor and tumor staging, and splenomegaly, results and safety in comparison to open splenectomy have not been clearly defined. **Controversy exists about the use of the laparoscope for these disorders**, since there is potential for spread of tumor or infection or massive bleeding during laparoscopic treatment. Laparoscopic splenectomy is being used increasingly for splenic tumors in selected patients. These disorders are therefore considered "relative contraindications" to laparoscopic splenectomy.

B. Patient Position and Room Setup

1. Most surgeons now use **the right lateral position** for splenectomy. This approach has also been called the "hanging spleen" method. In some circumstances, **a modified semi-frog-leg lithotomy position** may be useful (Fig. 37.1).
2. In the **right lateral position** (Fig. 37.2), the surgeon stands at the patient's side. Monitors are placed at the head and to the side of the patient. The patient is placed either in a true lateral position or at **a 45-degree angle, with the table rotated to attain a more lateral position**. In both positions, the patient is flexed at the waist to open the space between the costal margin and the iliac crest.
   a. Dissection of superior short gastric vessels and of the superior pole of the spleen may be difficult in the lateral position. Rotating the table to the left to a more supine position facilitates division of high short gastric arteries.

Table 37.1. Disorders treated by splenectomy.

Hematological disorders
  Idiopathic thrombocytopenic purpura (ITP)
  AIDS-associated ITP
  Hereditary spherocytosis
  Idiopathic autoimmune hemolytic anemia
  Felty's syndrome
  Thalassemia
  Sarcoidosis
  Sickle cell disease
  Gaucher's disease
  Congenital and acquired hemolytic anemia
  Thrombotic thrombocytopenic purpura

Miscellaneous diseases of the spleen
  Splenic artery aneurysm
  Splenic cysts
  Splenic abscesses*

Trauma*
  Acute rupture*
  Delayed rupture*

Splenic tumors
  Hodgkin lymphoma*
  Non-Hodgkin lymphoma*

Secondary hypersplenism

* Results of laparoscopic splenectomy not established.

    b.   The lateral position facilitates posterior dissection of the spleen and its hilum. It decreases the amount of splenic retraction required during the operation.

    c.   The 45-degree modification allows for quick repositioning of the patient and conversion to open operation if necessary.

3.   In the **modified lithotomy position**, the surgeon stands between the patient's legs with the monitor at the patient's head. Assistants and the scrub nurse are placed at the patient's sides. The anesthesiologist is placed to the side of and above the patient (Fig. 37.1).

    a.   This position provides excellent access to the spleen, stomach, body and tail of the pancreas, and splenic flexure of the colon. However, liver retraction necessitates an extralarge port site.

    b.   This position is excellent for patients requiring simultaneous laparoscopic splenectomy and cholecystectomy.

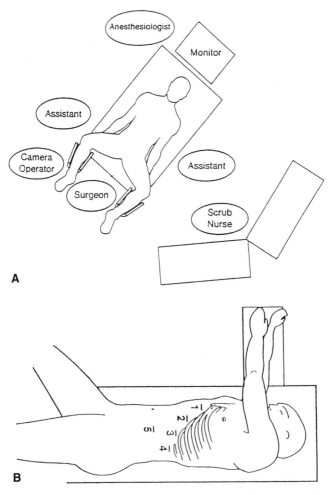

Figure 37.1. A. Right lateral position. B. Modified lithotomy position.

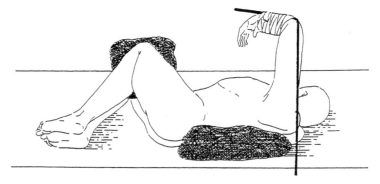

Figure 37.2. Patient positioned in 45-degree rotation. Table is further rotated to attain true lateral position, and the patient is flexed downward at the waist to open the space between costal margin and pelvis.

C. Trocar Position and Choice of Laparoscope

The location of trocar sites vary with the position chosen.

1. **In the right lateral position (Fig. 37.1).** Place the port for the laparoscope at the umbilical level or higher at the lateral rectus. It can be placed in the anterior axillary line as shown in the figure, but we prefer more medial placement, which places the camera away from the operating ports.

    a.   Place a 5-mm trocar in the midline just below the xyphoid.

    b.   Two trocars are placed on the left below the costal margin in the midclavicular and posterior axillary lines.

    c.   The most posterior trocar on the left is usually a 12-mm port for the stapling device. The other trocar can be a 5-mm instrument in most patients, but a larger port may facilitate removal in patients with difficult anatomy. It is now simple to upsize ports during the operation with most port systems.

2. **In the lithotomy position (Fig. 37.3).** Estimate the distance to the posterior left diaphragm using the laparoscope. A 10-mm port for the laparoscope is usually placed above the umbilicus in the midline. The exact distance above the umbilicus varies depending on body habitus.

Place two trocars on the left below the costal margin in the midclavicular and midaxillary lines.

Place two trocars on the right below the costal margin. Position varies by surgeon, but one port is usually placed in the subxyphoid region and the other in the midclavicular.

The size of trocars depends on the equipment available. At least one 12-mm port is required for the stapler (usually the lateral left port). The others may be either 5- or 10-mm ports depending on the size of the ultrasonically activated scissors and liver retractor used.

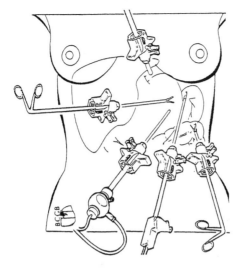

Figure 37.3. Port placement for laparoscopic splenectomy, lithotomy position.

3. **In either position**, visualization of the spleen and surrounding structures is improved by placing the patient in the reverse Trendelenburg (head up, feet down) position. The table may also be rotated to the right.

4. **A 30- or 45-degree laparoscope** is required to visualize the entire left upper quadrant of the abdomen and all surfaces of the spleen.

D. Performing a Laparoscopic Splenectomy

1. **Several strategies and devices** facilitate laparoscope splenectomy.

Laparoscopic splenectomy can be challenging. An assistant who is an experienced laparoscopic surgeon is helpful.

A 30- or 45-degree laparoscope is essential.

A suction-irrigation device is essential. A 5-mm tip suffices for most operations, but when there is bleeding, a 10-mm open-ended tip is useful for rapidly evacuating clot and visualizing the source of bleeding.

Use of multiple 12-mm ports allows flexibility in placement of the camera, instruments, and stapling device.

An ultrasonically activated scissors facilitates control of the short gastric vessels and splenic attachments. The device generally decreases operating time. A 5-mm device is optimal.

Frequent repositioning of the table facilitates visualization of important structures.

It is important to search for accessory spleens before beginning and at each stage of the splenectomy.

The operation proceeds in a similar manner regardless of position used.

2.   First, mobilize the **splenic flexure of the colon** with electrocautery, clips, or an ultrasonically activated scissors.

a.   Retract the splenic flexure of the colon inferiorly and to the patient's right side. Divide the lateral attachments of the colon.

b.   Divide the splenocolic ligament to mobilize the lower splenic pole. Secure vessels with clips or the harmonic scalpel.

3.   Next, divide the **gastrosplenic ligament**. Retract the stomach inferiorly and to the right with a Babcock clamp. A small opening is made in the gastrosplenic ligament entering the lesser sac. The ligament is then divided by progressing superiorly along the greater curvature of the stomach, dividing short gastric vessels in turn.

a.   Although short gastric vessels can be divided with cautery and clips, the author prefers the ultrasonically activated scissors because clips are sometimes accidentally dislodged and may interfere with placement of the vascular stapler later in the operation.

b.   Reposition the Babcock clamp frequently to maintain visibility. This is especially important for the short gastric vessels to the upper pole of the spleen.

c.   Gentle retraction of the upper pole of the spleen will aid in visualizing and dividing the highest short gastric vessel.

d.   Reposition the angle of the laparoscope to optimize visualization of the vessels and to avoid other instruments as you proceed.

4.   Continue by performing dissection posterior to the spleen, dividing the splenorenal and splenophrenic attachments. Use a grasper or suction tip to retract the spleen to the right as the dissection progresses.

5.   Identify the **hilum of the spleen**. Adipose tissue and/or remaining posterior attachments of the spleen often obscure the hilum and must be carefully dissected until the splenic vein is seen. Create a space in front of and behind the vein, and visualize the distal pancreas.

6.   Divide the **splenic vein** with the vascular stapler, while avoiding injury to the pancreatic tail.

Pass an endoscopic lineal stapling device with a vascular cartridge through a left, posterior lateral port site. Pass the stapler cephalad along the left colic gutter so that it lies perpendicular to the vein.

Open the stapler, carefully place it across the entire vein, and close it. Ensure correct placement prior to closure. **Opening the device for repositioning without firing it is dangerous** and may tear the vein, causing bleeding.

Fire the stapling device, then open and remove it. Check the staple line for bleeding, which is unusual if the device is applied correctly. If bleeding occurs, control it with cautery, clips, sutures, or reapplication of the stapler.

7.   Divide the **splenic artery** with the stapler (see earlier).

a.   Depending on the splenic anatomy, two to five applications of the stapler may be required to divide all branches to the upper pole of the spleen.

b.   Some surgeons prefer to ligate splenic hilar vessels with individual sutures. This can be difficult and time-consuming, and does not seem to have an advantage. Vascular staples are secure, and bleeding from the staple line is rare.

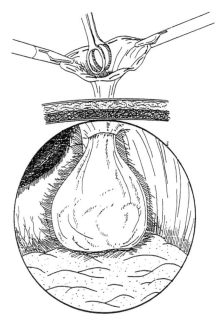

Figure 37.4. The plastic specimen bag has been retrieved through a large port site. A ring forceps is used to fragment the spleen and remove it piecemeal.

8. At this point, **posterior attachments of the upper pole of the spleen** often remain. Divide attachments using the stapler, cautery, or the ultrasonically activated scissors.

9. Once the splenic blood supply has been divided, the spleen can be safely retracted to visualize these remaining attachments.

Posterior attachments may require retraction of the spleen anteriorly and to the right. This may be facilitated by rotating the table to the right.

10. When the spleen is free, place it in a **large plastic bag**, and retrieve the bag through one of the large port sites (Fig. 37.4).

   a. Morcellize the spleen using a Kocher clamp and/or ring forceps.
   b. Remove the spleen in pieces, suctioning blood from the bag as needed. Place the bag on tension during morcellization, but take care to avoid damaging the bag.

11. After removing the spleen, **reinsert the port** and examine the left upper quadrant to ensure that there is no hemorrhage. The operation is concluded in the usual fashion.

F. Complications

Complications of laparoscopic splenectomy are the same as for the open operation. Although length of hospital stay and the time to full recovery is decreased, it is not clear that laparoscopic surgery is safer than open splenectomy. Laparoscopic splenectomy has the least benefit in patients with severe hematological disorders and/or medical comorbidities that, in themselves, necessitate prolonged hospitalization. A potential exists for increased intraoperative bleeding and need for transfusion.

1. **Hemorrhage**
    a. **Cause and prevention.** The spleen is a pulpy organ that is easily injured during retraction. The hilar vessels are delicate and can be torn. Laparoscopic splenectomy requires excellent visualization of important structures, careful dissection, and rapid control of bleeding. Any coagulation deficits should be corrected before surgery. Patients with ITP should be treated medically to optimize platelet counts. Patients with refractory thrombocytopenia may require platelet transfusion, which should be delayed until after the splenic aretery and vein have been divided.
    b. **Recognition and management.** Monitor the operative field carefully for hemorrhage during and after splenectomy. Hemorrhage is the most common reason for conversion to open operation. Hemorrhage must be controlled rapidly with cautery, clips, or sutures, or the operation should be converted to an open procedure. It is prudent to set a limit for blood loss. If the limit is reached without end to the splenectomy in sight, conversion to open operation is justified.
2. **Postsplenectomy sepsis**
    a. **Cause and prevention.** Warn all patients about this potential complication, and instruct them to contact their physician promptly if they develop febrile illnesses. Prompt treatment of bacterial illnesses with antibiotics is essential. Patients should receive preoperative vaccination against pneumococcal and *Hemophilus* organisms.
    b. **Recognition and management.** Physicians should be aware of postsplenectomy sepsis. Prompt recognition and aggressive treatment of bacterial infections is required.
3. **Failure to control the primary disease**
    a. **Cause and prevention.** Splenectomy will not improve every patient in which it is indicated. Careful selection of patients after assessment of all risks and benefits is important. During discussions of the operation, patients should be informed about expected results and the possibility of failure. Failure to recognize and remove an accessory spleen may result in persistent manifestation of the patient's disease. Each operation should include a careful search for accessory spleens. They should be removed when found.

b. **Recognition and management.** Patients with persistent disease require evaluation for accessory spleen. Accessory spleens can usually be visualized with a liver–spleen nucleotide scan. Removal of the accessory spleen is necessary and may be performed laparoscopically. If no accessory spleen is found, treatment is medical and should involve a hematologist who is an expert with the disorder.

4. **Injury to adjacent organs (stomach, colon, or pancreas)**

   a. **Cause and prevention.** Injury to adjacent organs occurs during dissection of splenic attachments and division of vessels to the spleen, or by tearing the organ during retraction. Careful dissection, exact application of instruments, staples, and clips, and gentle retraction are required to avoid these problems during laparoscopic splenectomy.

   b. **Recognition and management.** Ideally, injury is recognized intraoperatively and can then be directly repaired (either laparoscopically or by conversion to open operation). Unrecognized injuries become manifest as prolonged postoperative ileus, intraabdominal fluid collections, or postoperative abscess. Postoperative fluid collections and abscesses are often amenable to percutaneous drainage and antibiotic therapy. Measure the amylase concentration on any fluid drained from the abdomen to exclude pancreatic injury. If adequate drainage is obtained, infection can be controlled and fistulae will close. Failure of percutaneous drainage is an indication for reoperation.

5. **Subphrenic abscess**

   a. **Cause and prevention.** Subphrenic abscess is a well-known complication of splenectomy. It may occur as an isolated complication or be caused by an injury to an adjacent organ (see earlier).

   b. **Recognition and management.** Subphrenic abscess may causes persistent postoperative fever, elevated white blood count, and postoperative ileus. Subphrenic abscess can be diagnosed by computed tomographic (CT) scan of the abdomen. Subphrenic abscess is treated with antibiotic therapy and percutaneous drainage of the abscess. If the abscess is not amenable to or successfully treated by percutaneous drainage, operative drainage is indicated.

F. Selected References

Arregui M, Barteau J, Davis CJ. Laparoscopic splenectomy: techniques and indications. Intern Surg 1994;79:335–341.

Cadiere GB, Verroken R, Himpens J, Bruyns J, Efira M, DeWit S. Operative strategy in laparoscopic splenectomy. J Am Coll Surg 1994;179:668–672.

Cuschieri A, Shimi S, Banting S, Velpen GV. Technical aspects of laparoscopic splenectomy: hilar segmental devascularization and instrumentation. J R Coll Surg Edinb 1992;37(6):414–416.

Delaitre B. Laparoscopic splenectomy: the "hanged spleen" technique. Surg Endosc 1995;9:528–529.

Friedman RL, Fallas MJ, Carroll BJ, Hiatt JR, Phillips EH. Laparoscopic splenectomy for ITP: the gold standard. Surg Endosc 1996;10:991–995.

Gigot JF, Healy ML, Ferrant A, Michauz JL, Njinou B, Kestens PJ. Laparoscopic splenectomy for idiopathic thrombocytopenic purpura. Br J Surg 1994;81:1171–1172.

LeFor AT, Melvin S, Bailey RW, Flowers JL. Laparoscopic splenectomy in the management of immune thrombocytopenic purpura. Surgery 1993;114:613–618.

Phillips EH, Caroll BJ, Fallas MJ. Laparoscopic splenectomy. Surg Endosc 1994;8:931–933.

Poulin EC, Thibault C. Laparoscopic splenectomy for massive splenomegaly: operative technique and case report. Can J Surg 1995;38(1):69–72.

Rege RV, Merriam, LT, Joehl RJ. Laparoscopic splenectomy. Surg Clin North Am 1996,76(3):459–468.

Robles AE, Andrews HG, Garberolgio C. Laparoscopic splenectomy: present status and future outlook. Intern Surg 1994;79:332–334.

Schlinkert RT, Mann D. Laparoscopic splenectomy offers advantages in selected patients with immune thrombocytopenic purpura. Am J Surg 1995;170:624–627.

Yee JCK, Akpata MO. Laparoscopic splenectomy for congenital spherocytosis with splenomegaly: a case report. Can J Surg 1994;38(1):73–76.

Yee LF, Carvajal SH, de Lorimier AA, Mulvihill SJ. Laparoscopic splenectomy: the initial experience at University of California, San Francisco. Arch Surg 1995;130:874–879.

38. Lymph Node Biopsy, Dissection, and Staging Laparoscopy

Lee L. Swanström, M.D., F.A.C.S.

A. Indications

Laparotomy is commonly used to perform biopsies on nodal tissue, to perform therapeutic lymphadenectomies, and to perform palliative gastrointestinal bypasses. Image-guided percutaneous biopsy is a less traumatic but significantly less accurate alterative. Most recently, laparoscopy has been shown to be an accurate, less invasive staging method and, in some cases, a procedure to allow extended lymphadenectomies for improved survival. The role of surgical node biopsy is rapidly evolving as introduction of new imaging modalities such as positron emission tomograp scans and endoscopic ultrasonography become more widely available and increasingly accurate as staging tools. New evidence indicates that there may be a survival benefit from both a more aggressive policy of en-bloc lymphadenectomy and the use of laparoscopy vs open procedures. Current **indications** for the use of laparoscopy for intra-abdominal node dissections or biopsies are listed in Table 38.1.

B. Patient Preparation, Positioning, and Setup

Informed consent for all procedures should include not only a discussion of the procedure, its risks, and alternatives, but also further treatment options for various scenarios. Patient and surgeon should reach consensus on how to proceed with surgical cancer treatment depending on possible findings of the laparoscopic staging procedure. This allows the surgeon to proceed with an orderly plan of treatment that is consistent with the patient's wishes (e.g., to perform a formal resection under the same anesthesia, to attempt palliation, or to do nothing further) all depending on the intraoperative findings.

The details of preparation depend upon the anticipated site of dissection, duration of surgery, and associated pathology. Here are some general guidelines.

1. Place a **Foley catheter** for iliac node dissection, pelvic dissection, or long cases.
2. Retrogastric biopsy or other upper abdominal procedures require an orogastric tube.
3. Formal bowel preparation is advisable for para-aortic lymph node dissection as both the transabdominal and the retroperitoneal approaches involve extensive colon manipulation.

Table 38.1. Tumor sites for which laparoscopic lymph node biopsy or dissection has been reported, grouped by purpose of laparoscopic intervention.

Purpose of intervention	Tumor site
Staging (including sentinel node biopsy)	Ovary
	Uterine cervix
	Endometrium
	Prostate
	Bladder
	Testis (including germ cell)
	Hodgkin lymphoma*
Determination of resectability for cure	Esophagus
	Stomach
	Pancreas
	Hepatobiliary
	Unknown retroperitoneal masses
Therapeutic lymph node dissection	Colon**
	Stomach**
	Nonseminomatous testicular
	Uterine cervix or endometrium

* Also see Chapter 12 for more details on staging laparoscopy for Hodgkin lymphoma.
** As part of resection.

4. Patients with malignancy are at high risk for deep-vein thrombosis (DVT), and the effects of position and pneumoperitoneum may contribute to intraoperative venous stasis. **Anti-DVT prophylaxis** is extremely important.

5. A single dose of **antibiotics** is given immediately preoperatively, usually a first-generation cephalosporin.

6. Patient position and monitor setup in the operating room varies for these cases.
   a. Position the patient supine with the legs spread for **upper abdominal node biopsies, dissections, or Hodgkin staging** (Fig. 38.1). Arms can be tucked or secured to arm boards at less than a 90-degree angle.
   b. **Para-aortic dissections** can also be done in this position (with the arms tucked), but are more commonly done through a retroperitoneal approach with the patient positioned in the lateral decubitus position (Fig. 38.2). This position requires a beanbag with the patient positioned over the table break to allow lateral flexion. Attention to padding of the axilla, arms, and legs is critical to prevent neuropraxia. The monitors should be placed at the head and foot of the table.

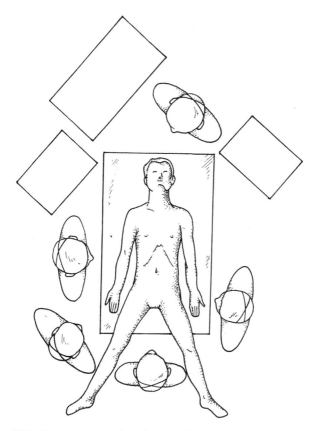

Figure 38.1. Room setup and patient position for upper abdominal node dissection.

c. For **iliac and low pelvic node dissection** the patient lies supine with both arms tucked (Fig. 38.3).

d. Laparoscopic staging procedures for **gynecologic and urologic malignancies** are often done in full lithotomy position, to allow access to the urethra or vagina for biopsy, hysterectomy, placement of a uterine elevator or endoscopy (hysteroscopy, cystoscopy, or sigmoidoscopy). The laparoscopic monitors are placed at the patient's feet.

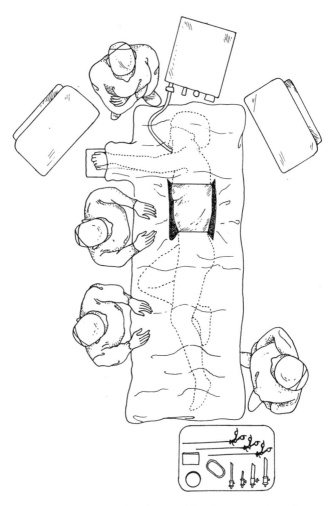

Figure 38.2. Room setup and patient position for retroperitoneal para-aortic node biopsy.

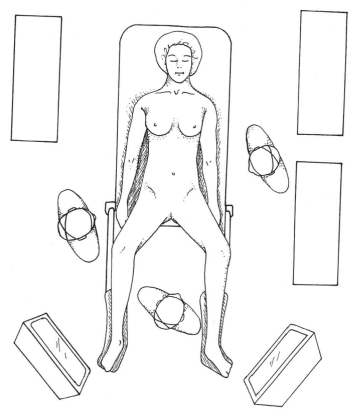

Figure 38.3. Room setup and patient position for iliac node dissection.

C. Access Ports and Equipment for Laparoscopic Node Biopsy

Simple biopsy can often be performed with three ports (two 5 mm and one 10 mm), but more formal retroperitoneal node dissections may require up to six ports (three 10 mm and three 5 mm). Recent developments in "minilaparoscopy," utilizing scopes, ports, and instruments between 1.5 and 3 mm in diameter, have permitted even less invasive access for at least staging and diagnosis. Placement obviously varies according to the area being sampled. Instruments that are typically needed are listed in Table 38.2.

Table 38.2. Instruments for laparoscopic node biopsy and dissection.

Angled laparoscope (3 to 10 mm)	5- or 10-mm endoclip applier
Atraumatic graspers (Glassman)	Specimen retrieval sac
Maryland dissector	Ultrasonically activated scissors*
Laparoscopic ultrasound probe	Dissecting balloons*
Endoscopic Metzenbaum scissor	Needle holders*

*Not needed in all cases.

D. Technique of Retrogastric Dissections

Retrogastric dissection is approached much the same as for a laparoscopic antireflux procedure.

1. Position the patient on a split leg table with arms out on arm boards, as previously noted (Fig. 38.1) and in reverse Trendelenburg position.
2. Place the initial trocar 3 cm above the umbilicus in the midline, the second (10-mm) trocar in the left midclavicular line, and the third (5-mm) in the right midclavicular line (Fig. 38.4).
3. Use a **25- to 50-degree angled laparoscope** to carefully perform a complete peritoneoscopy, which should include inspection of the pelvic cul-de-sac, Morrison's pouch, and the diaphragm. This is done to rule out any carcinomatosis that may obviate a more extended procedure.

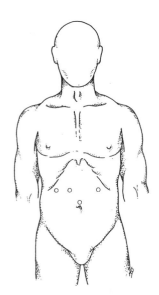

Figure 38.4. Trocar placement for upper abdominal dissection.

4. Next use **laparoscopic ultrasound** to assess the liver, portahepatic, celiac, and retrogastric nodes. Any nodes identified as enlarged should be targeted for biopsy.
5. If no adenopathy is noted, or the findings are equivocal, open the avascular portion of the gastrohepatic omentum and retract the lesser curvature of the stomach to the patient's left. This gives good access to the **celiac nodes** at the base of the patient's right crus. It also allows access to the head of the pancreas and the nodal tissue overlying this area as well as those immediately superior to the portal vein (Fig. 38.5).
6. Grasp the selected node(s) with an atraumatic grasper, and coagulate lymphatics and small feeding vessels with electrocautery or ultrasonic scissors.
7. Access the **retrogastric nodes** by dividing the gastrocolic omentum and entering the lesser sac behind the stomach. Take care when dividing the gastrocolic omentum to avoid injury to the gastroepiploic vasculature (Fig. 38.6).
8. Inside the lesser sac, divide the avascular adhesions between stomach and pancreas and use an atraumatic fan retractor to elevate the stomach. This retractor is best held by a table-mounted retractor holding system.

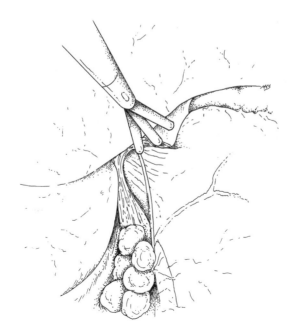

Figure 38.5. Exposure of the celiac nodes.

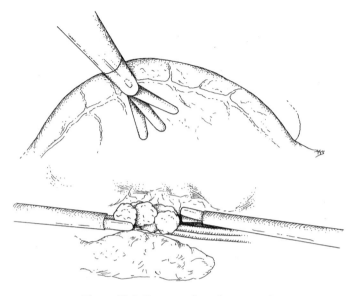

Figure 38.6. Retrogastric nodes exposed.

9. Node-bearing tissue also lies along the superior border of the splenic vein and pancreas and adjacent to the superior mesenteric vein and artery.
10. For simple staging, grasp and excise isolated nodes.
11. For more extended therapeutic dissections, the paraceliac and porta-hepatic nodes are usually dissected as one contiguous mass.
12. Node tissue between the superior mesenteric vein and splenic hilum is next removed in continuity.
13. The nodal tissue is placed in a specimen bag and removed through a trocar site (which may be enlarged if necessary).
14. A closed suction drain can be left in the field when an extensive node dissection is performed. This may control any postoperative lymphatic leakage. No drain is needed for simple biopsy.

E. Staging for Hodgkin Disease

Laparoscopic staging of Hodgkin lymphoma typically involves biopsy of multiple node-bearing areas and solid organ tissue. This indication has enjoyed some renewed interest with the ability to do it laparoscopically because it yields greater sensitivity and specificity than is possible with imaging techniques while minimizing patient morbidity and length of hospital stay. Chapter 13 contains some information about Hodgkin staging. The discussion here will focus on the specific techniques of lymph node biopsy.

1. Position the patient supine with legs spread.
2. Five trocars are used (three 5-mm trocars and two 10-mm trocars).
3. Perform laparoscopic ultrasonography to identify any obvious retroperitoneal masses (Fig. 38.7).
4. Perform a biopsy on any grossly (or ultrasonographically) visible nodes.
5. Obtain mesenteric nodes.
    a. Gently elevate the midjejunum with atraumatic graspers and use sharp and blunt dissection to dissect out mesenteric nodes, which are usually visible under the visceral peritoneum.
    b. The ultrasonic coagulating shears are useful for control of the lymphatic and vascular supply to the nodes.
    c. Single nodes can be withdrawn through the 10-mm port, labeled, and fixed in formalin for pathologic assessment. One node from each area should also be sent fresh to allow touch-prep slides to be made.
    d. Obtain nodes from the transverse colon mesentery in the same way. The omentum should be swept into the upper abdomen while

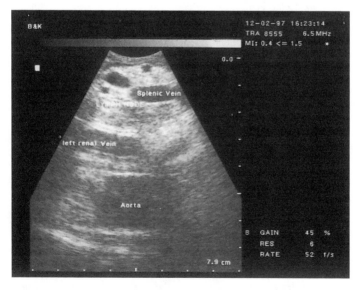

Figure 38.7. Ultrasonic image of retroperitoneal nodes.

the transverse colon is being elevated to allow mesenteric node sampling.

6. Access para-aortic nodes by carrying the dissection down to the root of the mesentery adjacent to the ligament of Treitz.
7. A wedge liver biopsy is performed (see Chapter 13).
8. Finally, a laparoscopic splenectomy is performed (see Chapter 37).

F. Para-aortic Node Dissections

A formal para-aortic node dissection is usually indicated for staging or therapy of endometrial or cervical carcinomas, or as a treatment for early-stage germ cell tumors of the testicle. A formal dissection is best approached with retroperitonoscopy.

1. Place the patient in the **lateral decubitus position** on a beanbag with the midabdomen positioned over the table break.
2. **Flex the table** so that the lateral abdominal musculature is stretched taut.
3. **Take care to prevent nerve injury.** An axillary roll must be carefully positioned, the uppermost arm supported, and abundant padding placed between the flexed legs.
4. **Gain access** by a direct cut down to the preperitoneal plane in the mid-clavicular line 2 to 3 cm lateral to the umbilicus. Use blunt finger dissection to establish the working space. Introduce a dissecting balloon (Origin MedSystems, Menlo Park, CA) and advance it posteriorly. Insufflate between 800 and 1600 mL into the balloon (with the scope in place to observe the resulting dissection). Stop the dissection when the aorta is visualized (Fig. 38.8).
5. Use insufflation at 10 to 15 mm Hg to maintain the created space and insert **additional ports** (5 and 10 mm) under direct vision. Additional dissection can be done to allow full access to the aorta between the hypogastric takeoff and the renal artery.
6. **Node sampling** is done throughout the entire area, with the nodes either removed individually or placed in a tissue bag, which is removed at the end of the procedure.
7. Take care to **avoid injury** to the lumbar sympathetics, anterior spinal nerve roots, and ureters.
8. While efforts are made to remove most of the nodes on the ipsilateral side of the tumor, it is also wise to **cross the midline** and sample nodes from the contralateral side.
9. For therapeutic dissections, take the nodes **in continuity** as much as possible. This may be combined with an ipsilateral iliac node dissection.
10. **No drains** are placed, and at the conclusion of the procedure the retroperitoneum is allowed to deinsufflate, the trocars are withdrawn, and fascias are closed for the larger port sites.

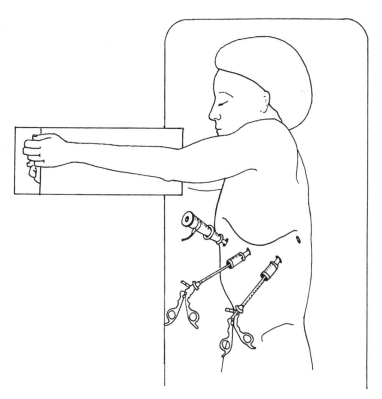

Figure 38.8. Trocar placement for retroperitoneal aortic node dissection.

G. Iliac Dissection

Iliac dissection can be performed either transabdominally or properitoneally. There is no clear-cut advantage of one approach over the other. Dissection is usually bilateral for prostate, cervical, or vulvar cancers, and unilateral (ipsilateral) for other malignancies confined to one side of the patient.

1. Room setup is the same for both approaches, with a single monitor at the foot of the bed.
2. Place the patient supine with arms tucked at the side.
3. The surgeon stands on the side opposite the initial dissection (Fig. 38.3).
4. Three ports are used for both approaches (two 10 mm and one 5 mm).
5. Place the laparoscope through a trocar in the subumbilical site.
6. For the **transperitoneal approach**, the trocars are placed as shown in Figure 38.9.

a. Incise the peritoneum overlying the iliac artery in a longitudinal fashion and dissect the edges of the peritoneum back medially and laterally.

b. The lymphatic tissue lies medial to the iliac artery and vein and within the obturator fossa (Fig. 38.10)

c. Dissect out the nodal tissues in continuity, beginning at the femoral ring and working from top to bottom.

d. Take care not to injure the obturator nerve, which marks the posterior boundary of the obturator fossa. A minimum of electrocautery should be used in this area.

e. Continue the dissection to the iliac bifurcation. Frozen section is usually obtained when doing nodes for prostate cancer, and if positive, there is no need to perform the contralateral node dissection.

f. There is debate about closing the resulting peritoneal defect. If left open, there is a risk of bowel adhesions to this area. If closed, a lymphocele could form potentially, compromising the iliac vein. If the peritoneum is closed, a closed suction drain may be advisable.

7. The preperitoneal approach utilizes the same technique used for a totally extraperitoneal hernia repair (see Chapter 40).

a. Enter the preperitoneal space via an infraumbilical port.

b. Create the initial entry into the preperitoneal space by finger dissection.

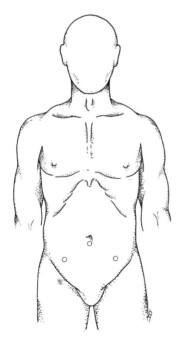

Figure 38.9. Trocar placement for transperitoneal iliac node dissection.

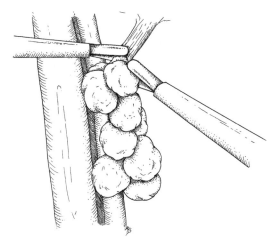

Figure 38.10. Exposure of iliac nodes.

c. Pass a dissecting balloon or trocar into the space. If a dissecting balloon is not used, the pressure of insufflation can be turned up (20 mm Hg) and the preperitoneum space dissected bluntly using the laparoscope.

d. When this space is developed, additional trocars may be placed along the abdominal midline (Fig. 38.11). The same dissection as the transabdominal approach is then performed. A drain is not

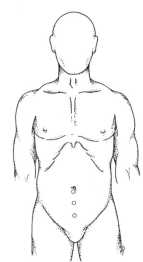

Figure 38.11. Trocar placement for preperitoneal node biopsy.

usually placed, but the patient should be counseled to watch closely for extremity swelling.

H. Complications

1. **Diffuse bleeding from a peritoneal biopsy site**
   a. **Cause and prevention.** Cancer patients frequently bleed from simple biopsies because of hypocoagulability (from decreased platelet counts, anti-inflammatory medications, clotting factor depletion, etc.) or portal hypertension secondary to hepatic or extrahepatic tumor involvement. Obtain a coagulation panel before surgery and correct any abnormalities. Look for clinical signs of portal hypertension (ascites, spider veins, history of variceal gastrointestinal bleeds, etc.) during preoperative assessment; this may represent a relative contraindication for the surgery.
   b. **Recognition and treatment.** Bleeding from a biopsy site is usually recognized at the time of biopsy and should be treated by judicious electrocautery. If this fails, a thrombogenic material can be inserted and pressure applied for 5 to 10 minutes. If bleeding continues, an endoscopically placed figure-of-eight suture tied intracorporally will almost always control the bleeding. Rarely an extended node dissection will result in diffuse bleeding over a wide area. The laparoscopic argon beam coagulator can be useful in these circumstances.

   Always check the security of hemostasis by lowering the insufflation pressure to less than 10 mm Hg at the end of the procedure. In spite of this, delayed bleeding can occur and postoperative lymph node dissection patients should be carefully watched for the first 24 hours for signs of bleeding (tachycardia, increasing pain, dropping hematocrit, flank discoloration from a retroperitoneal bleed). Treatment of delayed bleed depends on the hemodynamic stability of the patient. Stable patients with mild symptoms may require fluids and/or blood, check of coagulation factors, and administration of appropriate factors if indicated. Unstable patients should be returned to the operating room without delay for a laparoscopic or open exploration.

2. **Bleeding from a liver biopsy**
   a. **Cause and prevention.** Cancer patients are at increased risk of bleeding. Patients with severe coagulopathy or known portal hypertension who have to have a liver biopsy should have blood products given before surgery to correct anemia and normalize coagulation indices. Maximal medical treatment (diuretics) should also be undertaken to control ascites.
   b. **Recognition and treatment.** Bleeding from the site of a liver biopsy is hard to miss. Needle biopsy site bleeding is almost always controllable with cautery. Oozing is controlled with a monopolar device set on a high pure coagulating setting. This allows arcing of the current and prevents the resulting eschar from pulling away with the probe. High-pressure bleeds require a lower setting and direct contact of the

probe to apply pressure and heat simultaneously. Recalcitrant bleeding may require 15 to 20 minutes of direct pressure, argon beam coagulation, or injection of fibrin glue into the needle tract.

Bleeding from the exposed surface of a wedge resection should be controlled with a woven oxidized cellulose material and pressure. If this fails, the argon beam coagulator is useful.

3. **Chylous ascites**
   a. **Cause and prevention.** Rarely, disruption of major lymphatic channels can lead to a massive lymphatic leak and chylous ascites. Clip or ligate large lymph ducts before division, and perform all extended dissections with ultrasonic coagulating shears or electrocautery.
   b. **Recognition and treatment.** Sometimes division of a major lymph channel is recognized at the time of the dissection when milky chyle appears. Identify the ends of the duct and ligate, cauterize, or clip it. Chylous ascites may present many weeks after the surgery with increasing abdominal distention and discomfort (rarely pain). Treatment almost always involves reexploration, identification of the severed duct, and ligation.

4. **Lymphocele**
   a. **Cause and prevention.** Minor lymphatic leaks within the peritoneal cavity are seldom a problem because of the absorptive capacity of the peritoneum. When a leak occurs within a confined retroperitoneal space, a lymphocele may result. Lymphoceles may be asymptomatic, or they may present with pain or unilateral extremity swelling. They can occasionally obstruct venous outflow, and have even been implicated in major venous thrombosis. It may be prudent to leave a temporary drain in the preperitoneum if it is closed or to leave this space open to the peritoneal cavity.
   b. **Recognition and treatment.** Ipsilateral extremity swelling, a palpable mass, and diffuse back pain are signs of a possible lymphocele. Ultrasound is the test of choice to make the diagnosis. Treatment usually requires operative intervention via a laparotomy or laparoscopy, with the goal of opening the retroperitoneum, controlling obvious lymph leaks, and either draining the space with closed suction drains or leaving it open to the peritoneal cavity. Percutaneous drainage is seldom more than a temporizing maneuver and could lead to secondary infection. A lymphangiogram may be needed for the rare patient with a persistent leak.

5. **Port site tumor implantation.** There have been reports of tumor implantation in the retrieval port site after dissections for malignancies. Prevention of such occurrences depends on meticulous technique (avoiding node disruption) and use of a tough, impermeable specimen retrieval bag.

I. Selected References

Adachi Y, Kamakura J, Mori M, Maehara Y, Sugimachi K. Role of lymph node dissection and splenectomy in node positive gastric carcinoma. Surgery 1994;116(5):837–841.

436   L.L. Swanström

Childers JM, Balserak JC, Kent J, Surwit E. Laparoscopic staging of Hodgkin's lymphoma. J Laparoendosc Surg 1993;3(5):495–499.

Das S. Laparoscopic staging pelvic lymphadenectomy: extraperitoneal approach. Semin Surg Oncol 1996;12(2):134–138.

Gregor H, Sam CE, Reinthaller A, Joura EA. Port site metastases after laparoscopic lymph node staging of cervical carcinoma. J Am Assoc Gynecol Laparosc 2001;8(4): 591–593.

Holub Z, Jabor A, Kliment L, Lukac J, Voracek J. Laparoscopic lymph node dissection using ultrasonically activated shears: comparison with electrosurgery. J Laparoendosc Adv Surg Techniques A 2002;12(3):175–180.

Kavoussi LR, Sosa E, Chandhoke P, et al. Complications of laparoscopic pelvic lymph node dissection. J Urol 1993;149(2):322–325.

Kim JC, Gerber GS. Should laparoscopy be the standard approach used for pelvic lymph node dissection? Curr Urol Rep 2001;2(2):171–179.

Kitagawa Y, Ohgami M, Fujii H, et al. Laparoscopic detection of sentinel lymph nodes in gastrointestinal cancer: a novel and minimally invasive approach. Ann Surg Oncol 2001;8(9 Suppl):86S–89S.

Klotz L. Laparoscopic retroperitoneal lymphadenectomy for high risk stage I nonsemanomatous germ cell tumor. Urology 1994;43(5):752–756.

Mehler L. Indications for laparoscopic surgery in cases of gyncologic malignancies. Intern Surg 1996;81(3):266–270.

Namieno J, Koito K, Higashi J, Sato AN, Uchino J. General pattern of lymph node metastases in early gastric cancer. World J Surg 1991;20(8):996–1000.

Parkin J, Keeley FX Jr, Timoney AG. Laparoscopic lymph node sampling in locally advanced prostate cancer. Br J Urol Int 2002;89(1):14–17; discussion 17–18.

Spirtos NM, Eisenkop SM, Schlaerth JB, Ballon SC. Laparoscopic radical hysterectomy (type III) with aortic and pelvic lymphadenectomy in patients with stage I cervical cancer: surgical morbidity and intermediate follow-up. Am J Obstet Gynecol 2002;187(2):340–348.

Uyama I, Sugioka A, Fujita J, et al. Completely laparoscopic extraperigastric lymph node dissection for gastric malignancies located in the middle or lower third of the stomach. Gastric Cancer 1999;2(3):186–190.

Vasiley SA, McGonigle KF. Extraperitoneal laparoscopic para-aortic lymph node dissection. Gynecol Oncol 1996;61(3):315–320.

39.1 Laparoscopic Live Donor Nephrectomy

Aloke K. Mandal, M.D., Ph.D.
Michael J. Conlin, M.D.

A. Introduction

1. Since Ratner and Kavoussi described the technique in 1995, **laparoscopic live donor nephrectomy (LLDN)** has become the preferred technique for the procurement of live donor renal allografts at most transplant centers. Table 39.1.1 summarizes its development.

2. **Live donor renal transplantation**—whether from related or unrelated donors—is associated with improved outcomes compared with cadaveric renal transplantation. According to the United Network for Organ Sharing (UNOS), in 2002, 42% of all kidney transplants performed in the United States were from live kidney donors.

3. Compared to the open live donor nephrectomy (OLDN), **LLDN shortens length of stay, accelerates return to work, reduces disincentives to live donation, and provides comparable graft survival rates**. Because of these advantages of LLDN over OLDN, 3589 (69%) of all live donor nephrectomies in 2002 in the United States were done laparoscopically, and 70% of all transplant centers now provide LLDN.

4. LLDN has been performed in obese donors, donors with previous abdominal surgery, and donors with anomalous renal vasculature. After assuring that the risks of losing one kidney are minimal to the prospective donor, **the major contraindication** to LLDN becomes surgeon inexperience. Enthusiasm for this procedure must be tempered by **4 perioperative donor deaths** following LLDN reported to UNOS between 1999 and 2002. In addition, there has been one donor in a persistent vegetative state after hemorrhage and hypotension during LLDN.

5. Two approaches LLDN will be described in this section: **"purely laparoscopic" LLDN** and **"hand-assisted" LLDN**. In both instances, the kidney is obtained through a **transabdominal approach** that is familiar to most surgeons. Although not discussed in this chapter, **retroperitoneal (posterior) approaches** also have been described.

6. **LLDN of the right kidney** requires special consideration.

Table 39.1.1. Development of laparoscopic live donor nephrectomy.

Historical perspective
- 1990: Feasibility of laparoscopic nephrectomy demonstrated in pig model.
- 1991: First laparoscopic nephrectomy for disease
- 1995: First LLDN performed.

Evidence-based advantages of LLDN
- Decreased analgesic requirements
- Decreased length of stay
- Decreased recovery time
- Increased rates of live kidney donation

B. Preoperative Evaluation

1. The donor, who is a healthy individual and undergoes this operation as a magnanimous act, should be educated on the indications, short-term risks, and long-term risks of the operation. **At our program, concerns addressed at the initial visit, in descending order of importance, include safety of the donor, utilization of the kidney for transplantation, and ability to perform the operation with minimally invasive techniques.**
2. The screening evaluation is a multistep process, which includes histocompatibility testing and donor risk assessment for kidney disease, cardiovascular disease, and occult malignancies. A pregnancy test should be performed in women of childbearing age. Also, because of the risk of infectious transmissions from the donor to the recipient, microbial screening also is done on the donor.
3. A number of radiographic evaluations are performed to assess the renovascular anatomy of the prospective live donor (Table 39.1.2).

Table 39.1.2. Preoperative renal imaging.

Renal ultrasound
- Preliminary screen if the donor is genetically related to a recipient with polycystic kidney disease

Nuclear medicine
- Calculates glomerular filtration rate of left and right kidneys

Three-dimensional, spiral computed tomography
- Provides accurate imaging of renal arteries
- Better delineation of venous anatomy than can be obtained with conventional angiography
- Calculates right and left renal volumes

4.   Mechanisms should be in place so that the donor can opt out of live kidney donation in a confidential manner at any time during the evaluation process.

C. Anesthetic and Intraoperative Management

1. **Anesthesia**
    a.   **Nitrous oxide is avoided** to prevent bowel distention, which invariably obstructs the operative field.
    b.   Newer anesthetic techniques have been shown to facilitate recovery after minimally invasive techniques and should be applied to LLDN.
2. **Intravenous fluid administration**
    a.   The increased intraabdominal pressure (15 mm Hg) from pneumoperitoneum required for LLDN decreases renal blood flow, impairs creatinine clearance, and can lead to oliguria.
    b.   **Intravascular volume expansion with crystalloid at a rate of 15 mL/kg/h reverses the changes in renal blood flow and urine output.**
    c.   Aggressive intravenous volume expansion should begin prior to creation of the pneumoperitoneum.

D. Approaches to the Left Kidney

1. **Patient position and room setup**
    a.   Place the patient in a modified **right decubitus position** with the left side up (Fig. 39.1.1). Protective rolls or cushions are placed under the right flank, under the right axilla, and between the legs. The right (bottom) leg is flexed while the left leg is straight. The right arm is extended on an arm board and secured. The left arm is positioned parallel to the right, suspended on a board, and secured. The table is flexed to maximize the distance between the costal margin and the iliac crest; a kidney rest may be used depending on the surgeon's preference; and the patient's torso and legs are secured to the table with 2-in. cloth tape.
    b.   The surgical prep should extend from the nipple to the anterior superior iliac spine, and from the right side of the midline to the spine.
    c.   The surgeon and first assistant stand facing the patient's abdomen (i.e., on the right side of the patient). A second assistant can stand on the left side of the patient.
    d.   Two monitors are located near the head of the table on either side of the patient.
2. **Purely laparoscopic approach: trocar placement and choice of laparoscope**

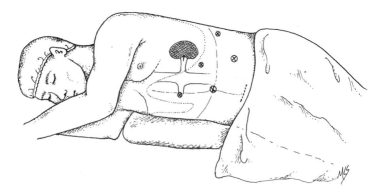

Figure 39.1.1. Patient position and placement of trocars in purely laparoscopic left live donor nephrectomy. Placement of the hand port and laparoscopic ports for hand-assisted laparoscopic live donor nephrectomy is shown.

a. **A transverse 10-mm skin incision is made in the left lower quadrant, and a Veress needle is inserted into the peritoneal cavity.** The incision is centered two thirds of the way from the umbilicus along an imaginary line between the umbilicus and the anterior superior iliac spine, above and medial to the anterior superior iliac spine. After insufflation to an intra-abdominal pressure of 15 mm Hg, a 0-degree laparoscope through a 10-mm port is placed through an optical trocar such as the VisiPort (U.S. Surgical, Norwalk, CT). **The 10-mm port passes through the oblique muscles and into the peritoneal cavity.** The 0-degree laparoscope initially remains in the left lower quadrant so that the remaining ports can be placed under direct vision.

b. Place a **5-mm trocar** in the **upper midline** between the xiphisternum and the umbilicus.

c. A **10-mm or, preferably, 15-mm trocar** also is placed in the midline just below the umbilicus. The 15-mm port allows for introduction of the large specimen pouch (Endo-Catch, U.S. Surgical, Norwalk, CT).

d. A **fourth** (5-mm) **trocar** often is placed along the lateral wall, in the midaxillary line at the level of the umbilicus for retraction.

e. An **optional, left subcostal 10-mm trocar** can be inserted 2 cm inferior to the eleventh rib along the midclavicular line. This port especially is helpful for retraction for surgeons with minimal experience in this procedure.

f. The trocars should be at least 5 cm or, more optimally, 10 cm away from each other.

g. After successful trocar placement, the 0-degree laparoscope is removed from the left lower quadrant site. A 30-degree laparoscope is placed in the infraumbilical port site. The surgeon operates through instruments placed in the upper midline and left lower quadrant ports. Atraumatic graspers or laparoscopic vascular DeBakey forceps (Snowden-Pencer) are placed in the upper midline port. Laparoscopic Metzenbaum scissors or a laparoscopic dissector (Surgiwand, U. S. Surgical, Norwalk, CT) connected to the electrocautery is placed in the left lower quadrant port for sharp and blunt dissection, respectively.

3. **Hand-assisted approach: trocar placement and choice of laparoscope (Fig. 39.1.1)**
   a. The hand assist device is placed through a **6- to 8-cm periumbilical incision in the midline**. Most new devices allow placement of a laparoscopic port directly through the hand port to allow insufflation of the abdomen. This technique permits very safe open entry into the abdomen and placement of laparoscope ports under direct vision.
   b. **A 10-mm trocar** is placed in the **upper midline** above the hand port. This will provide access for the 30- or 50-degree laparoscope.
   c. **A second 12-mm trocar is placed in the left lower quadrant**, which will allow use of the endovascula stapling device later.
   d. An additional **5-mm trocar** can be placed in the left lateral wall if necessary. This can be used to place a laparoscopic Kitner or atraumatic grasper to assist with retraction of the kidney, but often is not necessary.
4. **Exposure of the left kidney (Fig. 39.1.2)**

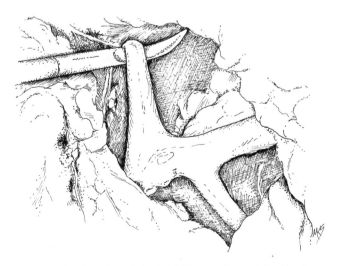

Figure 39.1.2. Identification of the left kidney and gonadal vein after medial mobilization of the colon and spleen.

a.   The left colon is lifted anteriorad and mediad either with an atraumatic grasper through the upper midline port (purely laparoscopic approach) or with the left hand in the periumbilical incision (hand-assisted approach). **Appropriate retraction of the colon is critical to identification of the plane between the mesentery and Gerota's fascia.** This portion of the dissection is a combination of blunt and electrocautery with laparoscopic Metzenbaum scissors or the Surgiwand. Care is made to keep the mesentery intact. Any defects in the mesentery should be closed, to prevent internal hernia and subsequent bowel obstruction. Also, the posterior and lateral attachments of the kidney to the abdominal wall are left intact to keep the kidney in a fixed position.

b.   The attachments between the colon and spleen are left intact. The plane of dissection is carried to the attachments between the spleen and lateral abdominal wall so that the spleen can drop mediad, which facilitates exposure of the renal hilum.

c.   With further medial mobilization of the colon and mesocolon, the gonadal vein is identified and traced to where it drains into the renal vein. **After identification of the gonadal vein, the colon is dissected off of the retroperitoneum inferiorad to the level of the iliac vessels.**

d.   At this point, **the anterior surface of the renal vein is dissected away from surrounding tissues**.

5.   **Dissection of the renal vessels**

a.   The gonadal vein then is dissected on its anterior and medial surfaces to its junction with the renal vein. **To preserve the ureteral blood supply, the gonadal vein is not dissected away from the ureter.** This dissection best is carried out with the Surgiwand or with laparoscopic DeBakey vascular forceps, which have a gentle curve that aids in circumferential dissection of blood vessels.

b.   The **anterior surface of the renal vein** is exposed with scissors or the hook electrocautery of the Surgiwand device. **This process exposes the adrenal, lumbar, and gonadal veins where they drain into the left renal vein.** A right-angle dissector or the DeBakey forceps is used to further dissect these venous branches.

c.   Two proximal and two distal clips are placed on the gonadal, lumbar, and adrenal veins prior to transection. A right-angle clip applier is used. **Care is taken to ensure that the clips will not interfere with subsequent placement of the endovascular stapling device.** If there is concern about the location of these clips, the renal vein side of the venous branches can be controlled with the Ligasure-Lap (Valleylab) or a harmonic scalpel.

d.   **The renal artery is identified just lateral and inferior to the transected lumbar vein.** From the level where the gonadal vein and any lumbar veins were transected from the renal vein, the inferoposterior border of the renal vein bluntly is dissected away from the surrounding tissue. **The combination of anterior mobilization of the gonadal vein with the ureter and dissection of**

the inferior border of the renal vein exposes the lymphatic and ganglionic tissue overlying the renal artery and aorta.

e.   Blunt dissection with the suction device of the Surgiwand and selective use of the hook electrocautery exposes anterior surface of the proximal part of the renal artery. This dissection proceeds cautiously to the aortorenal junction.

f.   Next, **the dissection proceeds to the upper pole of the kidney, and arguably this is the most difficult portion of the case**. Using the superior border of the renal vein where the adrenal vein had been transected as it entered the renal vein, *the surgeon* identifies a plane between the adrenal gland and the upper pole of the kidney and dissects the upper pole of the kidney away from the surrounding structures. During the upper pole dissection, the adrenal artery may be identified. Upper pole renal arteries (whether segmental or anomalous) must be identified and preserved. Finally, the upper pole of the kidney is more medial and posterior than would be expected. This realization should prevent any contusions or lacerations of the upper pole.

g.   After the upper pole of the kidney has been freed completely, it can be place on the anterior surface of the spleen. The kidney then is freed laterad and "flipped" mediad to expose the posterior surface of the vessels. Further posterior dissection often is necessary. Intermittently, this dissection should be interrupted and the kidney placed in its anatomic position to prevent kinking of the renal vasculature and subsequent ischemia.

6.   **Transection of the ureter and preparation for delivery of the kidney**

a.   The kidney, renal artery, and renal vein are completely freed from all attachments. Also, the surgical team should ensure that the recipient operation is proceeding normally.

b.   The ureter is freed from the surrounding tissues posteriorad off the psoas muscle and laterad up to the lateral border of the lower pole of the kidney.

c.   **At the level of the iliac vessels, the gonadal vein is divided between clips, and the ureter is clipped on the distal end before division with scissors.** Copious urine should be seen draining from the cut end of the ureter.

d.   **Division of the renal vessels is rehearsed with the entire surgical team to ensure that all instruments are available and working.** Extra vascular loads for the endovascular stapling devices should be in the room.

e.   **A second table is made ready for flushing of the kidney.**

f.   Heparin (2000 units) is administered intravenously.

7.   **Periumbilical delivery of the kidney: purely laparoscopic and hand-assisted approaches**

a.   The kidney is extracted through a 5- to 6-cm incision. This incision provides excellent cosmetic results and minimal postoperative pain. **Incisions smaller than 5 cm place the kidney at increased risk for injury during extraction.**

b. **For the purely laparoscopic approach, the 30-degree laparo-scope is removed from the infraumbilical position and placed in the left lower quadrant.** This switch is made so that the stapler is pointed posteriorad and laterad, to avoid injury to the superior mesenteric artery or the duodenum. For the hand-assisted approach, the laparoscope remains in the upper midline position.

c. For the purely laparoscopic approach, the infraumbilical port site is extended inferiorad or is converted into a periumbilical incision by superior extension. **The periumbilical incision has improved cosmesis, since half of the length can be placed in the recess of the umbilicus, and is technically easier, since most patients have maximal abdominal subcutaneous fat below the umbilicus.** During the extension of the skin incision, the 15-mm port is left in place. (If a 10-mm port was used rather than a 15-mm port, then the fascial incision is extended to the length of one skin incision and. A pursestring suture is placed in the peritoneum around the port. The port then is replaced with the Endo-Catch, and the pneumoperitoneum is maintained by cinching the pursestring suture around the sleeve of the bag.)

d. With anterior retraction, three surgical clips or an endovascular stapling device (GIA or TA) are placed on the **renal artery** just distal to the aortorenal junction. The TA endovascular device places only three rows of staples and allows inspection of the staple line prior to division of the vessels. The lack of distal staples will gain close to 0.5 cm of length on the vessels. Roticulating stapling devices are preferred.

e. Next, the **renal vein** is ligated with an endovascular stapling device (GIA or TA) and transected. In the purely laparoscopic approach, grasping the vein with the DeBakey forceps and retracting anteriorad prior to application of the stapling device can gain further length on the renal vein.

f. The kidney then is delivered through the periumbilical incision. For the purely laparoscopic approach, a large specimen retrieval bag then is placed through the 15-mm port. The kidney can be placed on the spleen to allow room to deploy the bag. Once the metal frame for the bag has been opened completely, the kidney along with the ureter is placed completely in the bag. The bag is closed using the pursestring. The kidney is removed inside the pouch after the fascial and peritoneal incisions have been extended to the length of the skin incision. For the hand-assisted approach, the kidney is delivered through the hand port without need for a specimen pouch.

8. **Pfannenstiel incision for delivery of the kidney: purely laparo-scopic approach**

a. More experienced surgeons have advocated use of the Pfannenstiel incision, especially in small individuals.

b. **A 5-cm Pfannenstiel incision provides better cosmetic results, provides for more working space in small individuals, allows for insertion of the retrieval bag before division of the renal**

vessels, and can be used for medial retraction of the colon early on in the case with either a fan retractor or the metal sleeve of the bag.

c.   If a Pfannenstiel incision is used, the left subcostal port site is superfluous.

9.   **After removal of the kidney**

a.   The kidney immediately is placed in an ice bath. Any staple lines are transected, and the renal allograft is perfused with cold preservation solution. The warm ischemic time, which is the time from when the renal artery was ligated to when the kidney was perfused with cold preservation solution is recorded and should be less than 3 minutes.

b.   **The operative site is inspected for areas of bleeding. Staple lines and surgical clips on vessels are inspected for hemostasis.**

c.   Next, all fascial defects from 10-mm or larger port sites should be closed, since there have been cases of herniation and bowel obstruction through these fascial defects. The fascial incision is closed with interrupted 0 polydioxanone or polyglyconate sutures. (In the purely laparoscopic approach, the incision is closed first, to restore the pneumoperitoneum prior to inspecting the operative site.)

d.   **Infiltration with a half-and-half mixture of 0.5% bupivicaine and 2% lidocaine of the fascia, subcutaneous fat, and skin at all port and incision sites greatly facilitates postoperative pain control.** If a left subcostal port site was used, then the periosteum of the tenth and eleventh rib and corresponding intercostal space also should be anesthetized.

D. Approaches to the Right Kidney

1.   **Special considerations**

a.   The left kidney from a live donor is preferred for renal transplantation because of the longer renal vein.

b.   In OLDN, the right kidney traditionally is selected when anatomic variations of the left kidney are noted on preoperative donor angiography.

c.   **Right LLDN is much more challenging than left LLDN.** Retraction of the liver, a short and thin renal vein, and the presence of friable venous branches draining into the inferior vena cava in proximity to the right renal vein all contribute to increased technical difficulty.

d.   Accordingly, **right LLDN is performed only if there is a clear advantage for the donor to retain the left kidney**. Anomalous left renal vasculature is not a contraindication to left LLDN.

e.   Because of increased technical difficulty, only experienced surgeons with advanced laparoscopic skills should perform this procedure. **The other major contraindication to right LLDN is a duplicated right renal vein**, since there is a higher incidence of renal vein thrombosis with these allografts.

f. Because of the shortened renal vasculature of the right kidney, the recipient operation also is modified. Specifically, **the recipient left iliac vein is mobilized completely by dividing all posterior branches and then transposed laterad to the left iliac artery**. This maneuver provides a tension-free venous anastomosis.

2. **Purely laparoscopic right donor nephrectomy: patient positioning and trocar placement (Fig. 39.1.3)**

a. The patient is placed in a modified left decubitus position with the table maximally flexed.

b. A laparoscope is placed through a **10-mm infraumbilical port**.

c. A **5-mm upper midline port** allows for placement of laparoscopic instruments for dissection and retraction.

d. A **10-mm right lower quadrant port** allows for placement of dissecting instruments and eventually insertion of the laparoscopic stapler for division of the right renal vein in a plane parallel to the inferior vena cava.

e. A **15-mm port is placed at level of the subsequent Pfannenstiel incision**. In this position, a fan retractor or metal sleeve of the retrieval bag without deployment of the bag can be used for medial retraction of the right colon.

f. Another **5- or 10-mm lateral port** placed in the midaxillary line at the level of the umbilicus can provide retraction of the liver with laparoscopic Kitner, atraumatic grasper, or expandable fan. Alternatively, a **5-mm epigastric** port, just below the xiphisternum also can be used to retract the liver.

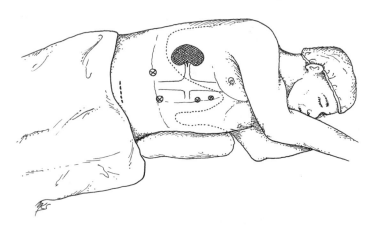

Figure 39.1.3. Patient positioning and trocar placement for purely laparoscopic right LLDN.

3. **Hand-assisted right donor nephrectomy: port and trocar placement**
    a. **Port placement mirrors are like those described for the hand-assisted left LLDN, except that the ports are 2 to 4 cm lower on the right to permit visualization under the liver. In addition, a 5-mm epigastric port can be placed just below the xiphisternum** for retraction of the liver.
    b. For right-handed surgeons, hand-assisted LLDN of the right kidney may be easier approach, since the left hand in the hand port can actively retract and hold structures while the right hand, which is in a more superior position, uses various laparoscopic instruments for dissection.

4. **Exposure of the right kidney**
    a. The first major challenge is **retraction of the liver**. A Kitner dissector, atraumatic grasper, or expandable fan all can provide retraction of the liver. If fractured, the liver can be a source of significant bleeding.
    b. The **right colon** is retracted anteriorad and mobilized mediad. The **duodenum** also is mobilized mediad. The duodenal mobilization should be kept to a minimum, just enough to expose the right kidney and the inferior vena cava.
    c. The right kidney thus is exposed, covered by Gerota's fascia.

5. **Dissection of the renal vasculature**
    a. After the right kidney has been identified, the **inferior vena cava is exposed**. As mentioned earlier, several small anterior branches draining into the right renal vein or the inferior vena cava in proximity of the right renal vein can be avulsed easily during mobilization of the colon and duodenum. A **harmonic scalpel** or **Liga-Sure** device may be helpful in ligating and transecting these branches so that surgical clips do not interfere with subsequent use of an endovascular stapling device.
    b. In contrast to left LLDN, **the gonadal vein** is preserved or divided at a point quite distant from the renal vein to prevent placement of a surgical clip where the renal vein subsequently will be stapled. **Lumbar veins**—which are shorter, cross the right renal artery, and have limited mobility—are transected after posterior mobilization with a harmonic scalpel or with scissors between surgical clips and the Liga-Sure device.
    c. The **renal artery** is identified after the short lumbar veins have been divided. Then, the renal artery is mobilized posterior to the vena cava. After dissection of the lateral and posterior attachments of the kidney to the abdominal wall, the kidney is flipped to allow posterior dissection of between the anterior surface of the artery and the vena cava. In this manner, adequate length of renal artery is obtained.

6. **Delivery of the right kidney**
    a. As with left LLDN, the artery is divided before the vein. If necessary, additional length of the right renal artery can be obtained by flipping the kidney mediad prior to ligation and transection.

b. For the purely laparoscopic right LLDN, the stapler comes from the right lower quadrant rather than from the infraumbilical position to divide the renal vein in a plane parallel to the inferior vena cava and thereby increase renal vein length. Ligation with laparoscopic TA stapler with a vascular load followed by transection with laparoscopic Metzenbaum scissors provide more renal vein length than use of the endo-GIA stapler.

c. Alternatively, a modified Satinsky clamp that originally was developed for thoracoscopic procedures can be positioned on the inferior vena cava; then the renal vein is transected with scissors, and the cavotomy is closed laparoscopically with a 3-0 non-absorbable monofilament suture.

d. The kidney then is delivered from the Pfannenstiel incision inside a specimen pouch (purely laparoscopic approach) or through the periumbilical incision (hand-assisted approach).

e. **For the purely laparoscopic approach, if the renal vein is shorter than 3 cm on preoperative angiographic studies, then a transverse right subcostal incision 5 to 6 cm long, instead of the Pfannenstiel incision, is used with open division of the artery and vein.** The rectus abdominis muscle is split, not incised. Use of a Satinsky clamp allows for a cuff of vena cava to be provided with the renal vein.

E. Expected Results and Reported Complications

1. **The goals of the procedure are to ensure donor safety, provide an excellent renal allograft to the recipient, reduce postoperative pain, and decrease recovery time for the donor.**

   a. Operating room costs are slightly higher for LLDN than OLDN because of the need for specialized, disposable equipment; nevertheless, **hospital charges can be lower for LLDN because of reduced length of stay**.

   b. Quality of life data demonstrate a clear preference for LLDN over OLDN.

   c. In selected patients, a 23-hour stay following LLDN is possible.

2. **The learning curve**

   a. Most centers report an open conversion between 1 and 6%.

   b. Reports from Johns Hopkins Hospital and the University of Maryland suggest that **complication rates are reduced after the initial 70 to 130 cases**. Specifically, in a report of an initial 30 cases at a county medical center, there was an intraoperative open conversion rate of 13.3%. In addition, another 3 (11.5%) patients required a second operation because of hemorrhage or retained foreign body.

   c. Results comparing the hand-assisted with the purely laparoscopic method have been similar. The hand-assisted approach may be facilitate teaching of the procedure and is more readily mastered by surgeons without extensive laparoscopic experience. In such instances, it may provide an additional margin of safety to the donor.

3. **Hemorrhage and renovascular complications**
    a. **Cause and prevention.** Correct any preoperative coagulopathies. The dissection should consist of meticulous attention to hemostasis. Securely clip both ends of all vascular structures least twice prior to transection.
    b. **Renovascular complications** present a serious challenge because they jeopardize not only the safety of the donor but also the utility of the allograft. Initial identification of the gonadal vein and **limiting the circumferential dissection of the renal vein at the level of where the gonadal, lumbar, and adrenal veins drain into the left renal vein** will prevent injury of vascular structures up in the hilum. **The lymphatic and ganglionic structures surrounding the proximal renal artery and the aortorenal junction are quite thick.** Blunt dissection with selective use of the hook cautery of these structures with the Surgiwand is much safer than sharp dissection. During dissection, care must be ensured that the cautery does not arc against vascular structures. Prior to firing the endovascular stapler, all surgical clips should be away from the staple line. Vascular structures should be ligated individually. Misfiring of the endovascular stapler and dislodgment of surgical clips need to be anticipated.
    c. **Recognition and management**
        i.   Intraoperative hemorrhage is easily identified and may require conversion to an open procedure if hemostasis cannot be achieved.
        ii. Because preoperative angiography can miss anomalous renal vasculature, the surgeon always should have a high index of suspicion for **aberrant renal vasculature**. If the renal artery is not directly posterior and slightly caudad to the renal vein, then most likely there is an arterial anomaly. For example, if the renal artery is identified more caudad, then invariably an upper pole artery coming off the aorta exists. Similarly, if the renal artery is more cephalad, then a lower pole artery coming off the aorta or iliac artery should be suspected.
        iii. Postoperative hemorrhage is best detected by carefully monitoring the patient's vital signs and urine output.
4. **Ureteral complications**
    a. Soon after the initial report of LLDN, an increased incidence of ureteral complications was noted. The majority of these complications were secondary to ischemic necrosis of the ureter.
    b. **Ureteral complications are reduced significantly if the gonadal vein is not dissected away from the ureter.**
    c. Intraoperative placement of internal ureteric stents during the recipient operation also can minimize ureteral complications.
5. **Damage to intra-abdominal or retroperitoneal structures**

a. **Cause and prevention.** By limiting the dissection of the spleen, **injuries to the spleen and pancreas** are avoided. In right LLDN, fatty **livers** especially are prone to retraction injuries. The **adrenal vein** should be seen exiting from the adrenal gland to avoid damaging an accessory renal vein. During the dissection of the space between the superior border of the renal vein and the adrenal gland, segmental renal arteries should be identified and preserved. The **venous branches** can be quite large, with limited mobility, and can be a source of massive bleeding if avulsed. **Bowel injuries** also have been reported.

b. **Recognition and management.** Damage to the liver or spleen will present as intraoperative or postoperative bleeding. In the postoperative period, injuries to the pancreas or gastrointestinal tract may present as abdominal pain, fever, tachycardia, or leukocytosis. A strong index of suspicion is required.

Acknowledgments

UNOS Analyses prepared by the Scientific Registry of Transplant Recipients, February 19, 2003. Subsequent interpretations of these data are the responsibility of the authors alone.

F. Selected References

Buell JF, Hanaway MJ, Potter SR, et al. Surgical techniques in right laparoscopic donor nephrectomy. J Am Coll Surg 2002;195:131–137.

Chan DY, Fabrizio MD, Ratner LE, Kavoussi LR. Complications of laparoscopic live donor nephrectomy: the first 175 cases. Transpl Proc 2000;32:778.

Eger EI, Saidman LJ. Hazards of nitrous oxide anesthesia in bowel obstruction and pneumothorax. Anesthesiology 1965;26:61–66.

Flowers JL, Jacobs S, Cho E, et al. Comparison of open and laparoscopic live donor nephrectomy. Ann Surg 1997;226:483–490.

Hsu THS, Su L-M, Ratner LE, Kavoussi LR. Renovascular complications of laparoscopic donor nephrectomy. Urology 2002;60:811–815.

Johnson MW, Andreoni K, McCoy L, et al. Technique of right laparoscopic donor nephrectomy: a single center experience. Am J Transpl 2001;1:293–295.

Kuo PC, Johnson LB, Sitzmann JV. Laparoscopic donor nephrectomy with a 23-hour stay: a new standard for transplantation surgery. Ann Surg 2000;231:772–779.

London ET, Ho HS, Neuhaus AM, Wolfe BM, Rudich SM, Perez RV. Effect of prolonged intravascular volume expansion on renal function during prolonged CO_2 pneumoperitoneum. Ann Surg 2000;231:195–201.

Mandal AK, Cohen C, Montgomery RA, Kavoussi LR, Ratner LE. Should the indications for laparoscopic live donor nephrectomy of the right kidney be the same as for the open procedure? Anomalous left renal vasculature is not a contraindication to laparoscopic left donor nephrectomy. Transplantation 2001;71:660–664.

Mandal AK, Snyder JJ, Gilbertson DT, Collins AJ, Silkensen JR. Does cadaveric donor renal transplantation ever provide better outcomes than live-donor renal transplantation? Transplantation 2003;75:494–500.

Matas A, Leichtman A, Bartlett S, Delmonico F. Kidney donor (LD) morbidity and mortality (M&M). Am J Transpl 2002;2(Suppl. 3):138.

Michaliakou C, Chung F, Sharma S. Preoperative multimodal analgesia facilitates recovery after ambulatory laparoscopic cholecystectomy. Anesth Analg 1996;82:44–51.

Pace KT, Dyer SJ, Phan V, et al. Laparoscopic versus open donor nephrectomy. Surg Endosc 2003;17:134–142.

Pace KT, Dyer SJ, Stewart RJ, et al. Health-related quality of life after laparoscopic and open nephrectomy. Surg Endosc 2003;17:143–152.

Odland MD, Ney AL, Jacobs DM, et al. Initial experience with laparoscopic live donor nephrectomy. Surgery 1999;126:603–606.

Philosophe B, Kuo PC, Schweitzer EJ, et al. Laparoscopic versus open donor nephrectomy: comparing ureteral complications in the recipients and improving the laparoscopic technique. Transplantation 1999;68:497–502.

Ratner LE, Cisek LJ, Moore RG, Cigarroa FG, Kaufman HS, Kavoussi LR. Laparoscopic live donor nephrectomy. Transplantation 1995;60:1047–1049.

Ratner LE, Fabrizio M, Chavin K, Montgomery RA, Mandal AK, Kavoussi LR. Technical considerations in the delivery of the kidney during laparoscopic live-donor nephrectomy. J Am Coll Surg 1999;189:427–430.

Ratner LE, Montgomery RA, Maley WR, et al. Laparoscopic live donor nephrectomy: the recipient. Transplantation 2000;69:2319–2323.

Schweitzer EJ, Wilson J, Jacobs S, et al. Increased rates of donation with laparoscopic live donor nephrectomy. Ann Surg 2000;232:392–400.

Velidedeoglu E, Williams N, Brayman KL, et al. Comparison of open, laparoscopic, and hand-assisted approaches to live-donor nephrectomy. Transplantation 2002;74:169–172.

Wolf JS, Merion RM, Leichtman AB, et al. Randomized controlled trial of hand-assisted laparoscopic versus open surgical live donor nephrectomy. Transplantation 2001;72:284–290.

39.2 Laparoscopic Adrenalectomy

Ahmad Assalia, M.D.
Michel Gagner, M.D., FACS, FRCSC

A. Indications

1. **Laparoscopic adrenalectomy (LA)** is currently considered the preferred alternative to open adrenalectomy for the vast majority of patients with small and medium-sized benign functioning and nonfunctioning adrenal lesions (Table 39.2.1). The available data indicate that the largest experience has been with aldosteronomas followed by Cushing syndrome, nonfunctioning adrenal masses ("incidentalomas"), pheochromocytoma, and Cushing's disease. Other nonprevalent reported indications included myelolipoma, cysts, adrenal hemorrhage, androgen-secreting tumors, and ganglioneuromas.
2. Laparoscopic adrenalectomy has been successfully performed in several other conditions, including the following: but further experience is still required before the procedure can be used routinely.
    a. Neuroblastoma
    b. Congenital adrenal hyperplasia (CAH) in children
    c. Isolated adrenal metastases
    d. Masses larger than 10 to 12 cm
3. **Contraindications** to laparoscopic adrenalectomy include the following:
    a. Large invasive adrenocortical carcinoma: although limited experience with noninvasive malignant tumors yielded encouraging results, an initial laparoscopic approach is an acceptable option only in experienced hands at selected specialized centers
    b. Metastatic pheochromocytoma to periaortic nodes
    c. Untreated/uncorrectable coagulopathy
    d. Other contraindications for general anesthesia and laparoscopy

B. Operative Approaches

Several laparoscopic approaches to the adrenal glands are recognized:
1. **Lateral transabdominal** with the patient in the lateral decubitus position
2. **Anterior transabdominal** with the patient in the supine position
3. **Retroperitoneal endoscopic adrenalectomy** (lateral or posterior)

Table 39.2.1. Indications for laparoscopic adrenalectomy.

1. Functional adrenal cortical masses
 Cushing syndrome caused by benign cortisol-producing adenoma
 Cushing's disease after failed pituitary surgery, or after failure to control or
  to find an ectopic tumor producing adrenocortico tropic hormone
 Aldosterone-producing adenoma (Conn's syndrome)
 Rare virilizing/feminizing secreting tumors.

2. Functional adrenal medullary masses
 Benign adrenal pheochromocytoma

3. Nonfunctional adrenal masses
 Benign-looking incidentalomas (nonfunctioning adenomas) confined to the
  adrenal glands and meeting accepted criteria for adrenalectomy (size
  >4 cm at presentation or growth in follow-up)
 Benign symptomatic lesions
 Rare entities such as cyst, myelolipoma, and hemorrhage

Although no clear objective advantages of one surgical approach over the others have been conclusively shown, the lateral transabdominal approach is the preferred technique practiced by most surgeons, followed by the retroperitoneal approach. Table 39.2.2 shows the possible advantages and disadvantages of each approach. The two most common approaches (lateral transabdominal and retroperitoneal) will be described separately in Sections C and D.

C. Lateral Transabdominal Approach

The lateral transabdominal approach to the **left adrenal gland** will be described first, followed by the approach to the right adrenal.
 1. **Patient position and room setup**
    a. Place the patient in the **left lateral decubitus position** with the left side up (Fig. 39.2.1). Position a cushion under the right flank and a protective roll under the right axilla. The left arm is extended over a board and secured. The right arm is positioned parallel to the left, suspended on a board, and secured. Flex the table to maximize the distance between the costal margin and the iliac crest, and secure the patient's torso and legs to the table with a 2-in. cloth tape.
    b. The surgical prep should extend from the nipple to the anterior superior iliac spine, and from the midline anteriorly to the spine posteriorly.
    c. The surgeon and the first assistant stand facing the patient's abdomen (i.e., on the right side of the patient).
    d. Place two monitors near the head of the table.

Table 39.2.2. Surgical approaches in laparoscopic adrenalectomy.

Approach	Advantages	Disadvantages
Lateral transabdominal	• Less dissection, retraction, and better exposure • Appropriate for large tumors • Other intra-abdominal pathologies may be diagnosed and treated • The most practiced approach	• Change of position in bilateral adrenalectomy • Certain difficulty in cases of peritoneal adhesions
Anterior transabdominal	• No need for changing position in bilateral adrenalectomy • Appropriate for large tumors • Other intra-abdominal pathologies may be diagnosed and treated	• More dissection needed and much difficult exposure • Longer operative time? • More blood loss? • The least practiced approach
Retroperitoneal endoscopic	• No need for changing position in bilateral adrenalectomy (with jack knife position) • Potential advantage in previous upper abdominal surgery; obese and pregnant patients	• Small operative field: appropriate only for small tumors (<5–6 cm) • Inability to diagnose and treat concurrent intra-abdominal pathology • Lack of anatomical landmarks familiar to the average abdominal surgeon

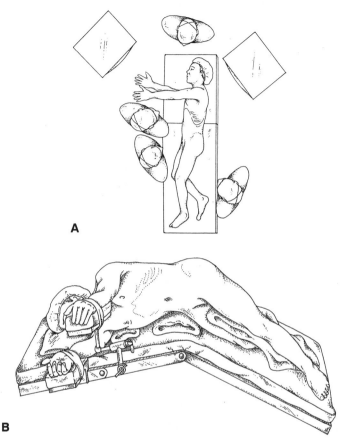

Figure 39.2.1. Patient position for laparoscopic transabdominal left adrenalectomy. A. Room setup for laparoscopic adrenalectomy. B. Placing the patient in the lateral decubitus position takes advantage of patient positioning to roll the viscera out of the operative field.

2. **Trocar placement and choice of laparoscope**
    a. **Although closed technique with Veress needle is possible, we prefer the open technique to access the abdomen and establish pneumoperitoneum. This is done at the left anterior axillary line,** approximately 2 cm below and parallel to the costal margin. Insufflate to 15 mm Hg and **place a 10-mm trocar** at the Veress insertion point.
    b. Insert a 10-mm **30-degree laparoscope** through this port.
    c. Place the **second 10-mm trocar** under the eleventh rib at the midaxillary line.

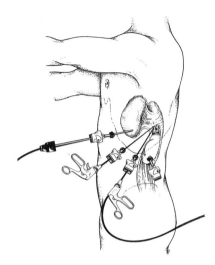

Figure 39.2.2. Placement of trocars in laparoscopic transabdominal left adrenalectomy. Three 10-mm trocars are usually placed initially; if a vascular stapler is needed, the middle trocar can be changed to a 12-mm port.

    d.   Place the **third 10-mm trocar** more medial and anterior to the first trocar. Position this trocar along the midclavicular line, lateral to the rectus muscle.

    e.   A **fourth trocar** (5 mm) may be inserted dorsally at the costovertebral angle to retract the spleen. This port is usually not necessary in patients with normal-size spleens.

    f.   The trocars should be at least 5 cm or, more optimally, 10 cm away from each other.

    g.   Place the laparoscope through the anterior-most trocar with the two middle trocars as the surgeon's operating ports (Fig. 39.2.2).

3.   **Left adrenalectomy**

    a.   Working with laparoscopic dissector and scissors, mobilize the splenic flexure medially to expose the lienorenal ligament (see Chapters 32, 33, and 37).

    b.   Incise the lienorenal ligament inferosuperiorly approximately 1 cm from the spleen. Stop the dissection when the short gastric vessels are visualized posteriorly behind the stomach. This maneuver allows the spleen to fall medially, exposing the retroperitoneal space.

    c.   If necessary, retract the spleen gently with an atraumatic retractor passed though the most posterior (fourth) trocar.

    d.   **Laparoscopic ultrasound** may be used as an adjunct to identify the adrenal gland, the mass within the gland, and the adrenal vein (see Chapter 13).

e. Grasping the perinephric fat, dissect the **lateral and anterior** part of the adrenal gland. Hook electrocautery or ultrasonic scalpel are useful instruments for this phase of the dissection.

f. Avoid grasping the adrenal gland or tumor directly, as the fragile tissue is likely to tear. Sometimes it is possible to grasp the connective tissue around the tumor or adrenal gland. At certain points in the dissection, the shaft of an instrument may be used to gently push the adrenal gland away from the region of interest, creating a space in which to work. The shaft of an instrument may also be used to elevate the adrenal gland.

g. Tilt the table to the **reverse Trendelenburg position**.

h. For **smaller adrenals (<5 cm)**, dissect the adrenal gland inferomedially. The **adrenal vein** may be identified early in the dissection, dissected using a right-angle instrument, and clipped with medium to large titanium clips, using three clips proximally and two clips distally. Continue the dissection superomedially, clipping adrenal branches of the inferior phrenic vessels.

i. For **larger glands** (>5 cm), dissect the adrenal gland superiorly, clipping the adrenal branches of the inferior phrenic vessels. Clip and divide the adrenal vein last (Fig. 39.2.3).

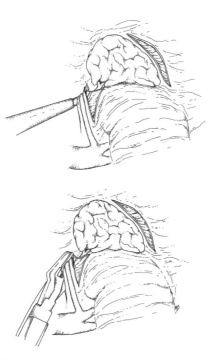

Figure 39.2.3. Division of left adrenal vein.

    j. Place the adrenal gland in an appropriately sized impermeable nylon bag. Remove the bag through the original trocar site by using a Kelly clamp to spread the abdominal wall musculature. The abdominal incision may have to be enlarged to remove the specimen (Chapter 8).

4. **Right adrenalectomy**

    a. **Patient position and room setup** are the reverse of those described for the left adrenal.

    b. **Trocar placement and choice of laparoscope**

       i. Access is gained using the open technique at the right anterior axillary line, approximately 2 cm below and parallel to the costal margin. Palpate the liver carefully to avoid the edge of the liver. **Place a 10-mm trocar for the 30-degree angled laparoscope** at this site.

      ii. Place three additional 10-mm trocars 2 cm below and parallel to the subcostal margin. Position one trocar in the right flank, inferior and posterior to the tip of the eleventh rib, and the other two more anterior and medial. The most medial trocar should be lateral to the edge of the ipsilateral rectus muscle.

     iii. The trocars should be at least 5 cm or, more optimally, 10 cm away from each other (Fig. 39.2.4).

     iv. The two most lateral trocars are the surgeon's operating ports.

     v. The most anterior port is used to place the fan retractor to retract the right lobe of the liver anteriorly.

    c. **Performing the adrenalectomy**

       i. The surgeon works with the laparoscopic dissector and scissors passed through the two most lateral ports.

      ii. Insert the fan retractor along the most anterior port and retract the right hepatic lobe anteriorly.

     iii. Lyse the **right lateral hepatic attachments** and the right triangular ligament up to the diaphragm.

     iv. **Laparoscopic ultrasound** may be of assistance in identifying the anatomy.

     v. Identify the **inferolateral edge** of the right adrenal gland and dissect inferiorly.

     vi. Tilt the table to the reverse Trendelenburg position.

    vii. For **adrenal glands less than 5 cm** in diameter, the right adrenal vein can be visualized early in the operation. Identify the right renal vein in the inferior most margin of the dissection. Along the lateral edge of the vena cava, the right adrenal vein is encountered and isolated using a right-angle instrument. Secure the vein proximally with three titanium clips and distally with two clips before transection. Clip and divide the adrenal branches of the inferior phrenic vein as the dissection proceeds superiorly (Fig. 39.2.5).

   viii. For **adrenal glands greater than 5 cm,** perform the lateral and superior dissection first, then dissect caudally along the

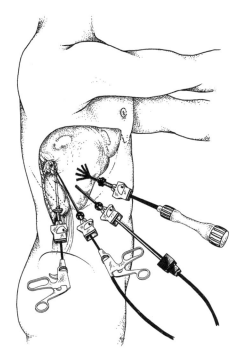

Figure 39.2.4. Trocar placement for transabdominal right adrenalectomy. Four 10-mm working trocars are used; if a vascular stapler is needed, one of these can be changed to a 12-mm port.

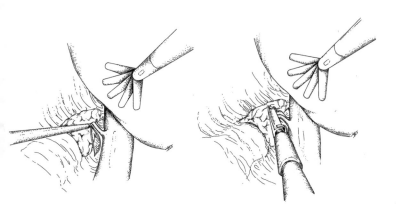

Figure 39.2.5. Division of right adrenal vein.

vena cava to identify the adrenal vein. Transect the vein as previously described.

ix.   A short fat right adrenal vein may require the vascular endoscopic stapler for secure division. Convert one of the 10-mm trocars to a 12-mm trocar and carefully pass the stapler, taking great care not to tear the vein.

x.   Place the adrenal gland in an impermeable nylon bag and removed via the original trocar.

D. Retroperitoneal Endoscopic Adrenalectomy: Posterior Approach

The lateral and posterior approaches are very similar except for positioning of the patient and the need for changing position in cases of bilateral adrenalectomy with the lateral position. Herein, the posterior approach is described.

1.   **Patient position and room setup**
   a.   Place the patient in the **prone jackknife position**, with the arms extended cephalad. Place support cushions longitudinally along the patient's torso and flex the table at the waist.
   b.   The **surgical prep** should extend from midscapula to the anterior superior iliac spines.
   c.   The **surgeon** stands on the side of the pathology.
   d.   The **first assistant** stands opposite the surgeon.
   e.   Place **two monitors** cephalad on each side of the table.

2.   **Trocar placement and choice of laparoscope**
   a.   Insert a balloon trocar into the retroperitoneal space 2.5 cm lateral to the twelfth rib. Inflate the balloon by pumping it 25 to 30 times.
   b.   Pass a 10-mm, **30-degree laparoscope** through the balloon trocar and inspect the retroperitoneum.
   c.   Exchange the balloon trocar for a standard 10-mm trocar.
   d.   Place a second **10-mm trocar medially**, just lateral to the ipsilateral erectus spinae muscles.
   e.   Place a third **10-mm trocar laterally** at the posterior axillary line. The most lateral and most medial trocars are the surgeon's operative ports (Fig. 39.2.6).

3.   **Performance of left adrenalectomy**
   a.   Identify the kidney and the adrenal gland.
   b.   Dissect along the inferomedial border of the gland, exposing the left renal vein.
   c.   Identify the adrenal vein, and clip and divide it.
   d.   Dissect and divide the remaining small vascular twigs.
   e.   Place the gland in an impermeable nylon bag and remove through the original trocar site.

4.   **Performance of right adrenalectomy**
   a.   Identify the kidney and adrenal gland.

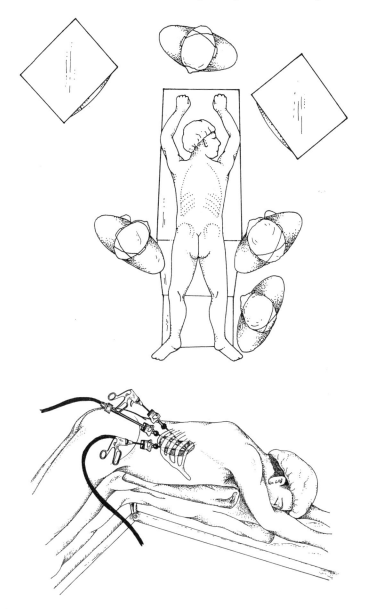

Figure 39.2.6. Placement of trocars in laparoscopic retroperitoneal adrenalectomy. Three 10-mm trocars are usually used. Bilateral adrenalectomies can be performed without repositioning the patient.

b. Dissect the adrenal gland attachments to the vena cava infero-medially, clipping all vascular elements.
c. Complete the dissection and remove the gland as described previously.

E. Complications

The available evidence suggests that laparoscopic adrenalectomy carries a mean morbidity rate of about 10%. Table 39.2.3 shows the different reported complications.

Bleeding is the most prevalent complication both intra- and postoperatively. This is not surprising considering that both adrenals are highly vascularized and situated in close proximity of major blood vessels. Together with organ injury, these two complications occurring frequently in laparoscopic adrenalectomy are discussed in this section.

Table 39.2.3. Complications of laparoscopic adrenalectomy.

Intraoperative
  Bleeding due to vascular injury:
    Adrenal vein
    Renal vein
    Inferior vena cava
    Others
  Organ injury
    Liver
    Kidney
    Spleen
    Pancreas
    Bowel
  Diaphragmatic injury
  Others

Postoperative
  Bleeding (intra-abdominal and abdominal wall)
  Wound (short and long term)
  Infectious
  Cardiovascular
  Pulmonary
  Gastrointestinal
  Urinary
  Thromboembolic
  Endocrine
  Others

1. **Hemorrhage**
    a. **Cause and prevention.** Experience with open adrenal surgery and intimate knowledge of anatomy are prerequisites for every surgeon attempting laparoscopic adrenalectomy. Correct any preoperative coagulopathies. The dissection should be meticulous, with special attention to hemostasis. Before clipping the adrenal vein, trace it back to the adrenal gland to avoid damaging an accessory renal vein. Securely clip the proximal portion of the adrenal vein at least twice.
    b. **Recognition and management.** Intraoperative hemorrhage is easily identified and may require conversion to an open procedure if hemostasis cannot be achieved. (See Chapter 6) Postoperative hemorrhage is best detected by carefully monitoring the patient's vital signs and urine output overnight and physical diagnosis of the abdomen.
2. **Organ injury**
    a. **Cause and prevention.** As with bleeding, the key for prevention is familiarity with anatomy and delicate technique. Care should be taken while dissecting along the superior aspect of a left adrenal gland to prevent injury to the tail of the pancreas. Retract liver and spleen gently to avoid injury and bleeding. High dissection in the abdomen may cause diaphragmatic injury, potentially leading to tension pneumothorax.
    b. **Recognition and management.** Damage to the liver or spleen will present as intraoperative or postoperative bleeding. Damage to the pancreas can present early as pancreatitis or later as pancreatic pseudocyst. These problems are usually self-limited but may require medical or surgical management. In case of injury to the diaphragm, closure with chest drainage will normally be sufficient.
3. **Others**
    Avoiding lengthy procedures will generally prevent severe hypercarbia and acidosis in cases of bilateral adrenalectomy. Appropriate pharmacologic blockade is mandatory before surgery for pheochromocytoma to avoid hypertensive crisis intraoperatively. Sufficient hormonal replacement is mandatory after bilateral adrenalectomy in Cushing's disease. Other complications are not specific to the procedure and, therefore, are not discussed here.

F. Selected References

Bax TW, Marcus DR, Galloway GQ, Swanstrom LL, Sheppard BC. Lapascopic bilateral adrenalectomy following failed hypophysectomy. Surg Endosc 1996;10:1150–1153.

Bonjer HJ, Lange JF, Kazemier G, et al. Comparison of three techniques for adrenalectomy. Br J Surg 1997;84:679–682.

Bonjer HJ, Sorm V, Berends FJ, et al. Endoscopic retroperitoneal adrenalectomy: lessons learned from 111 consecutive cases. Ann Surg 2000;232:796–803.

Brunt LM, Lairmore TC, Doherty GM, et al. Adrenalectomy for familial pheochromocytoma in the laparoscopic era. Ann Surg 2002;235:713–720.

Brunt LM, Moley JF, Doherty GM, et al. Outcome analysis in patients undergoing laparoscopic adrenalectomy for hormonally active tumors. Surgery 2001;130:629–634.

Duh QY, Siperstein AE, Clark OH, et al. Laparoscopic adrenalectomy. Comparison of the lateral and posterior approaches. Arch Surg 1996;131:870–875.

Fernandez-Cruz L, Saenz A, Benarroch G, Astudillo E, Taura P, Sabater L. Laparoscopic unilateral and bilateral adrenalectomy for Cushing's syndrome. Transperitoneal and retroperitoneal approaches. Ann Surg 1996;224:727–736.

Fernandez-Cruz L, Saenz A, Taura P, et al. Retroperitoneal approach in laparoscopic adrenalectomy: is it advantageous? Surg Endosc 1999;13:86–90.

Ferrer FA, MacGillivray DC, Malchoff CD, Albala DM, Shichman SJ. Bilateral laparoscopic adrenalectomy for adrenocorticotropic dependent Cushing's syndrome. J Urol 1997;157:16–18.

Gagner M. Laparoscopic adrenalectomy. Surg Clin North Am 1996;76:523–537.

Gagner M, Breton G, Pharand D, Pomp A. Is laparoscopic adrenalectomy indicated for pheochromocytomas? Surgery 1996;120:1076–1080.

Gagner M, Lacroix A, Bolte E. Laparoscopic adrenal in Cushing's syndrome and pheochromocytomas. N Engl J Med 1992;327:1003–1006.

Gagner M, Lacroix A, Bolte E, et al. Laparoscopic adrenalectomy: the importance of flank approach in lateral decubitus position. Surg Endosc 1994;8:135–138.

Gagner M, Pomp A, Heniford BT, Pharand D, Lacroix A. Laparoscopic adrenalectomy: lessons learned from 100 consecutive cases. Ann Surg 1997;226:238–247.

Gill IS. The case for laparoscopic adrenalectomy. J Urol 2001;166:429–436.

Henry JF, Sebag F, Iacobone M, et al. Results of laparoscopic adrenalectomy for large and potentially malignant tumors, World J Surg 2002;26:1043–1047.

Kebebew E, Siperstein AE, Clark OH, et al. Results of laparoscopic adrenalectomy for suspected and unsuspected malignant adrenal neoplasms. Arch Surg 2002;137:948–953.

Kebebew E, Siperstein AE, Duh QY. Laparoscopic adrenalectomy: the optimal surgical approach. J Laparoendosc Adv Surg Techniques 2001;11:409–413.

Siperstein AE, Berber E, Engle KL, et al. Laparoscopic posterior adrenalectomy. Technical considerations. Arch Surg 2000;135:967–971.

Staren ED, Prinz RA. Adrenalectomy in the era of laparoscopy. Surgery 1996;120:706–709.

Walz MK, Peitgren K, Neumann H, et al. Endoscopic treatment of solitary. Bilateral, multiple and recurrent pheochromocytomas and paragangliomas, World J Surg 2002;26:1005–1012.

Laparoscopy
VIII—Hernia Repair

40. Laparoscopic Inguinal Hernia Repair: Transabdominal Preperitoneal (TAPP) and Totally Extraperitoneal (TEP)

Muhammed Ashraf Memon, M.B.B.S., D.C.H., F.R.C.S.
Robert J. Fitzgibbons, Jr., M.D., F.A.C.S.

A. Indications

Laparoscopic hernia repair may be performed for the same indications as conventional (anterior) repair. The role of laparoscopic inguinal hernia repair in treatment of an uncomplicated, unilateral hernia is **unresolved**. Large, randomized, prospective trials will be needed to definitively settle the question of whether the added risks and costs are worth the benefits.

Transabdominal preperitoneal (TAPP) or totally extraperitoneal (TEP) laparoscopic inguinal herniorrhaphy may offer **specific benefits** in the following situations.

1. **Recurrent hernia.** Laparoscopic repair is a logical choice for patients with recurrent inguinal hernias. Conventional (anterior) repair for recurrent hernia is technically difficult because of scar tissue and distorted anatomy. It carries a failure rate as high as 30% in some series. The laparoscopic approach allows the repair to be performed through healthy tissue and may achieve a lower failure rate.
2. **Bilateral hernias.** Bilateral hernias can be repaired simultaneously without additional incisions or trocar sites.
3. **Patients undergoing another laparoscopic procedure.** A patient with an inguinal hernia can safely undergo laparoscopic herniorrhaphy following the completion of the primary laparoscopic procedure. For this to succeed:
   a. The primary procedure must not have created contamination by spillage of purulent material.
   b. Placement of additional trocars may be required. Hernia repair should not be performed using trocars in suboptimal positions. Access and appropriate angles for dissection are critical for laparoscopic surgery.

B. Patient Position and Room Setup: TAPP or TEP

1. Position the patient supine with arms tucked at the side. Extending the arms on arm boards may not allow enough room for the surgeon to comfortably operate.
2. The Trendelenburg position allows the bowel to fall away from the pelvis, providing excellent access.
3. The surgeon stands on the opposite side of the table from the hernia.
4. Placement of a Foley catheter is optional and depends on surgeon's preference.
5. Place a single video monitor at the foot of the operating table. Adjust the height of the monitor for comfortable viewing by both surgeon and assistants.

C. Transabdominal Preperitoneal (TAPP) Approach

1. Place the first trocar at the umbilicus. Optical systems have improved so much in the last several years that a 5-mm telescope may be sufficient for visualization. However this does make mesh introduction later in the procedure more difficult. Therefore, many surgeons still prefer a 10-mm cannula.
2. Place two additional trocars lateral to the rectus sheath on either side at the level of the umbilicus under direct vision (Fig. 40.1); 5-mm trocars are sufficient assuming no 10-mm instruments (e.g., a hernia stapler) will be required.
3. An angled laparoscope provides the best visualization of the inguinal region, which is somewhat anterior (Figs. 40.2 and 40.3).
4. Inspect both inguinal regions. Identify the median umbilical ligament (remnant of the urachus), the medial umbilical ligament (remnant of umbilical artery), and the lateral umbilical fold (peritoneal reflection over the inferior epigastric artery). If the median umbilical ligament appears to compromise exposure, divide it.
5. Use laparoscopic scissors to incise the peritoneum along a line approximately 2 cm above the superior edge of the hernia defect, extending from the median umbilical ligament to the anterior superior iliac spine.
6. Mobilize the peritoneal flap inferiorly using blunt and sharp dissection.
   a. Expose the inferior epigastric vessels, and identify the pubic symphysis and lower portion of the rectus abdominis muscle.
   b. Dissect Cooper's ligament to its junction with the femoral vein.
   c. Identify the iliopubic tract. Continue the dissection inferiorly, with care to avoid an injury to the femoral branch of the genitofemoral

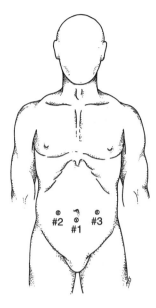

Figure 40.1. Trocar placement for TAPP.

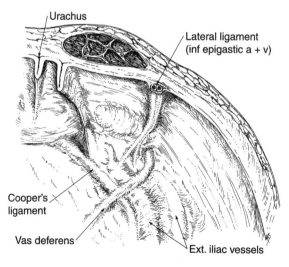

Figure 40.2. Male groin anatomy. In the female, the round ligament of the uterus leaves the pelvis at the internal ring.

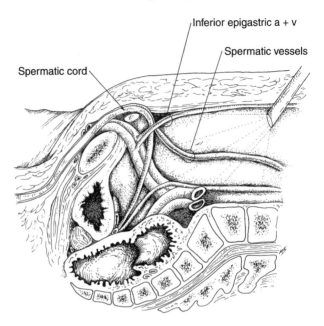

Figure 40.3. Anatomy of male pelvis as viewed by angled (30-degree) laparoscope.

       nerve and the lateral femoral cutaneous nerve, which usually enter the lower extremity just below the iliopubic tract.

    d.   Complete the dissection by skeletonizing the cord structures.

7. **Direct hernia.** Reduce the sac and preperitoneal fat from the hernia orifice by gentle traction (Fig. 40.4).

8. There are two options for **indirect hernias**:

    a.   A small sac is easily mobilized from the cord structures and reduced back into the peritoneal cavity.

    b.   A large sac may be difficult to mobilize because of dense adhesions between the sac and the cord structures due to the chronicity of the hernia. Undue trauma to the cord may result if an attempt is made to remove the sac in its entirety. In this situation, divide the sac just distal to the internal ring, leaving the distal sac *in situ*. This is most easily accomplished by opening the sac on the side opposite the cord structures and completing the division from the inside. Dissect the proximal sac away from the cord structures.

9. Next, place a large piece of mesh (at least 11 cm × 6 cm) over the myopectineal orifice so that it completely covers the direct, indirect, and femoral spaces (Fig. 40.5).

    a.   The mesh can be simply laid over the cord structures; or, a slit can be made in the mesh to wrap around the cord structures. Most

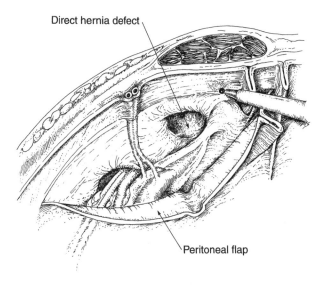

Figure 40.4. Mobilizing the peritoneal flap for a left direct inguinal hernia.

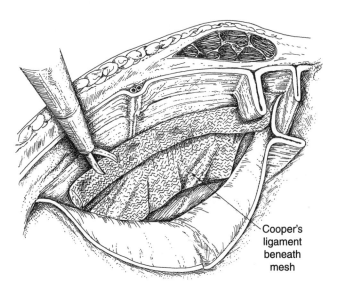

Figure 40.5. Placement of mesh. A large sheet of mesh is laid over the entire floor, covering the cord and all myopectineal orifices.

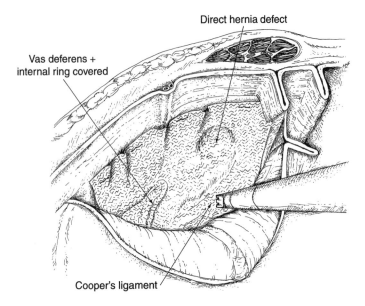

Direct hernia defect

Vas deferens +
internal ring covered

Cooper's ligament

Figure 40.6. Staple fixation of mesh. **Beware!** The lateral femoral cutaneous nerve and the genital branch of the genitofemoral nerve usually cross under the iliopubic tract lateral to the cord structures. Rarely, however, these nerves have been reported to enter the thigh above tract.

        surgeons now avoid the slit in the prosthesis because recurrences have been noted through these slits (even when they have been closed around the cord).

   b.   The large prosthesis allows the intra-abdominal pressure to act uniformly over a large area, thus preventing its herniation through the hernia defect in the abdominal wall.

10. Although not all surgeons think that stapling or tacking is necessary, most feel that the practice may prevent migration or shrinkage in some patients (Fig. 40.6).

   a.   Begin stapling/tacking along the superior border of the prosthesis.

   b.   Place staples horizontally along the superior border to minimize the chance of injury to the deeper ilioinguinal or iliohypogastric nerves.

   c.   Place staples/tacks at least 2 cm above the hernia defect beginning medially above the *contralateral* pubic tubercle and extending laterally to the anterior superior iliac spine.

   d.   Staple/tack the inferior border to Cooper's ligament medially. Again the opposite pubic tubercle marks the area to begin placing staples/tacks for the inferior border, and these are continued over the area of the ipsilateral pubic tubercle to the femoral vein. Do not place staples/tacks directly into either pubic tubercle because chronic postoperative pain (osteitis pubis) can result.

e. Affix the medial and lateral borders using vertically placed staples or tacks. This is the direction of the lateral cutaneous nerve of the thigh and the femoral branch of the genitofemoral nerve.

f. Lateral to the internal spermatic vessels, place all staples/tacks above the iliopubic tract. This avoids neuralgia from injury to the lateral cutaneous nerve of the thigh or the femoral branch of the genitofemoral nerve. It is useful to palpate the head of the stapler or tacking device through the abdominal wall with the nondominant hand. This ensures that stapling is done above the iliopubic tract (Fig. 40.7).

11. After stapling/tacking is complete, excise any redundant mesh.

12. Close the peritoneal flap over the mesh with staples, tacks, or continuous 3/0 Vicryl suture.

a. The goal should be to isolate the prosthesis from intra-abdominal viscera.

b. The authors do not feel that linear approximation of the peritoneum is necessary for all patients, especially if this results in a tenting of the peritoneum because of excessive tension required to approximate the two edges. The tenting effect may leave a space between the peritoneal flap and the prosthesis. Bowel might migrate into this space, resulting in bowel obstruction.

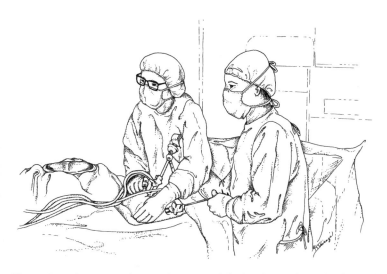

Figure 40.7. Surgeon using nondominant (left) hand to palpate the head of the stapler/tacking device through the anterior abdominal wall, thus verifying stapler/tacking device position relative to external landmarks and providing counterpressure.

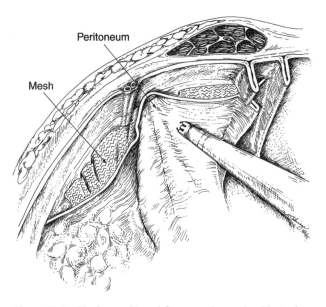

Figure 40.8. Closing peritoneal flap over the mesh with staples.

    c.   Occasionally, it is necessary to simply cover the mesh with the inferior flap, leaving exposed transversalis fascia.

    d.   Avoid excess gaps between staples; bowel can herniate or adhere to the mesh through these defects.

    e.   It may be helpful to decrease the pneumoperitoneum prior to flap closure (Fig. 40.8).

13.   Inject a long-acting local anesthetic such as bupivacaine into the preperitoneal space before closure, if desired, to decrease postoperative pain.

14.   **Bilateral hernias** can be repaired by using one long transverse peritoneal incision extending from one anterior superior iliac spine to the other.

    a.   Another option is to make two separate peritoneal incisions, preserving the peritoneum between the medial umbilical ligaments but still dissecting the preperitoneal space over the symphysis pubis. This has the theoretical advantage of avoiding damage to a patent urachus.

    b.   A large single piece of mesh measuring 30 cm × 7.5 cm can be stapled/tacked from one anterior superior iliac spine to the other anterior superior iliac spine.

    c.   Some surgeons prefer two separate pieces of mesh because of concern that placing the mesh across the bladder could interfere with bladder function. Also, it is technically easier to manipulate two pieces separately and tailor them more accurately to fit the preperitoneal space on either side.

D. Totally Extraperitoneal (TEP) Approach

1. Make the skin incision for the first trocar (10–12 mm) at the umbilicus. Open the anterior rectus sheath on the ipsilateral side and retract the muscle laterally to expose the posterior rectus sheath.
   a. Following the incision of the anterior rectus sheath, and retraction of the muscle laterally, insert a finger over the posterior rectus sheath, and gently develop this space.
   b. Insert a transparent balloon tipped trocar into this space directed toward the pubic symphysis. Place the laparoscope in the trocar. Under direct vision, inflate the balloon to create the extraperitoneal tunnel or space.
2. Place two additional trocars in the midline under direct vision: the second (5-mm) several centimeters above the pubic symphysis, and the third (5-mm) midway between the first and second (Figs. 40.9 and 40.10).

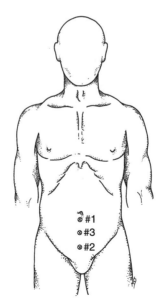

Figure 40.9. Trocar placement for TEP.

  a. Place these trocars by incising the skin with a scalpel; then use blunt dissection with a hemostat under direct vision.
  b. Avoid using a standard trocar, as inadvertent penetration through the narrow preperitoneal space into the peritoneal cavity may result.
3. Use an angled laparoscope to provide the best visualization of the inguinal region (which is somewhat anterior).
4. Complete the dissection of the preperitoneal space, placement of mesh and stapling/tacking in a similar manner to that described for TAPP procedure (Fig. 40.11).
5. Bilateral hernias can be repaired with the use of either a single large prosthesis or two separate pieces.

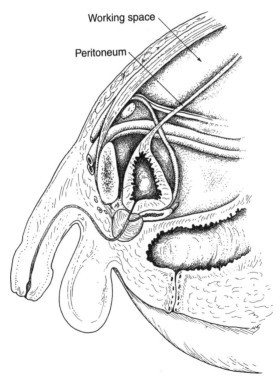

Figure 40.10. Sagittal view of extraperitoneal dissection. A space is developed between peritoneum and abdominal wall. Note that the bladder is mobilized downward.

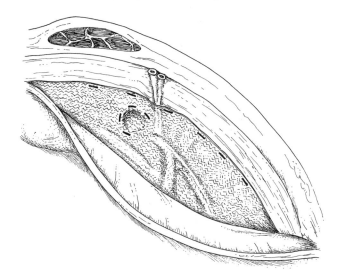

Figure 40.11. Mesh stapled in place using TEP approach.

F. Complications

Both the TAPP and TEP procedures are associated with any of the complications of laparoscopy, including major vascular injury, injury to hollow viscera, complications of pneumoperitoneum, or complications associated with anesthesia. This section describes several specific complications related to the laparoscopic herniorrhaphy.

1. **Vascular injuries**
   a. **Cause and prevention.** Injuries to the inferior epigastric and spermatic vessels are the most common vascular injuries reported during laparoscopic inguinal herniorrhaphy. Other vessels at risk include the external iliac, circumflex iliac profunda, and obturator vessels. Of course, vascular injury can occur during the initial trocar or Veress needle insertion as with any laparoscopic procedure. Inexperience, anatomic variations, and confusion during dissection, especially if the patient has had previous lower abdominal surgery, predisposes patients to vascular injuries. Use of the open laparoscopic technique for insertion of the initial cannula, meticulous dissection, and absolute identification of important landmarks are essential in preventing these injuries.
   b. **Recognition and management.** Bleeding is easily recognized at the time of surgery. Delayed bleeding may present with signs and symptoms of hypovolemia. All vessels in the inguinal region

except for the external iliacs can be safely ligated. Injury to the external iliac vessels requires immediate repair.

2. **Urinary tract complications**
   a. **Cause and prevention.** Urinary retention, urinary infection, and hematuria are the most common patient complications reported in the literature and are usually secondary to urinary catheterization, extensive preperitoneal dissection, general anesthesia, and/or administration of large volumes of intravenous fluids. Bladder injury is one of the more common complications of laparoscopic herniorrhaphy. It is most commonly seen in patients with previous "space of Retzius" surgery. **Previous surgery in this space (i.e., a prostate operation) should be considered a relative contraindication to laparoscopic hernia repair.** Renal and ureteral injuries have been seen with off-center trocar insertion. Careful technique should prevent these injuries.
   b. **Recognition and management.** Transient urinary catheterization and a short course of antibiotics usually solves problems with retention or infection. If a bladder injury is recognized during hernia repair, it should be repaired immediately either laparoscopically or via conventional laparotomy if necessary. A conventional herniorrhaphy without a prosthesis should then be performed to avoid the need to place a foreign body next to the bladder repair. A high index of suspicion is the key to the diagnosis of a missed urinary tract injury. Lower abdominal pain, distended bladder, dysuria, and hematuria should be promptly investigated. Other signs may include azotemia, electrolyte abnormalities, and ascites. Indwelling catheter drainage alone may suffice for retroperitoneal bladder injuries, but intraperitoneal perforations are best closed either laparoscopically or by a laparotomy.

3. **Nerve injury**
   a. **Cause and prevention.** The femoral branch of the genitofemoral nerve, the lateral cutaneous nerve of the thigh, and the intermediate cutaneous branch of the anterior branch of the femoral nerve are at risk of damage during laparoscopic herniorrhaphy because of (1) failure to appreciate the anatomy from the posterior aspect; (2) difficulty in visualizing the nerves preperitoneally; (3) variable course of the nerves in this region; (4) improper staple placement; or (5) extensive preperitoneal dissection. These problems have been almost eliminated by either use of onlay mesh without stapling or use of tacks.
   b. **Recognition and management.** Symptoms of burning pain and numbness usually develop after a variable interval in the postoperative period. If the neuralgia is present in the recovery room, immediate reexploration is the best course of action. When the symptoms are delayed in onset, the condition is usually self-limiting. In the majority of cases nonsteroidal anti-inflammatory agents are sufficient. Reexploration and removal of the offending staple may occasionally be required.

4. **Vas deferens and testicular complications**
   a. **Cause and prevention.** The majority of these complications are transient and self-limiting; they include testicular pain, testicular swelling, orchitis, and epididymitis. Testicular pain may be the result of trauma to the genitofemoral nerve or to the sympathetic innervation of the testis during dissection around the cord structures or during separation of the peritoneum from the cord structures. Testicular swelling may be secondary to narrowing of the deep inguinal ring, ischemia, or from interruption of lymphatic or venous vessels resulting from attempts at complete removal of a large indirect inguinal hernia sac. Transection of the vas deferens or testicular atrophy is seen in about the same incidence as conventional surgery. Avoiding excessive tightening of the deep inguinal ring, gently dissecting around the cord structures, and avoiding complete removal of large indirect hernia sacs will reduce vas deferens and testicular complications.
   b. **Recognition and management.** Most cord and testicular complications are treated by supportive care such as testicular support, limitation of activities, and analgesics. If the vas deferens is transected, the cut ends should be repaired with fine, interrupted sutures unless fertility is not a consideration. There is no treatment for unilateral testicular atrophy. The recommended treatment for bilateral testicular atrophy is the administration of parenteral testosterone usually by intramuscular injection.

5. **Complications related to the mesh**
   a. **Cause and prevention.** Migration of mesh, infection of mesh, mass lesions representing palpable mesh, adhesion formation, and erosion of the mesh into intra-abdominal organs have been reported following laparoscopic herniorrhaphy. Fixation of mesh prevents migration. The use of preoperative prophylactic antibiotics is recommended to prevent mesh infection. Adhesion formation is least likely to occur following the TEP procedure as the mesh is never in contact with intra-abdominal organs unless there are unrecognized perforations of the peritoneum. Following the TAPP procedure, adequate closure of the peritoneum over the mesh is the most important factor in preventing complications such as bowel herniating through large gaps and/or becoming adherent to exposed mesh. Minimizing trauma, avoiding infection, sparing the blood supply, and avoiding exposed mesh decreases the incidence of adhesion formation.
   b. **Recognition and management.** Mesh complications usually manifest themselves weeks to years following the repair in the form of small bowel obstruction, abscess, or fistula. These may respond to conservative management or may require formal laparotomy.

6. **Recurrence of the hernia**
   a. **Cause and prevention.** Recurrence may be due to a variety of mechanisms (Table 40.1). The authors feel that a thorough dissection of the preperitoneal space with identification of all the

Table 40.1. Potential mechanisms for recurrence.

Incomplete dissection
  Missed hernias
  Inadequate identification of landmarks
  Prosthesis rolls up rather than lying flat
Mesh too small
  Incomplete coverage of all defects
Migration of the mesh
Mesh slit and placed around cord
  Slit may be site of recurrence
Folding or invagination of mesh into defect
Displacement of mesh by hematoma

landmarks, followed by fixation of a large-size mesh that adequately covers and overlaps the entire myopectineal orifice without slitting or folding, is the best way to avoid recurrence.

b. **Recognition and management.** Recurrence is noted by patient or physician as a lump or pain in the groin. Either a repeat laparoscopic repair or a conventional repair will be needed to correct the recurrence.

7. **Miscellaneous complications**

a. **Cause and prevention.** Pubic and pelvic **osteitis** are usually caused by placing a staple into bone. Placing staples on the anterior and superior portion of Cooper's ligament or avoiding fixing mesh altogether prevents these complications. Groin **seroma** and **hematoma** usually result from extensive dissection or inadequate hemostasis. **Wound infection** may be prevented using meticulous sterile technique. **Port site herniation** can be prevented by fascial closure of any cannula site greater than 10 mm. There are now many disposable or reusable devices available to facilitate this.

b. **Recognition and management.** Pubic and pelvic osteitis are difficult to diagnose. The diagnosis is essentially one of exclusion. Simple measures such as anti-inflammatory agents and analgesia may be helpful. Groin hematoma or seroma may require evacuation or aspiration. Wound infection will require a course of antibiotics after drainage and may require removal of the mesh prosthesis if the infection extends to the groin. Port site herniation may require surgical intervention.

G. Selected References

Camps J, Nguyen N, Annibali R, Filipi CJ, Fitzgibbons RJ Jr. Laparoscopic inguinal herniorrhaphy: current techniques. In: Arregui ME, Fitzgibbons RJ Jr, Katkhouda N,

McKernan JB, Reich H, eds. Principles of Laparoscopic Surgery: Basic and Advanced Techniques. New York: Springer-Verlag, 1995;400–408.

Fitzgibbons RJ Jr, Camps J, Cornet DA, et al. Laparoscopic inguinal herniorrhaphy. Results of a multicenter trial. Ann Surg 1995;1:3–13.

Fitzgibbons RJ Jr, Zacker, K. Laparoscopic herniorrhaphy. In: Fischer JE, Nyhus LM, Baker RJ, eds. Mastery of Surgery. 4 edn. Philadelphia: Lippincott Williams & Wilkins, 2001.

Katkhouda N. Avoiding complications of laparoscopic hernia repair. Laparoscopic inguinal herniorrhaphy: current techniques. In: Arregui ME, Fitzgibbons RJ Jr, Katkhouda N, McKernan JB, Reich H, eds. Principles of Laparoscopic Surgery: Basic and Advanced Techniques. New York: Springer-Verlag 1995;435–438.

Lowham AS, Filipi CJ, Fitzgibbons RJ Jr, et al. Mechanisms of hernia recurrence after preperitoneal mesh repair. Traditional and laparoscopic. Ann Surg 1995;225:422–431.

Memon MA, Cooper NJ, Memon B, Memon MI, Abrams KR. Meta-analysis of randomized clinical trials comparing open and laparoscopic inguinal hernia repair. Br J Surg 2003;90:1479–1492.

Memon MA, Feliu X, Sallent EF, Camps J, Fitzgibbons RJ Jr. Laparoscopic repair of recurrent hernias. Surg Endosc 1999;13:807–810.

Memon MA, Fitzgibbons RJ Jr. Assessing risks, costs and benefits of laparoscopic hernia repair. Annu Rev Med 1998;49:63–77.

Memon MA, Fitzgibbons RJ Jr, Scott-Conner CEH. Laparoscopic inguinal hernia repair: transabdominal preperitoneal (TAPP) and totally extraperitoneal (TEP) repairs. In: Scott-Conner CEH, ed. Chassin's Operative Strategy in General Surgery. 3d ed. New York: Springer-Verlag, 2002;771–779.

Memon MA, Quinn TH, Cahill DR. Transversalis fascia: historical aspects and its place in contemporary inguinal herniorrhaphy. J Laparoendosc Adv Surg Techniques 1999;9:267–272.

Memon MA, Rice D, Donohue JH. Laparoscopic herniorrhaphy. J Am Coll Surg 1997;184:325–335.

Tetik C, Arregui ME. Prevention of complications of open and laparoscopic repair of groin hernias. In: Arregui ME, Fitzgibbons RJ Jr, Katkhouda N, McKernan JB, Reich H, eds. Principles of Laparoscopic Surgery: Basic and Advanced Techniques. New York: Springer-Verlag, 1995;439–449.

41. Laparoscopic Repair of Ventral Hernia

Gerald M. Larson, M.D.

A. Indications and Contraindications

1. **The general indication** for a laparoscopic repair of a ventral hernia is the presence of a hernia with a fascial defect 3 cm or greater in patients who would otherwise meet the criteria for a traditional open surgical repair. Small hernia defects less than 3 cm in diameter are readily repaired by standard techniques, and the laparoscopic approach usually offers no advantage to the patient. Abdominal wall hernias in the midline or in the upper and lower quadrants are equally accessible by the laparoscopic approach. Special conditions include the following.
   a. **The incarcerated hernia** can be repaired laparoscopically if one can obtain a good laparoscopic view of the hernia and its contents, dissect the adhesions, and reduce the hernia.
   b. In the **multiply operated abdomen**, the extent and density of adhesions are the main determinants of the operative time and difficulty of laparoscopic ventral hernia repair. Adhesion formation is unpredictable; therefore, multiple previous operations do not preclude the laparoscopic approach, provided an entry point for the first trocar can be obtained and a pneumoperitoneum safely established.
   c. **Swiss-cheese hernias** (multiple small defects) are actually a good indication for the laparoscopic approach because the number of fascial defects and extent of hernia formation are often greater than expected. The laparoscopic approach allows a clear delineation of all defects, so that the mesh prosthesis can be tailored accordingly.
2. **Contraindications** to laparoscopic repair of ventral hernia include the densely scarred abdomen (in which it is impossible to safely introduce a trocar or establish a pneumoperitoneum), and the acute abdomen with strangulated or infarcted bowel.

B. Patient Preparation and Room Setup

1. Place the patient supine on the operating table. Tucking the patient's arm on the surgeon's side improves mobility for the team, especially for hernias in the lower abdomen.

2.   For most midline hernias, the surgeon stands on either the patient's left
     or right with the video monitor positioned on the opposite side so that
     the surgeon's view on the screen is parallel to and in line with the
     laparoscopic view of the procedure within the abdomen.
3.   The assistant stands opposite the surgeon, and a second monitor is
     placed in a suitable position.
4.   In addition to the standard preoperative preparation, consider bowel
     prep if an incarcerated hernia with colon involvement is suspected.

C. Trocar Position and Choice of Laparoscope (Fig. 41.1)

1.   The author prefers open access with a Hasson cannula because of the
likelihood of adhesions and bowel fixed to the abdominal wall. Place the first
cannula well away (2 or 3 in.) from the nearest border of the hernia, in the midline
if possible. Establish pneumoperitoneum and insert an angled (30- or 45-degree)
laparoscope. Establish pneumoperitoneum and insert a laparoscope (0 degree) to
facilitate insertion of the other trocars.

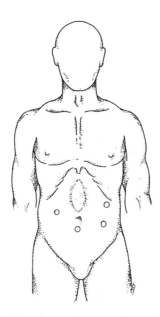

Figure 41.1. Demonstration of port placement for repair of a ventral hernia
in the upper abdomen. Place the first trocar in the lower midline, 2 or 3 in.
inferior to the ventral hernia. Ventral hernias in the lower abdomen require
placement of the camera port in the upper abdomen.

2.   Place one 10-mm and one or two 5-mm trocars as far laterally as possible. This will give a second port for the laparoscope to improve the view for dissection and also help insertion and placement of the mesh prosthesis. Specific port placement will depend on the size and location of the hernia. Establishing pneumoperitoneum through a midline trocar facilitates safe placement of lateral trocars and minimizes the risk of injury to the colon. It is more difficult to place the initial trocar in a left lateral location because it is necessary to dissect through the three muscle layers rather than the linea alba only; moreover, the air seal is not always tight, and one is concerned about proximity to the colon.

Some surgeons use a direct vision trocar in the left upper quadrant as the initial port. This is another option to the open or Veress needle technique, and my experience with these trocars has been good.

3.   Start the dissection with grasping forceps and scissors to first take down the adhesions, reduce the hernia, and outline the defect in the fascia. The scope can be placed in any port to improve exposure and the surgeon's view.

4.   For an optimal view and exposure it is best that the working ports be as far away from the hernia defect as possible. Since the mesh will overlap the defect by 3 to 4 cm, a very lateral or inferior position of the trocar site maximizes the view and efficiency of the instruments when one is unrolling the mesh and placing the tacking sutures to hold the mesh in place.

5.   For most of the dissection, an angled (30- or 45-degree) laparoscope is preferred.

6.   An extra 5-mm port may be necessary in the opposite side of the abdomen to assist with the dissection and then to position and tack the mesh to the muscle–fascia layer later in the procedure.

7.   Trocar position is to some extent a matter of surgeon's choice and preference, and must be modified for hernias in various locations.

    a.   Some surgeons may choose to stand on the patient's right, but the principles just described would apply.

    b.   For patients with subcostal hernias, the second and third trocar sites may move from the extreme lateral position to a more central inferior position in the abdomen, which will give good access to the length and breadth of the hernia defect.

D. The Technique of Laparoscopic Hernia Repair

Laparoscopic hernia repair is an intra-abdominal, intraperitoneal repair that uses a mesh prosthesis to secure and cover the hernia defect. The hernia defect itself is not closed. The mesh is anchored and held in position with transfascial mattress sutures (2-0 or 0) at each corner of the repair; usually four mattress sutures, but for larger hernias eight or more mattress sutures placed at 5- to 6-cm intervals, is appropriate. The sutures are tied through a small stab incision in the skin and tied subcutaneously. In between the mattress sutures the mesh is tacked or stapled to the abdominal wall fascia at 1-cm intervals with special hernia staples or spiral tacks.

An important principle is that the mesh must be tailored or trimmed so that it is 3 cm wider than the hernia defect on all four sides, thus permitting the prosthesis to be anchored and held in place to the solid musculofascial layer (Fig. 41.2). The mesh should be placed under some tension when it is sewn into place.

1. The first objective of the operation is to expose the hernia defect.
   a. Begin by dissecting the small bowel, omentum, and adhesions from the abdominal wall to expose the hernia defect (Fig. 41.3).
   b. External pressure applied to the abdominal wall and to the hernia assists in maintaining orientation and identifying the edge of the hernia. Frequently more than one defect is present.
   c. A variety of instruments aid in the dissection: standard grasping and dissecting forceps, sharp scissors, bowel clamps, and Babcock forceps all may be useful. The ultrasonic scalpel can be invaluable for dividing tissue and avoiding bleeding. Dissecting forceps and scissors should have electrocautery attachments.

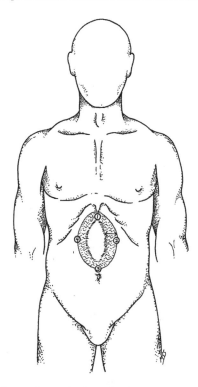

Figure 41.2. Cut the mesh prosthesis to the desired size and mark its intended location on the anterior abdominal wall. The shaded area indicates the approximate outline of the ventral hernia, and the mesh is indicated by crosshatches. The mesh should extend beyond the hernia defect by 3 cm or more on all sides. This 3-cm cuff will be used to anchor the mesh to the solid tissue surrounding the defect for the repair.

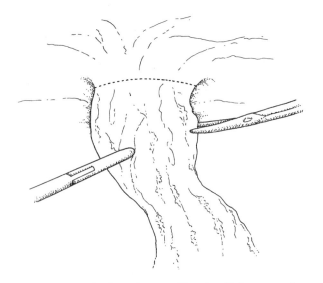

Figure 41.3. Laparoscopic view of a ventral hernia with incarcerated omentum. The hernia contents must be dissected free from the abdominal wall to expose the hernia defect.

2. Identify the edge of the defect by one of several methods.
    a. Push an intra-abdominal instrument against a palpating finger on the abdomen and mark the position of the edge.
    b. Pass needles through the abdominal wall, and confirm the position of the hernia defect relative to the needles by visual comparison.
3. Mark the edges of the defect on the skin with a marking pen.
4. Four types of mesh are currently available—a polypropylene mesh, an expanded polytetrafluoroethylene prosthesis (Gore-Tex Dual mesh), the Bard Composix mesh, and now a biologic mesh derived from porcine small intestine (Surgisis, Wilson Cook Biotech). Choice is largely a matter of personal preference. Select a piece of appropriate size and tailor the mesh prosthesis to allow a 3-cm cuff or margin lateral to the fascial defect in all directions. Mark the mesh with a colored pen so that it is readily obvious which side faces the fascia and which side faces the viscera. It is also helpful to mark the corners of the mesh 1, 2, 3, and 4 (unless the defect is circular) to maintain the proper orientation when the mesh is being tacked in place (Fig. 41.4).
5. Roll the mesh around a grasping forceps and insert it into the abdomen.
6. Horizontal mattress sutures, passed through the mesh and all layers of the abdominal wall, anchor the four corners of the mesh to solid portions of the musculofascial layer.

a.   Either a short Keith needle or a specially designed suture passer may be used.

b.   Use 2-0 braided or monofilament nonabsorbable suture for the suture passer. Heavier sutures do not pass easily.

c.   Make a small incision in the skin. This will allow the suture to be tied subcutaneously.

d.   Pass the suture through the abdominal wall (out to in), through and through the mesh (horizontal bite), and then back through the abdominal wall (in to out).

e.   Tie the sutures subcutaneously.

f.   The suture passer has a grasping jaw to carry a suture through a small skin incision through the abdominal wall (and solid fascia) into the abdomen and through the mesh. The suture is released, and the passer is removed and reinserted through the same skin site so that it will grasp the suture 1 cm away from the last entry point in the mesh and create a 1-cm mattress suture.

7.   For hernias measuring 3 to 5 cm, four anchoring sutures located at 90-degree intervals around the defect are adequate. For hernias larger than 5 cm, the author prefers to place eight of these mattress sutures using the suture passer technique and then supplementing the fixation of the mesh to the abdominal fascia with either a stapler or a spiral tacker in between at 1-cm intervals. The interval distance is important

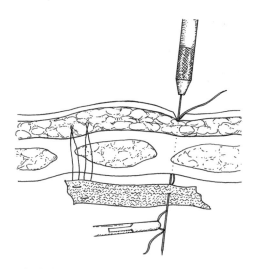

Figure 41.4.   Method of mesh fixation with a suture passer. Use the suture passer to introduce the suture through the musculofascial layer, the mesh, and then back out through all layers as a mattress suture. Use four to eight mattress sutures to anchor the mesh, depending on the size of the hernia and the surgeon's preference. Knot the sutures subcutaneously. Use hernia tackers or staples to fix the mesh to the abdominal wall between the mattress sutures.

so that bowel has no entry point between the clips, which could cause an obstruction.

8. The horizontal bite through the mesh is important. This allows the mesh to act as a pledget, thus preventing the suture from cutting through the fascia.

9. Close the trocar sites and small skin incisions in the usual fashion.

E. Complications

Complications include trocar site wound infection, urinary retention, and postoperative ileus. Dissection of adhesions and manipulation of bowel may result in injury (see Chapter 10.2, Previous Abdominal Surgery).

Recurrence is the complication unique to hernia repair. The risk can be minimized by adhering to sound surgical principles, clearly identifying all fascial defects, and placing the mesh properly with solid fixation to sound tissue. The mesh must be sufficiently large, and it must be sutured under some (but not excessive) tension.

The **wound infection** rate should be no greater than for other laparoscopic procedures of similar magnitude. Infections can generally be treated by opening the wound. This must be done in a timely fashion so that the anchoring sutures are not jeopardized.

Mechanical bowel obstruction may result from internal herniation of bowel between anchoring sutures or clips. This may require laparotomy for repair.

F. Selected References

Heniford BT, Ramshaw BJ. Laparoscopic ventral hernia repair. Surg Endosc 2000; 14(5):419–423.

Holzman MD, Puret CM, Reintgen K. Laparoscopic ventral and incisional hernioplasty. Surg Endosc 1997;11(1):32–35.

Larson GM. Ventral hernia repair by the laparoscopic approach. Surg Clin North Am 1999;1329–1340.

LeBlanc KA. The critical technical aspects of laparoscopic repair of ventral and incisional hernias. Am Surg 2001;67:809–812.

MacFadyen BV, Arregui ME, Corbitt JD. Complications of laparoscopic herniorrhaphy. Surg Endosc 1993;7:155–158.

Park A, Gagner M, Pomp A. Laparoscopic repair of large incisional hernias. Surg Laparosc Endosc 1996;6(2):123–128.

Temudom T, Siadati M, Sarr MG. Repair of complex giant or recurrent ventral hernias by using tension-free intraparietal prosthetic mesh (Stoppa technique): lessons learned from our initial experience (fifty patients). Surgery 1996;120(4):738–744.

Laparoscopy
IX—Pediatric Laparoscopy

42. Pediatric Minimally Invasive Surgery: General Considerations

John J. Meehan, M.D.

A. Indications

As with adult minimally invasive surgery, the indications for surgery have not changed simply because a new technical modality is available for treatment.

1. Laparoscopy has been applied to the following procedures and indications:
   a. Appendectomy
   b. Cholecystectomy
   c. Contralateral exploration during inguinal hernia repair
   d. Pyloromyotomy
   e. Fundoplication
   f. Splenectomy
   g. Adrenalectomy
   h. Laparoscopic assisted anorectal pull-through
   i. Ovarian cystectomy
   j. Undescended testicle
   k. Resection of Meckel's diverticulum
2. Thoracoscopy has been used in the following situations:
   a. Lung biopsy
   b. Congenital diaphragmatic hernia repair
   c. Resection of pulmonary sequestration
   d. Repair of tracheoesophageal fistula
   e. Empyema drainage and decortication
   f. Spinal exposure for scoliosis
   g. Pleurodesis
   h. Blebectomy

B. Contraindications

Absolute contraindications to laparoscopy in children are similar to those in adult patients, and include the following:

1. Uncorrected coagulopathy
2. Hemodynamic instability
3. Dense intra-abdominal adhesions

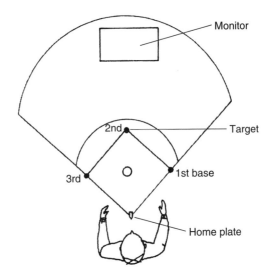

Figure 42.1. Position the trocars and monitors using the baseball analogy. The camera is at home plate, instrument ports are at first and third bases, and the target lesion is at second base. Place the monitor directly in the surgeon's line of sight.

C. Patient Position and Preparation

Ergonomic principles are crucial in planning any minimally invasive surgery. In pediatric surgery, these principles are even more important owing to the smaller abdominal or thoracic environment inside the pediatric patient.

A laparoscopic case can be considered with reference to a baseball field.

1. The camera is placed at home plate.
2. The working ports are typically located at first and third bases, and the target area of interest is located at second base (Fig. 42.1).
3. Positioning the monitors is just as important as patient positioning. Place these in a location similar to center field, directly behind the target second base area, so the surgeon can view the operation standing straight in line with the target area.
4. Accessory ports and assistants come in from the lateral fields (foul ground) as necessary.

D. Instrument and Port Size

Technology continues to make possible rapid improvements in laparoscopic instruments. The type of procedure performed usually dictates the size of the ports. For example, cholecystectomies and splenectomies still require at least one larger port (10 or 12 mm) to extract the specimen. If removal of a specimen is not required, then all ports can be downsized. Although 5-mm instruments are the most popular, 3-mm instruments are now rigid and durable enough to perform many advanced maneuvers. There are also 2-mm instruments available, but these devices are bit more flimsy and their popularity has been limited.

Advanced devices to assist in performing minimally invasive surgery have also been manufactured. Linear staplers and endoscopic specimen bags are available for 10-mm ports, while argon beam coagulators are now being produced in 5-mm sizes.

Most procedures are performed utilizing either a 3- or 5-mm telescope and viewing angles of 0, 30, and 70 degrees. Even smaller scopes are available, but the optical resolution declines with size.

E. Access to the Abdominal Cavity

Selection of trocar sites is critical to a safe and well-performed procedure. The umbilicus is used in many abdominal procedures, and the resultant scar is well hidden. Other port sites are chosen based on the target area and the principles of ergonomics discussed in Section C.

As usual, the site is prepped and draped in a sterile manner. Additional attention should be used when cleaning the umbilicus, which often a harbors dirt and other contaminants. A small incision can be made either superiorly or inferiorly around the umbilicus. The choice between inferior and superior is usually of minimal consequence but can give a slight advantage in small or large patients.

The smaller anterior-to-posterior diameter in a child highlights the need for exercising extreme caution while placing trocars. Typically, access is gained by inserting a Veress needle under controlled guidance or performing a facial incision just large enough to accept a Hasson blunt-tipped trocar. Both methods are effective and are used frequently.

1. To gain access using a Veress needle, anterior retraction on the abdominal wall is critical in placing the first trocar safely.
   a. Accomplish this by simply pinching the skin and lifting up.
   b. Alternate techniques include use of a piercing towel clamp or a monofilament suture to lift and retract the abdominal wall anteriorly.
2. To gain access using a Hasson cannula, make a small fascial incision and insert the blunt-tipped cannula into the abdomen under direct vision.
   a. Secure the cannula with an 0 or 2-0 Vicryl suture.
   b. This suture can be left in place at the end of the case to close the fascia.
   c. It is important not to make the trocar incisions too large or leakage of carbon dioxide (CO_2) from around the trocar can hinder the progress of the case. This is particularly true in small children with thin abdominal walls, since there is a minimal fat layer to create a seal around the trocars.

Once the trocars have been placed, reinsufflate the abdomen with CO_2. As in adults, the maximum abdominal pressure can usually be set to 12 to 15 cm H_2O in most children. Smaller patients may not tolerate a pressure this high. In particular, infants and newborns may only tolerate 7 to 8 cm of pressure. Decreased venous return from high intra-abdominal pressures can rapidly cause cardiac compromise, and decompression should be performed immediately simply by opening a port.

Close all trocar sites larger than 5 mm. Occasionally, 5-mm sites will also require fascial closure, but 2- and 3-mm sites usually do not.

Close the skin with 4-0 or 5-0 Vicryl suture.

43. Pediatric Laparoscopy:
Specific Surgical Procedures

John J. Meehan, M.D.

A. Appendectomy

1.   General considerations. Laparoscopic appendectomy is becoming more and more frequent for treating acute appendicitis in both pediatric and adult patients. In small thin children, many surgeons still prefer the open technique because the procedure can be performed through a small incision, which may be only 2 to 3 cm in length. Laparoscopic exploration, however, gives excellent visualization and gives the surgeon a better view for effectively irrigating the right gutter, right lower quadrant, and deep pelvis. A Foley catheter is recommended if a trocar is planned for the suprapubic location.

2.   Positioning and trocar placement. Position the patient supine. Three trocars are required and either of two popular techniques can be used for their placement (Figs. 43.1 and 43.2). Although the two methods are equally effective, we prefer the trocar placement outlined in Figure 43.1. In this arrangement, the video tower is off to the right of the operating table and the surgeon and assistant both stand on the patient's left. Surgeon and assistant may need to be on opposite sides of the table in the other method (Fig. 43.2), requiring two video towers.

Choice of specific trocars depends on how the appendix and mesoappendix will be divided and secured.

a.   Use of an endoscopic stapler requires a 10-mm port at the umbilicus.

b.   This allows use of an endoscopic retrieval bag for specimen removal through the same port.

c.   Alternatively, a 5-mm Liga-Sure or harmonic scalpel can be used to seal and cauterize the mesoappendix. The appendix can then be ligated doubly with endoloop sutures or even free ties if preferred. This technique offers the advantage of using a smaller 5-mm port.

3.   Details of operative procedure. Surgical technique is similar to that employed in adults (see Chapter 30), and will be summarized here.

a.   First, explore the abdomen and confirm the suspected diagnosis. The diagnosis is often evident after the first trocar has been placed.

b.   Once the diagnosis has been confirmed, place the remaining trocars.

c.   If there is purulent fluid, irrigation and suction may be performed first. Place the patient in a slight reverse Trendelenburg position to help pool all the purulent fluid in the pelvis and minimize contamination of the remaining abdominal cavity.

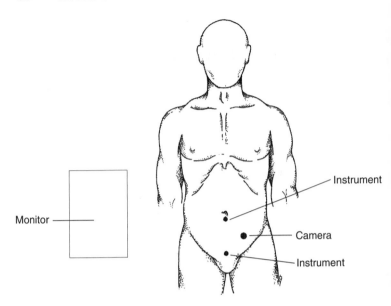

Figure 43.1. Trocar sites for laparoscopic appendectomy (preferred placement) with a single monitor to the right of the operating table. Surgeon and assistant stand to the left.

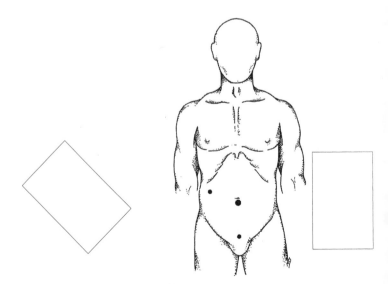

Figure 43.2. Trocar sites for laparoscopic appendectomy (alternate placement) with two monitors. Surgeon stands to the left, assistant may need to stand to the left.

d. Once the free fluid has been adequately drained, tilt the table in a slight Trendelenburg position and roll it to the left. These maneuvers will effectively roll the bowel away from the right lower quadrant and improve visualization.

e. Take any adhesions down bluntly or with cautery until the appendix is free from the retroperitoneum.

f. Demonstrate the mesoappendix and dissect the appendiceal artery with a curved dissector.

g. The mesenteric vessels may be secured with an ultrasonic dissector or a stapler. A reticulating stapler is particularly helpful.

h. After securely dividing the mesoappendix, amputate the appendix with a stapler or ligate it with a pretied suture ligature and divide it. If pretied ligatures are used, we recommend using two loops on the patient side near the base of the appendix, followed by one on the specimen side.

i. Amputate the appendix and remove it through the umbilical port.

B. Cholecystectomy

1. General considerations. Laparoscopic cholecystectomy is very similar in pediatric patients to the corresponding adult procedure (see Chapters 14–20). In addition to symptomatic cholelithiasis, other causes of cholecystitis in children include the following:
    a. Cystic fibrosis
    b. Sickle cell anemia
    c. Chronic use of total parenteral nutrition

2. Patient positioning and trocar placement
    a. Position the patient supine.
    b. For most patients, four trocars are used, placed in a manner similar to that used in adults (Fig. 43.3). However, slight modifications of the trocar placement may be required in smaller patients.
    c. The umbilical port is typically 10 mm to permit successful retrieval of the specimen at the conclusion of the case. All other ports are either 3 or 5 mm.
    d. Angle the upper midline port such that the trocar enters the abdomen to the right of the falciform ligament. The other working port is in the right midclavicular line, and the retracting port is placed along the right flank.

3. Details of procedure (see Chapter 14)
    a. Grasp the gallbladder through the retracting port and push it cephalad and over the liver to expose the porta hepatis.
    b. Use a grasper through the midclavicular port to retract the more proximal portion of the gall bladder laterally and the majority of the dissection is carried out from the midline port.

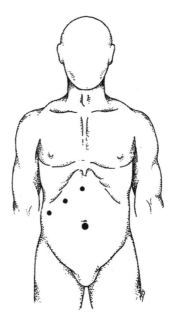

Figure 43.3. Trocar site placement for pediatric laparoscopic cholecystectomy is similar to the adult procedure.

   c.   Begin the dissection laterally and proceed medially, to safely identify structures.

   d.   Identify the cystic duct, and clip and divide it.

   e.   If a cholangiogram is desired, only partially divide the duct to facilitate cannulation (see also Chapter 16).

       i.   Bring a cholangiogram catheter into the field and introduce it into the proximal cystic duct.

      ii.   Place a clip lightly over the proximal duct and catheter to prevent leakage from the open ductomy, taking care not to occlude the catheter.

     iii.   After completing the cholangiogram, remove the temporary clip, retrieve the catheter, and secure the proximal and distal cystic ducts with the clip applier. Complete the division of this structure.

   f.   The cystic artery is usually located in close proximity to the duct. Clip and divide it in a similar fashion.

   g.   Next remove the gallbladder retrograde using hook cautery.

   h.   Remove the specimen through the umbilical port site. Occasionally, the incision will need to be extended or dilated slightly to retrieve the specimen if large stones are present.

C. Laparoscopic Splenectomy

1. General considerations. Postsplenectomy sepsis is far more common in children than in adults. Whenever possible, preoperative vaccinations for *Pneumococcus*, *Meningococcus*, and *Haemophillus* should be completed.
2. Patient positioning and trocar placement. Flexibility in trocar placement is important and should be arranged for on a case-by-case basis. Smaller patients and larger spleens may require the surgeon to make adjustments when selecting the optimal location for the ports.
    a. Place the patient either in a right lateral decubitus position or supine with a bump under the left hip to elevate the left side about 30 to 45 degrees.
    b. Positioning the patient over the break in the table and flexing the table a small amount can help, particularly if the lateral decubitus position is desired.
    c. Place trocars as shown in Figure 43.4.
3. Details of procedure (see Chapter 37)
    a. First take down the splenic attachments including the splenocolic, splenorenal, and splenophrenic ligaments. This can be accomplished with either a hook cautery or an ultrasonic dissector. The ultrasonic dissector is preferred as there may be small vessels hidden within these attachments.
    b. Divide the short gastric vessels in a similar fashion, reserving dissection of the splenic hilum for last.

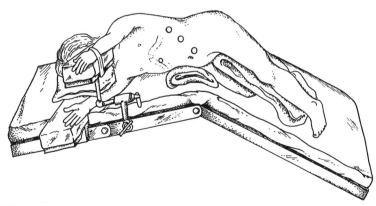

Figure 43.4. Patient position and trocar sites for pediatric laparoscopic splenectomy. Note that the patient is in the lateral position, and the operating table has been flexed to increase the distance between costal margin and superior iliac crest.

   c.   Elevate the spleen using a retractor passed through the accessory port.

   d.   Completely mobilize the spleen.

   e.   Dissect and control the splenic hilar vessels, using an endoscopic stapler with a vascular load or with clips. Some surgeons may be prefer to ligate these vessels with either silk or Vicryl sutures.

   f.   Ligate the artery first, then the vein, to reduce congestion of the spleen during these final steps.

   g.   Alternatively, both vessels can be taken together with a stapler. The risk of arteriovenous fistula seems to be more theoretical than real, as this complication has rarely been reported.

   h.   Removal of the spleen will require morcellation. This tedious procedure is a bit easier if ringed forceps are used.

D. Laparoscopic Pyloromyotomy

The use of laparoscopic surgery for the treatment of hypertrophic pyloric stenosis has been widely criticized. Opponents claim that the small incision required for the open technique invalidates the need to perform the procedure laparoscopically. Despite the controversy, many surgeons now perform the procedure laparoscopically as quickly as the open technique and with similar results. With 3-mm instruments, very small incisions can be made.

1.   Patient positioning and trocar placement

   a.   Position the patient supine.

   b.   Place a small roll to slightly hyperextend the spine, allowing better access to the pylorus.

   c.   Place three trocars, preferably 3 mm, as shown in Figure 43.5. The working port should be just to the left of midline and the camera at the umbilicus. Position the third port so the pylorus can be grasped and held in place as the myotomy is performed. This trocar should be slightly superior to the liver edge and directly lateral to the pylorus. By placing the trocar in this location, the grasping instrument is also used as a liver retractor by sweeping the liver superiorly and then grasping the pylorus and duodenum.

2.   Details of procedure

   a.   The myotomy is made from the working port in the standard fashion with either the cautery or a sharp knife. Until recently, an arthrotomy knife was adequate for this incision. However, laparoscopic pylorotomes are now manufactured and are ideal for this situation. Most are only about 2 mm in depth (Fig. 43.6A).

   b.   Use blunt dissection to spread the muscle with a laparoscopic pyloromyotomy spreader (Fig. 43.6B, C).

   c.   Confirm completeness of the pyloromyotomy by using graspers with gentle traction through the two working ports.

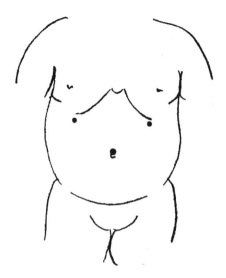

Figure 43.5. Trocar sites for laparoscopic pyloromyotomy.

E. Laparoscopic Fundoplication (see also Chapter 21)

1. General considerations. The Nissen, Toupet, and Thal fundoplications have all been incorporated into pediatric laparoscopic practice. The Nissen fundoplication is probably the most popular and consists of a full 360-degree wrap.

Variations of the original Toupet procedure currently performed include everything from a 180-degree posterior wrap to a 270-degree posterior wrap.

The Thal fundoplication is a 180-degree anterior wrap that reconstructs the angle of His.

Each technique has its own set of complications and failure rates.

2. Patient positioning and trocar placement. The general principles of laparoscopic surgery are nearly identical for all fundoplications.

    a.   Position the patient in a slight to moderate reverse Trendelenburg position to allow the bowel to fall into the pelvis.

    b.   Most importantly, bring the patient down to the foot of the bed as far as possible.

    c.   Infants and small children can have their legs taped over small rolls, while larger children will require a lithotomy position.

    d.   The surgeon should stand at the foot of the bed; the assistant is usually toward the patient's right, but still at the foot of the bed.

    e.   Place ports as shown in Figure 43.7. The camera is placed at the umbilicus. The working ports are placed along the left and right

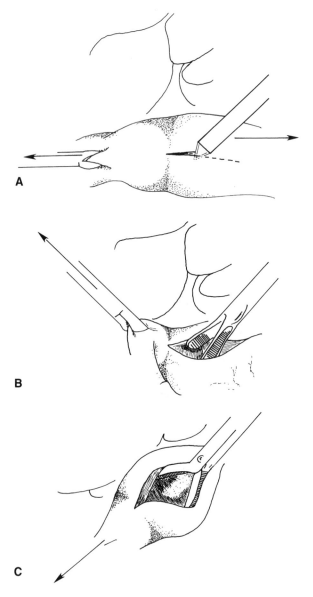

Figure 43.6. A. The myotomy is created with a laparoscopic myotome. Make this incision relatively shallow. Traction is applied by a grasper through the right-hand port. B. A pyloromyotomy spreader is used to divide the hypertrophied circular muscle fibers. C. This division is continued through the hypertrophied segment, but not onto the duodenum.

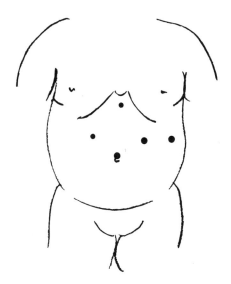

Figure 43.7. Trocar site placement for laparoscopic fundoplication.

midclavicular lines. A fourth port can be placed along the right anterior axillary line and used for liver retraction.
f.   Bring a fan or snake retractor into the field and use it to elevate the
     liver anteriorly. This retractor can be fixed to the table using a table-
     mounted clamp such as a Martin arm. This will free up the assistant
     during the case.
g.   A fifth port is sometimes required. Place this along the left anterior
     axillary line to assist in retracting the stomach inferiorly.
3. Details of procedure (see also Chapter 21)
a.   The anesthesiologist passes an appropriately sized bougie.
b.   Takedown of the short gastric vessels can help mobilize the fundus but
     is optional in many cases depending on the laxity of the fundus. This
     can be accomplished with many devices such as hook cautery, ultra-
     sonic scalpel, or a Liga-Sure device.
c.   Once the stomach has been adequately mobilized, incise the peri-
     toneum overlying the gastroesophageal junction vertically and iden-
     tify the esophagus and vagus nerve.
d.   For a posterior wrap (Nissen or Toupet), create a window behind the
     esophagus by blunt dissection. Slip the bougie back up the esophagus
     to make the dissection easier. This posterior window should be
     adequate in size to accept the fundus, but care should be taken to
     avoid overdissection, with a resultant hiatal hernia or creation of a
     pneumothorax.

e. Pass the stomach through the window to confirm that an adequate amount of stomach will be available for the wrap.

f. Before creating the wrap, reapproximate the crura with a permanent suture such as silk or Ethibond.

g. Have the anesthetist pass the bougie back down into the stomach. Pass the stomach back behind the esophagus to create the wrap. A minimum length of 2.5 to 3 cm is required for an adequate wrap. This usually takes three interrupted permanent sutures at the 12 o'clock position for the Nissen procedure and two sets of 3 interrupted permanent sutures at the 4 and 10 o'clock positions for the Toupet.

h. To create a Thal fundoplication, suture the fundus anteriorly in either a running or interrupted technique with reconstruction of the angle of His.

i. Complete the fundoplication, regardless of specific technique, by securing the wrap to underside of the diaphragm with two permanent sutures. This helps prevent a slipped wrap.

j. If a gastrostomy is desired, position the tube high enough from the pylorus to prevent gastric volvulus.

F. Laparoscopic Surgery for Undescended Testicles

The laparoscope can be a valuable tool to determine whether a testicle exists in a child with an empty scrotum and nonpalpable testis.

1. Port placement is the same for either a staged or primary orchidopexy. A 30-degree scope is inserted through an umbilical port. Working ports are slightly inferior to the umbilicus and 5 cm lateral to the midline in both directions, as shown in Figure 43.8. The visualization is excellent and the testicle is often easily found at the internal ring or nearby.

   a. If the testicle is adequate in size, the vessels will also appear normal in caliber.

   b. Occasionally, a vas is seen entering the canal and only rudimentary strands of vessels are seen, yet nothing is palpable within the inguinal canal. This is usually indicative of a prenatally torsed or absent testicle, and inguinal exploration with orchiectomy of the remnant is indicated.

   c. Rarely, no vas or vessels are seen entering the internal ring, and this warrants exploration to find the missing gonad. The gonad could reside anywhere from the internal ring all the way up the inferior pole of the ipsilateral kidney, and this entire tract should be explored. This can be accomplished laparoscopically.

2. Once the gonad has been found and viability determined, a decision must be made whether this gonad can be safely brought down to the scrotum during the current operation or whether a staged

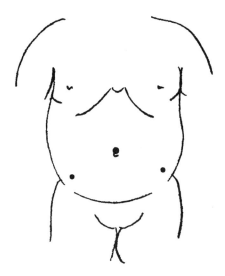

Figure 43.8. Trocar site placement for surgery for undescended testicle.

procedure will be required. If the testicle is at the internal ring, it is reasonable to attempt an orchiopexy during this time, and an inguinal incision with mobilization should be done in the standard fashion.

3.   If the testicle is too far from the inguinal canal, then a staged procedure should be selected. Ligate and divide the vessels to the testicle close to the gonad. That concludes the operation for the first stage. The patient can then undergo mobilization laparoscopically 3 to 6 months later, after the gonad has had an opportunity to develop an adequate secondary blood supply from the vas.

a.   During the second procedure, develop a wide strip of peritoneum with electrocautery as a flap on three sides, preserving the vas, testicle, and the peritoneum around them.

b.   This mobilized peritoneal flap with the vas and testicle on it is then brought up through the inguinal ring via a standard inguinal incision and brought down to the scrotum for the orchidopexy.

G. Contralateral Exploration for Inguinal Hernia

Controversy continues to surround exploration for a possible contralateral hernia in children less than 6 months of age. The risk of causing injury during an open exploration of an inguinal canal prompted laparoscopists to come up with a new way of determining the presence or absence of a contralateral hernia with minimal risk to the patient. Laparoscopic contralateral exploration offers an alternative and is performed in the following fashion:

1. The operation begins with a standard open exploration of the symptomatic side.
2. After isolating and dividing the hernia sac, a 2- or 3-mm trocar is placed into the sac.
3. Insufflate with 5 to 10 cm of pressure.
4. Insert a 70-degree scope to visualize the contralateral internal ring. A 30-degree scope may suffice in some cases.
5. After the determination has been made, allow the abdomen to desufflate and ligate the ipsilateral hernia sac in the usual fashion.
6. If a hernia is present, the contralateral side can be explored and a standard open repair performed immediately.
7. If no hernia is present, the risk of damaging the contralateral vas, vessels, and testis has been averted and nothing further is required.

H. Ovarian Torsion, Ovarian Cyst, and Ovarian Teratoma

Laparoscopy is an excellent method to evaluate ovarian pathology. Just about all ovarian operations can be performed using three ports as shown in Figure 43.9. Torsed ovaries are easily detorsed, and the cause for the torsion should be sought. An ovarian cyst is often the culprit, and excision of the cyst can be accomplished with the hook cautery. Incidentally discovered cysts greater than 5 cm in diameter should also be excised because of the risk of torsion. Teratomas can be excised using hook cautery and blunt dissection along the plane between the teratomas and normal ovary. Although ovarian teratomas are benign, contralateral ovarian biopsy should be performed for suspicious lesions.

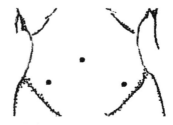

Figure 43.9. Trocar site placement for ovarian cystectomy.

I. Meckel's Diverticulum

The choice of trocar is a matter of surgeon's preference for this anomaly. We recommend setting the trocars similar to an appendectomy, with the camera inferior and to the left of the umbilicus with the suprapubic and umbilical ports used as the working ports. A 10-mm port is helpful for the umbilical port and can be used for a stapling device. Alternatively, the diverticulum can be brought directly through the umbilical incision once the omphalomesenteric vessels have been ligated or cauterized. An extracorporeal resection can than be performed, either with a stapler or excision with a standard hand-sewn closure.

J. Laparoscopic Pull-Through and Other Colon Resections

About 80% of patients with Hirschsprung's disease have the transition zone located in the rectosigmoid region. A transanal primary pull-through is all that is required, and abdominal incisions can be avoided in most of these cases. However, patients with intermediate or long segment disease will need more extensive colon mobilization.

The principles outlined here can also apply for total colonic aganglionosis or even diseases such as familial adenomatous polyposis or ulcerative colitis, where a total proctocolectomy is required.

1. Trocar site placement will vary, depending upon the extent of planned resection. In general, if a longer segment of colon needs to be removed, plan your trocar sites so that the camera can be switched from port to port if necessary. For example, a total colectomy can be achieved by combining the intra-abdominal mobilization with a transanal dissection in most cases.
2. The camera can be placed at the umbilicus and the working ports as shown in Figure 43.10.
3. Roll the patient away from the site you are working on to allow the bowel to fall out of the way.
4. Take colonic biopsy samples immediately after trocar placement in cases of Hirschsprung's disease, to determine extent of aganglionosis.
5. Take the retroperitoneal attachments with electrocautery.
6. Sequentially secure the mesentery with either an ultrasonic dissector or Liga-Sure device. Alternatively, a stapler can be used if a colon resection is required in older children with a thicker mesentery. These devices are brought in through a trocar in the left upper quadrant for the left colon and the right upper quadrant for the right colon.
7. After one half of the colon has been completely taken down, the camera is redirected to the contralateral side, and the surgeon moves to the opposite side of the table. The transverse colon is usually floppy and mobile enough to permit the majority of it to be taken down from either angle.

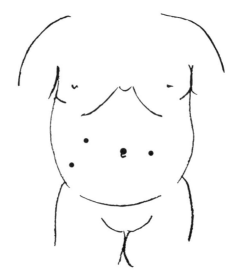

Figure 43.10. Trocar site placement for laparoscopic pull-through and other colon resections.

8. Be prepared to move the camera and working instruments from port to port.
9. The perineal dissection can be accomplished transanally at any time, although many surgeons prefer to do this first, since the length of mobilization achieved from this approach can be quite impressive.
   a. This leaves the surgeon with the problem of maintaining insufflation if abdominal exploration is performed after the transanal dissection has been completed and the peritoneal reflection entered.
   b. Remedy this by simply placing lap pads or sponges through the anal opening, thereby occluding the carbon dioxide leak through the anal canal.
10. After adequate mobilization of the colon, pull the bowel through the anus and perform the anastomosis in the usual fashion.
11. In cases of total proctocolectomy with ileoanal pull-through, a **J**-pouch may be desired.
    a. The terminal ileum will have to be divided just proximal to the ileocecal valve.
    b. This can be done intracorporeally or perhaps even extracorporeally if it reaches the anus.
    c. Construct the pouch by folding the final 10-cm segment of ileum back on itself and aligning it with two or three silk sutures intracorporeally.

d.   Use a stay stitch in the apex of the **J** to pass the new pouch through the open anal canal.
e.   Make an enterotomy at the apex of the **J** pouch and construct the ileoanal anastomosis using interrupted Vicryl sutures.
f.   Pass a stapler into the open ileoanal anastomosis, firing across the open proximal limb and the distal blind limb to create the reservoir.

44. Complications

John J. Meehan, M.D.

Most complications occur as a result of the operation itself and are independent of the decision to perform a procedure with a minimally invasive approach. However, a number of complications are specific to minimally invasive surgery and others may be at an increased risk. The complications discussed in this chapter are intended to highlight some of the issues surrounding minimally invasive surgery but are by no means complete.

A. General Complications

1. **Veress needle injuries.** If properly done, the Veress needle is a safe and effective method for starting a pneumoperitoneum. It also has the advantage of avoiding the annoying continual loss of pneumoperitoneum, which may occur from an open incision that was too generous. However, vascular and visceral injuries have occurred in all age groups as a result of Veress needle placement. Many surgeons have abandoned the Veress needle entirely and prefer to use an open technique with a Hasson trocar, a videoscopic trocar, or direct visualization. If a Veress needle is preferred, some guidelines should be followed:
   a. After making the skin incision, bluntly dissect the subcutaneous tissue away until the fascial layer is visualized.
   b. Using upward traction on the abdominal wall, a small nick in the fascia with an 11 blade or cautery will facilitate Veress needle placement without apply significant force.
   c. Once the needle is safely in the abdominal cavity, a "click" sound should be audible, indicating that the sharp needle tip has retracted and the blunt tip is now protruding from the tip of the device.
   d. Confirm location of the needle by sweeping the needle in a plane parallel to the operating room table. It should sweep around unimpeded and be easily visible distending the abdominal wall.
   e. A second confirmation test can be performed by injecting saline through the Veress needle port. It should flow easily without resistance. Keep the abdominal wall held upward under traction while doing this and then disconnect the syringe from port on the Veress needle. The remaining fluid in the Veress needle should fall into the abdomen, confirming proper location.

    f.   Careful inspection of the entire abdomen should be carried out once the telescope is inserted into the peritoneal cavity. Injuries should be treated immediately.

2.   Trocar site hernias

    a.   These complications may show up at any time following a laparoscopic case. Owing to the risk of incarceration, all trocar site hernias require repair.

    b.   This complication may be reduced by closing fascia on all incisions greater than 3 mm.

3.   Abdominal wall hemorrhage

    a.   This complication is rare in children. Most are self-limited and require no intervention. Occasionally, a trocar site will need to be reopened and the offending vessel ligated.

4.   Abdominal wall crepitus

    a.   This occurs as a result of leakage of carbon dioxide into the preperitoneal or subcutaneous space. It is often unduly alarming to families and requires no intervention. It should dissipate in 24 to 36 hours. If abdominal wall erythema and fever coincide with the crepitus, then the possibility of necrotizing fasciitis should be entertained and may require emergent resection and broad-spectrum antibiotics. Fortunately, this is exceedingly rare.

B. Complications of Specific Surgical Procedures

1.   Laparoscopic appendectomy

    a.   **Wound infection.** Even in open operations, wound infections are less common in children than in adults following appendectomy. However, wound infections still occur and may require reopening the incision. Antibiotics may be necessary if cellulitis develops, but simply opening the wound usually suffices. Extracting the specimen in a retrieval may reduce, but certainly will not eliminate, this potential complication.

    b.   **Intra-abdominal abscess.** This can occur in either open or laparoscopic appendectomy. It is markedly more common in perforated appendicitis than nonperforated, but either is possible. Patients present with an ileus, fever, diarrhea, constipation, or continued vomiting. A computed tomography (CT) scan is the best method for evaluating this but is of little value until at least 5 to 7 days following the initial procedure. Small collections usually disappear with continued antibiotic coverage. Large collections can be handled with percutaneous drainage under ultrasound or CT guidance. Reexploration is rarely required. The risk of abscess formation may be reduced by copious irrigation and suctioning during the initial procedure but can still occur despite all the most aggressive efforts.

    c.   **Appendiceal stump leak.** This complication usually presents similar to an abscess. Signs pointing to a leak over an abscess include a fistula that has developed through a trocar site or fecal material that is returned during an attempted percutaneous drainage of a fluid collection that was erroneously thought to be a simple abscess. Although exploration and closure of the appendiceal stump can be accomplished laparoscopically, the approach is best determined on a case-by-case basis. The cause of this complication is often unknown, and it is rare if a stapler is used. It may be related to an improperly secured endoloop. However, if the ligation of the appendiceal stump is performed on an area with questionable viability, then the selection of an endoloop or a stapler is irrelevant and a leak is at high risk for occurring. Placing two endoloops on the proximal stump may help reduce the risk of this complication.

2. Cholecystecomy
   Bile duct injury. The common bile duct could be injured in either a child or an adult in a similar manner. Careful identification of all pertinent structures will reduce this complication. Primary repair may be acceptable with a small incomplete injury. A Roux-en-Y choledochojejunostomy via an open technique is recommended for transaction or significant injury. Keep in mind that a child's bile duct may be too small for a **T**-tube.

3. Splenectomy
   a. **Bleeding.** Bleeding may occur from a number of sources including the splenic artery, splenic vein, or short gastrics. Exploration to determine the cause is required if significant postoperative bleeding is suspected.
   b. **Retained accessory spleen.** A surgeon should explore the left upper quadrant and omentum to search for any accessory spleens in the same manner as an open procedure. All accessory spleens should be removed at the initial operation. Missing an accessory spleen will often require reexploration.
   c. **Pancreatic injury.** Identification of the tail of the pancreas is obvious in some cases and difficult in others. The pancreas can be injured during dissection or ligation of the splenic vessels. Stapling across the tail of the pancreas should be sufficient to repair most injuries. A drain may be required.
   d. **Gastric injury.** This injury may occur during cauterization of the short gastrics. Recognition at the time of the initial procedure is important and primary repair will often suffice. This can be accomplished by simply oversewing the injury. Post operatively, sepsis or large volumes of free intra-abdominal air may point to this complication if it was not recognized during the initial procedure. If necessary, an upper gastrointestinal (GI) series with Gastrografin will confirm the injury. Exploration is warranted.
   e. **Colon injury.** Similar to a gastric injury, primary repair of a colon injury will suffice if this occurs. Contamination can be handled with irrigation and suction. A colostomy should be considered if contamination or injury is extensive.

f. **Inability to retrieve the specimen**. Surgeons often find that the most difficult part of a laparoscopic splenectomy is removing the specimen. Morcellating the specimen can be tedious, and the bag may rip. Options include retrieving the specimen through an extended trocar incision or dividing the specimen in pieces in the right upper quadrant. Irrigation of the right upper quadrant is important if any splenic elements are spilled during the attempted removal.

g. **Postsplenectomy sepsis**. This overwhelming and potentially fatal complication is more likely to occur in younger patients, particularly those less than 5 years of age. Patients present with a rapid onset of fever and full-blown sepsis. Broad-spectrum antibiotics and fluid resuscitation should be started immediately. Preoperative immunizations for pneumoccocus and *Haemophilus influenzae* should be given whenever possible and soon following surgery if it cannot be given ahead of time. These vaccinations have been instrumental in markedly reducing this complication. Daily prophylactic penicillin should also be given for young patients until the age of 18.

h. **Shoulder pain**. This is uncommon in children and usually represents diaphragmatic irritation. Occasionally, a fluid collection and abscess may be the cause. A fever will often accompany the latter. Most of these symptoms resolve within a few days. Investigation via CT scan is indicated if the problem persists or worsens.

4. Pyloromyotomy

a. **Mucosal tear**. This complication is more likely to occur near the pyloroduodenal junction from a myotomy that was carried too far distally. If suspected, the anesthetist can insufflate air through an orogastric tube and the surgeon can inspect the myotomy for bubbling. Repair should then be performed with a Vicryl suture and omentum tacked over the injury. Complete closure of the entire myotomy may be necessary if the injury is large. In this case, a second myotomy 90 to 180 degrees away from the first will be required. This may be difficult to reach laparoscopically and opening may be required.

b. **Inadequate pyloromyotomy.** Postoperatively, many infants with hypertrophic pyloric stenosis continue to vomit even if the pyloromyotomy was done properly. Swelling at the pylorus may have a role. We do not routinely investigate continued vomiting in the first 48 hours following a pyloromyotomy. However, patients with persistent vomiting should undergo an upper GI series to determine the potential cause. An inadequate pyloromyotomy will require reoperation. Prevention can be achieved by assuring independent movement of the two halves of the pylorus during the initial surgery.

5. Fundoplication

a. **Gastric volvulus.** This can occur from a gastrostomy placed too close to the pylorus. Patients will present with gastric distention and shock. This requires fluid resuscitation, antibiotics, and emergent exploration. The stomach should be detorsed and the gastrostomy site relocated.

b. **Esophageal tear.** This may occur from either a bougie that is too large or from overdissection at the hiatus.

c. **Slipped wrap.** This complication may occur from many possibilities including overdissection of the hiatus, wrap breakdown, and poor healing. Recurrent reflux, obstruction, pain or any combination of these symptoms may occur and reexploration is often necessary.

d. **Gas-bloat syndrome.** Many patients who require a fundoplication are aerophagic. Significant volumes of air may be swallowed with no release of the gastric air volume. Usually this problem is self-limited. This can be overcome by "burping" the stomach by venting a gastrostomy tube if present. If a gastrostomy tube is not present, one can be placed later if this continues to be a severe problem. Another cause may be related to poor gastric emptying, and this should be investigated with a radionuclide gastric emptying study. Pyloromyotomy may be required for patients with delayed gastric emptying.

6. Undescended testicle

   Atrophic testis. The risk of a testis degenerating after vessel ligation is well known regardless of the approach. An orchiectomy may be required if the testicle has completely degenerated.

7. Contralateral hernia exploration

   Hernia sac tearing. Care should be taken when placing or removing the trocar through the ipsilateral hernia sac to explore the contralateral side. When the inspection is complete, close inspection should identify any injury. Pursestring closure of the hernia sac proximal to the tear should be performed.

8. Ovarian cystectomy

   a. **Bleeding.** Although rare, bleeding may require exploration and cauterization.

   b. **Postoperative torsion.** This complication is rare but should be suspected in anyone with persistent lower abdominal pain. Ultrasound with Doppler will confirm the diagnosis and exploration can be done laparoscopically.

9. Meckel's resection

   a. **Leak.** A leak should be handled like all other intestinal leaks, and exploration will usually be required.

   b. **Obstruction.** Improper closure or simple adhesions may cause a bowel obstruction. Conservative measures with a nasogastric tube and fasting the patient are acceptable to see whether a partial obstruction will resolve on its own. Many will require eventual exploration.

10. Pull-through procedures

    a. **Enterocolitis.** Enterocolitis is a common pre- and postoperative problem for children with Hirschsprung's disease. An appropriate pull-through will certainly markedly reduce—but not eliminate—the risk of enterocolitis. The difficult chore of the surgeon is to determine the cause of the underlying postoperative illness. Enterocolitis, anastomotic stricture, ischemic bowel, cuff abscess or stricture, and simple gastroenteritis may all appear with similar symptoms. Abdominal distention, fever, sepsis, and inability to pass stool are more indicative of enterocolitis. Explosive passage of stool is often found on rectal examination. Rectal irrigations up to 3 or 4 times a day will improve these patients dramatically. Antibiotic coverage is recommended until normal bowel diameter is reestablished on plain film.

b. **Ischemic bowel.** Other symptoms may point to bowel ischemia. This may occur from excessive tension on pull-through or over-mobilization of the mesentery. These patients can present with a wide variety of symptoms including diarrhea, bloody stool, or overt sepsis. If the symptoms are mild, a colonoscopy can be performed to evaluate the mucosa of the pull-through segment. Patients who present with severe symptoms may have a necrotic section and will require exploration.

c. **Anastomotic stricture.** These patients present with symptoms similar to enterocolitis but are usually not as sick. The diagnosis is usually obvious on rectal examination and dilatation with Hegar dilators (to about 12 or 13 for infants) is usually sufficient. Rectal dilatations can be performed by the family at home for several weeks if necessary.

d. **Cuff abscess/cuff stricture.** The cuff created during a Soave endorectal pull-through should be divided at the time of the initial operation to avoid this complication from occurring. Abscesses can be drained transrectally or percutaneously.

45. Pediatric Thoracoscopy

John J. Meehan, M.D.

A. Empyema

Thoracoscopy has dramatically changed our treatment of empyema in the past 10 years. Children seemingly languished in hospitals for weeks while trying to recover from pneumonias that were complicated by an empyema. The previous strategy of waiting to see whether these fluid collections would resolve, reserving operations for only the worst collections, has been replaced with early intervention and drainage at the first sign of collection.

The pleural fluid that develops from a parapneumonic process is thin early and becomes more viscous with each passing day. Chest-tube or catheter drainage is often ineffective. Since the size of the incision for a 3- or 5-mm scope is no larger than a chest-tube incision, thoracoscopy with irrigation and drainage is a very effective way of reexpanding a trapped lung.

1. Single-lung ventilation is usually not necessary, as a carbon dioxide (CO_2) insufflation pressure of just 5 to 8 cm is adequate to keep the lung down for adequate visualization.
2. Place the first trocar along the midaxillary line, usually through the fifth or sixth intercostal space.
3. If the fluid is very thin with no significant loculations, irrigation and drainage may be accomplished through the same trocar by removing the camera and inserting a suction-irrigator.
4. When loculations are thick, we prefer to use at least two trocars. Additional trocars can be placed two to three rib spaces away from the camera.
    a. Although it is important to break down as many loculations as possible, it is not usually necessary to peel off all the fibropurlent material on the chest wall or pleural surface.
    b. Copious irrigation and drainage usually suffice for complete lung reexpansion once the adhesions have been taken down completely, and the majority of the rind can be left behind.
    c. Excessive rind removal may lead to an air leak from the lung.
5. Leave a small chest tube in place postoperatively through one of the trocar sites. Usually, suction for 24 hours followed by another 24 hours on water seal is all that is required. Removal of the tube after this point is usually safe, and recurrences are rare.

B. Lung Biopsy

Thoracoscopic lung biopsy can be accomplished for lesions in the periphery of the lung. Central lesions usually require needle biopsy guided by computed tomography.

1. With the patient in a decubitus position, place a trocar along the mid-axillary line in the fifth or sixth intercostal space.
2. Insufflation of the chest to a pressure of 5 to 8 cm negates the need for single-lung ventilation.
3. Depending on the location of the lesion, place a second port for grasping and a third port, usually 10 mm in size, for the stapling device and to allow retrieval of the specimen.
4. It is important to plan this port site far enough away from the lesion to allow for the stapler to open adequately, as well as for articulation if such a stapler is being used. Several firings of the stapler are often required, and a vascular-loaded stapler is preferable, since a better seal is formed.
5. A chest tube is left in place through a selected trocar site.

C. Repair of Tracheoesophageal Fistula

Several surgeons have ventured into repair of a tracheoesophageal fistula using a minimally invasive approach. The initial results are too preliminary to permit one to arrive at any conclusions, but the prospects have potential. Since the anatomy can be quite variable, we strongly recommend an echocardiogram and bronchoscopy prior to exploration. We will describe repair of the most common of these anomalies, the proximal esophageal atresia with distal tracheoesophageal fistula.

1. The trocar placement is shown in Figure 45.1, and a transpleural approach is required.
2. After the pleura has been incised, the azygos vein is dissected and ligated with a sealant device such as a Liga-Sure. Clips can be used as an alternative.
3. Once the azygos vein has been divided and is out of the way, dissection of the mediastinum will demonstrate the proximal esophagus, the distal esophagus, the trachea, and the fistula.
4. Division of the fistula should be accomplished in a piecemeal fashion to minimize the leak from the trachea is limited. Closure of the trachea is accomplished with polydioxanone or Vicryl sutures in an interrupted fashion with each successive division of the fistula until the division of the fistula is complete and the closure of the trachea secure.
5. Mobilize the distal and proximal esophagus as far as necessary to create an anastomosis. Traction sutures may be necessary on the tip of either of these structures to help facilitate the mobilization.
6. Once adequate mobilization has been achieved, perform an interrupted anastomosis with 5-0 suture.

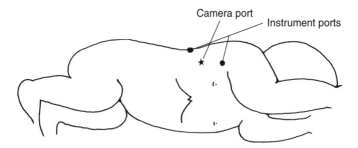

Figure 45.1. Patient position and trocar placement for repair of tracheoesophageal fistula.

    a.   Each suture must include mucosa to avoid stricture.
    b.   The first suture may not bring the two ends together adequately, but this will be overcome with subsequent suture placement.
    c.   The repair should be performed in an interrupted fashion.
    d.   Place the knots on the inside of the lumen for the back row.
    e.   Have the anesthesiogist gently slide a feeding tube or nasogastric tube past the completed back row of the anastomosis and down into the distal esophagus. The surgeon may have to help guide the tube with a grasper.
    f.   Complete the front row of sutures over the tube with the knots on the outside of the esophagus.
  7. A chest tube is probably more important in this technique (compared with the open technique), since the approach is transpleural.
  8. A swallowing study is preferred about 5 to 7 days postoperatively, and the chest tube can be removed once there is no evidence of a leak.

D. Repair of Congenital Diaphragmatic Hernia

A congenital diaphragmatic hernia (CDH) can be repaired either thoracoscopically or laparoscopically. The world experience with these two techniques is also rather untested, and it is too early to say which way, if either, is better.

The proponents of the thoracoscopic technique claim the visualization is better. This is probably true, since you are clearing the viscera from view when approaching from the chest instead of pulling it into the field, as occurs when you approach from the abdomen. However, the closure of the defect is a little more difficult when approached from the chest, since the rigid chest wall may not allow for a good angle for intracorporeal suturing along the most posterior and lateral edge, the location where almost no diaphragm is present and where recurrences are invariably found.

Patient selection may have a large impact on the success rate for these techniques. **Currently, we do not recommend using either of these techniques for** neonates who are on extracorporeal membrane oxygenation or who are marginal on ventilators in the neonatal intensive care unit. The insufflation of CO_2 in the chest or abdomen may further compromise an already tenuous patient, and a lengthy minimally invasive procedure may not be in the best interest of the patient unless he or she is stable from a cardiopulmonary standpoint.

1. **Laparoscopic CDH repair**
    a. Position the patient in a 45- to 90-degree lateral decubitus position with the head of the bed raised to allow for the viscera to fall out of view.
    b. Trocar placement is similar to a laparoscopic splenectomy, and three trocars may be all that is required.
    c. A fourth trocar may be necessary for retraction if the bowel or spleen is in the way.
    d. Use atraumatic graspers to gently reduce the viscera back into the abdomen. If the spleen is herniated into the chest, reduce it by grasping attachments near the hilum without grasping the hilar vessels themselves. When the inferior pole of the spleen comes into the abdomen, the rest usually slips in with gentle traction.
    e. See item 2 for repair.

2. **Thoracoscopic CDH repair**
    a. This is our preferred approach. Reduction of the viscera is easily accomplished using this method, and the visualization is excellent.
    b. It is very important to be sure the working trocars are placed relatively close to the defect; otherwise suturing on the most lateral aspect will be quite difficult.
    c. Allowing just the tip of the trocar inside the chest cavity will buy you a little more working room for needle drivers.
    d. Close the defect with horizontal mattress or even simple sutures.
    e. Patch closure has also been accomplished by some institutions using prosthetic material. The material is brought in through a 5-mm trocar, unrolled, and sewn in place in an interrupted fashion.

E. Pulmonary Sequestration

Extralobar sequestrations are easily removed thoracoscopically. These may be associated with a CDH and almost invariably have a single pedicle that needs to be ligated.

1. Place the patient in a lateral decubitus position.
2. Place the first trocar in the sixth intercostal space along the midaxillary line.
3. Secondary trocars are placed slightly inferior and 4 cm anteriorly and posteriorly from the camera port.

4. Carefully grasp the sequestration through one port and ligate the aberrant vessels with either a clip applier or pretied ligature. We recommend the use of two clips or ties on the patient side, since this vessel comes directly from the aorta.
5. Divide the vessel and remove the specimen through one of the trocar sites. It may be necessary to slightly extend the trocar site to accomplish this.

46. Pediatric Robotic Surgery

John J. Meehan, M.D.

Robotic surgery facilitates safe performance of minimally invasive procedures in children, as in adults, by providing wrist articulation and three-dimensional vision, and by negating tremors.

Several operations, such as cholecystectomies, fundoplications, and splenectomies, have already been reported in children by many institutions. Pediatric surgeons at the University of Iowa have performed more advanced procedures such as adrenalectomies, colon and small bowel resections, and total proctocolectomies. The complexity of cases is rapidly growing as more centers are adding these devices to their surgical suites. Table 46.1 shows the procedures performed at the University of Iowa using robotic technology.

A. Equipment

Initially, two major companies produced robotic devices. The Zeus system, produced by Computer Motion, which had the advantage of much smaller instruments and easier access to the patient while the case was proceeding, was particularly useful for pediatric surgeons. However, the Da Vinci system, produced by Intuitive Surgical, had the advantage of better optics and a user-friendly interface that more closely mimicked the movements of open surgery. In the summer of 2003, Intuitive Surgical and Computer Motion merged and combined their technologies. The newly formed company is supporting both systems, and the pooling of resources is expected to have a positive impact on development as well as support of the equipment these two companies had been making separately.

B. Advantages of Robotic Surgery

Robotic surgery provides several specific advantages over conventional laparoscopic and thoracoscopic surgery.

1. Robotic surgery adds **wrist articulation**. The biggest limitation to laparoscopic and thoracoscopic surgery has been the inability to perform complex maneuvers with the basic instruments currently available. Nevertheless, many surgeons have become quite good at performing complex procedures. Adding wrist action can make a huge impact on the ability to perform more complex tasks. By simply adding a wrist to the instrument, dissecting around structures becomes much easier. Suturing and tying knots become similar to

Table 46.1. Pediatric robotic procedures performed at the University of Iowa.

Cholecystectomy
Fundoplication
Heller myotomy
Paraesophageal hernia repair
Meckel's resection
Hemicolectomy
Total proctocolectomy with pull-through
Ladd's procedure
Mesenteric cyst excision
Adrenalectomy
Splenectomy
Neuroblastoma resection
Kasai portoenterostomy
Ovarian teratoma excision
Ovarian cystectomy
Partial lung resection
Mediastinal mass resection
Chest wall mass resection
Abdominal mass resection

instrument tying during an open technique. These advances have made robotic surgery a valuable tool in surgical applications.

2. Second, the stereoimaging camera system recreates a **three-dimensional visual field** that regains the depth perception lost in standard laparoscopy.

3. The surgeon has **complete control of camera placement and movement** during a case, and no additional assistant or scrub nurse is required for the camera movement.

4. **Tremors** from instrument movement—which none of us admit that we have but all of us do—**can also be eliminated**, as this type of random rapid movement is not translated from the robotic controls down to the instrument arms.

C. Limitations

The biggest limitation of robotic devices is the obvious matter of cost. In today's healthcare environment, with limited resources, the high price tag of the equipment and replacement instruments will limit their use. As with many other new technologies, however, the price of these devices should fall as new competitors emerge and production increases. Other specific limitations include the following.

1. **Lack of tactile feedback.** It is often stated that the surgeons' best eyes are their hands. Admittedly, even laparoscopic surgery markedly reduces this valuable information during a case. With the current robotic instruments, no tactile feedback is available whatsoever. Surgeons must rely on visual clues from the image display to appreciate the strength at which they are holding tissue or tying knots. Suturing, although much easier technically, can actually be frustrating when the suture breaks from too much tension applied during knot tying. These obstacles can be overcome with practice.

2. **Static, focused field.** In conventional laparoscopic surgery, the camera can be moved from port to port to get better visualization of a structure. The camera is designed to be inserted only through the center arm and cannot be moved to another port. In addition, once the robot has been docked to the trocars, the patient's bed cannot be moved. If the position is inadequate, the robot must be undocked from the trocars and the patient or table repositioned before the robot can be redocked to the trocars.

3. **Relatively large instruments and cameras.** The smallest Da Vinci instruments available were 8 mm until just recently. The 5-mm instruments now available have seen limited use to date, however. An assistant must take instrument changes. This takes a few moments and can slow the tempo of a case. The 12-mm Da Vinci camera offers excellent optics, but its huge size make it difficult to use in smaller patients. A new 5-mm two-dimensional robotic scope has recently become available.

4. **Robot size.** The Da Vinci, for example, is about 6 feet in height and takes up an enormous amount of space. The robot can dwarf even adult patients, and access for small patients, particularly neonates, can be difficult during a case. This is problematic for the surgeon, the assistant, as well as the anesthesiologist. Careful planning with the entire team with regard to robot location, operating table location, and patient positioning is crucial before bringing the patient into the operating room. Most importantly, all team members need to be flexible and ready to make adjustments when positioning the patient.

D. The Future

Despite the limitations of robotic surgery, this advanced technology is quickly becoming more and more useful in minimally invasive surgery. The variety of available instruments should expand as the diameter of the instruments decreases. Today's bulky machines will almost certainly become smaller and smaller as engineers design new and exciting ways to recreate complex maneuvers with robotic surgical technology.

Other advances such as instrument change on command features and the ability to change the camera from port to port are on the wish list of many surgeons who use robotic surgery. As more companies design equipment and more hospitals purchase the devices, the cost of surgical robots should decrease. This would allow more adult and pediatric surgeons to use this technology to treat their patients with minimally invasive techniques that otherwise seemed too cumbersome for standard laparoscopic instruments.

Part 2 Flexible Endoscopy

Flexible Endoscopy
I—General Principles

47. Flexible Endoscopes: Characteristics, Troubleshooting, and Equipment Care

Bipan Chand, M.D.
Jeffrey L. Ponsky, M.D., F.A.C.S.
Carol E.H. Scott-Conner, M.D., F.A.C.S.

A. Characteristics of Flexible Endoscopes

Flexible endoscopy provided a quantum leap in the area of diagnosis and therapy of the aerodigestive tract.

1. **Optical properties.** Two types of flexible endoscope are currently in use, and they transmit the image differently.

   a. **Fiberoptic endoscopes** are based upon fiberoptic light transmission technology. Light is conveyed through a bundle of fine glass fibers, each smaller than a human hair (60–70 μm in diameter), packed tightly together.

      i. Each individual fiber is clad in a wrapping of greater optical density, creating a reflective layer that causes light to bounce back and forth within the fiber with little loss of light. This cladding does not transmit light itself, creating a dark rim around the portion of the image produced by each fiber and accounting for the characteristic newsprint like image produced by fiberoptic endoscopes (Fig. 47.1).

      ii. Thousands of fibers are packed tightly together in a bundle, each carrying a small parcel of light to or from a portion of the viewing area.

      iii. One bundle of fibers carries light into the examined organ, and a second bundle transmits the image from the organ interior to the viewing optic.

      iv. The latter bundle must have all the fibers arranged in a "coherent bundle" (i.e., in the same spatial arrangement at both ends of the fiber, causing the portion of the total image that each carried to be in its proper position).

      v. Major disadvantages with flexible fiberoptic endoscopes include fragility. When individual fibers break, light transmission is decreased and the visual image develops dark spots (corresponding to the broken fibers).

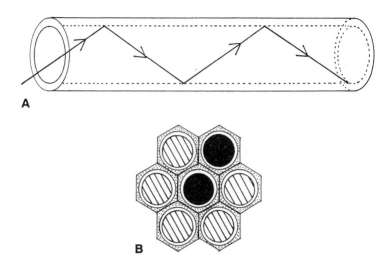

Figure 47.1. A. Internal reflection is assured by cladding each fiber with a coating of high refractive index. Virtually all light is reflected back and forth within the fiber with little loss. B. The image produced by a fiberoptic endoscope is composed of a multitude of images transmitted by each individual fiber. Broken fibers do not transmit light, resulting in black dropouts in the image.

    vi. These endoscopes are generally direct-viewing endoscopes; therefore the endoscopist looks directly into an eyepiece. An optical beam splitter allows a second observer to view the image. Alternatively, a small video camera may be placed on the end of the endoscope and the image viewed on a video screen. The addition of sidearms and external video screens introduces optical interference, which reduces visual clarity.

  b. **Videoendoscopy** applies video technology to endoscopy, with significant improvements in image quality and endoscope durability. An increasing number of the endoscopes in use today are videoendoscopes.

    i. Light is transmitted to the tip of the endoscope through a fiberoptic bundle, as in the endoscopes described earlier.

    ii. However, the viewing fiberoptic bundle is replaced with a charge-coupled device (CCD) chip camera, placed at the tip of the endoscope. This chip carries a digital image back to a video processor, which displays an image on a color monitor.

    iii. The CCD chip camera uses a dense grid of photocell receptors, each of which generates a single pixel on the monitor. Resolution depends on the density of receptor packing on the chip camera.

  iv. Some videoendoscopes use a single color (e.g., black-white) CCD chip and create color images by rapidly cycling through a color wheel. Newer videoendoscopes use three-color CCD chips and provide the most accurate color resolution.

  v. Most videoendoscopes incorporate an automatic iris in the system to decrease the problem of glare due to tissue reflection.

  vi. Videoendoscopes have the advantage of allowing the entire personnel to view the field. The CCD chip also allows for smaller scope diameters to transmit the same quality image.

2. **Channels.** Flexible endoscopes provide one or more instrument channels (2–3 mm) for passage of diagnostic and therapeutic instruments as well as for suctioning. Air and water insufflation channels permit distention of the bowel and cleaning of the lens.

3. **Instrument tip control.** Tip deflection is controlled by rotating wheels on the headpiece. The larger wheel allows for 12 and 6 o'clock manipulation, while the smaller wheel allows for 3 and 9 o'clock maneuvering. The shaft of the instrument may also be torqued in a clockwise or counter-clockwise manner to change direction. Locks are provided, but for most purposes, the wheels should be allowed to move freely (Fig. 47.2).

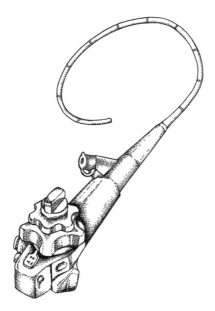

Figure 47.2. Rotating wheels on the headpiece of the endoscope control tip deflection. Instruments may be passed through an access port, which is kept capped when not in use (to prevent loss of insufflation and splashing of fluids).

4. **Illumination and image capturing.** Illumination is provided by an external source, either a xenon arc or a halogen-filled tungsten filament lamp. Modern endoscopes also include electronic systems to capture still images and record video footage.

B. Equipment Setup

The equipment for flexible endoscopy is generally arranged on a multiple-level cart, which allows access to all the equipment and easy mobility. The cart generally includes a monitor, video processor, light source, water bottle, and image printer (Fig. 47.3).

1. A fiberoptic cable connects the endoscope to the light source. This umbilical cable also contains connectors for suction, water, and air insufflation.
2. Air and water are introduced through a common channel by depression of a trumpetlike valve on the control head of the scope.
   a. Partial depression of the valve insufflates air and distends the viewed lumen.
   b. Complete depression of the valve forces air backward into the attached water bottle, forcing a stream of water to the tip of the instrument. This washes the lens.
   c. Depression of an adjacent trumpet valve enables suctioning of air or fluid at the tip of the instrument.
   d. Insufflation, irrigation, and suction should be tested prior to each use of the endoscope.
3. Common problems include sticky valves, lack of water in the water bottle, failure to secure all connections, or leaks in the valve apparatus.
4. To avoid pitfalls during the procedure, become well versed in the construction and function of the particular endoscopic system in use. All endoscopes are not constructed in the same manner. Accurate assessment of problems arising during a procedure often allows rapid resolution.
5. Adopt a standard approach to equipment setup. Problems commonly arise when one or another step is forgotten.
   a. Choose the appropriate size (length and diameter) and type of endoscope for the intended purpose. Both pediatric and adult upper gastrointestinal endoscopes are available.
   b. Connect the umbilical cable of the endoscope to the light source.
   c. Turn on all electronic equipment on the cart, even if use of a particular item (e.g., videocasette recorder) is not planned. The connections of the various pieces of equipment may require that all be on for any to work properly.
   d. Ensure that the water bottle is filled with clean water.
   e. Connect the hose from the water bottle to the side of the umbilical cable, near where it enters the light box. Generally the fittings are

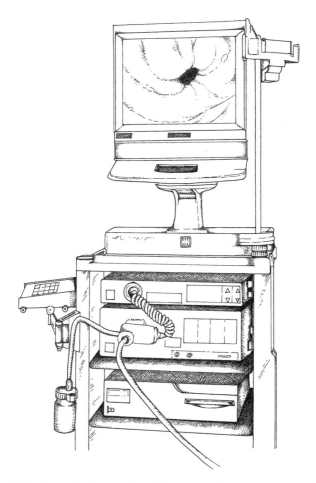

Figure 47.3. Cart with video monitor, light source, video processor, water bottle, and image printer. A keyboard allows entry of patient and physician names, patient number, date, and any additional documentation desired.

        arranged with a Luer-Lok or other mating set of connectors, so that the hose can only connect to one place.

f.   Connect suction to the remaining site on the umbilical cord.

g.   Obtain a cup or basin of water and test insufflation (by insufflation of air under water and observing bubbles), water irrigation (with the tip of the endoscope out of the water), and suction (by aspirating the water from the cup). If any of these functions are sluggish or nonfunctional, first check the connections. (See Section C, Troubleshooting, for additional tips.)

     h.   Take the light source off standby and aim the tip of the endoscope into the cupped fingers of one hand. A sharp image of the fingers should be seen on the monitor.

     i.   Check the tip deflection controls and verify that any locking devices are "off" so that the tip is free to move.

     j.   Verify that any additional items that may be required (such as biopsy forceps, polypectomy snares) are available, of appropriate size, and in good working order.

C. Troubleshooting

A systematic approach to identifying the problem, followed by creative measures to circumvent or repair the difficulty, will usually permit satisfactory completion of the examination. As mentioned previously, attention to detail during the setup phase can help minimize problems during the examination. Common problems and solutions are listed in Table 47.1.

Table 47.1. Common problems with flexible endoscopes and suggested solutions.

Problem	Check the following
No light at distal end	1. Light source plugged in and turned on
	2. Light source ignited
	3. Not in "standby" mode
	4. Lens at distal tip is dirty
	5. Bulb burned out
Out of focus	1. Adjust focus ring
	2. Fiberoptic scope—clean lens
No irrigation	1. Water bottle contains water
	2. Water bottle connected to umbilical cord
	3. Connection tight
	4. Lid of water bottle screwed on tightly
	5. Power turned on
	6. Valve stuck or occluded
No insufflation	1. Umbilical cord firmly seated into light source and screwed in if necessary
	2. Power turned on
	3. Valve stuck or occluded
Clogged valve or nozzle	1. Take valve apart and clean
	2. Flush channel of endoscope with cleaning solution, followed by clean water
Difficulty passing instrument	1. Check tip angulation; decrease angulation and try again
	2. Ensure that the instrument is fully closed
	3. Check size of instrument relative to instrument channel; try smaller diameter instrument

D. Equipment Care

Flexible endoscopes are expensive and relatively fragile. Attention to care is important.

1. The light fibers are fragile and easily broken. Coil the endoscope into gentle curves, rather than folding it in acute angles. Do not drop the endoscope, allow a wheeled cart to roll over it, or allow the patient to bite down on the endoscope.

2. Avoid extreme angulation of the tip wherever possible. Do not force biopsy forceps or other instruments down the channel when the tip is sharply angulated, as damage to the biopsy channel may result.

3. Ensure that polypectomy snares and sclerosing needles are fully withdrawn into the sheath before passing through the channel. Lubricate instruments with a suitable lubricant to facilitate passage.

4. The outer coating of the endoscope is delicate, particularly in the region near the tip. A rubber sheath, designed to flex as the tip bends, covers this region of the endoscope.

5. After each use, wash off any gross contamination and suction water through the endoscope. Do not allow blood, mucus, stool, or other foreign matter to dry on the endoscope or in the channels or valves.

6. Endoscopes are rarely actually sterilized. Generally high-level disinfection with a chemical agent (such as gluteraldehyde) is used. Disinfection does not work well when foreign matter (mucus, blood, enteric contents) are present. Therefore, the endoscope must be mechanically cleaned before disinfection. Many endoscopy suites use automated cleaners that rapidly wash, disinfect, and rinse the endoscope. Ultrasonic cleaners are available in some units.

7. Ethylene oxide gas sterilization is an option, but it requires an overnight cycle. Newer methods of sterilization and newer endoscopes that are more tolerant of sterilizing conditions are being developed. Be careful to follow the manufacturer's instructions for sterilization to avoid potentially severe damage to the endoscope.

E. Selected References

Bordelon BM, Hunter JG. Endoscopic technology. In: Greene FL, Ponsky JL, eds. Endoscopic Surgery. Philadelphia: WB Saunders, 1994;6–18.

Kawahara I, Ichikawa H. Fiberoptic instrument technology. In: Sivak MV, ed. Gastroenterologic Endoscopy. Philadelphia: WB Saunders, 1987;20–41.

48. Endoscope Handling

Bipan Chand, M.D.
Jeffrey L. Ponsky, M.D., F.A.C.S.

A. Room Setup

The endoscopy suite should have oxygen, suction, and monitoring devices. It should be sufficiently large to allow free movement around the gurney. Most endoscopic examinations are performed in rooms or suites specially designed for the purpose. Occasionally endoscopy is done at the bedside in the intensive care unit, in the operating room, or in some other location.

Take a few minutes to consider the room layout and the proposed endoscopic examination before bringing the patient into the room or setting up the equipment.

1. The nature of the examination influences patient position and room setup.
   a. For **upper gastrointestinal endoscopy**, the patient will be positioned with the left side slightly down. The endoscopist faces the patient; standing at the patient's left side near the head of the bed. This provides easy access to the mouth and oropharynx.
   b. For **colonoscopy or flexible sigmoidoscopy**, the patient is usually positioned in the left lateral decubitus position with the hips flexed and the knees brought up toward the chest. The endoscopist stands facing the back of the patient, just below the patient's buttocks. This generally puts the endoscopist on the opposite side of the gurney and requires an inverse room setup.
   c. If **both an upper gastrointestinal endoscopy and a colonoscopy**, or flexible sigmoidoscopy, are to be done on the same patient, it is often worthwhile to take the time to reverse the position of the patient (head to foot) on the gurney, or turn the gurney around, rather than deal with a less-than-optimal room setup for one of the two examinations.
2. The primary video monitor should be placed across from the endoscopist, in a direct line of sight. The endoscopy cart must be close to the intended working area. The majority of dedicated endoscopy suites have an additional screen behind the endoscopist for the assistant to view.

B. Manipulation of the Endoscope

Some endoscopists use both hands to manipulate the controls of the endoscope, and ask an assistant to advance and withdraw the endoscope. However,
significantly greater control can be attained if the endoscopist manipulates the
controls with the left hand and advances or withdraws the endoscope with the
right hand. This is the method described here. There are no left-handed endoscopes, and this method is used by both right- and left-handed endoscopists.
Specific techniques useful for performing various endoscopic examinations are
given in the sections that follow.

1. Stand in a comfortable position, facing the patient and the video
   monitor (Fig. 48.1).
2. If the endoscope is a direct-viewing fiberoptic endoscope, hold it
   comfortably up to your eye. Avoid a hunched-over posture, which
   contributes to back and neck strain. Always try to keep the shaft of
   the endoscope in a straight line.
3. Cradle the endoscope in the upper palm of the left hand. Rest the controls between the thumb and forefinger. Endoscopists with small hands
   will need to experiment to find a comfortable position that will allow
   access to all controls. The key is to keep the hand rotated so that the
   thumb can manipulate the control wheel.

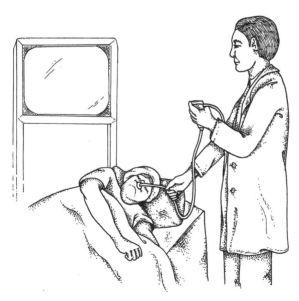

Figure 48.1. Stand comfortably, facing the patient and the video monitor. Generally the video monitor will be across the gurney from the endoscopist, directly
in the endoscopist's line of sight.

4. The index and long fingers work the two trumpet valves and thus control suction, insufflation, and cleaning of the lens. The ring and little fingers hold the control handle firmly against the palm.

5. The thumb of the left hand manipulates the large control wheel on the right side of the scope. This wheel anglaes the scope tip in an up or down direction.

6. The endoscopist's right hand works the small outer wheel, which controls right and left motion of the instrument tip. There are locking brakes associated with each control knob so that a position may be held while the hand is removed to perform another function.

7. While the control knobs provide motion at the tip of the endoscope, experienced endoscopists know that equal if not more vital directional control is provided by rotation and elevation of the scope's control head in concert with gentle torsion of the scope shaft. These often imperceptible maneuvers of the endoscopist occur throughout the procedure, and in combination with tip control allow complex manipulations to be performed. An accomplished endoscopist is rarely motionless during a procedure, but continually makes a complex "endoscopic dance."

8. Try to maintain the endoscope in a relatively straight or only slightly curved path. Minor deflections of the tip combined with gentle torsion and gentle advancing motions will allow the endoscope to traverse bends (Fig. 48.2). In contrast, sharply angulating the tip may prevent advancement and promote paradoxical tip motion (where the target actually gets farther away). Never use force to advance the endoscope.

C. Documentation of Findings

Early endoscopes provided visualization of the gastrointestinal tract but lacked the ability to record images for documentation or discussion. Cameras soon were developed that utilized film to record endoscopic images. Some models, such as the "gastrocamera," were designed specifically for this purpose and sacrificed visualization for the ability to record. These are primarily of historic interest.

Modern endoscopes enjoy the ability to record and document findings in a variety of formats. While cameras are still available for fixation to the viewing optic of fiberoptic systems, newer video endoscopes produce a digital signal that can be recorded on film, videotape, or computer disk. The images can then be incorporated into reports or teaching programs. With the digital format, large numbers of images can be stored in a small environment. Some problems have developed as individuals have attempted to transmit images across different systems. The electronic formats of all systems are not the same, and communication can be difficult. International standards for digital transmission of images are under development.

It is important that the practicing endoscopist record important findings to allow the entire healthcare team to appreciate the patient's pathology and to

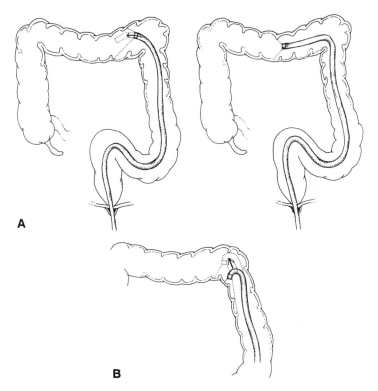

Figure 48.2. A. Minor tip deflection with gentle advancement and mild torsion allows the endoscope to traverse bends while maintaining a gentle curve. B. Sharp angulation of the tip (like a candy cane) hinders advancement and may result in paradoxical motion, where the target gets farther away rather than closer, or contribute to perforation.

permit comparison with subsequent (or previous) examinations. The simplest way to do this is to print an image for inclusion in the patient's medical record. Some endoscopy units keep separate files for teaching or research purposes. Many use specialized forms designed for each examination. Whatever system is employed, the record should be clear and easily interpretable.

D. Selected References

Cooper GS. Indications and contraindications for upper gastrointestinal endoscopy. Gastrointest Endosc Clin North Am 1994;4:439–454.

Jane PK. Technique of upper gastrointestinal endoscopy. Gastrointest Endosc Clin North Am 1994;4:501–521.

Mellinger JD, Ponsky JL. Endoscopic evaluation of the postoperative stomach. Gastrointest Endosc Clin North Am 1996;6:621–639.

Van Dam J, Chak A, Sivak MV. Technique of upper gastrointestinal endoscopy. In Gastroenterologic Endoscopy. Sivak MV ed., 2nd edition. Philadelphia: WB Saunders, 2000.

Van Dam J, Brugge WR. Endoscopy of the upper gastrointestinal tract. N Engl J Med 1999;341:1738–1748.

Lightdale CJ ed. Advances in endoscopic ultrasound. Gastrointest Endosc 2002;56: S1–S97.

Zaman A, Hahn M, Hapke R, Knigge K, Fennerty MB, Katon RM. A randomized trial of peroral versus transnasal unsedated endoscopy using an ultrathin videoendoscope. Gastrointest Endosc 1999; 49:279–284.

49. Monitoring, Sedation, and Recovery

Bipan Chand, M.D.
Jeffrey L. Ponsky, M.D., F.A.C.S.

A. Monitoring

Continuous patient assessment by a second trained individual is crucial and allows the endoscopist to concentrate on the examination. The levels of consciousness, responsiveness, and pain should be watched closely. The degree of sedation and analgesia represents a continuum from minimal sedation to general anesthesia. The amount of sedation to be achieved is individualized to the patient and the procedure to be performed. Moderate sedation and analgesia, also termed conscious sedation, are used for most patients undergoing upper and lower endoscopy. This level of sedation allows the patient to maintain his or her airway and still respond to verbal and physical stimulation. Deep sedation may require airway support and is usually used when one is performing longer or more invasive procedures. General anesthesia involves control of patient ventilation and may be used for pediatric patients or patients intolerant to deep sedation.

Most endoscopy units use a special form on which pulse, blood pressure, medications, and other measures can be recorded. Continuous monitoring of the following parameters is commonly used and generally recommended:

1. Pulse (usually by electrocardiograph)—rate and rhythm
2. Blood pressure (usually with periodic recordings)
3. Pulse oximetry

Even when conscious sedation is not used, bowel distention from insufflation may decrease ventilation. It is important to remember that oxygen saturation is not always an accurate reflection of ventilation, and depression of respiration with hypercapnea may occur despite adequate oxygen levels. Capnography is cumbersome and not readily available; hence, it is not currently the standard. All monitoring devices must be supplemented by constant nursing observation of the patient's ventilation, discomfort, and state of consciousness.

Because hypoxemia is common, many endoscopists routinely administer supplemental oxygen, via nasal cannula, during endoscopy and recovery. Care must be taken not to depress respiration if the patient suffers from chronic obstructive pulmonary disease.

Suction must be available, and resuscitation equipment should be conveniently located.

Monitoring must continue into the recovery phase (see Section C).

Table 49.1. Characteristics of conscious sedation.

Conscious sedation is a state of minimally depressed consciousness in which the patient:
- Retains protective airway reflexes
- Responds appropriately to physical stimuli and verbal commands
- Maintains continuous communication with caregivers

B. Sedation and Analgesia

Safe and effective administration of conscious sedation is as important as the endoscopy itself. While some endoscopic procedures can be performed without any sedation, most patients prefer to have intravenous sedation to facilitate the intervention. The characteristics of conscious sedation are enumerated in Table 49.1. Most agents used for conscious sedation also produce amnesia. This is regarded as desirable and facilitates patient acceptance of repeat examinations if necessary. The Joint Commission on Accreditation of Healthcare Organizations (JCAHO) regards sedation with certain medications, such as midazolam, to be anesthesia.

Table 49.2. Agents commonly used for conscious sedation during endoscopy.

Name of drug	Advantages	Disadvantages
Diazepam (Valium)	1. Reduces anxiety 2. Causes amnesia 3. Minimal cardiovascular effects 4. Relatively flat dose–response curve	1. Pain on injection 2. High incidence of chemical phlebitis
Midazolam (Versed)	1. More rapid onset 2. Less pain on injection 3. More amnesia	1. Significantly more potent, requiring dose adjustment 2. Avoid combination with narcotic agents
Propofol	1. Rapid onset 2. Fast recovery 3. Easily titratable 4. Deeper sedation	1. Minimal levels of analgesia 2. Cardiopulmonary depression
Fentanyl	1. Analgesic effect 2. Fast onset	1. Respiratory depression
Meperidine (Demerol)	1. Analgesic effect	1. Minimal amnesia 2. Cardiopulmonary depression

Prior to administering sedation for endoscopy, an intravenous line must be obtained. The intravenous line is used for administration of agents used for conscious sedation and is crucial if resuscitation is required. Agents commonly used for conscious sedation during endoscopy are listed in Table 49.2. A combination of sedative and analgesic are used in most patients. Deeper sedation has been performed using the agent propofol, which also has a faster onset and faster recovery. All of these agents can be administered by an endoscopist who is also certified for advanced cardiac life support.

C. Recovery

Monitoring (and recording information) should continue until the patient has fully recovered from the procedure. The benzodiazepine antagonist flumazenil has been used after endoscopy in an attempt to shorten recovery time. Flumazenil rapidly reverses the central effects of diazepam or midazolam but may not completely reverse the respiratory depression. Resedation may occur after 1 to 2 hours. Patients should be cautioned against driving and should be released into the care of a responsible accompanying person.

D. Selected References

Andrus CH, Dean PA, Ponsky JL. Evaluation of safe, effective intravenous sedation for utilization in endoscopic procedures. Surg Endosc 1990;4:179–183.

Arrowsmith JB, Gerstman BB, Fleischer DE, Benjamin SB. Results from the American Society for Gastrointestinal Endoscopy/US Food and Drug Administration collaborative study on complication rates and drug use during gastrointestinal endoscopy. Gastrointest Endosc 1991;37:421–427.

Bartelsman JFWM, Sars PRA, Tytgat GNJ. Flumazenil used for reversal of midazolam-induced sedation in endoscopy outpatients. Gastrointest Endosc 1990;36:S9–S12.

Council on Scientific Affairs, American Medical Association. The use of pulse oximetry during conscious sedation. JAMA 1993;270:1463–1468.

Holzman RS, Cullen DJ, Eichhorn JH, Philip JH. Guidelines for sedation by nonanesthesiologists during diagnostic and therapeutic procedures. J Clin Anesth 1994; 6:265–276.

Keeffe EB, O'Connor KW. 1989 A/S/G/E survey of endoscopic sedation and monitoring practices. Gastrointest Endosc 1990;36:S13–S18.

Lewis BS, Shlien RD, Wayne JD, Knight RJ, Aldoroty RA. Diazepam versus midazolam (Versed) in outpatient colonoscopy: a double-blind randomized study. Gastrointest Endosc 1989;35:33–36.

McCloy RF, Pearson RC. Which agent and how to deliver it? A review of benzodiazepine sedation and its reversal in endoscopy. Scand J Gastroenterol Suppl 1990;179:7–11.

Flexible Endoscopy
II—Upper Gastrointestinal Endoscopy

50. Diagnostic Upper Gastrointestinal Endoscopy

John D. Mellinger, M.D., F.A.C.S.

A. Indications

1. Diagnostic upper gastrointestinal endoscopy, or esophagogastroduodenoscopy (EGD), may be indicated for symptom evaluation, malignancy surveillance, and in several special circumstances (Table 50.1).
2. Therapeutic EGD is appropriate for acute upper gastrointestinal bleeding, foreign body ingestion, polyp removal, dilation of stenoses, placement of feeding or drainage catheters, eradication of esophageal varices, and palliative therapy of obstructing neoplasms (see Chapters 51–57).

B. Patient Preparation

1. Do not permit the patient to eat or drink for 6 to 8 hours before routine elective EGD. This minimizes aspiration risks associated with a sedated procedure and facilitates a complete and unhampered examination.
   a. Consider a **longer period of preparation** (NPO, and/or liquid diet) if gastric outlet obstruction or impaired gastric motility is anticipated.
   b. If retained ingested material, secretions, or blood are likely, consider **preprocedural gastric aspiration or lavage**.
2. **Obtain informed consent** for the procedure. This includes a discussion of specific complications as well as anticipated outcomes and their general frequency. Review alternative therapies, the information to be gained from the proposed study, and anticipated practical impact on the patient's care. If a new technique is likely to be employed, frank discussion of experience with the new method is in order.
3. Apply monitoring devices (see Chapter 49) and ensure that a secure intravenous line is in place. Use of ultrathin endoscopes (5-mm diameter), which may be passed transorally or transnasally, may facilitate performance without sedation and decrease or eliminate the need for advanced monitoring and intravenous access.
4. Have the patient **remove dentures**.

Table 50.1. Indications for EGD.

Indication	Specific examples
Symptoms	• Dyspepsia* • Dysphagia • Odynophagia • Pyrosis* • Nausea and vomiting
Malignancy surveillance	• Barrett's epithelium • Gastric polyps • Familiar polyposis syndromes • Gastric ulcer • Esophageal ulcer • Marginal (postgastrectomy) ulcer
Other circumstances	• Occult gastrointestinal bleeding • Cirrhosis (to evaluate varices) • Malabsorption (for small intestine biopsy)

*If persistent, recurrent despite medical management, or associated with other gastro-intestinal symptoms or signs such as weight loss.

5. **Topical anesthesia** is usually employed prior to EGD. Effective topical anesthesia facilitates intubation and comfort of the otherwise neurologically intact patient (especially when sedation is not employed) and may allow a smaller amount of sedation to be used.
    a. Deliver the topical agents to the posterior pharynx by spray or gargle, rather than to the oral cavity and tongue only.
    b. Topical anesthetics take a few minutes to work. Use this time to check the endoscope (see Chapter 47) and verify that all items that might be needed (such as biopsy forceps) are available.
    c. Test the patient's gag response before attempting endoscopy. This is a good indicator of patient tolerance.
    d. Several applications of topical anesthesia may be required.
    e. Topical agents are probably of marginal importance when deeper conscious sedation is required.

C. Performance of Diagnostic Upper Gastrointestinal Endoscopy: Normal Anatomy

1. Place the patient in the left lateral decubitus position with a pillow under the head.
2. Place a bite block between the teeth.
3. Lubricate the endoscope with water-soluble lubricant and hold it in front of the patient's mouth. The initial insertion is best done under visual guidance.

a. Hold the endoscope in the right hand, approximately 20 to 30 cm from the tip.

b. This facilitates passage through the upper esophageal sphincter without the need to release and regrasp the instrument. If the endoscope is held farther back, it may buckle.

c. Position the endoscope in front of the mouth in such a way that a simple deflection of the large (up/down) control wheel with the thumb of the left hand moves the tip to the desired curve (inferiorly in the axis of the patient's midline).

d. Rotate the instrument with the right hand to orient this downward deflection in the appropriate axis.

e. Next, straighten the instrument, pass it through the bite block, and insert it to the level of the posterior pharynx.

f. Maintain the endoscope in the midline of the pharynx, and deflect the tip inferiorly by repeating the maneuver as just rehearsed. Attention should now shift to the video monitor. The base of the tongue and epiglottis will be seen anteriorly.

g. Advance the endoscope slowly and smoothly to minimize gagging, using torque with the right hand to accomplish right/left movements and left thumb deflections to make anterior/posterior adjustments. Visualize the laryngeal cartilages and vocal cords, and advance the scope in the midline immediately posterior to the arytenoid cartilages (Fig. 50.1).

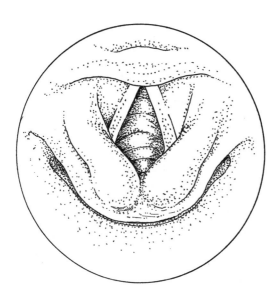

Figure 50.1. The esophageal opening is recognized as a simple slit at the base of the triangle formed by the glottis, just behind the arytenoid cartileges. The two piriform sinuses lie on each side of the esophageal opening.

h. Passage through the upper esophageal sphincter is facilitated by having the patient swallow, which relaxes the sphincter.
    i.   Often the simple presence of the instrument in this area will initiate a swallow and allow passage through the upper esophageal sphincter.
    ii. If the patient is not too deeply sedated, asking him or her to perform a swallow may achieve the same.
    iii. If gentle pressure in the appropriate midline position does not achieve the desired result, withdraw the scope and repeat the maneuver; lateral deflection into the piriform sinus area can easily occur and lead to injury if increasing pressure is applied.
i. Alternative techniques, such as placing two fingers in the patient's mouth to guide the endoscope and keep it in the midline, are especially useful for patients who are under anesthesia.
j. If an endotracheal tube is in place, it is crucial that someone hold the endotracheal tube to prevent accidental dislodgment. It may be necessary to deflate the balloon to allow the endoscope to pass.

4. Advance the endoscope slowly down the length of the esophagus, again using torque and limited deflection of the up/down control wheel to allow preservation of a luminal view at all times. Never advance the endoscope without a visible lumen (Fig. 50.2).

5. Watch for peristaltic activity, distensibility, and mucosal appearance. Measure the distance from the incisors to the squamocolumnar junction (where the white esophageal epithelium abruptly gives way to pink gastric mucosa). Identify the location of the diaphragm by asking the patient to sniff. Visible contraction of the diaphragm will produce extrinsic compression of the esophagus.

6. As soon as the endoscope enters the stomach, step back from the table and allow the instrument to assume an unrestrained, straightened posture. This is often best accomplished by completely letting go of the scope with the right hand as one steps back.

7. With the patient on the left side, this will typically orient the instrument in the stomach such that the greater curve will be at the 6 o'clock position, the lesser curve at 12 o'clock, and the anterior and posterior walls to the left and right, respectively (Fig. 50.3). Insufflate sufficient air to obtain a good view, and note rugal folds, peristaltic activity, and distensibility. Avoid overdistention, as this may trigger pylorospasm.

8. Continue to advance the endoscope down the length of the stomach, maintaining upward deflection of the tip in a gentle curve to preserve an antegrade view and hug the lesser curvature (Fig. 50.4).

9. Advance the endoscope to the pylorus and carefully note the pyloric channel and duodenal bulb. Often some of the best views of the bulb are achieved prior to pyloric intubation via such an antegrade view. Make very fine maneuvers of the deflection wheels to hold the

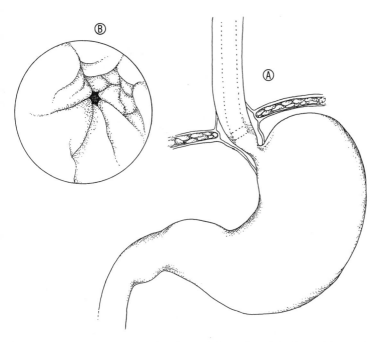

Figure 50.2. A. The endoscope is advanced down the relatively straight esophagus until the lower esophageal sphincter is identified. B. The lower esophageal sphincter often coincides with the transition from squamous epithelium (white) of the esophagus to mucosa (pink) of the stomach.

pylorus in the center of the visual field as gentle continued advancement of the scope allows it to pass into the proximal duodenum (Fig. 50.5).

10. Rarely, application of a brief period of suction will allow the pylorus to be drawn over the scope if it seems unwilling to otherwise admit the same, provided the suction is applied as the tip of the scope sits immediately in front of the opening of the pyloric channel.

11. Carefully visualize the duodenal bulb before advancing the instrument further. The posterior bulb is often the most challenging area to visualize well. Inspection of this area can be achieved by withdrawing the endoscope and using torque and fine deflections of the tip to achieve an adequate view (Fig. 50.6).

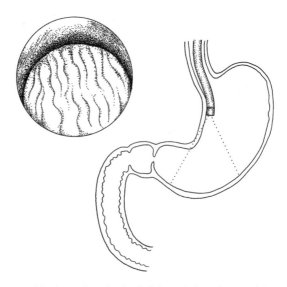

Figure 50.3. With the patient in the left lateral decubitus position, the endoscopist facing the patient, and the scope relaxed as described in the text, entry into the stomach will generally give a view oriented with the lesser curvature at 12 o'clock, the greater curvature at 6 o'clock, anterior at 9 o'clock, and posterior at 3 o'clock.

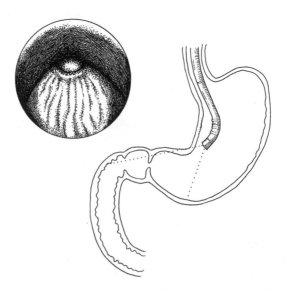

Figure 50.4. As the endoscope is advanced, the lumen is kept in view. A gentle upward deflection of the tip helps the endoscope hug the lesser curvature.

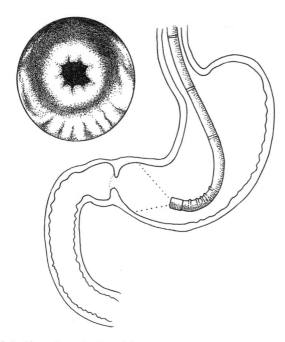

Figure 50.5. The pylorus is viewed from the gastric antrum. The endoscope is gently advanced while keeping the pylorus directly in the center of the visual field. Sometimes the pylorus will be observed to open and close. Position the endoscope ready to pass through the pylorus when it opens.

12. Advance the endoscope as far into the second portion of the duodenum as luminal visualization permits (Fig. 50.7).
   a. In some cases, full introduction into the second and third portion of the duodenum is easily achieved in this fashion.
   b. More commonly, the posterior sweep of the duodenum requires some further maneuvering. In such settings, the luminal view is lost as the duodenum turns posteriorly near the junction of its first and second portions.
   c. Deflect the tip of the instrument slightly upward with the left thumb on the larger control wheel and simultaneously rotate the left wrist 90 degrees clockwise. This is best accomplished with the right hand completely off the endoscope.
   d. Next, pull back on the endoscope to straighten it and achieve further advancement of the tip. This "paradoxic motion" occurs as the instrument moves from the looped, greater curvature position in the stomach (which usually follows initial antegrade intubation), to a lesser curve or "short stick" position.

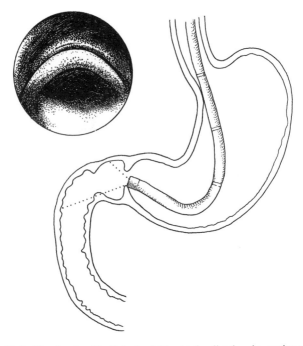

Figure 50.6. The duodenal bulb lacks folds. At the distal and superior aspect is the superior duodenal fold, which marks the entrance to the second portion of the duodenum.

    e.   Further antegrade intubation can also be accomplished after this maneuver, if deeper duodenal entry is desired.

13. As the endoscope is withdrawn, carefully inspect all areas.

14. Position the endoscope with its tip in the gastric antrum and retroflex it.

    a.   Deflect the tip of the instrument upward, using the left thumb on the larger control wheel, while simultaneously rotating the left wrist 90 degrees counterclockwise. Frequently an "owl's eye" view of both pylorus and cardia may be seen as the tip crosses the incisura to look directly back at the cardia (Fig. 50.8).

    b.   This maneuver is easily accomplished with the right hand off the endoscope.

    c.   Manipulate the endoscope with the right hand (torque, advancement, withdrawal) to obtain optimal visualization of the incisura, cardia, fundus, and remaining proximal stomach. Grasp the endoscope 10 to 20 cm from the patient's mouth to allow a wide range of movements to be done with fluid motions.

    d.   Often the "gastric lake" of dependent fundic fluid is seen from this vantage point, and should be suctioned to allow complete inspection. Suction of fluid is most efficient when the meniscus of the fluid surface is oriented transversely across the endoscopic field of visualization. In this position, the suction port (at 6 o'clock in the visual field) is located completely under the fluid, while a luminal view is preserved above the same. Short bursts of suction at a lower setting minimize capturing of the gastric mucosa in the port, which requires repositioning before continuing the suction process. By proceeding in this fashion, fluid evacuation can be accomplished efficiently while continuing dynamic inspection of the lumen.

15. Return the endoscope to its normal (straight, antegrade) position and gradually remove it, reinspecting all areas as the instrument is removed.

16. Suction excess air after the stomach is reinspected during withdrawal. Carefully inspect the esophagus, hypopharynx, and larynx during removal.

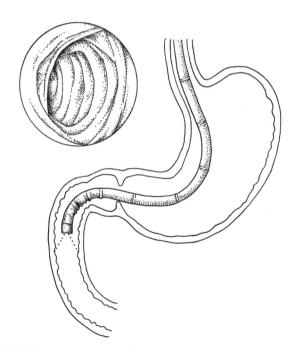

Figure 50.7. The second portion of the duodenum is recognized by its concentric semicircular folds.

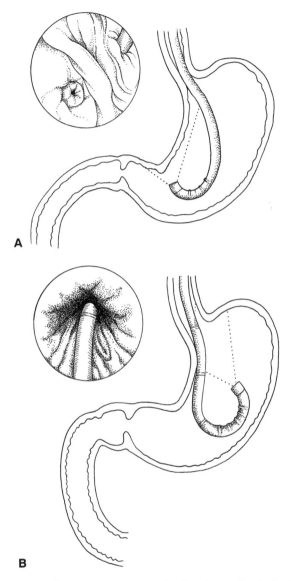

Figure 50.8. Retroflex the endoscope to visualize the cardia. A. Perform this maneuver by deflecting the tip sharply back. An owl's eye view of both pylorus and cardia may be seen as the tip crosses over the incisura. B. As the cardia is identified, move the tip in a circular manner to inspect the entire cardia. Pull the endoscope back to bring the tip (now sharply retroflexed) closer to the area of interest.

Table 50.2. Anatomic alterations associated with specific surgical interventions.

Disease category	Anatomic changes	Surgical procedures
Gastroesophageal reflux	• Augmentation of the cardia	• Fundoplication
Peptic ulcer disease	• Gastric outlet alteration • Partial absence of stomach	• Pyloroplasty • Gastroduodenostomy • Gastrojejunostomy • Antrectomy with Billroth I, Billroth II, or Roux-en-Y reconstruction
Neoplasia	• Partial or complete absence of stomach	• Subtotal or total gastrectomy, varying reconstructions
Morbid obesity	• Gastric partitioning • Gastric bypass	• Vertical banded gastroplasty • Gastric bypass

D. The Postoperative Stomach

The postoperative stomach offers some special challenges worthy of brief mention. Foregut disease states, which may prompt surgical intervention and the associated anatomic changes, are listed in Table 50.2. As a general rule, the endoscopist does not need to change the technique of the examination because of these alterations, other than being sensitive to, and able to recognize and identify specific problems related to, their presence. Preendoscopic review of prior operative reports or contrast studies can be invaluable, particularly in patients with multiple previous operations.

A few additional techniques assist the endoscopist in these special situations. These techniques, in conjunction with a sound understanding of anatomy and the basic maneuvers described in Section C, will enable the endoscopist to conduct the postoperative exam with the same facility as in the normal anatomic setting. When difficulty is encountered or anticipated, consider one or more of these special techniques:

1. **Longer but small caliber instruments**, such as a pediatric colonoscope, are useful for accessing the jejunal limbs after gastrojejunostomy (Fig. 50.9).
2. A **side-viewing duodenoscope** may facilitate visualization of the proximal stomach when a small, surgically reduced pouch precludes normal retroflexion.
3. **Vital staining** or other special tests are used to visualize subtle mucosal changes (Lugol's solution, methylene blue), or to monitor postvagotomy parietal cell function (pH indicators).
4. Change the **position of the patient** to avoid retained material (bezoars), or to place the area being intubated in a more dependent location.

558   J.D. Mellinger

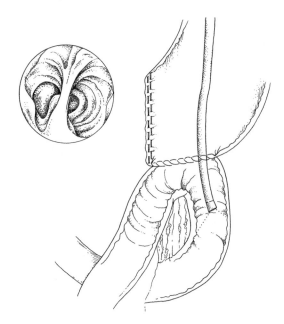

Figure 50.9. A pediatric colonoscope facilitates intubation of the jejunal limbs, particularly the afferent limb, after gastrojejunostomy.

E. Tissue-Sampling Techniques

Biopsy and brushing techniques are an important adjunct to endoscopic visualization in the conduct of upper gastrointestinal endoscopy. Brush cytology, forceps biopsy, large-particle biopsy, and chromoscopic techniques enhance the diagnostic yield beyond that provided by endoscopic inspection alone.

Cytology is particularly useful in the evaluation of fungal and viral infections of the foregut and is also an acceptable way to evaluate for *Helicobacter pylori* infection. It can add 10% to the diagnostic yield of biopsy alone in the evaluation of upper gastrointestinal malignancy. Brush cytology for malignancy is 85% to 90% sensitive and close to 100% specific in the foregut setting. In touch cytology, a standard biopsy sample is processed by rolling it on a slide and then fixing and staining the same for cytologic review. This technique has been shown to be a useful adjunct to biopsy alone when evaluating for infectious organisms including *Candida*, *Helicobacter*, and *Giardia*.

Standard biopsy techniques offer high diagnostic yields for a number of foregut pathologies, provided the disease is manifested at the mucosal level. Appropriate targeting of the tissue being sampled can be important in optimizing diagnostic yield. In the setting of evaluation for *H. pylori*, it has been shown that diagnostic yields are comparable from all areas of the stomach, and virtually all infected patients can be identified by a combination of three biopsy samples, obtained from the prepyloric antrum, lesser curve near the incisura, and greater curve body. With malignant ulcers, yields are highest with multiple biopsies (7–10), obtained from the rim of the ulcer as well as its base. Such approaches, particularly when combined with brush cytology and salvage cytology of material retained in the endoscope biopsy channel following forceps biopsy, allow documented diagnostic accuracies of 100% with malignant gastric ulcers.

1. Perform **brush cytology** by passing a sheathed brush through the endoscope biopsy channel.
    a. Position the sheath adjacent to the area to be sampled and extend the brush.
    b. Vigorously move the sheath–brush complex to and fro across the area being evaluated. This dislodges cells onto the brush.
    c. Retract the brush back into the sheath to prevent sample loss while the sheath is being withdrawn through the endoscope biopsy channel.
    d. The material obtained is then processed onto slides for cytologic evaluation.
    e. Washing the brush itself in balanced salt solution may allow recovery of additional material for pathology review.

2. **Forceps biopsy** provides sufficient tissue (generally limited to the mucosa) for histologic examination. Several kinds of biopsy forceps are available, and it is important to choose the proper type for the intended purpose.
    a. **Spiked forceps** have a tiny needle like projection between the jaws of the forceps to facilitate obtaining multiple samples on a single pass of the forceps. The endoscopist's ability to grasp tissue that is oriented tangentially to the endoscope may be enhanced by helping the forceps to firmly engage the tissue to be sampled.
    b. **Large cupped forceps**, or jumbo forceps as they are often called, require a therapeutic-size endoscope with a 3.7-mm biopsy channel. These instruments typically provide a larger mucosal specimen but do not usually allow submucosal sampling.

3. **Endoscopic mucosal resection** is sometimes useful when larger areas of mucosa are to be sampled or excised. This allows more complete removal of areas of suspicious mucosal pathology. It is particularly applicable in the setting of early gastric cancer, where it is used in concert with endoscopic ultrasound evaluation.
    a. **Inject saline** underneath the target lesion to elevate the mucosa and produce an easier target to snare. Hypertonic saline prolongs the effect.
    b. Resect the target lesion with a **standard snare technique**.
    c. The technique may be modified by using two small-caliber endoscopes simultaneously. This allows the first endoscope to provide forceps traction after injection, while the second endoscope applies the snare around the base of the lesion.
    d. Another modification utilizes a single cap-fitted endoscope capable of applying suction to the tissue, which is snared after being drawn into the cap.

4. **Large-particle biopsy** allows submucosal tissue sampling in the setting of infiltrative submucosal pathology not amenable to standard mucosal biopsy techniques. The risk of perforation is higher with such techniques, and other alternatives for submucosal evaluation and sampling are becoming available via endoscopic ultrasound (see Section F).

   a. Use a **therapeutic, two-channel endoscope**. Pass a snare down one channel and a biopsy forceps down the second.

   b. **Open the snare** and place it over the area to be sampled.

   c. **Pass the biopsy forceps** through the snare. Pick up and elevate both mucosa and submucosa, thus allowing the snare to incorporate a deeper level of tissue than would otherwise be possible.

5. **Chromoscopic techniques** are briefly mentioned because of their particular utility in the postoperative setting. Probably underutilized in the United States, chromoscopy can be employed along with magnification video endoscopy to enhance detection of neoplastic and preneoplastic mucosal abnormalities.

   a. **Lugol's solution** (typically ≥ 20 mL of a 1–2% solution applied directly via an endoscopic catheter) stains glycogen-containing tissue, which is present in normal esophageal squamous mucosa. Areas of intestinal metaplasia, carcinoma, and inflammation stain negatively with this agent and may thus be more apparent for biopsy sampling after its application.

   b. **Methylene blue** is usually applied as a 0.5% to 1% solution in similar volume following application of a mucolytic agent, and is taken up selectively by absorptive epithelium, such as intestinal metaplasia.

F. Endoscopic Ultrasound

Endoscopic ultrasound (EUS) is an area of expanding significance in diagnostic upper gastrointestinal endoscopy. Current **areas of application** include the diagnosis and staging of upper aerodigestive tract neoplasia, diagnosis of submucosal pathology, and diagnosis of choledocholithiasis. A specially designed endoscope is required.

EUS-guided **fine-needle aspiration cytology** offers great promise in adding to the diagnostic potential of this modality and may make it a diagnostic procedure of choice in the setting of esophageal, gastric, pancreatic, and even pulmonary neoplasia. Its staging potential in these settings, particularly in view of this tissue-sampling capability, is increasingly being shown to be superior to radiologic methods such as computed tomography. EUS is also showing promise in the diagnosis and monitoring of submucosal pathology such as stromal and neuroendocrine lesions, and varices.

With continuing technologic improvements, including the availability of instruments capable of combined luminal visualization and EUS, through the scope's high-frequency/high-resolution probes, Doppler capability, therapeutic echoendoscopes with elevator-equipped biopsy channels, and improved tissue-sampling instrumentation, EUS is poised for increasing importance and utilization in the years ahead. Factors that may limit its application include instrument cost, a steep learning curve required for meaningful interpretation (50–100 cases), and the need for further studies documenting significant and cost-effective changes in patient management based on its use. References in Section G give further information on this emerging diagnostic tool.

G. Selected References

Cooper GS. Indications and contraindications for upper gastrointestinal endoscopy. Gastrointest Endosc Clin North Am 1994;4:439–454.

Jane PK. Technique of upper gastrointestinal endoscopy. Gastrointest Endosc Clin North Am 1994;4:501–521.

Lightdale CJ, ed. Advances in endoscopic ultrasound. Gastrointest Endosc 2002; 56:S1–S97.

Mellinger JD, Ponsky JL. Endoscopic evaluation of the postoperative stomach. Gastrointest Endosc Clin North Am 1996;6:621–639.

Van Dam J, Brugge WR. Endoscopy of the upper gastrointestinal tract. N Engl J Med 1999;341:1738–1748.

Van Dam J, Chak A, Sivak MV. Technique of upper gastrointestinal endoscopy. In: Sivak, MV, ed. Gastroenterologic Endoscopy. 2nd ed. Philadelphia: WB Saunders, 2000.

Zaman A, Hahn M, Hapke R, Knigge K, Fennerty MB, Katon RM. A randomized trial of peroral versus transnasal unsedated endoscopy using an ultrathin videoendoscope. Gastrointest Endosc 1999;49:279–284.

51. Upper Gastrointestinal Endoscopy After Bariatric Surgery

Bruce David Schirmer, M.D., F.A.C.S.

A. Indications

Flexible upper gastrointestinal endoscopy is an important diagnostic and therapeutic procedure that is frequently indicated for symptoms of upper gastrointestinal problems following bariatric surgery. The bariatric surgeon is well advised to become proficient at flexible upper endsocopy because it is an important tool to be used by the surgeon to optimize postoperative outcomes. Specific indications include the following:

1. Symptoms of postoperative esophagogastric obstruction
2. Upper gastrointestinal bleeding
3. Known anastomotic stenosis
4. Epigastric or upper abdominal pain
5. Gastroesophageal reflux
6. Inability to tolerate food postoperatively after gastric restrictive surgery
7. Symptoms or signs suggesting potential erosion of a gastric band into the lumen of the stomach
8. Concern of a gastric staple line dehiscence
9. Preoperative investigation of the anatomy after previous gastric surgery when intial or revisional bariatric surgery is planned
10. Weight regain or poor weight loss after previous restrictive bariatric surgery

Therapeutic upper endoscopic procedures, which may be performed for several of the foregoing indication at the time of flexible endoscopy, include **balloon dilation** for stenoses or obstructions, **injection therapy, heater probe,** or **bicap electrocautery** for treatment of upper gastrointestinal (GI) bleeding, and **feeding tube guidance** for temporary nasoenteric or nasogastric feeding tubes or guidance of **percutaneous endoscopic gastrostomy** for more permanent feeding tube placement when the distal stomach is accessible. Chapter 29 deals with laparoscopic guidance of jejunostomy feeding tubes when the distal stomach is not endoscopically accessible.

Endoscopic retrograde cholangiopancreatiography (ERCP) is performed with a flexible side-viewing scope that allows visualization of the ampulla of Vater and imaging of the biliopancreatic tree. ERCP may be indicated in patients after bariatric surgery in the following situations:

1. Clinical and or radiographic picture suggesting choledocholithiasis
2. Postoperative suggestion of biliary obstruction after cholecystectomy done at the time of bariatric surgery

3. Postoperative pancreatitis in a patient with known gallstones
4. Obstructive jaundice of unknown etiology

The ability to perform ERCP after bariatric surgery depends on the operation performed, and whether endoscopic access to the duodenum is feasible. With restrictive gastric banding of all types, and short limb Roux-en-Y gastric bypass, ERCP is possible. Following all malabsorptive operations, as well as Roux-en-Y gastric bypass where the Roux limb length is 150 cm or longer, the endoscope cannot reach the duodenum. ERCP is discussed in complete detail later (see Chapter 61) and will not be described further in this chapter.

B. Patient Positioning and Room Setup

1. Place the patient comfortably in the left lateral position, after first obtaining intravenous access and informed consent.
2. The surgeon should stand facing the patient, near the head.
3. The assisting nurse should stand behind the patient. The assisting nurse's primary responsibility is monitoring the patient. Secondary responsibility is administration of medications for conscious sedation, and third responsibility is assisting in passage of instruments down the flexible endoscope. For complex therapeutic procedures, such as ERCP or difficult dilations, a second nurse to focus on assisting with the passage of instruments is mandatory.
4. The patient is equipped with monitoring devices for electrocardiography, blood pressure, and oxygen saturation (oximeter) during the procedure. Standard equipment for safe administration of conscious sedation is available.
5. Two video monitors are ideal: one at the patient's foot and one at the head. The monitor at the head is part of the tower that includes the flexible endoscope and image recording equipment.

C. Instrumentation

1. Choose the appropriate flexible endoscope. Thinner scopes with narrower working channels are appropriate for diagnostic procedures, while thicker therapeutic scopes with larger working channels are appropriate for known therapeutic procedures. Before starting the procedure, confirm that the scope's channels for suction and air insufflation are in working order.
2. Inflatable balloon catheters of 18- to 20-French size should be available if a dilation may be performed.
3. If the procedure is being performed for bleeding, the surgeon should have at least one and preferably two methods for endoscopic hemostasis present. These include an injection catheter for injecting epinephrine in the bleeding site, a heater probe with appropriate unit to

provide energy, and a bicap electrode probe with appropriate electrosurgical unit for energy.

5. Biopsy forceps are routinely available for all procedures for sampling lesions visualized.

D. Technique of Sedation and Scope Passage

1. Preoperative Topical Anesthesia

Flexible upper endoscopy is performed only after the patient has had adequate and thorough topical anesthesia for the hypopharynx. A variety of agents are available for this, including viscous Xylocaine (our current agent of choice) and aerosol sprays of cetacaine or benzocaine. Benzocaine is rarely associated with the induction of methemoglobinemia and tends to leave white residual deposits in the esophagus, which the inexperienced eye can confuse with those seen for thrush. After adequate topical anesthesia has been achieved, the patient is placed in the left lateral position and conscious sedation is initiated.

2. Conscious Sedation

The principles of conscious sedation is a subject for significant lengthy reports. However, the key principles are summarized in the list that follows. This is not meant to be a comprehensive coverage of the subject. All surgeons who perform flexible endoscopy should be privileged and appropriately credentialed by their institution in the procedure of conscious sedation.

1. Preprocedure history to document patients at high risk for oversedation (such as those with sleep apnea) or any history of problems with conscious sedation. A review of medications that could influence efficacy of the sedative medications given is advisable, as well.

2. Preprocedure physical with special attention to airway.

3. Use of one or at most two sedating drugs, for which pharmacologic reversal is available. Drugs should be short acting and have a short half-life. A combination of an analgesic narcotic and a sedative works well. Our usual choices are Versed (with flumazecon available for reversal) and fentanyl (with narcan for reversal).

4. Medications should be given in a titrated fashion, beginning with a low dose that is certain not to produce oversedation.

5. There should be constant patient monitoring for the sedative effects of the drugs, with special attention to oxygen saturation levels measured by pulse oximetry.

6. Available equipment for resuscitation (pharmacologic as noted above) and airway management.

7. Liberal use of supplemental oxygen for most patients to enhance safety of preventing hypoxia.

8. Careful postprocedure monitoring of patients until reversal of sedation is clear.
9. Special caution in the frail, elderly (these two less likely after bariatric surgery) or patients with known hypoventilation syndromes (not uncommon in bariatric surgery populations).

3. Scope Handling

a. Hold the scope in the left hand, with the ring and little fingers forming a **V** in which the base of the scope head is placed. The thumb, index, and middle fingers are thus positioned to move the two wheels of the scope which direct the tip in horizontal and vertical axes.
b. The right hand grasps the scope itself at a point about 6 to 10 in. from the incisors. Initially the scope is held about 10 in. from the tip for introduction and initial passage.
c. The index and middle fingers can press the suction and air/irrigation valves of the scope as needed.

4. Scope Passage

a. Place a bite block between the patient's teeth, and pass the scope through it.
b. Passage of the scope is done via a direct visualization or blind technique. Since the direct visualization technique is necessary for patients under general anesthesia, if only one technique is to be learned, this is the one.
c. **Direct visualization.** Pass the scope gently over the tongue, the tip pointed downward toward the epiglottis. Advance the scope slowly and sufficiently to clearly visualize the epiglottis and the vocal cords. Pass the scope at the 6 o'clock position relative to the cords, under the inferior fold in the tissue. This allows the scope tip to pass posterior to the cords and epiglottis, into the hypopharynx. As the scope is advanced just past the cords, the upper esophageal sphincter may cause slight resistance to the passage of the scope. As long as the scope is passed using firm but gentle pressure, not to excess, directly through the center of the tissue fold that represents the convergence of the upper esophageal sphincter, the sphincter will usually relax and the scope pass with minimal difficulty. At times, if slight resistance is met, the patient may be asked to swallow. If the patient is not excessively sedated and is cooperative, this greatly assists in passage of the scope. If resistance is encountered, maintain mild continuous pressure for a few seconds, at which time almost always the scope will then pass without difficulty. Continued resistance is an indication to withdraw the scope to the point where the vocal cords and epiglottis are clearly

again visible and centered in the scope's visual field; then repeat the process.

d. **Blind technique.** This is not recommended for beginners. More experienced endoscopists sometimes prefer to introduce the scope by a blind technique. The scope, held in the right hand, is passed through the bite block and over the tongue. The left index finger pulls the tongue forward, just to the left of the midline of the tongue. The scope is passed directly to the right of the left index finger, positioning it in the midline of the hypopharynx. With gentle forward pressure on the back of the tongue and a split second later passage of the scope with the right hand, a relaxation from the tongue retraction is produced sufficient to allow the scope tip to pass blindly into the upper esophagus past the upper sphincter. With this technique, any significant resistance is cause for cessation of the attempt to pass the scope and a reattempt. Multiple failures at this approach should be followed by introduction of the scope under direct visualization.

E. Technique of Diagnostic Upper Endoscopy

1. Scope Advancement Down Esophagus

Now advance the scope down the esophagus under direct visualization. Assess the esophagus for lesions, especially esophagitis, which could indicate obstruction (most likely) or postprocedure gastroesophageal reflux disease (less likely). In postbariatric surgery patients, when the end of the esophagus is reached, the endoscopist must pass the scope through the gastroesophageal junction area very slowly and carefully, unlike the normal anatomy patient for whom this maneuver may be done with increased speed and with less caution for visualizing structures until the stomach is entered. The reason for this is that postbariatric patients will usually have a restrictive pouch created from the proximal stomach, which may be only 2 cm long at most. Suction, air insufflation, and scope manipulation are used to clearly visualize the proximal gastric pouch and its mucosa.

2. Visualization of the Gastric Pouch/Proximal Stomach

Visualize the pouch for lesions including gastritis, ulcers, and openings. Assuming the anatomy of the previous bariatric surgery is known, the endoscopist should identify either the anastomosis of the gastric pouch with the jejunum (gastric bypass) or the passage into the lower stomach (banding). If more than one opening exists, it signifies a break in a previously placed gastric staple line, and a resulting gastrogastric fistula. The true anastomosis or passage to the distal stomach should be differentiated from the staple line break. The anastomosis is assessed for patency, size, and the presence of marginal ulcers in its vicinity. For banding patients, the integrity of the mucosa is confirmed if there is any suspicion of band erosion.

3. Visualization of the Postanastomotic Intestine or Distal Stomach

Pass the scope beyond the gastric pouch into either the intestinal limb (jejunum for gastric bypass, ileum for biliopancreatic diversion) or the distal stomach (for banding). Assess the distal stomach for lesions. Retroflex the scope to view the proximal gastric anatomy from the distal stomach. Patients who have undergone duodenal switch operations should have the integrity of the stomach sleeve confirmed, and the scope is passed through the duodenoileostomy anastomosis into the ileum. The anastomosis is assessed as before.

4. Documentation and Biopsy

The appropriate anatomic areas of concern based on preoperative symptoms are now documented by pictures taken using the flexible scope. Such photos are often quite valuable in clinical management for the patient, should a second endoscopy be required, especially if the endoscopist is not the same or a period of time has passed and recollection of the exact anatomy is not certain.

Biopsy is performed on any lesions in question, with the biopsy forceps passed down the working channel of the scope. Most forceps are "double-bite" action, meaning two samples of tissue may be taken before the forceps are withdrawn, each sample fitting in one of the two cuplike jaws of the biopsy forceps.

5. Assessment for Failure of Sustained Weight Loss

Diagnostic upper endoscopy is indicated in situations of poor weight loss or weight regain after previous bariatric surgery. In such situations, the surgeon endoscopist should be focused on documenting the existing anatomy, and whether the previous operation was anatomically appropriate for the production of weight loss. The integrity of staple lines of the proximal gastric pouch should be confirmed. The size of the pouch (not excessively large) should be documented. The presence of any other abnormalities that would preclude maintenance of weight loss should be documented. Finally, the anatomic justification for performing a reoperative procedure should be determined. Any surgeon contemplating reoperative bariatric surgery is well advised to perform not only flexible upper endoscopy but also obtain radiographic contrast studies of the upper gastrointestinal anatomy of potential patients.

F. Technique of Endoscopic Balloon Dilation

If the endoscopist encounters an anastomotic stricture or a gastric outlet obstruction, the cause should be determined by visual assessment.

1. The most common cause for anastomostic stricture after Roux-en-Y gastric bypass (RYGB) or biliopancreatic diversion (BPD) is post-operative stricture from one of several factors, such as technical error, tension, poor blood supply, or foreign body reaction to foreign material used in creating the anastomosis.
2. A marginal ulcer, if present, should be identified. When present, it must be assumed that the ulcer or the scarring secondary to the ulcer, is at the cause of the stenosis.
3. For gastric outlet obstruction after banding, the most common cause is slippage of the band after laparoscopic adjustable gastric banding (LAGB) or concentric hypertrophy for fixed bands such as after vertical banded gastroplasty (VBG)
4. Any clearly visible foreign bodies, such as sutures bridging the anastomotic opening or staples protruding into the lumen of the anastomosis, should be removed with the biopsy forceps and scissors forceps if needed. For LAGB or VBG, the mucosa is assessed for signs of band erosion.
5. The endoscopist should attempt to pass the scope through the anastomosis, if passage is feasible based on the size of the opening. Small openings may sometimes allow passage of the scope if the decrease in the lumen is secondary to swelling and edema of the surrounding bowel wall.

1. Successful Passage of Scope Beyond Stricture

If the scope can be passed through the stricture, then the balloon catheter is passed into the lumen of the intestine or stomach beyond the anastomosis. The balloon is fully passed such that if it is beyond the end of the scope. Then the scope is slowly withdrawn backward, allowing the balloon to assume a position astride the stenosis, with a portion of the balloon proximal and distal to the stenosis. This method is the safest for balloon dilation, since it positions the balloon across the stenosis without blindly passing the tip through and beyond the stenosis. It is worth the effort to change to a smaller caliber scope if initial use of a larger bore therapeutic scope prevents passage through the stricture. Passage of the smaller caliber scope can be followed by initial balloon dilation with a smaller caliber balloon. This will usually allow sufficient dilation to permit immediate subsequent passage of a therapeutic scope and a second dilation with an even larger lumen balloon.

Once positioned across the stenosis, the balloon is insufflated using the pneumatic-controlled insufflator gun, to achieve full insufflation pressure. This is held in place for one minute, then released. Tight stenoses will usually form a "waist" in the balloon as it is insufflated.

The anastomosis is assessed for success of dilation. Repeat dilation is now performed with the same or a larger scope as needed. The goal is to dilate the opening to sufficient size to allow passage of a therapeutic scope if possible.

2. Unsuccessful Passage of Scope Beyond Stricture

If the scope cannot be passed beyond the anastomosis, the surgeon must be aware of the postanastomotic anatomy. Often when RYGB has been created, the Roux limb is brought up and an end-to-side anastomosis created with the proximal gastric pouch. This anatomic situation means that just beyond the anastomosis is the back wall of the jejunum. The endoscopist in this situation is ill advised to blindly pass the balloon catheter through the anastomotic opening, since the firm tip of the balloon catheter can easily perforate the back wall of the jejunum.

In this situation, the balloon catheter is carefully inserted only partially through the lumen of the stenosis, with the endoscopist being careful to stop passage if any resistance is met. Passage of the balloon catheter at a slightly angled right direction will usually help avoid immediate contact with the back wall of the intestine. The balloon is passed such that a portion of it is through the anastomosis. The endoscope is now withdrawn slowly, advancing the balloon out of the scope such that the balloon is completely out of the scope but the tip has not been pushed much further into the intestinal lumen.

Insufflation with part of the balloon into the anastomosis is performed. The balloon catheter in this situation will have a tendency to back out as it is insufflated, and the endoscopist must work to try and maintain a portion of it within the stricture to achieve a partial dilation.

Once a partial dilation has been achieved, attempts are again made to pass the scope through the anastomotic stenosis, with subsequent performance of another dilation as already described when the scope can be so passed.

3. Marginal Ulcer

If a marginal ulcer is present, the patient must be carefully dilated and the ulcer bed examined for the potential presence of a gastrogastric fistula. The latter condition usually only occurs after prolonged presence of a marginal ulcer, with considerable erosion of surrounding tissue into the distal stomach. The presence of such a fistula presents an anatomic situation that will require operative treatment to prevent the free reflux of acid and continued stenosis of the anastomosis, as well as the need to reseparate the proximal gastric pouch from the distal one for restrictive purposes.

Presence of a marginal ulcer without gastrogastric fistula is an indication to add empiric treatment for *Helicobacter pylori* after completion of the endoscopic treatment.

4. Multiple Dilations

Many patients with anastomotic stenosis after RYGB will be successfully treated with only one such endoscopic balloon dilation. However, roughly 50%, in our experience, will require more than one dilation. We have adopted a strategy of using either a second endoscopic dilation with a larger balloon, or a fluoroscopic-guided dilation, with an even larger balloon, for the second or subsequent dilations. Failure of dilations to produce adequate relief of obstruction, requiring surgical therapy, has, in our experience, been limited to those patients with marginal ulcer causing the stenosis.

G. Technique of Endoscopic Treatment of Upper GI Bleeding After Bariatric Surgery

Upper gastrointestinal bleeding after bariatric surgery is a relatively uncommon complication. It is almost never seen after LAGB or VBG, unless in the prolonged postoperative period associated with erosion of the band into the lumen of the stomach. In such cases, diagnostic endoscopy confirms the need for operative therapy to correct the problem. After RYGB, upper GI bleeding may occur in the first week after surgery due to bleeding from the recently created anastomosis. The use of low-molecular-weight heparin for prophylaxis versus venous thromboembolism may contribute to this condition, especially if the patient has a borderline iatrogenic coagulopathy. This should be corrected if documented. Upper GI bleeding after RYGB may occur a few weeks after surgery, associated with the development of marginal ulcer. The endoscopic treatment of bleeding from either a marginal ulcer or an anastomotic site is similar, and involves one of three techniques: all three techniques work well, and the endoscopist may choose the one with which he or she is most comfortable and familiar. Achievement of hemostasis is usually readily apparent by endoscopic inspection of the bleeding site.

1. Injection of Submucosal Epinephrine at Bleeding Site

a. Flexible upper endoscopy is performed, preferably with a therapeutic endoscope. The bleeding site is identified. This may be more difficult than expected, particularly if a significant-sized hematoma is present in the proximal gastric pouch or the lumen of the stomach. Depending on the anatomy and the temporal relationship to the bleeding relative to the operation, the endoscope itself may be used to evacuate the hematoma (a sometimes slow process) or an Ewald tube carefully passed to help remove the hematoma (more efficient but only feasible with well-healed staple lines and usually an accessible distal stomach).

b. The site of the bleeding is identified.

c. The injection catheter is passed and submucosal injections of epinephrine are used to cause contraction of the bleeding vessel. Injections are performed in a circular fashion around the site of the bleeding vessel, using 1 mL of epinephrine per injection. The epinephrine serves to constrict and contract the vessel to produce hemostasis. This is our preferred method, as it involves no energy and minimizes intestinal and gastric injury postprocedure.

2. Use of a Heater Probe

The endoscopist may choose to use a heater probe to achieve coagulation of the bleeding site. The probe is directly applied to the bleeding site, achieving hemostasis by tissue coagulation. This method does have a higher potential for delayed perforation at an anastomotic site than epinephrine injection.

3. Use of a Bicap Electrode

The endoscopist may instead opt to use a bicap electrode, which uses bipolar electrocautery to coagulate a bleeding site. This is also associated with some potential for tissue damage and subsequent perforation, but this danger is relatively low. Appropriate patient grounding is needed for this procedure.

H. Technique of Percutaneous Endoscopic Gastrostomy

The patient who develops excess weight loss after bariatric surgery, usually owing to psychological rather than anatomic factors, is a candidate for placement of a sustained enteral feeding access until the malnourishment and depression (which is usually present) can be successfully treated and reversed. A careful assessment for the reasons for the excess weight loss must precede the decision to place a feeding tube. If there has been excess malabsorption after a malabsorptive operation, then surgical correction is indicated. However, if behavioral issues, potentially reversible, are responsible, then the indication exists for placement of a feeding tube. Patients who have undergone VBG or LAGB are potential candidates for a **percutaneous endoscopic gastrostomy (PEG)** in the lower residual stomach.

The technique for PEG is summarized as follows:

1. Patient preparation as for therapeutic endoscopy, but patient in the supine position.
2. Passage of flexible endoscope into stomach, diagnostic endoscopy performed, stomach insufflated.
3. Point on abdominal wall (left upper quadrant to epigastric region) where maximum indentation of the inflated stomach occurs when external pressure is applied.
4. This point chosen for local anesthesia, needle catheterization, and threading of a guidewire into the lumen of the stomach.
5. Grasping the guidewire with a snare passed through the endoscope.
6. Pulling the wire out the mouth.
7. Threading the gastrostomy catheter over the guidewire until the tip of the catheter is visible through the skin of the anterior abdominal wall.
8. Grasping the catheter, enlarging the skin incision, and pulling the catheter out virtually all the way, until its inner bolster is flush against the anterior gastric wall.
9. Adjusting the outer bolster to maintain this pressure of the bolster in place.

I. Complications

1. **Perforation**
a. **Cause and prevention.** Endoscopic perforation results from too much force applied to a wall of the gastrointestinal tract. Perforation with upper endoscopy is rare, on the order of 0.1% for diagnostic upper endoscopy. This frequency increases with the number of difficult dilations performed; these have the highest potential for leakage at the dilated site if a full-thickness tear is made in the wall of the esophagus, stomach, or intestine.

   Use of excessive force in trying to push a scope through an anastomotic or strictured area. The endoscopist must use gentle but not excessive force in this situation, relying on balloon dilation instead to increase the luminal opening with pressure more evenly distributed over the surface of the balloon. If balloon dilation fails as well to open a strictured area, operative therapy will be needed and no further dilation attempts should be performed. This is an uncommonly encountered situation, however.

b. **Recognition and management.** The endoscopist should be prepared to test the patient postdilation for potential leaks. Some clinicians send patients for a Gastrografin swallow following a dilation; others do this selectively. Signs of perforation after upper endoscopy include upper abdominal pain, which is normally not present after the procedure. Persistent pain, especially if accompanied by fever, is a very worrisome sign for potential perforation. Persistence of such pain warrants a plain abdominal film. Presence of free air in the peritoneal cavity is diagnostic for a perforation. If no free air is seen, or if it is and the site of perforation is unclear, a Gastrografin swallow is next indicated to define the site and severity of the perforation.

c. Treatment is normally operative, but nonoperative treatment of minor contained perforations of the esophagus has been described in patients undergoing pneumatic balloon dilation for achalasia. There is no documentation of conservative therapy for leaks after dilation for stenosis following bariatric surgery. If in doubt, operative therapy is recommended. A gastric or gastrojejunal anastomotic perforation may be treated with a laparoscopic approach to oversew and drain the perforation site. If the perforation is in the midst of severely scarred tissue, and obstruction remains despite the perforation, then resection of the stenosis is indicated, and this may require open surgery for optimal results.

Resection is greatly preferred unless precluded by condition of the intestinal tissue itself (e.g., intestinal loops virtually "frozen" by severe intra-abdominal adhesions). Proximal diversion may require placement of a feeding tube for administration of an elemental formula or even total parenteral nutrition. Occasionally bypass of the leaking anastomosis may be feasible; adequate diversion of the enteric stream should be assured by this technique to prevent likely releakage. Do not attempt to restore intestinal continuity for at least 3 months. It is prudent to wait longer if severe inflammation and adhesions were encountered at the second operation. These management principles are no different from those followed when an open small bowel resection results in leak.

2. **Bleeding**

a. **Cause and prevention.** Bleeding after upper endoscopy is unusual and occurs less frequently than perforation. Injury of a mucosal surface by the endoscope is the mechanism of postendoscopic bleeding. The cause is excessive torque or pressure on the surface of an organ, resulting in tearing and hemorrhage of the mucosal surface. Simple care to appropriate technique is the simple rule to prevent this complication.

Rarely the endoscopist will encounter esophageal or gastric varices on endoscopy. This would be most unusual in the setting after bariatric surgery, since patients with cirrhosis and portal hypertension are normally not considered candidates for bariatric surgery. Postoperative pancreatitis with splenic vein thrombosis could result in gastric varices. Gastric varices could be a source of postendoscopic bleeding if the endoscopist were to disrupt one of the varices with the scope while maneuvering it through the stomach. Prevention of this complication is through diligent attention to not passing the scope against the surface of gastric varices, if they are present. Biopsies should be cautiously taken of lesions, which could potentially represent varices or other venous structures.

b. **Recognition and management.** Upper gastrointestinal bleeding after endoscopy is usually manifested by hematemesis. On occasion, the patient will have only melena without hematemesis. The latter is more common with duodenal bleeding or lower gastric bleeding below a partial barrier such as an inflatable band. However, most bleeding that occurs as a result of scope trauma will present with regurgitation of some of the blood and hematemesis. The temporal sequence of the bleeding will often suggest that the etiology is related to the procedure, and thus is iatrogenic. Monitoring patients after upper endoscopy is mandatory. Such monitoring has several purposes. One is to ensure that the effects of conscious sedation have adequately reversed. Another is to be vigilant for alterations in vitals signs that would suggest a complication of the endoscopy. Bleeding may manifest itself initially as unexplained tachycardia or hypotension, which may precede hematemesis. Suspicion of bleeding with such vital sign changes is important to allow early recognition of the problem.

c. **Management of upper GI bleeding** after endoscopy includes appropriate fluid and blood product resuscitation, and a repeat endoscopy to determine the site and source of the bleeding. An Ewald tube may be needed to evacuate the stomach of hematoma. Once the site has been identified, many bleeding sources can be appropriately treated through the use of endoscopic energy sources, such as heater probe or bicap forceps. Injection of an epinephrine solution into the bleeding site endoscopically via a needle passed down the working channel of the endoscope is another option for management of the bleeding. Bleeding of a significant volume that cannot be stopped with endoscopic or conservative means requires emergent surgery or emergent radiologic embolization. The former is favored over the latter for upper GI bleeding, since embolization is technically difficult and may not produce hemostasis owing to the rich blood supply of the stomach.

3. **Excessive sedation/reaction to medication**

a. **Cause and prevention.** Conscious sedation has as its major drawback the potential for oversedation and compromise of respiratory function. This is more likely to happen in the patient population at risk for oversedation, including the frail, elderly, small in stature patient, or the patient with sleep apnea, no matter how large. It is the latter patient that is most likely to be represented among patients undergoing upper endoscopy after bariatric surgery. The cause is overmedication with sedative or narcotic medications, relative to that patient's tolerance on that day. Prevention of this problem is by titration of sedative medications during conscious sedation, always giving small incremental doses until the desired cumulative effect is achieved. Conscious sedation is always appropriately performed with patient monitoring of vital signs, including oxygen saturation. A drop in oxygen saturation is a harbinger that any further sedation could be followed by precipitous further drop in oxygen saturation and then respiratory arrest.

b. **Recognition and management.** When the patient is appropriately monitored for vital signs and oxygenation using pulse oximetry, deterioration of the oxygen saturation is the first sign of impending oversedation. Careful clinical observation coupled with this objective evidence are the obvious ways of early recognition. Delay in recognition could prove detrimental or fatal when one is treating a respiratory arrest. Management of mild hypoxia begins with the application of supplemental oxygen via nasal cannula or other reliable delivery method. Stimulation by voice or touch, commands to breath deeply, and the use of supplemental oxygen are often adequate to reverse the earliest stages of oversedation. However, any more profound oversedation must be treated by the additional intravenous administration of an appropriate reversal agent. This is naloxone in the case of oversedation with narcotic agents and flumazecon in the case of oversedation with benzodiazepams. After the administration of such reversal agents, the team should be in the process of preparing to intubate the patient and follow advanced cardiac life support system protocol for resuscitation if the intravenous reversal agent does not produce immediate reversal of the oversedation. Intubation, airway control, and assisted ventilation are required for the most severe cases of oversedation or reaction to medications.

4. **Aspiration**
   a. **Cause and prevention.** The patient undergoing upper endoscopy is at risk for aspiration at the initiation of flexible upper endoscopy. This is a result of a full stomach, usually due to distal obstruction or less commonly bleeding. The patient may vomit in response to the scope being introduced, and aspiration can easily occur. Occurrence of the problem is usually clinically obvious. Any patient who vomits during endoscopy and has uncontrolled fluid or secretions in the area of the epiglottis must be viewed as having aspirated until proven otherwise. Decompression of the suspected full stomach is the best means of prevention of aspiration. In addition, careful and thorough topical sedation of the hypopharynx to limit gagging, maintenance of the patient on his or her side with good access to the mouth for immediate suctioning of any regurgitated material, and performance of such suctioning are all adjunct methods of preventing or limiting the amount of aspirated material. However, gastric decompression remains the single best method of prevention whenever possible. Finally, if the patient is considered an aspiration risk, much less conscious sedation should be used so that the patient is in a more awake state to help protect his or her own airway.

   b. **Recognition and management.** Aspiration is usually a readily observable and dramatic event, associated with copious vomiting in the setting of a patient sedated and unable to protect his or her airway. If there is question about whether aspiration has indeed occurred, then flexible bronchoscopy should be performed to examine the tracheobronchial tree for signs and evidence of aspiration. Management of aspiration is through bronchoscopy and lavage to cleanse the airways of obvious contaminating materials and liquids, followed by intravenous administration of broad-spectrum antibiotics, hospitalization, and careful monitoring of respiratory and ventilatory status to determine whether these are compromised. The patient with mild aspiration in otherwise good health may require only supplemental oxygen, while the patient in poor health or with significant aspiration may require intubation with full ventilatory support as treatment.

J. Selected References

Ahmad J, Martin J, Ikramuddin S, et al. Endoscopic balloon dilation of gastroenteric anastomotic stricture after laparoscopic gastric bypass. Endoscopy 2003;35:725–728.

Bell RL, Reinhardt KE, Flowers JL. Surgeon-performed endoscopic dilatation of symptomatic gastrojejunal anastomotic strictures following laparoscopic Roux-en-Y gastric bypass. Obes Surg 2003;13:728–733.

Erenoglu C, Schirmer BD, Miller A. Flexible endoscopy in the management of patients undergoing Roux-en-Y gastric bypass. Obes Surg 2002;12:634–638.

Huang CS, Forse RA, Jacobson BC, Farraye FA. Endoscopic findings and their clinical correlations in patients with symptoms after gastric bypass surgery. Gastrointest Endosc 2003;58:859–866.

Kretzschmar CS, Hamilton JW, Wissler DW, et al. Balloon dilation for the treatment of stomal stenosis complicating gastric surgery for morbid obesity. Surgery 1987; 102:443–446.

Vance PL, de Lange EE, Shaffer HA Jr, Schirmer B. Gastric outlet obstruction following surgery for morbid obesity: efficacy of fluoroscopically guided balloon dilatation. Radiology 2002;222:70–72.

Verset D, Houben JJ, Gay F, et al. The place of upper gastrointestinal endoscopy before and after vertical banded gastroplasty for morbid obesity. Dig Dis Sci 1997; 42:2333–2337.

Wayman CS, Nord HJ, Combs WM, Rosemurgy AS. The role of endoscopy after vertical banded gastroplasty. Gastrointest Endosc 1992;38:44–46.

Wolper JC, Messmer JM, Turner MA, Sugerman HJ. Endoscopic balloon dilation of late stomal stenosis: its use following gastric surgery for morbid obesity. Arch Surg 1984;119:836–837.

52. Therapeutic Upper Gastrointestinal Endoscopy

James P. Dolan, M.D.
John G. Hunter, M.D.

A. Endoscopic Polypectomy

1. Indications

Polypectomy is less commonly applied in the upper gastrointestinal (GI) tract than in the colon. This is because true adenomas are unusual in this location. The majority of upper GI polyps are submucosal and most (75%) are inflammatory in origin. A minority (15–25%) of these lesions have malignant potential, and the biopsy of dominant masses is indicated to exclude early gastroesophageal malignancy. If polyps are sessile, multiple, or larger than 2 cm, an operative approach to their removal should be considered.

2. Technique

    a. A **diathermy snare** is effective for esophageal or gastric lesions amenable to excisional biopsy.
        1. Use a forward-viewing endoscope.
        2. Pass the snare loop over the polyp and tighten the snare around its stalk.
        3. Excise the lesion with a blend of cutting and coagulation electrocautery.
        4. Gastric polyps may be less pedunculated and therefore require a two-channel endoscope for their manipulation and excision (see Chapter 50).
    b. **Endoluminal gastric surgery** may be an alternative for excision of gastric lesions not amenable to snare excision (see Chapter 26).
        1. This employs laparoscopic instruments and techniques to work within the stomach.
        2. Specialized trocars are placed through the abdominal wall into the stomach. The number and orientation of trocars depends on the position of the pathology.

3. While a flexible endoscope may be used to guide endoluminal surgery, a rigid laparoscope introduced through an intragastric trocar, from outside the body, optimally facilitates the procedure.
4. Resection of mucosa-based polyps is facilitated by submucosal injection of saline to elevate the lesion.
5. Submucosal lesions may be "shelled out" and the mucosa closed over the defect.
6. If there is visible mucosal redundancy around a mucosal-based polyp, an endostapling device may be used to transect below the polyp and provide for control of bleeding.

B. Dilatation

1. Indications

Upper gastrointestinal strictures are dilated to improve passage of food and saliva. Dilatation should be preceded by a precise diagnostic evaluation, including endoscopy and biopsies, to define the underlying pathology and to **exclude unrecognized malignancy**. Dilatation is most commonly applied to peptic esophageal strictures and may also be beneficial in cases of gastric outlet obstruction from ulcer disease or stenosis after gastroenterostomy or pyloroplasty. The objective of esophageal dilatation is to resolve dysphagia. Patients who can accept a 44-French dilator are able to swallow most foods.

2. Technique

a. **Mercury-filled rubber bougies (or dilators)** are useful in cases of simple, straight strictures. **Maloney dilators** have a tapered end and are well tolerated and easy to use, while the **Hurst dilators** have a blunt tip.
   1. The patient may be treated in the sitting position. More commonly, the left lateral decubitus position is used.
   2. Most patients require only topical anesthetic spray; however, small doses of midazolam or meperidine should be available, since dilatation may cause discomfort.
   3. Determine the initial caliber of the stricture by passing successively larger dilators until resistance is appreciated.
   4. Dilate the lumen 6- to 10-French beyond this point, using only mild force to advance the dilators.
   5. Use fluoroscopy liberally, especially for patients with narrow strictures or large hiatal hernias.
   6. Schedule repeat sessions at 1- to 3-week intervals until dysphagia is resolved. Overzealous dilatations increase the risk for esophageal perforation.

   b. **Wire-guided dilators** (Savary dilators) are more rigid than Maloney or Hurst dilators and are preferred for tight, tortuous strictures. Fluoroscopy is always indicated in this setting.

      1. Place a guidewire across the stricture and into the stomach using an endoscope.

      2. Pass graded dilators over the wire with fluoroscopic control.

      3. Do not dilate a stricture more than 6- to 10-French at any one session, with repeat dilations at 1- to 3-week intervals until dysphagia is resolved.

   c. **Hydrostatic balloons** may be used to dilate upper GI strictures under endoscopic visualization. Thus, fluoroscopy is not required. Since the endoscopist cannot "feel" the stricture, he or she must estimate its diameter. The balloon is inflated with water to a predetermined pressure. The dilator may be passed theough a 2.8-mm biopsy channel on the endoscope, although the 3.5-mm working channel is the preferred conduit. Frequently it is necessary to use progressively larger balloons and multiple procedures.

C. Palliation of Upper Gastrointestinal Malignancies

1. Indications

Endoscopic palliation is indicated when resection or other therapy has failed or is impracticable. The most common site is esophageal, and obstruction is the most common indication for endoscopic intervention. Occasionally bleeding or tracheoesophageal fistula requires endoscopic control. There are several methods currently used for palliation of malignant esophageal obstruction. Perforation, the most feared complication of palliative dilatation, stenting or ablation, occurs at a rate between 0.01% and 0.25%.

2. Techniques

   a. In cases of advanced esophageal cancer with short life expectancy, **dilatation** (see Section B) alone may afford satisfactory relief of dysphagia.

   b. Usually, more lasting relief is needed. Endoscopic or radiographic placement of rigid plastic or expandable wire **stents** across malignant esophageal strictures will achieve more durable alleviation of symptoms. Both rigid and self-expanding metal stents are available.

      1. Stents are directed into position over an endoscope or an inner guide tube placed across the stricture.

2. Rigid stents are manually pushed into position across the stricture. These stents are more economical but are accompanied by a 5% to 10% incidence of perforation during placement and a 15% incidence of early migration.
3. Rigid prostheses are not easily tolerated for proximal esophageal strictures owing to discomfort and airway compression. For these reasons, more expensive self-expanding wire stents have gained popularity.
4. Self-expanding wire stents are more easily delivered across tight strictures because of their narrower profile before expansion, and they are less prone to migrate because they engage the tumor with outward force.
5. Problems with tumor ingrowth have been lessened by the use of urethane coating and wire coils.

c. **Laser ablation** of bulky esophageal tumors offers effective palliation of dysphagia in 70% to 80% of patients after three to five sessions. Although once a popular option for palliation, this modality is currently not widely utilized owing to the introduction of effective stenting devices. In some instances, though, it remains a viable option for palliative care.
1. Prophylactic antibiotics and intravenous sedation are usually required for the procedure.
2. Visualize the tumor and direct an endoscopic laser at the intralumenal component of a tumor to heat and vaporize the obstructing tissue and restore a 10- to 12-mm lumen. Use a neodymium-yttrium-aluminum-garnet (Nd:YAG) or a potassium-titanium dioxide-phosphate (KTP) laser.
3. If the anatomy permits, traverse the tumor with the endoscope and treat during withdrawal. Antegrade treatment is associated with a higher perforation rate.
4. Complications such as perforation, bleeding, and fistula are reported in 5% to 20% of cases.
5. Laser units are expensive and require special training and attention to safety in their use.

D. Foreign Body Removal

1. Indications

Most **foreign body** ingestions occur in children between 1 and 5 years of age and are usually coins. Impacted food is the most prevalent esophageal foreign body in adults. Up to 90% of objects will pass through the gastrointestinal tract spontaneously. Approximately 10% will require endoscopic removal. Urgent endoscopy is usually not necessary if the patient is able to handle secretions. Urgent removal is indicated if secretions cannot be cleared, if there is respiratory distress, or if the foreign body is a sharp object. Sometimes ingestion of carbonated beverages or administration of nitrates or calcium-channel blockers will result in clearance of a retained esophageal food bolus. Otherwise, rigid or flexible endoscopy will allow successful retrieval in 99% of cases.

Swallowed foreign bodies that have cleared the esophagus usually proceed uneventfully through the alimentary tract. Thus most foreign body ingestions that do not result in esophageal impaction can be managed by watchful waiting. Sharp, large, or potentially dangerous foreign objects may need to be removed from the stomach or duodenum.

2. Technique

A rigid endoscope permits better suction and easier fragmentation of the bolus, but a flexible instrument is safer in high-risk patients. Improvements in instrumentation have made flexible endoscopy the procedure of choice for most endoscopists.

1. Most impacted food can be pushed into the stomach with the expectation that it will then pass normally.
2. Retrieve other foreign bodies with apolypectomy snare or foreign body removal forceps (tenaculum or alligator forceps).
3. Use a small-caliber fiberscope with an overtube to overcome many of the drawbacks of flexible endoscopy.
4. Remove sharp foreign bodies (such as open safety pins) with the point trailing. This may necessitate pushing the object into the stomach where it can be turned around and positioned properly for removal.
5. After removing foreign object, especially impacted food boluses, make a careful search for underlying pathology.
6. Maintain a high index of suspicion for associated perforation. Carefully inspect the mucosal surfaces after removal.

E. Emerging Technologies

In recent years, the field of upper gastrointestinal endoscopy has seen the introduction of new technologies for the treatment of numerous conditions. These include:

1. Photodynamic and thermal therapy for the treatment of esophageal Barrett's dysplasia.
2. Submucosal "lifting" and thermal snaring of areas of Barrett's mucosa.
3. Endoscopic, full-thickness, gastric plication devices for the treatment of gastroesophageal reflux disease (GERD).

These new applications are showing promise in the treatment of upper gastrointestinal disease. However, outcomes from their application are awaiting the results of long-term data.

F. Selected References

Beger HG, Schwarz A, Bergmann U. Progress in gastrointestinal tract surgery: the impact of gastrointestinal endoscopy. Surg Endosc 2002;16(12):1514–1518.

Chuttani R, Kozarek R, Critchlow J, et al. A novel full thickness plicator for treatment of GERD: an animal model study. Gastrointest Endosc 2002;56(1):116–122.

Ponec RJ, Kimmey MB. Endoscopic therapy of esophageal cancer. Surg Clin North Am 1997;5:1197–1217.

Schwesinger WH. Laser treatment of esophageal and gastric lesions. Surg Clin North Am 1992;3:581–595.

Trus TL, Fink AS. Interventional and therapeutic upper gastrointestinal endoscopy. In: Eubanks WS, Swanstrom LL, Soper NJ, eds. Mastery of Endoscopic and Laparoscopic Surgery. Philadelphia: Lippincott Williams & Wilkins, 2000;123–132.

Wo JM, Waring JP. Medical therapy of gastroesophageal reflux and management of esophageal strictures. Surg Clin North Am 1997;5:1041–1053.

Wolfsen HC. Photodynamic therapy for mucosal esophageal adenocarcinoma and dysplastic Barrett's esophagus. Dig Dis 2002;20(1):5–17.

53. Variceal Banding

Gregory Van Stiegmann, M.D., F.A.C.S.

A. Indications

Documented hemorrhage from esophageal varices is the traditional indication for endoscopic treatment of bleeding esophageal varices. Prophylactic treatment of large varices that have not bled is now also an appropriate indication for endoscopic band ligation.

1. Perform **diagnostic upper gastrointestinal endoscopy** as soon as possible after the patient who presents with an upper gastrointestinal hemorrhage has been resuscitated and is hemodynamically stable. If bleeding from varices is suspected, an intravenous vasoactive agent such as octreotide (50 μg IV bolus, then 25–50 μg/h IV) should be started prior to endoscopy. If bleeding from varices is confirmed this drug should be continued after endoscopic treatment for 3 to 5 days. In addition, if bleeding from varices is confirmed, broad-spectrum antibiotic treatment (e.g., fluoroquinolone given intravenously and then switched to orally) should be started and continued for 7 days. Antibiotic therapy has been shown to diminish the incidence of recurrent bleeding as well as other serious infections in cirrhotic patients.

2. Confirm hemorrhage from varices by observing:
   a. Actively bleeding varices
   b. A varix with a fibrin plug ("cherry red spot" or pigmented protuberance)
   c. The presence of varices with no other identifiable source of upper gastrointestinal bleeding

B. Patient Positioning, Room Setup, and Special Considerations in the Bleeding Patient

1. Place the awake sedated patient in the left lateral decubitus position.
2. Adequate monitoring, suctioning, and resuscitation apparatus must be readily available, particularly in patients who are actively bleeding.
3. Patients who are combative, encephalopathic, or are bleeding briskly may require **endotracheal intubation**. This protects the airway and allows sufficient sedation for the procedure to be performed.

C. Technique of Endoscopic Variceal Band Ligation

Both endoscopic band ligation and sclerotherapy (see Chapter 54, Sclerotherapy of Variceal Bleeding) are effective techniques for management of bleeding varices. This section describes endoscopic ligation performed with a "multiple-fire" device.

1. Intubated patients may be treated in the left lateral or supine position (see Chapter 49).
2. Attach the ligating device to the endoscope.
   Care must be exercised when introducing the multifire ligating devices into the esophagus to avoid damage to the hypopharynx. Ligate the most distal esophageal varices first, usually beginning at or just caudad to the gastroesophageal junction.
   a. Perform subsequent ligations at the same level or more cephalad.
   b. Treat actively bleeding patients in the same manner, unless a bleeding site is identified. In this case, that site is ligated first, either by placing the band on the rent in the varix or by ligating proximal and distal to the rent. Subsequent ligations are performed as before until all varices in the distal esophagus have been ligated at least once.
3. Identify the target lesion and advance the endoscope under direct vision until the banding cylinder is in full 360-degree contact with the target.
4. Activate endoscopic suction, drawing the lesion into the banding chamber (Fig. 53.1). When the target has filled the chamber, as witnessed by a complete redout, pull the trip wire to securely fix the latex O-ring around the base of the target.
5. Repeat ligation treatments aimed at eradication of varices are conducted at 1- to 3-week intervals until varices in the distal esophagus have been obliterated. Elective repeat treatments are performed on an outpatient basis.

D. Complications of Endoscopic Band Ligation

Complications of endoscopic ligation directly related to endoscopic ligation are infrequent. Bleeding from ligation site ulcers occurs in up to 8% of patients. Shallow ulcers occur at each treated site when the ligated tissue bolus sloughs (usually 3–6 days following ligation) and are not preventable. There is some evidence that sucralfate or acid blocking agents may decrease this risk. If bleeding recurs, diagnosis and treatment entail repeat endoscopy and repeat ligation or sclerotherapy. Many treatment ulcer bleeding episodes are self-limited.

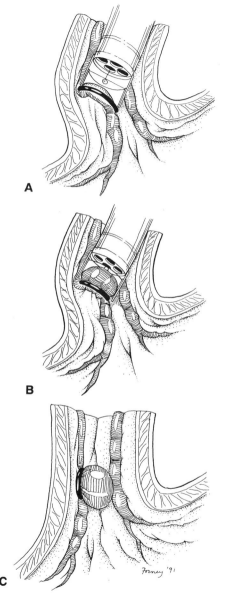

Figure 53.1. A. The endoscopist makes contact with the varix to be ligated. B. The varix is aspirated into the ligating device using endoscopic suction, and the elastic band is ejected from the ligator to ensnare the varix. C. The ligated varix. (Reprinted with permission from Springer-Verlag. World J Surg 1992;16:1034–1041.)

E. Selected References

Banares R, Albillos A, Rincon D, et al. Endoscopic treatment versus endoscopic plus pharmacologic treatment for acute variceal bleeding: a meta-analysis. Hepatology. 2002;35(3):609–615.

Bernard B, Grange JD, Khac EN, Amiot X, Opolon P, Poynard T. Antibiotic prophylaxis for prevention of bacterial infections in cirrhotic patients with gastrointestinal bleeding: a meta-analysis. Hepatology 1999;29:1655–1661.

Stiegmann GV. Motion-prophylactic banding of esophageal varices is useful: arguments for the motion. Can J Gastroenterol 2002;16(10):689–692.

Tait IS, Krige JE, Terblanche J. Endoscopic band ligation of oesophageal varices. Br J Surg 1999;86(4):437–446. Review.

54. Sclerotherapy of Variceal Bleeding

Choichi Sugawa, M.D.

A. Indications and Results

Endoscopic sclerotherapy (ES) and variceal banding (VB) (Chapter 53) are currently accepted as primary treatment modalities for bleeding esophageal varices. When variceal hemorrhage is found to be the cause of bleeding by initial diagnostic endoscopy, the patient is best served if the endoscopist proceeds to definitive control of bleeding with ES or variceal banding.

Indications for ES are similar to those for banding and (1) actively bleeding varices, (2) nonbleeding varices with stigmata of bleeding (an erosion, clot, or red or brown elevations on the surface of the varix), and (3) nonbleeding varices without any other lesion or source of bleeding. Prophylactic ES in patients who have not yet experienced variceal hemorrhage is controversial. There are both positive and negative reports on this. In a recent meta-analysis of five studies, Imperiale et al. (2001) found prophylactic esophageal variceal banding to significantly reduce the rate of initial hemorrhage, and bleed-related mortality in comparison to controls. In Japan, prophylactic ES or variceal banding is standard procedure. Currently, we do not perform prophylactic ES. Prophylactic VB should be considered for selected patients with large nonbleeding esophageal varices who are not candidates for β-adrenergic blockers.

Sclerotherapy controls acute variceal bleeding in 75% to 95% of patients. Most clinical reports show that ES reduces recurrent bleeding from esophageal varices. Hospital mortality rates of 25% to 30% have been reported. There have been a few controlled studies indicating that ES of esophageal varices, compared with medical therapy, improves overall survival. Several prospective randomized controlled trials have compared VB with ES. In all studies, VB and ES were equally effective in controlling active bleeding, but complications were significantly lower with VB in all studies. Rebleeding rates and mortality rates in VB were lower in some studies. Some of the drawbacks of VB include a restricted endoscopic view, especially in patients wth endotracheal intubation, and blood pooling within the hood mechanism.

B. Contraindications

There are no contraindications to the use of ES in the acute phase of hemorrhage. Endoscopy should be performed after adequate resuscitation. In case of massive bleeding, we usually intubate the patient to prevent aspiration, which is relatively common in massively bleeding patients. With torrential bleeding, a

Blakemore or Minnesota tube may be necessary for 12 to 24 hours before attempting sclerotherapy. In patients with advanced liver disease and severe variceal hemorrhage it is reasonable to initiate therapy with intravenous octreotide (25–50 μg bolus, then 25–50 μg/h continuous infusion) on admission and continue for a few days. The majority of patients stop bleeding and urgent endoscopy can be performed safer and easier.

C. Technical Considerations

1. **Timing and preparation.** Perform ES at the earliest possible time in a patient's hospital course. ES can be done in the endoscopy examination room or in the intensive care unit. An expert endoscopist and a skilled assistant should be available, since emergency endoscopy requires the utmost skill and clinical judgment. Carefully monitor the bleeding patient during the procedure.
2. **Endoscopy.** Videoendoscopes are preferred for ES. The author uses a double-channel or large, single-channel videoendoscope for acute upper gastrointestinal bleeding, but switches to a single-channel endoscope for elective sclerotherapy or band ligation. The author does not use an overtube or balloon cuff to tamponade the injection site.
3. **Needle (injector).** Single-use disposable sclerotherapy injectors are available from several manufacturers. These provide a catheter or sheath with a 23- or 25-gauge needle capable of advancing 5 mm beyond the end of the catheter.
4. **Sclerosant.** Geography and operator preference determine the choice of sclerosant. In the United States, three effective sclerosing agents are available (Table 54.1).
5. **Volume of sclerosant.** The volume of sclerosant varies according to the type of sclerosant used, the number, size, and length of varices, and the presence of active bleeding. The average volume injected per puncture is 1 to 3 mL, although larger varices will require more volume. The total volume of solution injected during the first proce-

Table 54.1. Sclerosing agents available in the United States.

Sodium morrhuate	
Sodium tetradecyl sulfate	• 0.75–1.5% solution, or • 1% in combination with 33% ethanol and 0.3% normal saline
Ethanolamine oleate	• Used extensively in Europe and Japan • Most expensive agent • Author's sclerosant of choice

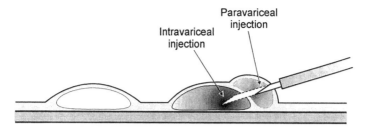

Figure 54.1. In intravariceal injection, the sclerosant is injected directly into the varix. In paravariceal injection, sclerosant is injected in the surrounding tissues.

dure varies from 10 to 20 mL, depending on the size and number of varices.

6. **Injection site.** The sclerosant may be injected into the varix (intravariceal) or in the tissue adjacent to the varix (paravariceal) (Fig. 54.1).

D. Technique of Variceal Injection

This section describes the technique of intravariceal injection. This is the method most commonly used.

1. **Pass the injection needle** through the biopsy channel of the endoscope and advance it into view.
   a. **Choose a target** for injection. Begin the injections at two or three points in each line of varices at 2- to 3-cm intervals, from just above the gastroesophageal junction up to the proximal esophagus. Successful obliteration of varices in the distal esophagus usually eliminates the proximal varices or at least decreases their size.
   b. **Advance the needle** out of the sheath and pass it directly into the lumen of the varix.
   c. In most cases, the injections are made in a direction tangential to the varix (Fig. 54.2).
   d. An assistant performs the injection while the endoscopist controls the position of the needle within the varix.
   e. The goal of the **intravariceal injection** is to introduce the sclerosant directly into the lumen of the varix, resulting in acute variceal thrombosis.

2. If a site of active variceal bleeding is seen, begin injections distally, continue proximally, and finally into and around the site until bleeding is controlled.

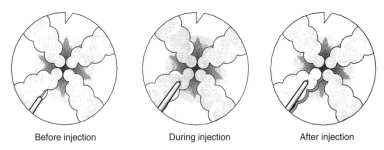

Before injection   During injection   After injection

Figure 54.2. The injections begin just above the gastroesophageal junction and progress up into the proximal esophagus.

    a.   Usually 6 to 9 mL of sclerosant are injected (2–3 mL for three or four injections).

    b.   Then inject the other varices.

    c.   The author injects sclerosant directly into the varices and removes the needle slowly while injecting to tamponade the injection site (Fig. 54.1).

3.   **Bleeding gastric varices** are difficult to treat endoscopically, and results are not as good as ES of esophageal varices. Injection of a large volume of sclerosant or bucrylate into gastric varices has been described. There are two types of gastric varix: junctional and fundics.

    a.   **Junctional varices** are gastric varices seen as an extension of esophageal varices and without extension into the fundus. These are treated with standard intravariceal sclerotherapy from the proximal, connecting, esophageal varices.

    b.   **Fundic varices** are gastric varices confined to the fundus, with channels extending distally to the gastroesophageal junction.

        i.   In patients with fundic varices, the author performs sclerotherapy only on varices that are bleeding or have stigmata of bleeding, using the retroflexed view. The author's preference is to inject 2 mL of sclerosant into the varices, with a total of 6 mL to 9 mL of 5% **ethanolamine oleate**.

       ii.   **Cyanoacrylate** has been used for the control of gastric variceal hemorrhage. Either isobutyl-2 or N-butylcyanoacrylate is mixed with Lipiodol and injected directly into the varices, producing a virtual acrylic cast of the varices. It appears to be quite effective, but major concerns include the lack of a licensed, deliverable agent and the potential for endoscopic damage.

    c.   **Control of gastric pH** with high-volume continuous intravenous infusion of H_2 blockers or oral omeprazole (20–40 mg every 12 hours) has been recommended to decrease the risk of bleeding from injection site erosions.

E. Injection Schedule and Timing of Therapy

After successful initial hemostasis by ES or VB, ES or VB is repeated during hospitalization. Number and intervals of injections for obliteration of varices differ according to the sclerosant and injection methods. The author injects two to four times electively, in 2- to 3-day intervals during hospitalization and repeats at 6- to 8-week intervals until the varices are believed to be obliterated. On average it takes three to four sessions to achieve obliteration of the bulk of varices.

Repeat outpatient sclerotherapy is necessary every 2 to 6 months to prevent rebleeding from residual or new varices. If bleeding vessels or varices are still apparent during follow-up examination, we usually perform ES, since it is difficult to treat these vessels by VB because scarring decreases the compliance of the wall, which in turn will result in inability to fully suction mucosa into the ligating cylinder. For the most part, recurrent bleeding is not as severe as the initial episode and can be controlled by repeat ES. Compliance with follow-up therapy and abstinence from alcohol abuse improve the prognosis. Patients who adhere to these recommendations but still have progressive liver failure may benefit from liver transplantation.

F. Complications

The complication rate is reported to be from 12% to 50%. Complications may be divided into major and minor ones. **Major complications** are severe bleeding, perforations, mediastinitis, adult respiratory distress syndrome, sepsis, and stricture formation. Major complications occur in about 2% to 3% of patients. Among the **minor complications** are fever, transient chest pain, odynophagia, and pleural effusion, which are usually transient and inconsequential. Esophageal ulcers are commonly seen a few days after injection and usually heal spontaneously.

G. Selected References

D'Amico G, Pagliaro L, Bosch J. The treatment of portal hypertension: a meta-analytic review. Hepatology 1995;22:332–355.

Fardy JM, Laupacis A. A meta-analysis of prophylactic endoscopic sclerotherapy for esophageal varices. Am J Gastroenterol 1994;89:1938–1948.

Grace ND, Diagnosis and Treatment of Gastrointestinal Bleeding Secondary to Portal Hypertension. The American Journal of Gastroenterology 1997;92: 1081–1091.

Imperiale TF, Chalasani N. A meta-analysis of endoscopic variceal ligation for primary prophylaxis of esophageal variceal bleeding. Hepatology 2001;33:802–807.

Kitano S, Iso Y, Koyanagi N, et al. Ethanolamine oleate is superior to polidocanol (Athoxysklerol) for endoscopic injection sclerotherapy of esophageal varices: a prospective randomized trial. Hepatogastroenterology 1987;34:19–23.

Knechtle SJ, Rikkers LF. Current management of esophageal variceal bleeding. Adv Surg 1999;33:439–459.

Lo GH, Lai KH, Cheng JS, et al. Emergency banding ligation versus sclerotherapy for the control of active bleeding from esophageal varices. Hepatology 1997;25(5):1101–1104.

Luketic VA, Sanyal AJ, Esophageal varices. I. Clinical presentation, medical therapy, and endoscopic therapy. Gastroenterol Clin North Am 2000;29:337–384.

Lyons SD, Sugawa C, Geller EF, Vandenberg DM. Comparison of 1% sodium tetradecyl sulfate to a thrombogenic sclerosant cocktail for endoscopic sclerotherapy. Am Surg 1988;54:81–84.

McKee RE, Garden OJ, Anderson JR, Carter DC. A trial of elective versus on-demand sclerotherapy in "poor risk" patients with variceal hemorrhage. Endoscopy 1994; 26:474–477.

Nakamura R, Bucci LA, Sugawa C, et al. Sclerotherapy of bleeding esophageal varices using a thrombogenic cocktail. Am Surg 1991;57:226–230.

Roberts LR, Kamath PS. Pathophysiology and treatment of variceal hemorrhage. Mayo Clin Proc 1996;71:973–983.

Sugawa C, Okumura Y, Lucas CE, Walt AJ. Endoscopic sclerosis of experimental oesophageal varices in dogs. Gastrointest Endosc 1978;24:114–116.

Sugawa C, Steffes CP, Nakamura R, et al. Upper GI bleeding in an urban hospital. Ann Surg 1990;212:521–527.

Veterans Affairs Cooperative Variceal Sclerotherapy Group. Sclerotherapy for male alcoholic cirrhotic patients who have bled from esophageal varices: results of a randomized, multicenter trial. Hepatology 1994;20:618–625.

55. Control of Nonvariceal Upper Gastrointestinal Bleeding

Choichi Sugawa, M.D.

A. Introduction

Early endoscopy has an important role in the evaluation and treatment of the patient with upper gastrointestinal bleeding. Definition of the precise appearance of the lesions by endoscopy gives important information about the prognosis, risk of rebleeding, and indications for surgery. There are several effective endoscopic modalities for the control of bleeding. This chapter describes several techniques currently used for endoscopic management of nonvariceal upper gastrointestinal bleeding.

B. Diagnosis

Although individual series vary, peptic ulceration generally is the most common cause of upper gastrointestinal bleeding, followed by acute erosive gastritis, esophageal varices, and Mallory-Weiss tears. Other sources include esophagitis, tumors, vascular malformations, and gastric varices. Before endoscopic hemostasis can be achieved, the exact sites of bleeding must be accurately identified and the visual field must be clear. Endoscopic hemostasis should be attempted only under the following circumstances: the precise bleeding site can be visualized, hemostatic devices can be accurately placed near the bleeding vessels, and hemorrhage is not torrential.

C. Indications

The strongest endoscopic predictor of persistent or recurrent bleeding is ongoing active bleeding at the time of endoscopy. The presence of a discrete protuberance within the ulcer crater is important. This is referred to as a "visible vessel" or "sentinel clot" (Fig. 55.1). Some pigmented protuberances (e.g., red, blue, purple) imply a high risk of rebleeding.

Indications for hemostasis include active bleeding from a peptic ulcer or ulcers with a sentinel clot. Mallory-Weiss tears, acute gastric mucosal lesions, and esophagitis usually cause only minor bleeding. If severe bleeding does occur in these lesions, there will be a discrete ulcer with either an arterial bleeder or

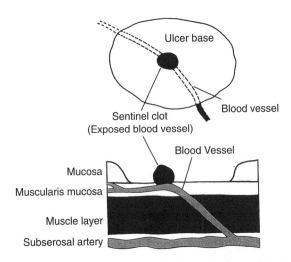

Figure 55.1. A visible vessel or sentinel clot on the base of the ulcer.

a sentinel clot. Multiple clinical and endoscopic risk factors can be used to predict the occurrence of continued or recurrent bleeding (Table 55.1).

Patients with high clinical and endoscopic risk factors need clinical intervention to control upper gastrointestinal hemorrhage, while patients with no risk factors can be treated as outpatients or triaged to early discharge.

Table 55.1. Clinical and endoscopic risk factors for continued or recurrent bleeding.

Clinical risk factors
    Patient history
        Age >60 years
    Coexistent major organ system disease
        In-hospital onset
        Admission hemoglobin <8.0
    Other clinical criteria
        Shock (systolic blood pressure <90)
        Transfusion requirements >5 U packed erythrocytes
        Coagulopathy

Endoscopic risk factors
    Endoscopic appearance
        Torrential hemorrhage
        Ulcer location in posterior bulb or high on lesser curvature
        Active spurting or oozing from base
        Pigmented protuberance (visible vessel)
        Adherent clot
    Doppler-positive lesion

Many terms have been used to describe mucosal and submucosal vascular lesions: telangiectasia, arteriovenous malformation, and angiodysplasia. Endoscopic distinction of these three lesions is seldom possible. Endoscopic treatment should aim at the submucosal level and avoid full-thickness burn. A small lesion can be easily treated directly by endoscopic hemostasis. With a larger lesion, treatment proceeds from the periphery to the center of the lesion.

D. Methods and Results

Several modalities are available for endoscopic control of hemorrhage. These include thermal devices (including electrocautery), injection therapy, clips, and other methods described here. The author has employed a variety of methods, but, because of laboratory and clinical experience, currently favors the use of epinephrine injection, heater probe, and multiple coagulation, sometimes in combination with epinephrine and a thermal modality.

1. **Thermal therapy.** Thermal devices are among the most commonly employed and effective. Localized heating causes tissue edema, shrinkage, protein denaturation, contraction of blood vessels, and tissue desiccation to achieve hemostasis.

    a. **Heater probe.** This device is preferable because of cost and portability, in addition to effectiveness. Probes are available in diameters of 3.2 and 2.4 mm. They are designed to allow the simultaneous application of heat and pressure (coaptive coagulation) (Fig. 55.2).

        i. Apply the heater probe to the bleeding vessel with firm pressure. The objective is to coapt the vessel walls (Fig. 55.3). The large-diameter probe (3.2 mm) is more effective.

        ii. When the vessel is occluded by pressure, apply three to four sequential pulses of 30 J each in tandem for a total of 120 J, with no cooling period between pulses.

        iii. Recommended techniques for heater probe hemostasis for different types of bleeding lesions are shown in Table 55.2. Fewer joules and total pulses are recommended for Dieulafoy's disease, Mallory-Weiss tears, and gastrointestinal angiomas.

    b. **Bicap (multipolar) endoscopic probe.** This electrocoagulation device has equally spaced microelectrodes along the side and over the tip, and can contact the bleeding lesion from any direction. The power unit incorporates a water pump, allowing water irrigation of the target area intermittently or constantly. Bipolar probes produce less damage compared with monopolar electrocoagulation or yttrium-aluminum-garnet (YAG) lasers.

        i. Press the probe against the bleeding site to find the precise point that tamponades bleeding.

        ii. When the exposed bleeding artery (sentinel clot with bleeding) is demonstrably occluded by pressure, apply heat to seal the vessel (Fig. 55.3).

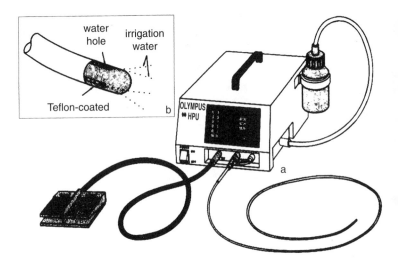

Figure 55.2. Heater probe power unit with foot pedal and large probe (Olympus Corp. Tokyo). Irrigation from the tip of the heater probe. Simultaneous tamponade and washing of a bleeding arterial lesion are feasible with the heater probe.

iii.   The optimal technique for bipolar electrocoagulation should include the use of the large (3.2-mm) probe, positioning of the tip of the endoscope en face as close as possible to the bleeding lesion, lower watt settings of 3 to 5 (i.e., 15–25 W), and prolonged periods of coagulation.

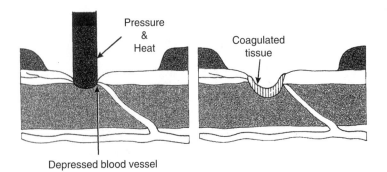

Figure 55.3. Simultaneous application of heat and pressure (coaptive coagulation).

Table 55.2. Techniques for heater probe hemostasis.

Lesion	Tamponade pressure	Setting (Js)	Pulses/ tamponade station	Site of hemostasis
Chronic peptic ulcer*	Very firm	30	4	Only on visible vessel
Acute ulcer or Dieulafoy's disease**	Firm	25	3	Only on bleeding point
Mallory-Weiss tear**	Moderate	20	2–3	Only on bleeding point
Gastrointestinal angiomas***	Gentle	10	1–2	Entire angioma

*Treatment of visible vessel (either actively bleeding or nonbleeding) only is recommended.
**Treatment of actively bleeding lesions only.
***For treatment of all angiomas in the bowel segment causing GI bleeding.
Source: Jensen (1992).

      iv. Multiple 2-second pulses given in rapid succession appear to be as effective as a single, long pulse of identical duration.

    c. **Laser photocoagulation.** The intense monochrome light energy produced by a laser can be directed through safe flexible light guides and effectively coagulate tissue. Currently there are two lasers suitable for endoscopic therapy: the neodymium:YAG (Nd:YAG) laser and the argon laser.

      i. The standard recommendation for use of the Nd:YAG laser is 80 W of energy over 0.5-second pulses from a distance of 1 cm.

      ii. Begin laser therapy at least 2 to 3 mm away from the visible arterial segment.

      iii. Depending on the distance (e.g., 0.5 cm), a lower and shorter setting may be required.

      iv. The control trials of ulcer hemostasis generally suggest that laser photocoagulation is effective treatment for both actively bleeding and nonbleeding visible vessels. The lasers are not portable, are extremely costly, and require a high level of training for both laser endoscopist and technician.

  2. **Injection therapy.** Injection sclerotherapy of esophageal varices has been shown to be relatively safe and effective in the control of bleeding esophageal varices (see Chapter 53). This technique has been expanded to include nonvariceal bleeding lesions. Injection therapy is simple, inexpensive, and readily available, and can be performed at the

time of diagnostic endoscopy. Injection therapy with saline or water provides effective hemostasis mainly by tamponade. Several other agents have been used.

a. **Epinephrine (1 : 10,000).** Epinephrine injection is more effective for immediate hemostasis and preferable to ethanol injection because of greater overall effectiveness, ease, and lessened tissue damage.

    i. This solution is made by mixing 1 mL of epinephrine (1 : 1,000) with 9 mL of normal saline (0.9%).

    ii. The total volume used ranges from 5 to 20 mL, with a larger volume used to stop spurting vessels.

    iii. Inject this solution directly around the blood vessel in three or four increments (Figs. 55.4 and 55.5).

    iv. Recent controlled studies concluded that endoscopic epinephrine injection was effective in stopping bleeding, and decreased the transfusion requirement and the need for emergency surgery. No complications were reported.

b. **Absolute ethanol**

    i. The total dose of 0.6 to 1.2 mL of 98% dehydrated ethanol (Abbott Laboratories) is injected through a 1-mL disposable plastic tuberculin syringe in amounts of 0.1 to 0.2 mL per injection.

    ii. Inject this solution at three or four sites surrounding the bleeding vessel, and 1 or 2 mm from the vessel, causing thrombosis, to dehydrate and fix the blood vessel (Figs. 55.4 and 55.5).

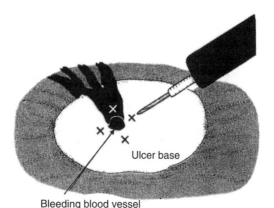

Ulcer base

Bleeding blood vessel

✕ Injection site

Figure 55.4. Epinephrine or ethanol is injected around and into the bleeding point at the base of the ulcer.

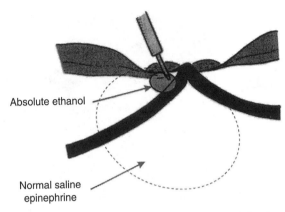

Figure 55.5. The principle of the hemostatic effect of epinephrine (tamponade) and ethanol (dehydration and fixation of tissue).

       iii. Permanent hemostasis with absolute ethanol injection reportedly has a success rate of greater than 90%. Ethanol injection is technically more difficult, as it calls for precise injection in small volumes.

   c. **Epinephrine followed by other sclerosing agents or thermal therapy**

       i. Epinephrine (1:10,000, 5–20 mL) is injected submucosally directly around the blood vessel to obtain initial hemostasis by compression and vasoconstriction.

       ii. To achieve definitive hemostasis by obliterating the vessel, 5 mL of 1% polidocanol or multipolar electrocoagulation or heater probe is applied into the blood vessel after initial injection of the epinephrine solution.

       iii. Research shows that application of further therapy after initial injection therapy improves the hemostatic results. Combination therapy with injection (typically with epinephrine 1:10,000) followed by bicap or heater probe therapy is now the method generally used to control upper gastrointestinal bleeding in the United States. The Injector Gold Probe (Microvasive Corp.) allows for both injection and cautery using a single injector-probe.

3. **Other therapies.** Many other forms of endoscopic therapy have been assessed for the treatment of bleeding ulcers.

   a. **Metallic clip** (hemoclip). Hemoclips (miniature metal clips) can be applied to bleeding vessels by a special flexible slip applicator through the biopsy channel of an endoscope. With recent improvements in the clip and applicator, this technique is easier to perform. It is very popular in Japan, where good results are

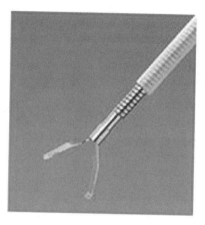

Figure 55.6. The Quick clip (Olympus, Tokyo) miniature metallic clip.

reported. Recently, a new disposable hemoclip has been available
with a redesigned delivery device (Fig. 55.6). It is an easy to use
a preloaded device (Quickclip, Olympus Corp.) Recent studies
that have compared the hemoclips to other techniques of controlling upper gastrointestinal bleeding have reported improved
outcomes with hemoclips.

b.   **Argon plasma coagulator.** Activated argon gas is currently
used by surgeons to promote hemostasis on the surface of the
diaphragm or the liver. Inert argon gas is delivered into the intestinal lumen through a small catheter in the biopsy channel of the
endoscope. Once the wire at the tip of the catheter is activated,
the argon gas becomes electrically energized, and an electric
spark is formed from the tip of the sheath to the intestinal wall.
This is a noncontact thermal modality. The argon plasma coagulator is an excellent modality to stop bleeding from superficial
lesions such as radiation proctitis, vascular malformations,
polypectomy-induced bleeding, and bleeding cancer.

E. Complications

Complications include perforation, induced acute hemorrhage, and delayed
hemorrhage. The incidence of perforation from endoscopic hemostasis has been
low, with rates of 1% to 2% commonly quoted. Induced bleeding can occur more
commonly during thermal therapy than during injection therapy. To prevent ulceration caused by the endoscopic therapy itself, it is desirable to limit the area and
depth of treatment as much as possible in clinical applications (see Chapter 58).

F. Selected References

Chung SCS, Lau JYW, Sung JJY, et al. A randomized comparison between adrenaline injection alone and adrenaline injection plus heat probe treatment for actively bleeding ulcers. Br Med J 1997;314:1307–1311.

Cooper GS, Chak A, Way LE, et al. Early endoscopy in upper gastrointestinal hemorrhage: associations with recurrent bleeding, surgery, and length of hospital stay. Gastrointest Endosc 1999;49:45–152.

Haber G, Dorais J, DuVall A, et al. Argon plasma coagulation: a new effective technique of noncontact thermal coagulation. Experience in 44 cases of GI angiomata. Gastrointest Endosc 1996;43:293.

Jensen DM. Endoscopic coagulation therapy. Part A: Heater probe. In: Sugawa C, Schuman BM, Lucas CE, eds. Gastroinstestinal Bleeding. New York: Igaku-Shoin, 1992; 298–313.

Laine L, Peterson WL Bleeding peptic ulcer. N Engl J Med 1994;331:717–727.

Lin HJ, Tseng GY, Perng CL, et al. Comparison of adrenaline injection and bipolar electrocoagulation for the arrest of peptic ulcer bleeding. Gut 1999;44:715–719.

Raju GS, Gajula L. Endoclips for GI endoscopy. Gastrointest Endosc 2004;59(2):267–279.

Soehendra N, Sriram PVJ, Ponchon T, Chung SCS. Hemostatic clip in gastrointestinal bleeding. Endoscopy 2001;33(2):172–180.

Steffes CP, Sugawa C. Endoscopic management of nonvariceal gastrointestinal bleeding. World J Surg 1992;16:1025–1033.

Sugawa C. Injection therapy for the control of bleeding ulcers. Gastrointest Endosc 1990;36:S50–S52.

Sugawa C, Fujita Y, Ikeda T, Walt AJ. Endoscopic hemostasis of bleeding of the upper gastrointestinal tract by local injection of ninety eight percent dehydrated ethanol. Surg Gynecol Obstet 1986;162:159–163.

Sugawa C, Steffes CP, Nakamura R, et al. Upper GI bleeding in an urban hospital. Ann Surg 1990;212:521–527.

56. Endoluminal Approaches to Gastroesophageal Reflux Disease

John D. Mellinger, M.D., F.A.C.S.
Bruce V. MacFadyen, Jr., M.D., F.A.C.S.

A. Indications

The indications for endoluminal treatments for gastroesophageal reflux disease (GERD) are similar to those for laparoscopic antireflux surgical procedures, with some added restrictions with regard to disease severity. Patients with documented pathologic reflux disease requiring ongoing therapy with proton pump inhibitors may be candidates for endoluminal therapy, particularly if they have incomplete control of symptoms on medication or are unwilling to continue long-term pharmaceutical management. In general, patients with complicated reflux disease, including Barrett's esophagus, erosive esophagitis, reflux associated stricture or dysphagia, and patients with large (≥2 cm) hiatal hernia, are considered more appropriate for surgical intervention. For some techniques, documentation of a modicum of residual pretreatment lower esophageal sphincter pressure (≥8 mm Hg) has also been advised.

Of the currently available endoluminal techniques, which broadly include radiofrequency induction of localized thermal injury, endoscopic suturing, and endoscopic submucosal injection/implantation, the radiofrequency technique (Stretta, Curon Medical, Sunnyvale, CA) has been most widely studied and applied, and is approved by the U.S. Food and Drug Administration (FDA). For this reason it will be the primary procedure herein discussed; other modalities being developed and studied are briefly reviewed at the end of this chapter.

B. Patient Preparation

1. Patients should be thoroughly evaluated prior to considering endoluminal therapy. Workup should include esophagogastroduodenoscopy (EGD) with biopsy, esophageal manometry, and 24-hour pH monitoring. Selective use of additional tests appropriate in the evaluation of GERD in select settings, including gastric emptying studies, contrast radiography, and evaluations to exclude nonforegut sources for symptomatology may also be necessary. Indications and contraindications as outlined should generally be followed in determining

whether a given patient is a suitable candidate for endoluminal treatment.

2. Informed consent discussion should include a detailed discussion of treatment options including lifesyle modification measures, continued pharmacologic management, and surgical treatment. Risks that should be reviewed would include esophageal or gastric perforation, bleeding, and complications of conscious sedation, which is required for a longer period with this procedure than for typical EGD. Complication rates of 0.15% to 0.6%, with mortality rates of 0.07%, are reported (the latter comprising two mortalities related to aspiration pneumonia described in early experience prior to organized clinical trials). Patients should also be apprised that while adverse long-term side effects are not reported, available follow-up in treated patients is less than 5 years, and on the order of 1 to 2 years in most published series. Finally, the practitioner's own level of experience with the procedure should be discussed openly with the patient.

3. NPO status for 8 hours prior to the procedure should be observed. Patients are generally treated on an outpatient basis. Intravenous catheters should be placed for administration of the agents chosen for conscious sedation, and standard monitoring techniques including electrocandiography, blood pressure, and pulse oximetry monitoring should be employed.

C. Stretta Technique

1. Patients are positioned in the left lateral decubitus position, as for EGD. Intravenous sedation is titrated to patient comfort. Because it is important for the patient to remain still through what amounts to a 45-minute procedure, deeper sedation and more frequent retitration of medication may be required than for standard EGD.

2. Diagnostic EGD is performed to delineate the distance of the squamocolumnar junction from the incisors. If contraindications to the procedure missed on prior EGD are identified such as enumerated earlier, the procedure is terminated. Otherwise, a guidewire is left in place in the gastric antrum as the endoscope is withdrawn. The Stretta catheter is introduced over the guidewire and positioned 1 cm above the squamocolumnar junction as dictated by the prior endoscopic measurement. The balloon on the catheter (30-French [Fr] size with balloon inflatable to maximum size 90 Fr, Fig. 56.1) is partially inflated to 2.5 psi, and four 22-gauge, 5.5-mm-length nickel-titanium electrodes are deployed. The needles are initially fully deployed to allow mucosal penetration and then partially retracted using a predetermined setting on the device.

Radiofrequency current (465 kHz) is then delivered by a generator with continuous mucosal cooling with nonconductive chilled water. Continuous feedback monitoring of the temperature of the tissue at the electrode tip, as well as impedance and mucosal temperature, is employed. If the mucosal temperature exceeds 50°C, the tip of the needle (muscle temperature) exceeds 100°C, or the impedance exceeds 100 ohms, the generator automatically shuts off power to that

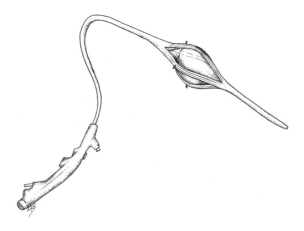

Figure 56.1. Stretta balloon catheter device.

particular needle. The treatment is continued for 90 seconds, after which the needles are withdrawn, the catheter rotated 45 degrees at the same depth of insertion from the incisors, and the needles redeployed for another 90 seconds of treatment to create a ring of 8 lesions at that particular location.

The catheter is then moved distally in 5-mm increments to create three more rings of 8 lesions each in similar fashion. After the creation of these 4 rings of treatment, the catheter is advanced distally into the stomach and inflated with 25 cm^3 of air, after which it is withdrawn until gentle resistance is felt at the level of the gastroesophageal junction (Fig. 56.2). The needles are deployed and 90-second treatments performed as described above.

The treatment is repeated at this level twice, rotating the catheter 30 degrees to the right and then to the left from the original position. A second pullback or retrograde treatment is done with the balloon inflated with 22 cm^3 of air. Thus a total of 6 rings are created, with 8 antegrade and 6 retrograde 90-second treatment periods across the region of the squamocolumnar junction (Fig. 56.3). Repeat endoscopy is done at the completion of the procedure to assess the appearance of the mucosa and junction. Total treatment time in the range of 45 minutes is typical.

3. Following the procedure, patients are recovered in normal fashion and discharged if stable by the usual postendoscopic criteria. Effects of the procedure are not immediate, and antisecretory medications are continued for 3 weeks following the procedure and then gradually weaned off. Patients are advised to avoid nasogastric tube placement or any unguided esophageal entubation for the first month after the procedure because of an anecdotal report of perforation possibly related to tube placement in the first month after a Stretta procedure. No dietary restrictions are advised.

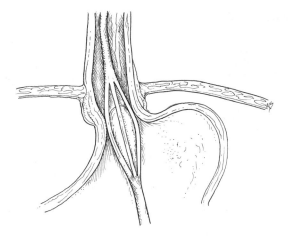

Figure 56.2. Catheter positioned appropriately.

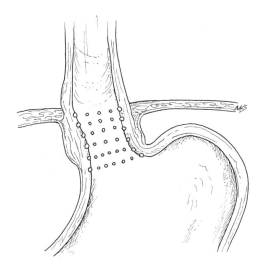

Figure 56.3. Desired pattern of radiofrequency lesions.

D. Outcomes

1. Described significant complications were outlined in Section B.2 in connection with informed consent. The FDA public database has shown a decreasing complication rate with increasing procedural experience nationally over the years 2000 to 2002.

2. Overall, studies have demonstrated that in properly selected patients, one can anticipate statistically significant improvement in GERD symptom and quality-of-life indices, diminished pharmacologic requirements, and decreased esophageal acid exposure as assessed by 24-hour pH monitoring after the procedure. A randomized, blinded, sham-controlled trial has shown that symptom score improvement is statistically significant within 6 months, continues to improve with 12-month follow-up, and that patients who cross over to the treatment arm accrue similar benefit after failing sham therapy. Follow-up available out to almost 3 years suggests that patients who benefit from the procedure continue to do so over time. Approximately two thirds of patients note relief of GERD symptoms within 2 months of the procedure, and approximately 90% note improvement at one-year follow-up. Less than 10% note no improvement following treatment.

3. It appears that at least part of the mechanism of action, in addition to effects on lower esophageal sphincter (LES) compliance, may be a dercrease in the number of transient LES relaxations after therapy; it is hypothesized that this may be due to partial denervation of the LES posttreatment.

E. Other Endoluminal Therapies

1. Endoscopic suturing techniques have been shown to decrease regurgitation symptoms and, perhaps somewhat less reliably, medication requirements. These treatments are technically more challenging and are done with overtube assistance. The technique takes over an hour to perform, and results to date do not appear to be as consistent as what has been described with radiofrequency treatment. The most common technique involves the use of an appliance placed on the end of the endoscope into which tissue is suctioned to allow suture purchase. After obtaining two such purchases, the endoscope is used as a knot pusher to secure the knot. Suture placement in longitudinal fashion along the lesser curve and placement circumferentially at the cardia appear to be of comparable efficacy.

Newer devices are being developed and tested that employ other techniques to minimize the challenge of suture tying, including the use of pledgets, T-fasteners, and mucosal retracting devices to facilitate adequate suture purchase.

2. Implantation via submucosal injection of inert substances for LES augmentation is yet another endoluminal therapy being evaluated. Historically, collagen was first tested for this purpose. More recent techniques involve the use

of inert biopolymers, polymethylmethacrylate microspheres, and an expanding submucosal hydrogel prosthesis. These techniques are technically the easiest of the current endoluminal therapies to apply, but further evaluation with regard to efficacy is needed before their potential utility can be defined.

F. Summary

Endoluminal approaches to GERD are in their infancy. To date, the radio-frequency approach has been best attested and evaluated. Injection techniques appear to be the simplest and least costly, whereas suturing techniques as currently available are technically the most demanding. All these techniques are being applied primarily in patients with disease that is medically manageable and are not advised for patients with more severe forms of GERD. The ideal technique would be applicable to patients with more advanced disease, and inexpensive, as well as readily learned and applied by practitioners, it would not alter the gastroesophageal junction in a way that hampered future surgical intervention, if required. It is likely that further development and eventual consensus will evolve with further study of these techniques and others perhaps yet to be developed.

G. Selected References

Corley DA, Katz P, Wo J, et al. Temperature controlled radiofrequency energy delivery to the gastroesophageal junction for the treatment of GERD (the Stretta procedure): a randomized, double-blind, sham-controlled, multi-center clinical trial. Gastrointest Endosc 2002;55:AB19.

Filipi CJ, Lehman GA, Rothstein RI. Transoral, flexible endoscopic suturing for treatment of GERD: a multicenter trial. Gastrointest Endosc 2001;53:416–422.

Lehman G. Endoscopic and endoluminal techniques for the control of gastroesophageal reflux: are they ready for widespread clinical application? Gastrointest Endosc 2000;52:808–811.

Swain P, Park P-O, Kjellin T, et al. Endoscopic gastroplasty for gastroesophageal reflux disease. Gastrointest Endosc 2000;51:AB144.

Triadafilopoulos G, Dibiase JK, Nostrant TT. The Stretta procedure for the treatment of GERD: 6 and 12 month follow up of the U.S. open label trial. Gastrointest Endosc 2002;55:149–156.

Triadafilopoulos G, Dibiase IK, Nostrant TT. Radiofrequency energy delivery to the gastroesophageal junction for the treatment of gastroesophageal reflux disease. Gastrointest Endosc 2001;53:407–415.

Wolfsen HC, Richards WO. The Stretta procedure for the treatment of GERD: a registry of 558 patients. J Laparosc Adv Surg Techniques 2002;12:395–402.

57. Percutaneous Endoscopic Feeding Tube Placement

Bipan Chand, M.D.
Carol E.H. Scott-Conner, M.D., F.A.C.S.
Jeffrey L. Ponsky, M.D., F.A.C.S.

A. Indications

Gastrostomy is indicated as a route for enteral feedings in patients with functioning gastrointestinal tracts who are unable to take oral nutrition. Gastrostomy may be indicated in patients with stroke, dementia, progressive neurological processes, severe psychomotor retardation, tumors of the upper aerodigestive tract, or severe facial trauma. Patients should demonstrate potential for extended survival with adequate nutrition. Critically ill patients with a low probability of survival are not appropriate candidates for percutaneous endoscopic gastrostomy (PEG) or other invasive methods of feeding tube placement. When the patient's status is uncertain, begin feedings via a nasoenteric feeding tube and continue this until it is likely that the patient will tolerate an invasive procedure and demonstrates a potential for extended survival.

Three basic routes for gastrostomy creation are now available: traditional surgical gastrostomy, laparoscopic gastrostomy (see Chapter 24, Laparoscopic Gastrostomy), and percutaneous endoscopic gastrostomy. There are advantages and disadvantages to each method (Table 57.1).

Two methods of PEG placement (the "push" and "pull" techniques) are in current use and will be described here. A simple modification allows placement of a feeding tube in the jejunum and will be considered in Section D.

B. The "Push" Technique for PEG Placement

The "push" method utilizes the Seldinger technique to place a Foley catheter in the stomach under endoscopic guidance. The Foley catheter balloon must remain inflated to maintain tube position. Dislodgment of the tube may result if the balloon is inadvertently deflated. The advantage of this method is that the endoscope need be passed just once. Ease of tube dislodgment is a major disadvantage, and the authors prefer the "pull" technique for this reason. Kits are available for each method.

1. Two trained individuals are needed: one to perform the upper gastrointestinal endoscopy and the second to perform the PEG insertion.

Table 57.1. Advantages and disadvantages of methods of gastrostomy formation.

Method	Advantages	Disadvantages
Surgical gastrostomy	• Secure fixation of stomach to anterior abdominal wall • Permanent tract may be created	• Requires laparotomy • May require general anesthesia
Laparoscopic gastrostomy	• Less invasive • May achieve secure fixation of stomach to abdominal wall • Visual selection of site of entry onto stomach	• Requires laparoscopic access • May require general anesthesia
PEG	• May be performed under local anesthesia • May be done in the endoscopy suite • Single puncture, no incision	• Requires patent upper gastrointestinal tract • Early dislodgment of tube may require laparotomy • Potential for injury to adjacent viscera unless technique carefully followed

Videoendoscopy allows all members of the team to visualize the procedure.

2. Place the patient on the endoscopy table in the supine position.
3. Prepare the upper abdomen in the usual fashion.
4. Topical anesthesia of the oropharynx may be supplemented with intravenous sedation to allow endoscopy. Local anesthesia will be infiltrated at the PEG site.
5. Introduce the endoscope into the stomach, perform a careful examination, and fully inflate the stomach.
6. Maneuver the endoscope so that its light is seen through the anterior abdominal wall. It may be necessary to turn off the room lights and use the X-illumination function of the videoendoscope to see this. Choose a point on the upper abdomen where the transillumination is easily seen. This transillumination indicates that the inflated stomach is closely apposed to the anterior abdominal wall without intervening tissue or viscera (e.g., the colon). The site will generally be just proximal to the incisura.
7. Gently depress the abdominal wall at the selected site. The endoscopist should easily see the wall indent (Fig. 57.1).

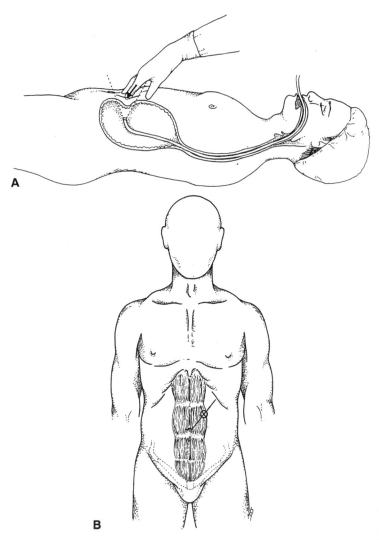

Figure 57.1. A. Transillumination and finger depression of the abdominal wall confirm juxtaposition of the inflated stomach and the anterior abdominal wall. B. The site selected will generally be approximately halfway between costal margin and umbilicus.

8. Next, use the Safe-tract method to confirm that no intervening bowel lies between the stomach and the anterior abdominal wall. This method utilizes the needle, syringe, and local anesthetic in the kit. Use the needle and syringe and pass it through the selected site while maintaining negative pressure. The endoscopist should see the needle enter the stomach at the same instance the assistant sees air within the syringe. If air is seen prior to entry into the stomach, the needle has passed through another lumen (most likely the colon). Once confirmation that no other bowel is between the stomach and abdominal wall, infiltrate the selected site with local anesthesia.

9. Use an 11 blade to make a skin incision 3 to 4 mm in length (large enough for easy passage of the catheter).

10. Remove the needle, guidewire, dilator, and sheath from the kit. Confirm that the Foley catheter passes easily through the sheath. Test the balloon of the Foley catheter.

11. Thrust the needle through anterior abdominal wall and well into the stomach and confirm this by endoscopic visualization.

12. Pass the guidewire through the needle and remove the needle.

13. Pass the dilator over the guidewire, followed by the sheath. Firm but gentle pressure and a twisting motion facilitate their passage. The technique is the same as that used for percutaneous insertion of venous catheters. Endoscopic visualization confirms passage of needle, wire, dilator, and finally the sheath into the stomach.

14. Occasionally the dilator or sheath will tent up the mucosa of the stomach rather than entering the stomach. The endoscopist can apply counterpressure with the closed tip of a biopsy forceps, or increase the insufflation of the stomach. The sheath must fully enter the stomach.

15. Lubricate the Foley catheter and slide it into the stomach through the sheath. Peel away the sheath and remove it. Inflate the balloon of the Foley catheter. Pull the catheter back until the stomach is just barely indented by pressure of the balloon and secure the catheter in place. Too much tension on the catheter may lead to pressure necrosis of the gastric wall; too little may allow leakage around the tube.

C. The "Pull" Technique for PEG Placement

1. Prepare the patient and select a site for PEG placement as described in Section B, items 1 to 8. Again use transillumination, finger indentation, and most importantly the Safe-tract technique to obtain proper location.

2. Make the skin incision a bit longer, generally around 1 cm in length. This appears to decrease the incidence of infection around the tube

site, as the tube will be pulled through mouth, esophagus, and stomach before exiting the skin.

3. The endoscopist should position an open polypectomy snare against the anterior stomach wall at the expected entry site.

4. Take the needle, braided suture, and catheter from the kit and confirm that all are in good working condition. The needle may have a short sheath over it.

5. Thrust the needle through the small skin incision and into the stomach. The needle should enter the stomach through the polypectomy snare. If the snare does not encircle the needle at this point, allow the endoscopist to reposition the snare. If the needle carries a sheath, confirm that the sheath has entered the stomach and withdraw the needle.

6. Look carefully at the braided suture and note that one end is doubled back upon itself, essentially sharply folded on itself. Insert this end through the needle (or sheath) and into the stomach.

7. Withdraw the needle. Allow the endoscopist to lasso the braided suture. The endoscopist should tighten the snare and withdraw endoscope, snare, and braided suture out through the patient's mouth (Fig. 57.2). Maintain control of the end of the braided suture so that it is not pulled completely into the stomach. The braided suture will generally have a knot or metal clip as a safeguard.

8. The PEG catheter is then handed off to the endoscopist. The PEG catheter has a tapered end that terminates in a suture loop. The endoscopist passes one loop through the other in such a fashion that the PEG catheter is securely fastened to the braided suture. The endoscopist then uses the snare to hold the flange of the PEG, allowing the endoscope to follow the PEG into the stomach. The catheter is generously lubricated with water-soluble lubricant.

9. Gently but firmly pull the braided suture back through the abdominal wall. The PEG catheter and endoscope will follow (Fig. 57.3). Stop and open the snare, releasing the flange, at the 20-cm mark on the endoscope. Remove the snare from the biopsy channel and continue to follow the PEG with the endoscope into the stomach. This technique allows the endoscope to gain reentry into the esophagus without difficulty.

10. After the tapered portion has exited the anterior abdominal wall, the rubber tube of the catheter will be seen. Some catheters have marks or are otherwise identifiable. Continue to pull gently but firmly until resistance indicates that the bumper of the PEG tube is engaged on the stomach wall.

11. The endoscopist, having followed the PEG into the stomach, visualizes the entry site and confirms hemostasis. Visual confirmation of adequate position of the bumper, which should be snug but not tight against the gastric wall, is the final maneuver prior to securing the catheter (Fig. 57.4).

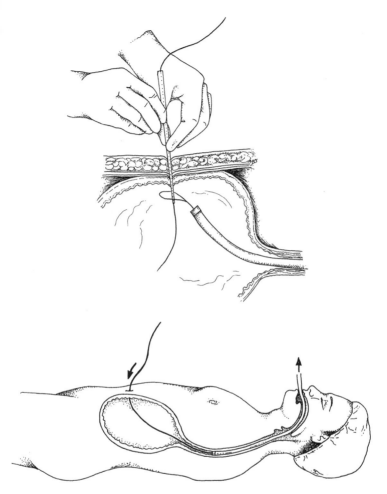

Figure 57.2. The braided suture is snared by the endoscopist and will be drawn back through the esophagus to exit through the mouth.

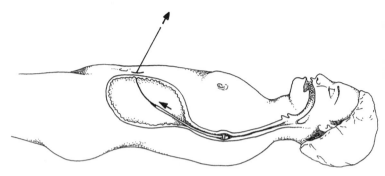

Figure 57.3. The PEG tube is pulled back into the stomach. Endoscopic verification of placement is essential.

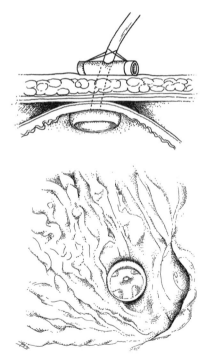

Figure 57.4. Endoscopic verification of adequate positioning of the bumper, which should be snug but not tight against the gastric wall.

D. Endoscopic Placement of Jejunal Feeding Tubes

The indications for feeding jejunostomies include the need for long-term enteral support, gastric dysmotility with paresis or pulmonary aspiration, or prior gastric resections precluding the placement of a PEG. Small-caliber feeding tubes may be placed through the pylorus under endoscopic or fluoroscopic guidance. The tube may be a nasoenteric feeding tube, or it may be placed adjacent to or through a PEG. First described is the placement of a feeding tube through a preexisting PEG.

1. Visualize the tube with an endoscope positioned in the stomach. Grasp the tube with an alligator forceps.
2. Advance the endoscope and feeding tube through the pylorus under direct vision.
3. Try to advance the tube as far into the duodenum as possible.
4. Position the patient with the head of the bed elevated and left side down.
5. Allow gravity to carry the tube farther down into the jejunum.
6. Confirm distal placement with fluoroscopy if possible.

The direct percutaneous endoscopic jejunostomy (PEJ) is another method of placing a feeding jejunal tube. This method entails using a longer endoscope, such as a pediatric colonoscope, and directly pushing the scope pass the ligament of Treitz as one would while performing a small bowel push endoscopy. In this method, fluoroscopy and utilization of the Safe-tract technique are mandatory. The method is in essence the same as the pull-type PEG.

1. Prepare the patient as described in Section B, items 1 through 4.
2. Pass the endoscope into the stomach, through the pylorus, through the duodenum and into the proximal jejunum.
3. Use fluoroscopy to identify the tip of the endoscope and then attempt finger indentation to confirm a likely position on the anterior abdominal wall. This is the most difficult part of the procedure, given that the small bowel is not as "fixed" as the stomach.
4. Once a potential site has been determined by finger indentation, utilize the Safe-tract technique to localize that segment of small bowel. It is crucial that this method be utilized in performing the direct PEJ. Occasionally a longer needle, such as a spinal needle, may be needed to perform this maneuver.
5. Once access has been gained into the small bowel, follow the pull-type PEG technique given earlier (Section C, items 5–11).
6. Finally, contrast is injected through the PEJ to confirm placement in the small bowel.

E. Selected References

Edelman DS. Laparoendoscopic approaches to enteral access. Semin Laparosc Surg 2001;8:195–201.

Gauderer MWL, Ponsky JL, Izant R. Gastrostomy without laparotomy: a percutaneous endoscopic technique. J Pediatr Surg 1980;15:872–875.

Ponsky JL, Aszodi A. Percutaneous endoscopic jejunostomy. Am J Gastroenterol 1984;79:113–116.

Ponsky JL, Gauderer MWL. Percutaneous endoscopic gastrostomy: a nonoperative technique for feeding gastrostomy. Gastrointest Endosc 1981;27:9–11.

Stellato TA, Gauderer MWL, Ponsky JL. Percutaneous endoscopic gastrostomy following previous abdominal surgery. Ann Surg 1984;200:46–50.

58. Complications of Upper Gastrointestinal Endoscopy

Brian J. Dunkin, M.D., F.A.C.S.

A. General Considerations

Flexible upper gastrointestinal endoscopy is a safe procedure with a complication rate well below 2% and a mortality rate of 0.004%. The incidence of complications increases when biopsy, polypectomy, or other invasive diagnostic or therapeutic maneuvers are performed.

Proper preparation for esophagogastroduodenoscopy (EGD) begins with a thorough history and physical examination. Both physician and patient should understand the indications for the procedure and possible complications. Patients who undergo EGD are frequently older and may have multiple medical problems or be taking medications that increase the risk of complications. General risk factors include advancing age, history of cardiac disease, or history of chronic obstructive pulmonary disease. Specific problems that are likely to be encountered and the manner in which they increase risk are given in Table 58.1.

1. **Cardiopulmonary complications.** Although the overall complication rate from EGD is low, 40% to 46% of serious complications are cardiopulmonary, related to hypoxemia, vasovagal reflexes, and relative hypotension.

    a. **Hypoxemia** is common. Up to 15% of patients experience a decrease in oxygen saturation below 85% during EGD.

        i. **Cause and prevention.** Hypoxemia is due to sedation and to encroachment upon the airway.

        ii. **Recognition and management.** Routine monitoring of oxygen saturation gives the diagnosis (remember that hypercarbia is usually present before oxygen desaturation is observed). Supplemental oxygen should be administered but may result in carbon dioxide retention if chronic obstructive pulmonary disease is present. Constant observation by a second individual who monitors vital signs, oxygen saturation, and level of consciousness (and reminds the patient to take periodic deep breaths) can help minimize this problem. A jaw thrust maneuver, performed by this assistant, will often improve airflow and oxygen saturation. Remove the endoscope if necessary.

    b. **Bradycardia**

        i. **Cause and prevention.** The vasovagal reflex from gastric distention or pressure against the stomach wall from the endoscope can trigger bradycardia and hypotension. Pre-

Table 58.1. Medical problems that may increase the risk of EGD.

Medical problem	Nature of complication
Valvular heart disease	Bacterial endocarditis
Diabetes	Hypoglycemia (due to NPO status)
Liver disease	Oversedation (inability to metabolize narcotics and benzodiazepines)
Depression	Hypertensive crisis (monoamine oxidase inhibitors react with meperidine)
Renal insufficiency	Oversedation, seizures (inability to excrete normeperidine, a meperidine metabolite)
Cardiac dysrhythmias	Dysrhythmia, hypotension
Obesity, chronic obstructive pulmonary disease	Hypoxemia, hypercarbia, carbon dioxide retention
Bleeding diatheses	Bleeding

treatment with atropine combats the bradycardia, but the resulting tachycardia may increase myocardial oxygen demand. Patients who are taking β-adrenergic-blockers may be unable to manifest a tachycardia in response to pain and hypovolemia. This relative bradycardia then contributes to hypotension (see item c).

    ii. **Recognition and management.** Continuous electrocardiographic monitoring allows early recognition. Evacuation of gastric air and reduction of gastric wall pressure from the endoscope is the first intervention. If this is unsuccessful, atropine is generally the drug of choice. Further management should follow advanced cardiac life support (ACLS) protocols.

  c. **Hypotension**

    i. **Cause and prevention.** Hypovolemia, cardiac dysrhythmias, myocardial ischemia, drug interactions, and oversedation are all potential causes. Monitoring, adequate hydration, and attention to medications and level of sedation are all crucial. Take a careful history, including medication usage, prior to EGD.

    ii. **Recognition and management.** Frequent blood pressure checks during the procedure and in the recovery phase will allow early detection. Administer a fluid bolus and search for other treatable causes (e.g., bradycardia).

2. **Medications that cause bleeding diatheses.** Many medications have the potential to cause bleeding problems. A list of common medications, problems, and suggestions for management follows.

  a. **Aspirin** irreversibly poisons platelets, and the effect lasts until new platelets have replaced the affected platelets. With an average life span of 10 days in the circulation, a significant replacement effect can be noted after about 7 days. Aspirin should be stopped 1 week prior to the procedure if possible. If therapy is performed, aspirin should not be restarted for another 14 days.

b. Other nonsteroidal anti-inflammatory drugs (NSAIDs) also inhibit platelet function, but the effect is variable and reversible. **Piroxicam** (Feldene) has an effect similar to aspirin in duration. Most other NSAIDs can be stopped 48 hours prior to the procedure.

c. **Warfarin** is another drug commonly encountered in the EGD patient. As in open surgery, there is no consensus about its periprocedure management. Anticoagulated patients undergoing diagnostic EGD alone are not at increased risk for bleeding. Those undergoing therapeutic EGD, however, may be. There are basically four options for management of anticoagulated patients undergoing therapeutic EGD: stop the warfarin with no parenteral anticoagulation coverage (heparin or low-molecular-weight heparin), stop the warfarin with parenteral anticoagulation coverage, continue warfarin at the usual dose, or continue at a reduced dose. In deciding which option to choose, it is important to assess the patient's risk for a thromboembolic complication when anticoagulation medication is withdrawn and to be clear on the indications for a therapeutic EGD. Patients at highest risk for thromboembolism are those with mechanical heart valves, coronary artery disease with persistent exertional angina, and overt arterial disease at more than one site, as well as those with a history of experiencing a thromboembolic event while anticoagulated. The risk–benefit ratio of the four anticoagulation options must be individualized for each patient.

d. **Ticlopidine** (Ticlid) is commonly given to patients with cardiovascular problems. It retards platelet aggregation. A single dose will effect the platelets for 4 to 36 hours. The bleeding time is maximally increased after 5 to 6 days of therapy and will take 4 to 8 days to normalize after stopping the drug. The drug should therefore be managed the same as aspirin. In an emergency situation, the time to normalization of the bleeding time can be decreased to less than 2 hours by administering intravenous methylprednisolone.

e. **Clopidogral** (Plavix) inhibits platelet aggregation and is frequently used in patients with cardiovascular or cerebralvascular disease. Inhibition of platelet aggregation can be seen within 2 hours of a single dose, with steady state reached at 3 to 7 days. This drug irreversibly inhibits platelet function and should be managed similar to aspirin.

3. **Infectious complications**

a. **Endocarditis, infection of prostheses (including joint prostheses), systemic infection.** Both diagnostic and therapeutic EGD have been demonstrated to cause bacteremia. Certain groups of patients are considered at risk and should receive antibiotics prior to endoscopic procedures (Table 58.2). Carefully seek any past

Table 58.2. American Society for Gastrointestinal Endoscopy (ASGE) recommendations for antibiotic prophylaxis for endoscopic procedures.

Patient condition	Procedure	Antibiotic prophylaxis
Prosthetic valve, history of endocarditis, systemic-pulmonary shunt, synthetic vascular graft <1 year old	Stricture dilation, varix sclerosis, ERCP for obstructed biliary tree	Recommended
	Other endoscopic procedures including EGD and colonoscopy (with or without biopsy or polypectomy), variceal ligation	Insufficient data to make firm recommendation; endoscopists may choose on case-by-case basis
Cirrhosis and ascites, immunocompromised patient	Stricture dilation, varix sclerosis, ERCP for obstructed biliary tree	Insufficient data to make firm recommendation; endoscopists may choose on case-by-case basis
	Other endoscopic procedures including EGD and colonoscopy (with or without biopsy or polypectomy), variceal ligation	Not recommended
Prosthetic joint or orthopedic prosthesis	All endoscopic procedures	Not recommended

ERCP: endoscopic retrograde cholangiopancreatography.

history of endocarditis, valvular heart disease, or recent valve or vascular replacement surgery. An acceptable **prophylactic regimen** for these high-risk patients is 2 g of parenteral ampicillin and 1.5 mg/kg gentamicin (up to 80 mg) 30 minutes before the procedure. This should be followed by a single 1.5-g dose of oral amoxicillin 6 hours after the procedure. One gram of parenteral vancomycin may be substituted for the preprocedure ampicillin, with omission of the post procedure amoxicillin in patients allergic to penicillin.

b. **Transmission of infection.** Strict adherence to proper disinfection procedures is important to avoid iatrogenic transmission of bacterial or viral infection.

i. *Pseudomonas aeruginosa* infections caused by contaminated scopes or water bottles have been frequently reported and have a high mortality rate.

<ul>
<li>ii. Contamination by *Salmonella*, *Helicobacter*, and *Mycobacterium* has also been documented.</li>
<li>iii. **Viral** infections have not been documented convincingly, and to date there has been no evidence of colonization of an endoscope with HIV and no reports of transmitting HIV to a patient from a contaminated scope.</li>
</ul>

4. **Aspiration.** Topical anesthesia, gastric distention, and sedation all increase the risk of aspiration during EGD. Yankauer suction must be available to clear secretions and emesis. Patient position is important: the left lateral decubitus position with the head slightly elevated reduces the risk of aspiration. Patients requiring emergent endoscopy or a supine position for the procedure (e.g., PEG placement) are less able to protect their airway. Consider intubation for patients undergoing EGD for bleeding or foreign body removal.

5. **Complications of conscious sedation.** Take a careful history with attention to patient allergies, medications, and comorbidities. Use the smallest amount of sedation that will provide the desired effect. Narcotics and benzodiazepines in combination are more likely to produce cardiopulmonary complications than either drug given alone. Flumazenil (reversibly inhibits benzodiazepines) and Narcan (reversibly inhibits opiate analgesics) should be readily accessible before the start of the procedure. Remember that these drugs have a shorter half-life than the benzodiazepine or narcotic being inhibited. **Therefore, a patient who is awake and responsive after receiving Narcan or flumazenil may again become unresponsive when the drug wears off.**

B. Complications of Diagnostic EGD

Mechanical complications of diagnostic EGD include esophageal perforation and dislodgment of teeth.

1. **Esophageal perforation**
   a. **Cause and prevention. The risk of esophageal perforation from diagnostic EGD is 0.03% and most frequently occurs at the cervical esophagus.** Risk factors include anterior cervical osteophytes, Zenker's diverticulum, esophageal stricture or web, or a cervical rib. Most cervical esophageal perforations occur during rigid endoscopy, or with blind passage of a flexible endoscope. Gentle passage under direct visual control is the best way to prevent perforation. Perforation can occur at any level at which there is a stricture or other pathology. Retching with an over-insufflated stomach and the endoscope occluding the gastroesophageal junction (GEJ) can result in Mallory-Weiss tears or esophageal perforation. Avoid this by adequate sedation, limiting insufflation, and removing the endoscope from the GEJ if the patient starts to retch.

b. **Recognition and management.** Cervical pain, crepitus, and cellulitis are all signs of a high esophageal perforation. Distal perforations cause chest pain. The diagnosis is confirmed by water-soluble contrast esophagram. **Cervical esophageal perforations** can usually be managed with antibiotics and withholding oral intake, or by cervical exploration and drainage. Rarely is primary repair or diversion necessary. **Distal esophageal perforation** may require immediate surgical drainage or repair.

2. **Dislodgment of teeth or dentures**

a. **Cause and prevention.** Avoid this problem by removing any dentures before introducing the scope. Place a bite block to protect the teeth and the instrument.

b. **Recognition and management.** The problem is usually recognized by the patient. Obtain a posteroanterior and lateral chest x-ray to exclude aspiration. Remove aspirated foreign bodies immediately (bronchoscopy). Ingested teeth will pass without incident. Ingested dental appliances may or may not, depending on size. Repeat endoscopy and removal may be needed (see Chapter 52, Section D, Foreign Body Removal).

C. Complications of Therapeutic EGD

1. **Therapeutic endoscopy for nonvariceal bleeding** is associated with few complications. One risk of major concern is **precipitation of bleeding** from a nonbleeding ulcer, but this occurs in only 5% of cases. Complications of specific modalities used for control of bleeding are as follows.

a. **Injection therapy.** Bleeding peptic ulcers can be controlled by injection of epinephrine with or without a sclerosant or cyanoacrylate. Plasma epinephrine levels increase four- to fivefold within minutes of injection of **epinephrine** but return to baseline within 20 minutes. These levels may be higher in patients with liver disease. Only one case of **asymptomatic hypertension and ventricular tachycardia** has been reported after epinephrine injection. Sclerosing agents can (rarely) cause **full-thickness necrosis, obstructive jaundice**, and **intramural hematoma**. Cyanoacrylate ("superglue") is nontoxic with minimal side effects and has been found to be efficacious in nonvariceal bleeding. The main risk with its use is damage to the endoscope from inadvertent application in the working channel.

b. **Cauterization (thermal therapy).** The use of heater probes, multipolar probes, and argon plasma coagulation (APC) all have low rates of treatment-induced bleeding and perforation. Monopolar cautery is generally avoided because of a high incidence of full-thickness injury.

c. **Other modalities.** Early experience with endoscopic clips demonstrates that they are safe and efficacious, but perhaps not as good as thermal therapy. Variceal band ligators have been used for Dieulafoy lesions with good success.

2. **Therapeutic EGD for variceal bleeding** has become commonplace with approximately a 90% success rate at controlling the initial bleeding episode. The primary complications are stricture, perforation, and bleeding.

   a. **Esophageal variceal banding (EVB).** The incidence of stricture (0%), perforation (0.7%), bleeding from ulceration at the banding site (2.6–7.8%), aspiration pneumonia (1%), peritonitis (4%), and mortality (1%) are all lower than with sclerotherapy. Chest pain is common after EVB and may be related to esophageal spasm. Historically, EVB had the additional risk of requiring the use of an overtube to facilitate multiple passes of the endoscope. This is not needed with multiband ligators and has subsequently eliminated the risk of perforation.

   b. **Esophageal variceal sclerotherapy (EVS).** Complications occur in 20% to 40% of cases with up to 2% mortality. The most common serious complications are stricture formation (11.8%), perforation (4.3%), bleeding from ulceration at the injection site (12.7%), and pneumonia (6.8%). Chest pain, pleural effusions, pulmonary infiltrates, and bacteremia can each occur in 44% to 50% of patients.

3. **Dilatation of strictures** is primarily performed for esophageal lesions, although dilatation of nonesophageal lesions is becoming more frequent and is associated with a very low complication rate. This section concentrates on the complication of esophageal dilatation. There are two methods of dilatation: placement of a guide-wire across the stricture (under endoscopic or fluoroscopic guidance) followed by advancement of a bougie dilator, and transendoscopic balloon dilatation with or without the use of a guidewire. These techniques appear to be equally safe and efficacious. The risk of developing a complication from endoscopic dilatation is more dependent on the underlying pathology than the technique of dilatation, provided proper technique is followed (see Chapter 52). **Perforation** is the most feared complication, with an overall incidence of 0.2% for all techniques and pathology (Table 58.3). Esophageal dilatation results in **bacteremia** in up to

Table 58.3. Type of stricture and risk of perforation following dilatation.

Type of stricture	Risk of perforation (%)
Benign peptic	0.1–0.3
Malignant	9–24
Radiation induced	0–3.6
Caustic	0–15.4 (0.8%/dilatation)
Anastomotic	0
Achalasia	0–6.6

50% of patients; prophylactic antibiotics should be given to prevent endocarditis (see earlier: Section A). **Hematemesis** occurs in 1 to 1.5% of patients but is usually self-limited; hemorrhage requiring transfusion is rare.

4. Endoscopic placement of **esophageal stents** is most commonly performed for palliation of obstructing tumors and is sometimes preceded by dilatation. Perforation is most frequently associated with the dilatation and it is therefore recommended to avoid dilatation unless absolutely necessary. Complications from the stent itself include erosion with perforation, bleeding, migration, tumor ingrowth with recurrent obstruction, food impaction, and aspiration. Stents placed in the very proximal or distal esophagus are associated with the highest rates of complication. Stents in the **cervical esophagus**, close to the upper esophageal sphincter, can cause difficulty with swallowing, globus, and predispose to aspiration. Those across the **GEJ** can cause gastroesophageal reflux with esophagitis and aspiration. The risk of **aspiration** is minimized by maintaining the patient in a "head-up" position or by using stents with antireflux valves. **Esophagitis** is managed with H_2-blocker therapy or proton pump inhibitors. **Recurrent obstruction** is minimized with the use of covered stents and treated with laser or argon plasma coagulator ablation of the tumor ingrowth, or placement of a second stent through the first.

D. Complications of Percutaneous Endoscopic Gastrostomy and Jejunostomy

Large cumulative retrospective studies have reported that 10 to 43% of both adult and pediatric patients have at least one complication following PEG placement.

Pneumoperitoneum is a frequent occurrence after percutaneous gastrostomy. This is the result of air escaping around the puncturing needle, wire, or tube. Routine x-ray films are unwarranted. Air in the abdominal cavity has been shown to last for up to 5 weeks after PEG placement. Patients found to have pneumoperitoneum after gastrostomy must be clinically evaluated. In the absence of abdominal tenderness, leukocytosis, or fever, there is no need for further evaluation.

Good **skin care** is important after gastrostomy. It is common to see a foreign body reaction around the tube with some exudate or granulation tissue. Swab the exudate away with hydrogen peroxide and leave the site open to air. Cauterize granulation tissue with silver nitrate. Avoid occlusive dressings; these may lead to skin maceration.

Other more significant complications are as follows.

1. **Wound infections** are common.
    a. **Cause and prevention.** Contamination with oral and gastric flora contribute to the incidence of wound infection (particularly with a "pull" and "push" technique). Wound problems can also result

from excess tension on the tube (causing pressure necrosis) and a small skin incision (which fails to allow egress of bacteria). The incidence is significantly decreased with a single prophylactic dose of antibiotic decreased (from 26% to 2% in one study).

b. **Recognition and management.** Signs and symptoms of wound infection include erythema around the gastrostomy tube site several days after the procedure, local tenderness, slight edema of the skin, low-grade fever, and leukocytosis. Incision and drainage of the area under local anesthesia most often resolves the problem. Failure to identify and treat this problem at an early stage can result in **necrotizing infections of the abdominal wall** and death.

2. **Buried bumper syndrome** (extrusion of the head of the tube from the gastric lumen into the subcutaneous tissue).

a. **Cause and prevention.** Excessive tension is the cause. Do not tighten up the bumper in an attempt to prevent leakage around the tube, and do not place dressings under the skin anchoring device. At all times, avoid excess pressure and tension.

b. **Recognition and management.** This condition may cause wound infection or leakage of gastric juice and feedings into the peritoneal cavity or subcutaneous tissues. Remove the gastrostomy tube, place the patient on nasogastric suction, and treat the patient with parenteral antibiotics until the gastrostomy tract inflammation and skin necrosis resolve.

3. **Leakage of feedings** into the peritoneal cavity is one of the most serious complications.

a. **Cause and prevention.** Leakage is usually the result of separation of the gastric and abdominal walls and often is due to necrosis of the gastric wall from excessive tension on the catheter. Premature dislodgment of the tube from the gastric lumen (before a tract has formed) or malposition of the tube during attempted reinsertion may also cause this problem.

b. **Recognition and management.** Patients who develop abdominal tenderness, fever, or leukocytosis should be evaluated for leakage and the resultant peritonitis. This is done by instilling water-soluble contrast material into the gastrostomy tube under fluoroscopic guidance. Intraperitoneal extravasation indicates something has gone awry. If the contrast study indicates that the head of the tube remains in the stomach and that the extravasation is around it, the tube can usually be salvaged by inserting a nasogastric tube, placing the PEG to drainage, and administering intravenous fluids and antibiotics. If the contrast study reveals complete separation of the gastric and abdominal walls with dislodgment of the tube from the stomach, the tube should be pulled from the abdominal wall and the treatment just described instituted. A patient whose PEG has been pulled out inadvertently less than 2 weeks from the time of insertion should be treated similarly. If at any time the patient's condition begins to deteriorate or signs of peritonitis worsen, exploratory laparotomy or laparoscopy with operative repair should be performed.

4. **Gastrocolic fistula** has rarely been known to occur after percutaneous gastrostomy.

    a. **Cause and prevention.** This fistula may be due to puncture of the colon at the time of gastrostomy or pinching of the colon between the gastric and abdominal walls with subsequent necrosis of the colonic wall and fistula formation. It is prevented by careful technique. Laparoscopic visualization (described in Chapter 24) may be useful in difficult cases.

    b. **Recognition and management.** This complication usually becomes apparent after several weeks with the development of severe diarrhea following feedings. It may be documented with an upper gastrointestinal series or barium enema. In nearly all cases, the condition may be treated by removing the gastrostomy tube. The fistula closes rapidly once the tube has been removed.

5. **Progressive enlargement of the stoma** around the gastrostomy tube may occur in some patients.

    a. **Cause and prevention.** Excessive tension, poor nutritional status, and excess movement of the tube at skin level can cause this problem. As previously mentioned, excess tension is to be avoided. Minimize tube mobility by securing the tube or using a stabilizing device.

    b. **Recognition and management.** The problem is easily recognized by leakage of gastric juice and feedings around the tube. Replacing the gastrostomy tube with a larger size provides only a short-term solution, as the tract generally continues to enlarge. A better solution is to remove the tube entirely and allow the tract to close. When the tract contracts, insert a new tube and stabilize it at the skin level.

6. **Neoplastic seeding** (to skin around the gastrostomy tube) has been reported when PEG placement for both oropharyngeal and esophageal cancers. This is not an issue when the gastrostomy is placed for palliation in a patient with limited life span. It should be kept in mind, however, when gastrostomy placement is planned prior to neoadjuvant therapy. There may be advantages to using an introducer technique in this setting, but this has not been tested.

E. Selected References

Arrowsmith J, Gerstman B, Fleisher D, et al. Results from the American Society for Gastrointestinal Endoscopy/U.S. Food and Drug Administration collaborative study on complication rates and drug use during gastrointestinal endoscopy. Gastrointest Endosc 1991;37:421–427.

ASGE Position Statement: The recommended use of laboratory studies before endoscopic procedures. Gastrointest Endosc 1993;39:892.

ASGE recommendations for antibiotic prophylaxis for endoscopic procedures. Gastrointest Endosc 1995;42(6):633.

Cook DJ, Guyatt GH, Salena BJ, et al. Endoscopic therapy for acute nonvariceal upper gastrointestinal hemorrhage: a meta-analysis. Gastroenterology 1992;102:139.

Jain NK, Larson DE, Schroeder KW, et al. Antibiotic prophylaxis for percutaneous endoscopic gastrostomy. A prospective, randomized, double-blind clinical trial. Ann Intern Med 1987;107:824–828.

Lee JG, Lieberman DA. Complications related to endoscopic hemostasis techniques. Gastrointest Endosc Clin North Am 1996;6(2):305–321.

Marks JM. Esophagogastroduodenoscopy. In: Ponsky JL, ed. Complications of Endoscopic and Laparoscopic Surgery. Prevention and Management. Philadelphia: Lippincott-Raven, 1997;13–28.

Ponsky JL, Dunkin BJ. Percutaneous endoscopic gastrostomy. In: Yamada T, ed. Textbook of Gastroenterology. Philadelphia: Lippincott-Raven, 1997.

Preclik G, Grune S, Leser HG, et al. Prospective, randomized, double blind trial of prophylaxis with single dose of co-amoxiclav before PEG. Br J Surg 1999;319:881–884.

Repici A, Ferrari A, DeAngelis C, et al. Adrenaline plus cyanoacrylate injection for treatment of bleeding peptic ulcers after failure of conventional endoscopic haemostasis. Dig Liver Dis 2002;34(5):349–355.

Silvis SE, Nebel O, Rogers G, et al. Endoscopic complications. Results of the 1974 American Society of Gastrointestinal Endoscopy Survey. JAMA 1976;235:928.

Flexible Endoscopy
III—Small Bowel Enteroscopy

59. Small Bowel Enteroscopy

Charles H. Andrus, M.D., F.A.C.S.
Scott H. Miller, M.D., F.A.C.S.

A. Indications

Small bowel endoscopy (enteroscopy) is generally used when other diagnostic modalities are inadequate.

1. **Occult gastrointestinal (GI) bleeding** is the most common indication.

   a. Five percent of GI bleeding is undiagnosed after esophagogastroduodenoscopy (EGD), colonoscopy, and contrast radiographic studies. Enteroscopy has been reported to diagnose the small bowel as the source of "obscure" GI bleeding in a range of 13% to 77% of cases with a median of 57%. The most commonly identified source is an angiodysplasia (synonyms: arteriovenous malformation [AVM], mucosal or vascular ectasia).

   b. Enteroscopy may be used preoperatively as well as intraoperatively to guide treatment. It provides localization of the bleeding source.

   c. In the comparison of the usefulness of enteroscopy in the diagnosis of occult GI bleeding sites, in 553 examinations (348 yielded positive reports) the overall positive yield by location was reported by Berner as follows: EGD, 103 (18%); push enteroscopy distal to EGD, 101 (18%); and sonde enteroscopy distal to push enteroscopy 144 (26%).

2. Evaluation of **small bowel tumors or polyps**

   a. Familial adenomatous polyposis and Gardner's syndrome
   b. Hamartomas as in Peutz-Jeghers syndrome
   c. Gastrointestinal stromal tumors (GISTs)
   d. Lymphoma, carcinoma, melanoma, and Kaposi's sarcoma
   e. Carcinoid

3. Assessment of **other small bowel pathology**

   a. **Crohn's disease.** While 70% of patients with Crohn's disease will have small bowel involvement, 30% will have **only** small bowel involvement. Owing to the distal small bowel distribution of Crohn's disease, the effectiveness of the enteroscopy method in diagnosing Crohn's disease is most probably dependent on the distance potentially traversed, the ability to perform biopsies, and the ability to visualize mucosal involvement due to associated stricture formation. While the relative invasiveness and availability of enteroscopic techniques will locally impact on the utilization of enteroscopy, the possible effectiveness of the entero-scopic methods in increasing potential of the identification of Crohn's disease are push, (retrograde ileoscopy), sonde, capsule, and intraoperative.

b. **Celiac disease.** In the endoscopic diagnosis of the loss or reduc-tion in folds for the diagnosis of subtotal villous atrophy: sensi-tivity 88%; specificity, 83%; positive predictive value, 65%; negative predictive value, 95%. While endoscopically visualized villous atrophy is suggestive of celiac disease, biopsy pathologic evaluation, identification of the presence of serum endomysial antibodies (EMA) and anti-gliadin antibodies (AGA), and diag-nostic confirmation by response to a gluten-free diet are most important and complementary. In the evaluation of malabsorption disease, push enteroscopy with biopsy has limited additional diagnostic value when compared with EGD with biopsy [2 of 16 = 12%; Cuillerier et al., 2001].

c. **Refractory sprue.** In one report, 5 of 8 enteroscopies revealed ulcerative jejunitis vs only 1 case of ulcerative gastritis.

d. **HIV-related GI disease**—Although upper GI pathology due to opportunistic infections like cytomegalovirus can usually be identified by EGD with biopsy, small bowel biopsy may be beneficial in patients with chronic severe diarrhea in the presence of HIV.

B. Technique of Enteroscopy

Several methods of small bowel endoscopy are available. Nonoperative enteroscopic methods, the push, sonde, and capsule techniques, are described here, as well as intraoperative endoscopy.

1. **Push enteroscopy.** This is the easiest and quickest of the methods, but it can reach only 60 cm beyond the ligament of Treitz as documented by concomitant radiological exam (range, 30–150 cm; median, 100 cm). (A longer push enteroscope may not facilitate a significant distal traverse of the small bowel [Benz et al., 2002]).

a. Use a pediatric colonoscope (135–145 cm) or a flexible entero-scope (165–200 cm). (e.g., Models SIF-100, XSIF-100, SIF-Q140 Olympus Corp., Tokyo).

b. Stop aspirin at least 5 days prior to enteroscopy.

c. Administer simethicone orally prior to endoscopy.

d. Employ a stiff overtube to straighten the scope from the mouth to the pylorus into the short (lesser curve) position in the stomach and thus prevent curling. (Use of an overtube provides a signifi-cantly deeper insertion of the enteroscope into the small bowel [Taylor et al., 2001]).

e. This technique requires two individuals: one to control the entero-scope deflection and one to control overtube placement and sta-bility and forward advancement of the scope.

Table 59.1. Push enteroscopy identification yield in occult GI bleeding.

Source	*n*	Source of bleeding identified
Chong	55	35 (64%)
Hayat	78	24 (31%)
Rossini	61	25 (41%)
Shackel	23	13 (57%)
Schmit	83	49 (59%)

(The push enteroscopy yield variability in occult GI bleeding in the literature may in part reflect lesions missed at the time of EGD that retrospectively were accessible by EGD [Pennazio and Rossini, 1996].)

   f.   Advance the enteroscope through the mouth and esophagus to just beyond the gastroesophageal junction.

   g.   Lubricate the overtube well and then advance the overtube over the scope into the proximal stomach.

   h.   Advance scope and overtube together through the pylorus.

   i.   Advance the enteroscope through the lumen of the small bowel under direct vision. Attempt to telescope the enteroscope through the small bowel as far as possible.

   j.   Completely evaluate the small bowel mucosa during enteroscope withdrawal.

   k.   If a mucosal source of bleeding is identified (e.g., angiodysplasia), heater probe ablation therapy is possible (e.g., of 23 treated patients, 7 rebled after treatment, and 3 of the original 23 continued to bleed).

   l.   Table 59.1 gives the results of five authors who identified source of bleeding with push enteroscopy.

2. **Sonde enteroscopy**

   a.   A 5-mm-diameter, 275-cm scope (e.g., Model SSIF VIII, Olympus Corp., Tokyo) is inserted transnasally and introduced through the pylorus by a piggyback technique with a pediatric colonoscope.

   b.   The scope has two internal channels:

       i.   One for air inflation of the small bowel

       ii.   One for balloon inflation

       iii.   No channel for biopsies or brushes

   c.   The technique consists of the placement of the scope through the pylorus with subsequent insufflation of the balloon and distal progression by peristalsis.

   d.   The distal position of the scope is confirmed by fluoroscopy. The average transit time through the entire small bowel is about 6 hours.

   e.   Once the scope has reached its most distal position, it is withdrawn with small bowel insufflation and the small bowel mucosa is examined during this withdrawal phase.

Table 59.2. Sonde enteroscopy identification yield in occult GI bleeding.

Source	n	Source of bleeding identified
Lewis*	22	17 (77%)
Morris	65	25 (38%)

*Same yield as by intraoperative enteroscopy in same patients.

    f.   Complete examination of the bowel during withdrawal is impossible owing to the inability to steer this scope and the variability to control the rate of withdrawal through the telescoped bowel.

    g.   Table 59.2 gives the results of two authors who identified the source of bleeding with sonde enteroscopy.

3.   **Mayo Clinic sonde technique** (prototype sonde small bowel enteroscope (Olympus, Corp., Tokyo, Model SIF VI KAI: 267.5 cm)

    a.   The enteroscope is introduced orally through an insertion tube and is positioned by fluoroscopy near the pylorus.

    b.   The scope is introduced through the pylorus under direct vision.

    c.   A guidewire is inserted through the inner channel (2 mm diameter) and the scope is advanced over the guidewire under fluoroscopic control.

    d.   The average duration of the procedure is about 4.5 hours. Approximately 85% of the reported procedures by this technique have reached the mid- to distal ileum.

    e.   Although a 2-mm channel is present, it is difficult to pass any instrument through the channel.

4.   **Intraoperative enteroscopy**

    a.   This technique is considered the best and most complete method of endoscopic small bowel evaluation.

    b.   Formal laparotomy is performed and adhesions (if present) are lysed so that the small intestine can be freely manipulated from the ligament of Treitz to the ileocecal valve.

    c.   Two trained individuals cooperate. One manipulates the bowel through the surgical incision. The second serves as endoscopist.

    d.   The endoscopist passes a standard colonoscope through the mouth into the stomach.

    e.   The surgeon manually directs the scope through the pylorus and around the sweep of the duodenum while the endoscopist advances the endoscope.

    f.   With continued advancement of the scope by the endoscopist, the surgeon manually telescopes the small bowel over the scope and it is advanced to the ileocecal junction.

    g.   With the operating room lights darkened, the scope is slowly withdrawn, with the rate of small bowel examination controlled by the surgeon. Manual occlusion proximal and distal allows insufflation of a selected segment without distention of the entire

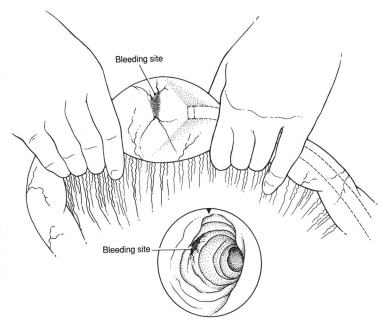

Figure 59.1. Manual compression proximal and distal to a selected segment allow insufflation. The lesion is visualized both by the endoscopist and by transillumination. (Reprinted with permission from Scott-Conner CEH, Dawson DL. Operative Anatomy. Philadelphia: Lippincott-Raven, 1993).

small bowel (Fig. 59.1). Ectasias and bleeding sites can be visualized by both the endoscopist directly and by the surgeon by transillumination.

h. Table 59.3 gives the results of four authors who identified GI bleeding in intraoperative enteroscopy.

Table 59.3. Intraoperative enteroscopy identification yield in occult GI bleeding.

Source	*n*	Source of bleeding identified
Douard	20	16 (80%)
Kendrick	70	52 (74%)
Lewis*	22	17 (77%)
Zaman	12	7 (58%)

*Same yield as by sonde enteroscopy in same patients, described in Table 59.2.

5. **Capsule endoscopy**
   a. The newest, revolutionary technique, which was approved by the U.S. Food and Drug Administrate in August 2001, is the M2A Capsule Endoscope (Given Imaging Limited, Yoqneam, Israel), which potentially will provide the most complete visual evaluation of the small bowel by the least invasive methodology. This technique is considered in additional detail in Chapter 60.
   b. This enteroscopy system consists of a single-use video transmitter capsule (11 mm × 26 mm capsule containing a miniaturized video system of a color camera with lens, radiofrequency transmitter, six light-emitting diodes, two batteries, and an antenna); a Sensor Array, which is taped to the abdomen; a DataRecorder, which is worn on a belt; and a RAPID workstation.
   c. After a fast of at least 12 hours, the patient drinks a solution of simethicone prior to swallowing the capsule. The patient is kept NPO for an additional 4 hours after swallowing the capsule, and the data collection period is approximately 8 hours.
   d. The video images are then reviewed on the Workstation monitor by the endoscopist.
   e. Comparison investigations in humans are now being reported. When compared with push enteroscopy in the same patients, the site of obscure bleeding was identified in 6 of 20 (30%) by push enteroscopy vs 11 of 20 (55%) by capsule endoscopy ($p = .0625$). More significantly, though, the capsule identified 5 of 14 sites distal to the small bowel range of the push enteroscope (Lewis and Swain, 2002).
   f. With its ability to traverse the entire small bowel, it can be concluded that capsule endoscopy is superior to push endoscopy distally, but it remains to be seen whether capsule endoscopy will supplant sonde enteroscopy, although such has been advocated by some (Waye, 2001).
   g. Because it is minimally invasive, capsule endoscopy is well tolerated and seems to be well accepted by patients.
   h. Table 59.4 gives the results of three authors who identified occult GI bleeding with capsule endoscopy.
6. **Biopsy and sampling techniques**
   a. When a pediatric or standard colonoscope are employed by the push technique, standard endoscopic biopsy forceps and brushes can be utilized.

Table 59.4. Capsule enteroscopy identification yield in occult GI bleeding.

Source	n	Source of bleeding identified
Ell	32	21 (66%)
Lewis	20	11 (55%)
Scapa	35	22 (76%)

b. When the sonde-type scopes are employed, a biopsy channel is absent or extremely small, preventing easy passage of biopsy sample, brush, or laser fibers.

C. Complications

1. **Epistaxis**
    a. **Cause and prevention.** Epistaxis can be caused by prolonged nasal irritation and may be minimized by frequent lubrication during the passage of the enteroscope.
    b. **Recognition and management.** Although the condition is easily recognized, complete prevention may not be possible.
2. **Pancreatitis**
    a. **Cause and prevention.** This is theorized to result from prolonged irritation to the ampulla of Vater. No prevention is known.
    b. **Recognition and management.** Pancreatitis is documented by standard chemical serologic markers. It is managed according to severity.
3. **Intestinal injury**
    a. **Cause and prevention.** Forceful or blind advancement of the overtube and/or scope may cause a Mallory-Weiss tear, mucosal stripping, or perforation. Advancement under direct vision to and through the pylorus and small bowel are the best ways to prevent such an occurrences.
    b. **Recognition and management.** Intestinal perforation can be recognized by the radiologic identification of free air and most probably will require operative management.
4. **Inability to advance the scope or to confirm the diagnosis.** By sonde methods, only 50 to 75% of the mucosa is visualized on the average, while by the push technique only 60 cm distal to the ligament of Treitz can be reached. In approximately 50% of patients who come to enteroscopy, it is not possible to definitively diagnose the site of GI bleeding.

D. Selected References

Axon ATR. Small bowel and duodenum: enteroscopy. In: Cotton PB, Tytgat GNJ, Williams CB, eds. Annual of Gastrointestinal Endoscopy 1989. London: Current Science, 1989;35–37.

Benz C, Jakobs R, Riemann JF. Does the insertion depth in push enteroscopy depend on the working length of the enteroscope? Endoscopy 2002;34:543–545.

Berner JS, Mauer K, Lewis BS. Push and sonde enteroscopy for the diagnosis of obscure gastrointestinal bleeding. Am J Gastroenterol 1994;89(12):2139–2142.

Cellier C, Cuillerier E, Patey-Mariaud N, et al. Push enteroscopy in celiac sprue and refractory sprue. Gastointest Endosc 1999;50(5):613–617.

Chong J, Tagle M, Barkin JS, Reiner DK. Small bowel push-type fiberoptic enteroscopy for patients with occult gastrointestinal bleeding or suspected small bowel pathology. Am J Gastroenterol 1994;89(12):2143–2146.

Cuillerier E, Landi B, Cellier C. Is push enteroscopy useful in patients with malabsorption of unclear origin? Am J Gastroenterol 2001;96(7):2103–2106.

Dickey W. Diagnosis of coeliac disease at open-access endoscopy. Scand J Gastroenterol 1998;33:612–615.

Dickey W. Endoscopy, serology and histology in the diagnosis of celiac disease. Dig Liver Dis 2002;34:172–176.

Douard R, Wind P, Panis Y, et al. Intraoperative enteroscopy for diagnosis and management of unexplained gastrointestinal bleeding. Am J Surg 2000;180:181–184.

Eisen GM, Dominitz JA, Faigel DO, et al. Enteroscopy (ASGE). Gastrointest Endosc 2001;53(7):871–873.

Ell C, Remke S, May A, Helou L, Henrich R, Mayer G. The first prospective controlled trial comparing wireless capsule endoscopy with push enteroscopy in chronic gastrointestinal bleeding. Endoscopy 2002;34(9):685–689.

Harewood GC, Murray JA. Diagnostic approach to a patient with suspected celiac disease—a cost analysis. Dig Dis Sci 2001;46(11):2510–2514.

Hayat M, Axon ATR, O'Mahony S. Diagnostic yield and effect on clinical outcomes of push enteroscopy. I. Suspected small-bowel bleeding. Endoscopy 2000;32(5): 369–372.

Kendrick M, Buttar N, Anderson M, et al. Contribution of intraoperative enteroscopy in the management of obscure gastrointestinal bleeding. J Gastrointest Surg 2001;5(2): 162–167.

Lahoti S, Fukami N. The small bowel as a source of gastrointestinal blood loss. In: Current Gastroenterology Reports. Vol 1. Part 5. Philadelphia: Current Science; 1999; 424–430.

Lee SD, Cohen RD. Endoscopy of the small bowel in inflammatory bowel disease. Gastrointest Endosc Clin North Am 2002;12:485–493.

Lewis BS, Swain P. Capsule endoscopy in the evaluation of patients with suspected small intestinal bleeding: results of a pilot study. Gastrointest Endosc 2002;56:349–353.

Lewis BS, Wenger JS, Waye JD. Small bowel enteroscopy and intraoperative enteroscopy for obscure gastrointestinal bleeding. Am J Gastroenterol 1991;86(2):171–174.

Lobo AJ, Axon ATR. Endoscopy of the small bowel and duodenum. In: Cotton PB, Tytgat GNJ, Williams CB, eds. Annual of Gastrointestinal Endoscopy, 1991. London: Current Science, 1991;33–39.

Morris AJ, Wasson LA, MacKenzie JF. Small bowel enteroscopy in undiagnosed gastrointestinal blood loss. Gut 1992;33:887–889.

Pennazio M, Rossini FP. Main issues in push enteroscopy. Ital J Gastroenterol Hepatol 1998;30:96–101.

Rossini FP, Arrigoni A, Pennazio. Clinical enteroscopy. J Clin Gastroenterol 1996; 22(3):231–235.

Scapa E, Jacob H, Lewkowicz S, et al. Initial experience of wireless-capsule endoscopy for evaluating occult gastrointestinal bleeding and suspected small bowel pathology. Am J Gastroenterol 2002;97(11):2776–2779.

Schmit A, Gay F, Adler M, Cremer M, Van Gossum A. Diagnostic efficacy of push-enteroscopy and long-term follow-up of patients with small bowel angiodysplasias. Dig Dis Sci 1996;41(12):2348–2352.

Schuman BM. Endoscopy of the small bowel and duodenum. In: Cotton PB, Tytgat GNJ, Williams CB, eds. Annual of Gastrointestinal Endoscopy 1988. London: Gower Academic Journals, 1988;29–35.

Seensalu R. The sonde examination. Gastrointest Endosc Clin North Am 1999;9(1):37–59.

Shackel NA, Bowen DG, Selby WS. Video push enteroscopy in the investigation of small bowel disease: defining clinical indications and outcomes. Aust N Z J Med 1998;28:198–203.

Shields SJ, Van Dam J. Endoscopic evaluation of the small intestine. Can J Gastroenterol 2002;16(3):178–183.

Shinya H, McSherry C. Endoscopy of the small bowel. Surg Clin North Am 1982;62:821–824.

Taylor ACF, Chen RYM, Desmond PV. Use of an overtube for enteroscopy—does it increase depth of insertion? A prospective study of enteroscopy with and without an overtube. Endoscopy 2001;33(3):227–230.

Waye JD. Enteroscopy. In: Cotton PB, Tytgat GNJ, Williams CB, eds. Annual of Gastrointestinal Endoscopy 1992. London: Current Science, 1992;61–65.

Waye JD. Endoscopy of the small bowel: push, sonde and intra-operative. Endoscopy 1994;26:60–63.

Waye JD. Small-intestinal endoscopy. Endoscopy 2001;33(1):24–30.

Wilcox CM. Role of endoscopy in the investigation of upper gastrointestinal symptoms in HIV-infected patients. Can J Gastroenterol 1999;13(4):305–310.

Wilmer A, Rutgeerts P. Push enteroscopy: technique, depth, and yield of insertion. Gastrointest Endosc Clin North Am 1996;6(4):759–776.

Yu M. M2A Capsule endoscopy. Gastroenterol Nurs 2002;25(1):24–27.

Zaman A, Sheppard B, Katon RM. Total peroral intraoperative enteroscopy for obscure GI bleeding using a dedicated push enteroscope: diagnostic yield and patient outcome. Gastrointest Endosc 1999;50(4):506–510.

60. Capsule Endoscopy

John D. Mellinger, M.D., F.A.C.S.
Bruce V. MacFadyen, Jr., M.D., F.A.C.S.
Gina L. Adrales, M.D.

A. Indications

Capsule endoscopy is a relatively new technique for gastrointestinal assessment, the optimal utilization of which continues to be elucidated. Early experience has suggested that it is a promising modality for the evaluation of the small intestine, specifically in the setting of obscure gastrointestinal bleeding. In such patients, average costs in excess of $30,000 per patient, spent on repeated admissions and interventions, without a definite diagnosis being made, have been documented. Traditional radiologic assessments of the small intestine, including enteroclysis studies, have diagnostic yields of less than 15% in such instances. While push enteroscopy (see Chapter 59) can allow visualization of much of the jejunum in experienced hands, and the terminal ileum is usually accessible colonoscopically, the remainder of the small bowel has remained relatively resistant to endoscopic assessment. Sonde enteroscopic techniques can allow ileal endoscopic imaging, but these are lengthy and uncomfortable and have not been widely accepted. In view of the expense and limitations of standard testing modalities, and the growing experience with capsule endoscopy, there now exists ample evidence to support the use of this technique in the diagnostic evaluation of the patient with obscure gastrointestinal bleeding of suspected small intestinal origin.

Initial concerns over its safety and utility in the setting of cardiac pacemakers have not been borne out in subsequent patient trials, and the device has been utilized in such settings. Capsule endoscopy is limited, however, in that it cannot be used in the presence of obstructive pathology. In addition, in patients with motility disorders, the battery life of the device can be exceeded before complete small bowel transit is accomplished. Review of the images obtained is time-consuming and labor intensive by virtue of sheer numbers (see Section B). Because of limitations in localization, and because neither biopsy nor intervention can be accomplished with the capsule, this form of endoscopy is not an appropriate substitute for the assessment of areas accessible to standard upper or lower endoscopic techniques.

B. Patient Preparation and Technique

Early reports suggested that a period of no oral intake of 8 to 12 hours was the only preparation required for adequate capsule endoscopic evaluation of the small intestine. Subsequent reports have suggested that formal bowel preparation with polyethylene glycol solutions followed by NPO status may improve visualization, although this has not been documented to the point of statistical significance. Erythromycin as a motility agent to facilitate rapid delivery of the device distal to the pylorus, and complete and efficient small bowel transit, has been investigated with some promise, given the limited battery life available with which to accomplish the examination.

The device itself is 11 mm × 26 mm in size and contains six light-emitting diodes, a lens, a color camera chip, two silver oxide batteries, a radiofrequency transmitter, and an antenna. The camera chip is a complementary metal oxide semiconductor (CMOS) chip, which requires less power than standard charge-coupled device (CCD) chips and can operate effectively at very limited levels of illumination. The capsule takes 2 pictures per second and transmits these via radiofrequency to a recording device, which the patient wears at the waist. Following the examination, the recording device is downloaded to a computer with software that allows image portrayal on the computer monitor screen. The capsule is passed naturally and is not retrieved. In a typical 8-hour exam, approximately 57,000 images are obtained. Multiple-view video streams may be useful in reducing the time required for image review. Seven skin sensors allow some localization capability based on signal strength at the time of image acquisition in the exam sequence. The interpreting physician reviews the images for pathology.

For patients with foregut dysmotility, endoscopic delivery systems have been utilized. Endoscopic suturing techniques have been evaluated to allow prolonged viewing of specific anatomic sites. Magnetic methods have been investigated to facilitate the retrieval of devices that are retained in the small intestine.

C. Utility and Outcomes

Clinical studies to date suggest that capsule endoscopy significantly improves the diagnostic yield in comparison to other techniques for evaluating patients with obscure gastrointestinal bleeding. Diagnostic rates in the 60% to 80% range for capsule endoscopy, compared with yields in the 30% range for push enteroscopy, are typical of the published literature to date. Studies comparing capsule endoscopy to operative enteroscopy have suggested that the latter does not improve the diagnostic yield over that achieved with the capsule examination. Some investigators have successfully used the localization information gathered on capsule endoscopy to allow more limited operative enteroscopy and/or laparoscopic small bowel resection. The possibility of false positive exams leading to subsequent nontherapeutic surgical intervention has been borne out as a relatively rare, but real possibility in patients evaluated with capsule endoscopy. In addition, it appears that capsule endoscopy significantly increases the diagnostic yield of incidental small bowel pathology (especially ulcers and nonbleeding angiodysplastic lesions). Thus, approximately half the lesions seen on capsule endoscopy lead to therapeutically useful changes in management strategy, while the remainder may be misleading with respect to the precise cause of obscure blood loss. The therapeutic-driving value of the exam appears to be optimal in patients with completely negative workups on other modalities and is less powerful when pathology is already suspected from prior workup.

D. Summary

In summary, the available data suggest that capsule endoscopy significantly improves the diagnostic yield in patients with obscure gastrointestinal blood loss. The procedure is nonetheless oversensitive from a therapeutic efficacy standpoint and can lead to nontherapeutic interventions based on incidental pathology or, rarely, false positive examination findings. It is therefore perhaps best applied in the patient with ongoing gastrointestinal bleeding occult to other standard examinations, in whom directed more invasive diagnostic evaluation such as operative enteroscopy, or therapeutic surgical intervention, may be both clinically justified and guided by capsule endoscopic findings.

It is likely that future developments and further study will refine and expand the utility of this novel tool in gastrointestinal practice. Preparation standardization, motility regulation, real-time imaging, improved localization capacity, capsule manipulation, and ultimately therapeutic delivery are all areas of potential future development.

E. Selected References

Adler DG, Gostout C, Knipshield M. Prospective, blinded comparison of video capsule endoscopy versus push enteroscopy in patients with gastrointestinal bleeding of obscure origin. Gastrointest Endosc 2003;57:AB164.

Appleyard M, Glukhovsky A, Swain P. Wireless-capsule endoscopy for recurrent small-bowel bleeding. N Engl J Med 2001;344:232–233.

Chong A, Taylor A, Miller A, Desmond P. Clinical outcomes following capsule endoscopy (CE) examination of patients with obscure gastrointestinal bleeding (OGB). Gastrointest Endosc 2003;57:AB166.

Ell C, Remke S, May A, et al. The first prospective controlled trial comparing wireless capsule endoscopy with push enteroscopy in chronic gastrointestinal bleeding. Endoscopy 2002;34:685–689.

Goldfarb N, Phillips A, Conn M, Lewis B, Nash D. Economic and health outcomes of capsule endoscopy. Dis Manage 2002;5:123–135.

Guda N, Molloy R, Carron D, Gleisner M, Vakil N. Does capsule endoscopy change the management of patients? Gastrointest Endosc 2003;57:AB167.

Flexible Endoscopy
IV—Endoscopic Retrograde
Cholangiopancreatography

61. Endoscopic Retrograde Cholangiopancreatography

Harry S. Himal, M.D.

A. Indications

For a long time examination of the extrahepatic biliary tree and pancreatic duct was possible only during laparotomy. In 1968 McCune, a surgeon, and his colleagues first reported the endoscopic visualization of the common bile and pancreatic duct. Since then, innovations and improvements in technology have resulted in the technique of endoscopic retrograde cholangiopancreatography (ERCP) becoming indispensable in the diagnosis of diseases of the biliary tree and pancreatic duct. The development of computed tomographic scans, endoscopic ultrasonography, percutaneous transhepatic cholangiography, and magnetic resonance imaging has not diminished the importance of ERCP. ERCP is used for three major purposes: visualization of the ampulla of Vater, radiographic study of the common bile duct (cholangiography), and radiographic study of the pancreatic duct (pancreatography). Specific indications are listed in Table 61.1, and representative radiographs are shown in Figures 61.1 through 61.6.

B. Facilities and Equipment

ERCP requires the following facilities and equipment:
1. An x-ray room capable of both fluoroscopy (to visualize which duct has been cannulated) and film or digital radiography. A room dedicated to ERCP is most convenient (Fig. 61.7).
2. The ERCP endoscope is a side-viewing instrument that allows accurate visualization of the ampulla of Vater (Fig. 61.8). Videoendoscopy is now considered standard for ERCP.
3. A variety of different catheters are used to cannulate the ampulla (Fig. 61.9).

C. Patient Preparation

1. **Explain the technique and possible complications** to the patient and obtain informed consent. A knowledgeable, informed patient will cooperate with the endoscopist so that the procedure can be done quickly and safely.

Table 61.1. Indications for ERCP.

- Visualization of ampulla of Vater
  Adenomas
  Carcinoma
  Surveillance in patients with polyposis syndromes

- Cholangiography (Figs. 61.1–61.4)
  Cholestatic jaundice of unknown cause
  Choledocholithiasis
  Cholangitis
  Carcinoma of the bile duct
  Bile duct stricture
  Bile duct injury

- Pancreatography (Figs. 61.5, 61.6)
  Chronic pancreatitis
  Pancreatic carcinoma
  Pancreatic ascites
  Pancreatic pseudocyst
  Pancreatic trauma
  Gallstone pancreatitis

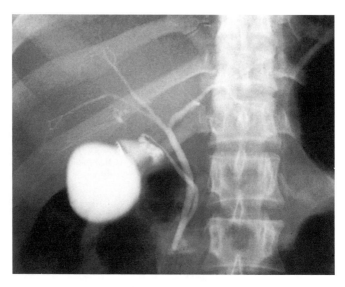

Figure 61.1. Normal cholangiogram obtained at ERCP. Note that gallbladder is also visualized.

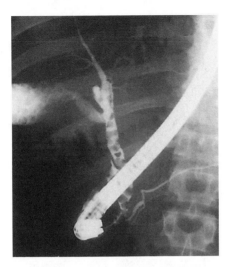

Figure 61.2. ERCP performed in patient with cholestatic jaundice in whom the differential diagnosis included both drug-induced and mechanical causes of jaundice. The cholangiogram demonstrates stones within the common bile duct.

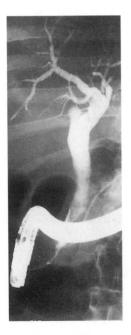

Figure 61.3. Common bile duct full of small stones and debris in a patient with cholangitis. Endoscopic sphincterotomy and removal of stones and debris resulted in clinical improvement.

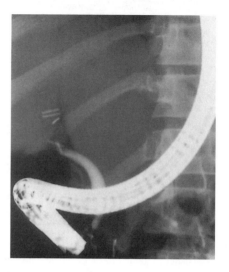

Figure 61.4. Common bile duct injury in a patient who had undergone laparoscopic cholecystectomy. Clips are seen across the proximal common bile duct.

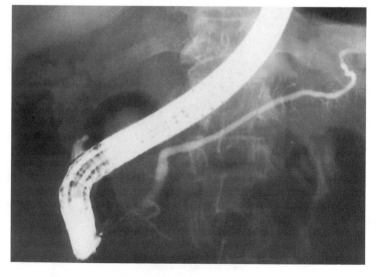

Figure 61.5. Normal pancreatogram obtained at ERCP.

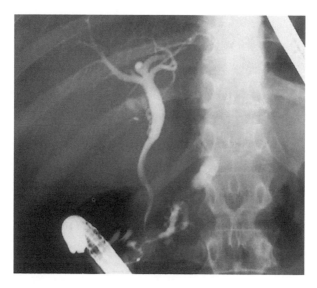

Figure 61.6. Pancreatic duct in a patient with chronic pancreatitis demonstrating dilatation and strictures. The common duct is also visualized and demonstrates extrinsic compression by the pancreatic mass.

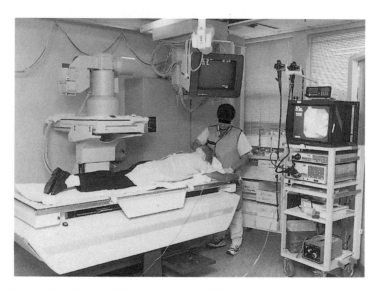

Figure 61.7. X-ray facilities to carry out ERCP include fluoroscopy. Note the position of the patient, endoscopic cart, and fluoroscopic monitor.

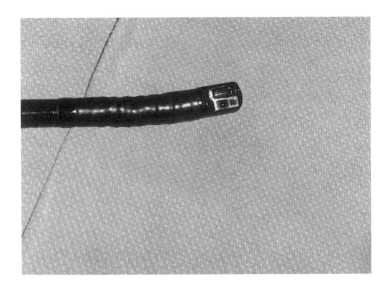

Figure 61.8. The side-viewing endoscope used for ERCP allows en face visualization, biopsy, and cannulation of the ampulla of Vater.

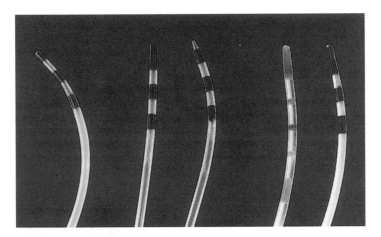

Figure 61.9. Catheters used for cannulation of ampulla of Vater.

2. The patient is **kept NPO for 6 hours prior** to the procedure. Diabetic patients on insulin should have an intravenous drip started.
3. If therapeutic ERCP (papillotomy, biopsy, stone extraction) may be required, evaluate the **coagulation status** of the patient. This is particularly important in jaundiced patients.
4. Patients with possible biliary obstruction, cholangitis, or choledocholithiasis should receive antibiotics directed at common biliary flora.
5. Anesthetize the oropharynx with topical anesthetic. The author prefers Xylocaine 4%.
6. Place a secure intravenous catheter in the right hand or arm.
7. Position the patient prone with the head turned to the right (Fig. 61.5).
8. Analgesia and conscious sedation facilitate the procedure (see Chapter 41). The author's preference is for intravenous meperidine, 25 to 50 mg, with intravenous diazemuls, 5 to 10 mg.
9. Appropriate monitoring includes pulse oximetry, heart rate, and blood pressure (see Chapter 49).
10. As soon as the endoscope is within the duodenum, give Buscopan (hyoscine butylbromide) intravenously, 20 to 40 mg, or 1 mg of glucagon hydrochloride, also intravenously, to decrease duodenal peristalsis.

D. Passing the ERCP Scope: Normal Anatomy

1. Introduce the endoscope gently through the mouth guard into the mouth and oropharynx. This is essentially a blind procedure, which is greatly facilitated by having the patient swallow.
2. Pass the endoscope gently down the esophagus into the stomach.
3. Once in the stomach, advance the endoscope toward the pylorus (Fig. 61.10). The side-viewing endoscope sometimes makes it difficult to traverse the stomach and identify the pylorus. Persistent maneuvering, combined with shortening of the endoscope by withdrawing to eliminate redundancy in the stomach, will ultimately prove successful. Frequently the presence of bile in the distal stomach will lead one to the pylorus, which is usually close by.
4. Use gentle rotation and pressure to pass the endoscope through the pylorus into the proximal duodenum (Fig. 61.11).
5. Turn the "up and down" and "right and left" dials both to their maximum clockwise extent and lock these controls.
6. Shorten the endoscope by pulling back. The ampulla of Vater should then be centrally visualized (Fig. 61.12). Make small adjustments in the locked dials so that the ampulla of Vater is seen en face.
7. Biopsy of the ampulla or selective cannulation of the pancreatic and common bile ducts may then be performed (Fig. 61.13).
8. The orifice of the pancreatic duct is at the 1 o'clock position and the orifice of the common bile duct is at the 11 o'clock position. Introduce the cannula into the orifice of the ampulla of Vater and gently inject 1 to 2 mL of 50% Hypaque dye (or alternative contrast medium

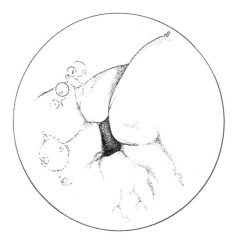

Figure 61.10. View of pylorus. Bubbles indicating bile provide a clue to the location of the distal stomach when orientation of the side-viewing endoscope is difficult.

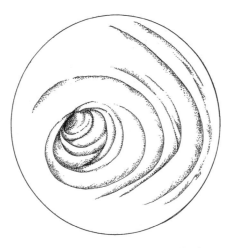

Figure 61.11. View of the proximal duodenum.

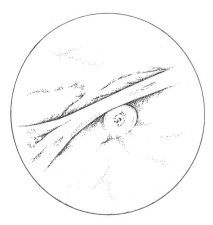

Figure 61.12. Endoscopic visualization of the ampulla of Vater. A transverse fold of mucosa overlying the ampulla is frequently seen, as shown here.

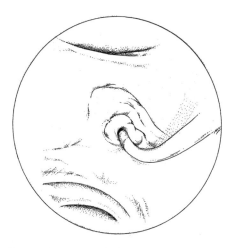

Figure 61.13. Cannulation of ampulla of Vater.

in patients allergic to Hypaque) while monitoring passage of contrast under fluoroscopy to identify the ductal anatomy. Further technical details of cannulation, cholangiography, and pancreatography are given in Chapter 63.

E. Selected References

Baillie J. Predicting and preventing post-ERCP pancreatitis. Rev Cur Gastroenterol Rep 2002;4:112–119.

Barron TH, Fleischer DE. Past, present and future of endoscopic retrograde cholangiopancreatography. Perspective on the National Institutes of Health Consensus Conference. Mayo Clin Proc 2002;77:407–412.

Bilbao MK, Dotter CT, Lee TG, Katon RM. Complications of endoscopic retrograde cholangiopancreatography (E.R.C.P.). Gastroenterology 1976;70:314–320.

Calleti G, Brocchi E, Agostini D. Sensitivity of endoscopic retrograde pancreatography in chronic pancreatitis. Br J Surg 1982;69:507–509.

Cameron JL. Chronic pancreatic ascites and pancreatic pleural effusions. Gastroenterology 1978;74:134–140.

Frick MP, Feinberg SB, Goodale RL. The value of endoscopic retrograde cholangiopancreatography in suspected carcinoma of the pancreas and indeterminate computer tomography results. Surg Gynecol Obstet 1982;155:177–182.

Gaisford WS. Endoscopic retrograde cholangiopancreatography in the diagnosis of jaundice. Am J Surg 1976;132:699–704.

Ghazi A, Washington M. Endoscopic diagnosis and management of diseases of the pancreas and hepatobiliary tract. Probl Gen Surg 1990;7:1610–1674.

Himal HS. The role of E.R.C.P. in laparoscopic cholecystectomy related cystic duct stump leaks. Surg Endosc 1996;10:653–655.

Himal HS. Common duct stones: the role of preoperative, intraoperative, and postoperative ERCP. Semin Laparosc Surg 2000;7:237–245.

Himal HS, Lindsay T. Ascending cholangitis: surgery versus endoscopic or percutaneous drainage. Surgery 1990;108:629–634.

Kozarek R, Gannan R, Baerg R, Wagonfeld J, Ball T. Bile leak after laparoscopic cholecystectomy: diagnostic and therapeutic application of endoscopic retrograde cholangiopancreatography. Arch Intern Med 1992;152:1040–1043.

Kullman E, Borch K, Lindstrom E, Ansehn S, Ilse I, Anderberg B. Bacteremia following diagnostic and therapeutic E.R.C.P. Gastrointest Endosc 1992;38:444–449.

Laraja RD, Lobbato VJ, Cassaro S, Reddy S. Intraoperative endoscopic retrograde cholangiopancreatography (E.R.C.P.) in penetrating trauma of the pancreas. J Trauma 1986;6:1146–1147.

Low DE, Mioflikier AB, Kennedy JK, Stiver HG. Infectious complications of endoscopic retrograde cholangiopancreatography. Arch Intern Med 1980;140:1076–1077.

McCune WS, Shorb PE, Moscowitz H. Endoscopic cannulation of the ampulla of Vater: a preliminary report. Ann Surg 1968;167:752–756.

Neoptolemos JP, Carr-Locke DC, London NJ, Bailey IA, James D, Fossard DP. Controlled trial of urgent endoscopic retrograde cholangiopancreatography and endoscopic sphincterotomy versus conservative treatment for acute pancreatitis due to gallstones. Lancet 1988;2:979–983.

O'Connor M, Kolars J, Ansel H, Silvis S, Vennes J. Preoperative endoscopic retrograde cholangiopancreatography in the surgical management of pancreatic pseudocysts. Am J Surg 1986;151:18–24.

Oi L. Fiberduodenoscopy and endoscopic pancreatocholangiography. Gastrointest Endosc 1970;17:59–62.

Sherman S, Lehman GA. E.R.C.P. and endoscopic sphincterotomy induced pancreatitis. Pancreas 1991;6:350–367.

Skude G, Wehlin L, Maruyama T, Ariyama J. Hyperamylasemia after duodenoscopy and retrograde cholangiopancreatography. Gut 1976;17:127–132.

Vennew JA, Bond JH. Approach to the jaundiced patient. Gastroenterology 1983;84:1615–1619.

62. Surgically Altered Anatomy and Special Considerations

Maurice E. Arregui, M.D., F.A.C.S.

A. Postgastrectomy

This section deals predominantly with the most difficult application of endoscopic retrograde cholangioponcreatography (ERCP), namely, ERCP that must be done after gastric resection with Billroth II reconstruction. Chapter 51 discusses issues related to ERCP scope passage after bariatric surgery.

Successful passage of the endoscope with cannulation of the ampulla is achieved in only 50% to 85% of patients with Billroth II anastomoses (in contrast to the 90% success rate that can be attained in patients with normal anatomy). This is due to both the difficulty in maneuvering through a variably long or angled afferent limb and the unusual position of the papilla once it is reached. Some endoscopists prefer to use a pediatric colonoscope or gastroscope; others prefer to use the duodenoscope. Specialized papillotomes are often required for therapeutic maneuvers. The indications for performing ERCP in patients with a Billroth II anastomosis are identical to those in patients with normal anatomy.

1. The **room setup**, **patient position**, topical anesthesia, sedation, and monitoring are the same as for patients with normal anatomy.
2. It is often useful **pass a gastroscope first** to better familiarize oneself with the anatomy.
3. **Enter the stomach** and identify the gastrojejunal anastomosis.
4. Pass the scope into one of the orifices.
5. It is often difficult to tell which is the afferent limb without fluoroscopy. Therefore, as the scope is passed, **check the position with fluoroscopy**.
6. If the scope goes into the pelvis, it is in the efferent limb. Bring the scope back into the stomach and enter the second orifice.
7. When the afferent limb is entered, maneuver the scope in a fashion similar to that used to maneuver a colonoscope through a tortuous sigmoid colon. Advance the scope for a distance and then retract it in an attempt to shorten the loop of jejunum. Sharp angles may be difficult to get around, and the shortening maneuver often helps to decrease an accentuated angle created by insufflating the bowel or excessive stretching of the bowel limb with the endoscope.
8. **Check the trajectory of the scope** with fluoroscopy to be certain that it is headed for the right upper quadrant (Fig. 62.1). An antecolic Billroth II may be more difficult to maneuver than a shorter retrocolic anastomosis.

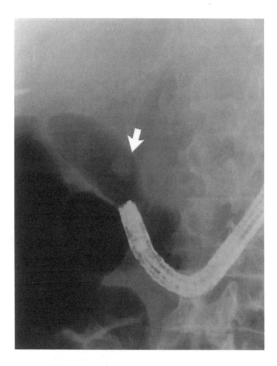

Figure 62.1. X-ray view of a gastroscope in the afferent limb of a Billroth II anastomosis. Insufflation of the duodenum shows a blind ending limb in the right upper quadrant. The ampulla (arrow) is seen in this air duodenogram.

9. When the **proximal duodenum** is entered, identify the blind proximal end and slowly pull the scope back until the papilla is identified.
10. Many prefer using the side-viewing **duodenoscope**. Passage with either scope is the same; because of the difference in perspective, however, passage of the duodenoscope is slightly more difficult.
    a. Because the papilla is viewed from below, the orientation and perspective is different.
    b. Rather than a typical en face papilla with the common bile duct oriented at the 11 to 12 o'clock position, the papilla is seen in the right upper portion of the viewing area with the common bile duct orifice at the 6 o'clock position (Fig. 62.2).
11. If a gastroscope or pediatric colonoscope is used, the papilla is oriented in a more tangential position in the lower left of the screen. Cannulation of the common bile duct with a straight-viewing scope is often very straightforward because the scope is often oriented in line with the common bile duct. A standard diagnostic cannula is used.

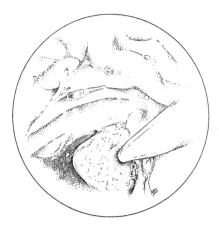

Figure 62.2. View of the ampulla through a duodenoscope. Cannulation requires positioning the catheter at a 6 o'clock location.

12. **Cannulation** with a duodenoscope can be more difficult owing to the unusual orientation of the common bile duct orifice at 6 o'clock (Fig. 62.3). Because of the curve of the duodenoscope, the cannula tip has a tendency to curve toward a more 12 o'clock to 9 o'clock position. A wire through the tip of the cannula may provide a straighter trajectory to allow cannulation at the 6 o'clock postion.

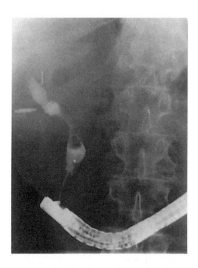

Figure 62.3. Cannulation of the bile duct using a duodenoscope. Contrast injection reveals a common bile duct stone.

13. **Technique of sphincterotomy** (see also Chapter 64). Once successful cannulation has been performed and a need for sphincterotomy established, the orientation of the duodenoscope and the papilla creates a challenge for the endoscopist.
    a. The advantage of the duodenoscope is the ability to maneuver the papillotome.
    b. Because of the orientation of the scope and the papilla compounded by the upward deflection of a standard papillotome, specialized sphincterotomes and techniques are often employed. For example, a Billroth II papillotome bows the wire outward, which allows orientation of the cutting wire toward the 6 o'clock position when one is using the duodenoscope.
    c. Alternatively, place a 7-French stent in the common bile duct and use a needle papillotome to cut the papilla over the stent.

B. Choledochoduodenostomy

Sump syndrome (characterized by cholangitis, liver abscess, or recurrent pancreatitis) is the most common indication for evaluation of a choledochoduodenostomy. Treatment consists of removal of debris and stones and possible sphincterotomy.

1. Either a thin-caliber gastroscope or a side-viewing duodenoscope may be used.
    a. Advance the gastroscope into the second portion of the duodenum. If the anastomosis is not stenotic, the scope can be advanced in directly. The technique is no different from standard gastroscopy.
    b. Pass the side-viewing duodenoscope as during standard ERCP.
2. Debris can be retrieved through the choledochoduodenostomy or the ampulla.
    a. If the choledochoduodenostomy is the route chosen, advance a gastroscope or small-caliber pediatric scope through the anastomosis.
    b. Pass wire baskets or balloon catheters through the channel of the scope to retrieve the stones or debris.
    c. If the anastomosis is stenosed, balloon dilation may be required prior to passage. No attempt should be made to use a sphincterotome to enlarge the anastomosis, as bleeding or perforation could result.
    d. Alternatively and preferably, the duodenoscope can be used to cannulate the common bile duct through the ampulla and sphincterotomy carried out using standard technique. Debris is removed with a balloon catheter or a wire basket. Performing a sphincterotomy may improve the dependent drainage and thereby reduce the chances for recurrence of the sump syndrome.

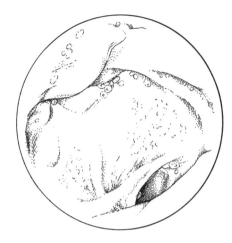

Figure 62.4. Endoscopic view of a choledochojejunal anastomosis in a patient who had a gastrointestinal bleed. A laparoscopic side-to-side choledochojejunostomy had been performed 2 months previously for an unresectable distal cholangiocarcinoma causing obstructive jaundice.

C. Choledochojejunostomy

Endoscopy is performed to evaluate bleeding or obstruction at the site of the anastomosis.

1. Use a **colonoscope or enteroscope**. Pass the scope in standard fashion through the pylorus and into the third portion of the duodenum. As in passage in a patient with a Billroth II anastomosis, the jejunum may be difficult to advance owing to the length and sharp angles encountered. Maneuver the scope in a to-and-fro manner to try to keep the length of the jejunum short. As in colonoscopy, pressure over the left upper quadrant or to the left of the umbilicus may prevent excess looping of the scope.

2. **Endoscopic treatment**. If the anastomosis is widely patent, the scope can be passed into the biliary tree, which is usually dilated in this group of patients (Fig. 62.4). If the anastomosis is narrowed, balloon dilation may be required for entry into the bile ducts.

D. Special Considerations

Anatomical variants or distortions unrelated to surgical alterations may make passage of a duodenoscope a challenge. These include cervical diverticula such as a Zenker's diverticulum, a paraesophageal hiatal hernia, or a large J-shaped stomach.

1. Cervical diverticula can be a special challenge for a side-viewing duo-denoscope with the risk of perforation. Passage of a gastroscope with careful maneuvering into the esophagus under direct visualization followed by passage of a guidewire or placement of an overtube will aide passage of the duodenoscope.
2. A large paraesophageal hiatal hernia can pose a difficult challenge to passage of the duodenoscope into the distal stomach. The scope will often curl in the intrathoracic stomach, making orientation and passage difficult. Passage of a gastroscope and placement of a long overtube into the antrum will allow passage of the duodenoscope.
3. A long J-shaped stomach may make it difficult to pass the duodeno-scope through the pylorus while the patient is in the prone position. Placing the patient in the lateral position with the right side up will often allow cannulation of the duodenum. The patient can then be placed back into the prone position for ERCP. If this does not work, passage of an overtube into the antrum may add enough stiffness to allow cannulation of the duodenum to complete the ERCP.

E. Selected References

Cotton PB, Williams CB. Practical Gastrointestinal Endoscopy. 2d ed. Oxford: Blackwell Scientific, 1982.

Marbet UA, Staider GA, Faust H, Harder F, Gyr K. Endoscopic sphincterotomy and surgical approaches in the treatment of the "sump syndrome." Gut 1987;28:142–145.

Nawras AT, Catalano MF, Alsolaiman MM, Rosenblatt ML. Overtube-assisted ERCP in patients with altered gastric and esophageal anatomy. Gastrointest Endosc 2002;56(3):426–430.

Osnes M, Rosseland AR, Aabakken L. Endoscopic retrograde cholangiography and endoscopic papillotomy in patients with a previous Billroth-II resection. Gut 1986;27:1193–1198.

Siegel JH. Endoscopic Retrograde Cholangio-Pancreatography. 1st ed. New York: Raven Press, 1992.

Siegle JH, Yatto RP. ERCP and endoscopic papillotomy in patients with a Billroth II gastrectomy: report of a method. Gastrointest Endosc 1983;29:117–118.

63. Cannulation and Cholangiopancreatography

David Duppler, M.D., F.A.C.S.

A. Cannulation and Cholangiopancreatography

1. After identifying the papilla, make certain that the patient is adequately sedated to minimize movement and that the duodenum is adequately paralyzed to stop peristalsis.

2. Keep the tip of the scope deflected to the right—this will usually aid in holding the proper position in the duodenum.

3. Observe the papilla for a few moments. Attempt to identify the orifice, and the likely orientation of the common bile duct and pancreatic duct. Usually, there is one orifice for both the pancreatic and bile ducts, with the ducts sharing a common channel of varying length. Occasionally, there are two orifices, the more superior of which is the orifice of the bile duct.

4. Advance the cannula toward the papilla with a combination of advancement of the cannula with the right hand, change in angle of the catheter using the elevator, and change in the position of the scope using the deflection wheels or by torquing the instrument. It is generally best to cannulate the duct of interest first. If this is the pancreatic duct, the cannula should approach the orifice of the papilla nearly at a right angle to the duodenal wall with the catheter approaching in a left-to-right orientation. For common bile duct cannulation, the cannula should be oriented in a more cephalad direction and approached from a right-to-left position (Figs. 63.1 and 63.2).

    a. In most situations, the pancreatic duct is the easier of the two ducts to cannulate. Once the cannula is within the orifice, inject a small amount of dye under fluoroscopic control. In opacifying the pancreatic duct, it is crucial to avoid distention of the pancreatic ductal system. Overinjection of the pancreatic duct (as evidenced by opacification of the secondary and tertiary branches of the duct) or repeated cannulations of the duct increase the risk of postprocedure pancreatitis.

    b. Bile duct cannulation is usually facilitated by advancing the scope past the papilla and deflecting the tip upward. This "tucked under" position often aligns the cannula with the axis of the common bile duct (Fig. 63.3). Direct the cannula toward the 10 to 12 o'clock position on the papilla. As the cannula enters the orifice of the papilla, lift the cannula with the elevator to advance the

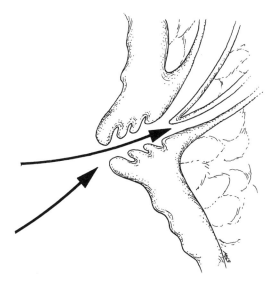

Figure 63.1. The proper cannulation angle for the pancreatic duct is nearly at right angles to the duodenal wall, while bile cannulation requires a more cephalad orientation.

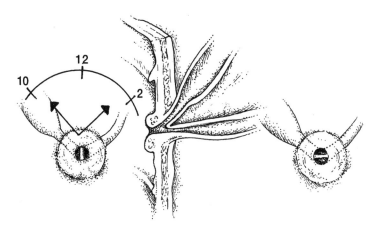

Figure 63.2. The septum separating the orifices to the pancreatic and bile ducts can be oriented in any direction from horizontal to vertical. When the papilla is viewed en face, the course of the bile duct is usually toward the 10 o'clock position and the pancreatic duct toward the 2 o'clock position, although some variation exists.

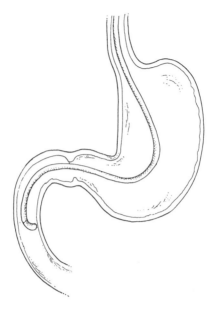

Figure 63.3. The "tucked under" position is usually obtained by advancing the endoscope slightly and deflecting the tip upward.

catheter along the roof of the papilla. This increases the likeli-hood of elective cannulation of the common bile duct (Fig. 63.4). Manually curving the cannula in a more cephalad orientation prior to its insertion will also enhance common bile duct cannu-lation, whereas leaving the catheter straight usually facilitates pancreatic duct cannulation.

c. If these maneuvers do not allow for selective cannulation of the appropriate duct, switching to a different type of cannula is some-times helpful. A tapered tip cannula is often helpful when the orifice of the papilla is quite small. A sphincterotome can be used to obtain a greater cephalad orientation of the catheter for selec-tive bile duct cannulation (Fig. 63.5).

d. Although injection of dye under fluoroscopic control with the cannula impacted at the papilla will often opacify the desired duct, free cannulation of the pancreatic duct usually can be facil-itated by advancing the catheter toward the 2 o'clock direction on the papilla. Withdrawing the scope slightly will also make the cannula approach a 90-degree angle with the duodenal wall, which will also improve the chances of free cannulation of the pancreatic duct.

e. Free cannulation of the common bile duct is also often facilitated by withdrawing the scope slightly after the common bile duct has

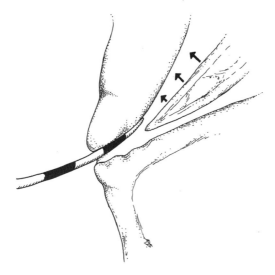

Figure 63.4. Lifting the cannula to insert it along the "roof" of the papilla increases the likelihood of entry into the bile duct.

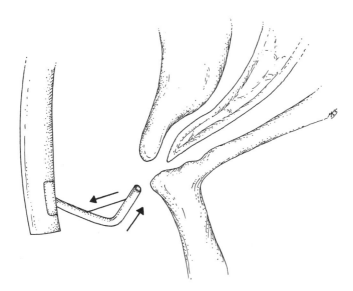

Figure 63.5. Sometimes bile duct cannulation requires orientation of the cannula in a cephalad direction. This can be accomplished by using a sphincterotome. Tightening the cutting wire bows the cannula upward and produces a more cephalad orientation for the tip of the cannula.

been opacified with contrast. This allows the catheter to change directions within the papilla, as the common bile duct often becomes more horizontal within the duodenal wall. If the sphincterotome is used for cannulation, this can also be accomplished by lessening the tension on the cutting wire, which will straighten the tip of the sphincterotome within the papilla. As the scope is withdrawn, it is sometimes necessary to slightly withdraw the cannula back into the scope to prevent excessive pressure on the papilla. Free cannulation of either duct can also be facilitated by the passage of a floppy-tipped guidewire, although care must be taken to avoid the use of excessive force with guidewires, as this can lead to false passages and perforations.

5. In opacifying the common bile duct, make the injection under fluoroscopic control and obtain exposures throughout the injection to provide both early filling and later phases. This facilitates detection of small stones and other more subtle abnormalities.

6. In a patient with an obstructed system, it is often helpful to attempt to aspirate bile initially, before adding contrast, to try to relieve some of the pressure within the system. This is especially important in a patient who may have cholangitis.

B. Special Considerations and Situations

1. **Duodenal diverticula** often make it more difficult to locate the papilla. The papilla is generally located along the inferior edge of the diverticulum, although it is occasionally located within the diverticulum itself.

    a. When two diverticula are present, the papilla is often located on the isthmus of tissue between the diverticula. Once again, time should be spent locating the papilla and observing it to identify the orifice.

    b. If the papilla cannot be identified, it is probably within the diverticulum. It can sometimes be brought into view by suctioning some of the air out of the duodenum, using the cannula to probe the edge of the diverticulum, putting pressure on the right upper quadrant of the patient's abdomen, or changing the patient's position. If the papilla is located within the diverticulum and cannot be easily approached with the cannula, it can sometimes be pulled outside the diverticulum with the cannula or with the use of a sphincterotome. Occasionally, if the diverticulum is large, the tip of the scope can be placed within the diverticulum to facilitate cannulation.

2. **Periampullary tumors** may distort the anatomy of the papilla. Patience is required to search the area slowly to identify the papillary orifice, which can be significantly elevated or depressed by the tumor.

The tumor also can distort the normal path of the pancreatic and bile ducts within the papilla, making free cannulation more difficult. Gentle probing of the tumor with the cannula will often lead to cannulation, but aggressive and forceful probing should be avoided because this will lead to bleeding and edema, which will further obscure the anatomy.

3. An **impacted stone within the papilla** will often turn the orifice of the papilla in a caudad orientation. This will usually require the "tucked under" position for successful cannulation.

4. **Cannulation of the minor papilla** may be indicated when the diagnosis of pancreas divisum is suspected or when a tumor involving the head of the pancreas precludes opacification of the proximal pancreatic duct.

    a. The minor papilla is usually located 1 to 3 cm proximal to the major papilla and slightly to the right.

    b. Approach the minor papilla at right angles to the duodenal wall using a tapered or ultratapered catheter.

    c. Once again, care should be taken to not overdistend the pancreatic ductal system.

5. **Precut papillotomy.** If selective cannulation of the common bile duct is not possible with any of the previously mentioned maneuvers, consideration should be given to performing a precut papillotomy. This is a blind maneuver in which the sphincter is cut prior to radiographic visualization. This procedure is associated with an increased risk of bleeding and pancreatitis. It should be used only when access to the common bile duct is considered mandatory, such as in patients with jaundice or cholangitis.

    a. Insert a precut papillotome or a needle-knife papillotome into the papillary orifice and make small, 1- to 2-mm cuts in the direction of the 10 to 12 o'clock position.

    b. In general, the precut sphincterotomy should not extend more than 5 mm, and then repeated attempts should be made to obtain a selective cannulation of the common bile duct.

    c. Avoid injection of dye in the impacted position after precut sphincterotomy, as this increases the risk of developing an intramural injection.

    d. Precut sphincterotomies should be performed only by endoscopists with significant experience in standard sphincterotomy.

6. Multiple attempts at cannulation often result in enough papillary trauma to induce edema and occasionally bleeding. This further decreases the likelihood of successful cannulation. If this has occurred, or if there has been an intramural injection of contrast, it is best to terminate the procedure with plans to repeat it 2 to 3 days later. One can expect an approximate 50% success rate with this second procedure. If unsuccessful, referral of the patient to a more experienced endoscopist or the use of other modalities for evaluating the pancreaticobiliary system should be considered.

C. Selected References

Farrell RJ, Howell DA, Pleskow DK. New technology for endoscopic retrograde cholan-giopancreatography: improving safety, success, and efficiency. Gastrointest Endosc Clin North Am 2003;13:539–559.

Laasch HU, Tringali A, Wilbraham L, et al. Comparison of standard and steerable catheters for bile duct cannulation in ERCP. Endoscopy 2003;35:669–674.

Maeda S, Hayashi H, Hosokawa O, et al. Prospective randomized pilot trial of selective biliary cannulation using pancreatic guidewire placement. Endoscopy 2003;35: 721–724.

64. Therapeutic Endoscopic Retrograde Cholangiopancreatography

Gary C. Vitale, M.D., F.A.C.S.
Stan C. Hewlett, M.D.
Carlos M. Zavaleta, M.D.

A. Biliary Sphincterotomy

Therapeutic endoscopic retrograde cholangiopancreatography (ERCP) has evolved over the last 30 years out of what was once an avant-garde endoscopic diagnostic test. Now, in an era of highly accurate imaging techniques (high-resolution computed tomography [CT], magnetic resonance imaging, magnetic resonance cholangiopancreatographic scans, etc.), diagnostic information can be obtained noninvasively; with minimal risk to the patient (see Chapter 61). ERCP is thus increasingly used as a therapeutic rather than diagnostic modality.

1. **Selective cannulation of bile duct.** Before endoscopic sphincterotomy, the common bile duct must be selectively cannulated with passage of the opacifying cannula or a guidewire up into the duct (deep cannulation). Selective biliary cannulation can be difficult in settings of inflammation (acute gallstone pancreatitis) and when the anatomy is unfavorable (tortuous common channel). If the pancreatic duct (PD) is accessible, placement of a PD stent can straighten out this channel and improve cannulation success. This should be considered as an alternative to precut papillotomy or percutaneous transhepatic (PTC) access when cannulation is clinically indicated (Fig. 64.1).

2. **Positioning the sphincterotome.** Place the sphincterotome in the orifice of the papilla with the "cutting" wire coming in contact with the papilla at the 11 to 12 o'clock position. Cutting in this position reduces pancreatitis and bleeding (Fig. 64.2). A wire-guided sphincterotomy is performed with the sphincterotome over a guidewire. This helps keep the sphincterotome from twisting and also allows the operator to advance the instrument in and out of the papilla during the course of the sphincterotomy.

3. **Cutting the papilla.** Bow the sphincterotome by tightening the wire. Using a blended current, with more cutting current than coagulation, apply short bursts of current, allowing the sphincterotome wire to cut slowly through the ampullary sphincter.

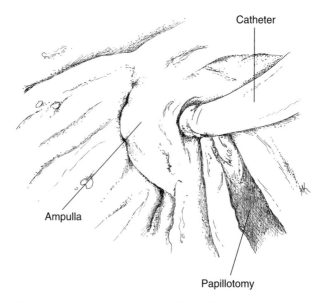

Figure 64.1. Endoscopic view of precut knife papillotomy above pancreatic duct stent performed for a difficult cannulation of common bile duct.

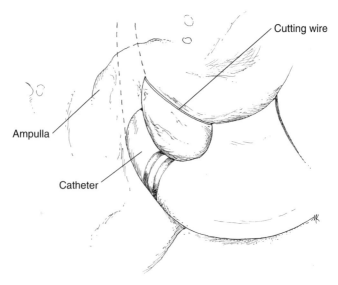

Figure 64.2. Technique for a sphincterotomy showing cutting wire in contact with the major papilla at 12 o'clock position.

a. The complete sphincterotomy should extend just to the inferior margin of the suprapapillary duodenal fold.

b. To avoid the "zipper effect" in which the sphincter is cut too fast, risking bleeding and perforation, the sphincterotome should not be bowed too tightly by the nurse during the sphincterotomy. It should be bowed just enough to press lightly into the tissue, letting the current do the cutting.

4. **Transhepatic (PTC)-guided sphincterotomy.** In cases in which the sphincterotome or the guidewire cannot be advanced into the bile duct, a transhepatic wire can be placed percutaneously into the duodenum. This wire can then be grasped endoscopically and brought out through the operating channel of the scope. A sphincterotome can then be passed over the guide wire and positioned for a standard sphincterotomy.

5. **Precut sphincterotomy.** In selected cases, a precut sphincterotomy may be performed. The precut knife is used to directly cut the papilla to gain access to the biliary tree. There are two techniques used. In the first, the cut is made beginning at the orifice of the ampulla and is extended superiorly along the apex of the ampulla. In the second, the cut is begun on the superior aspect of the infundibulum (bulge) of the papilla and extended inferiorly with short, deepening cuts into the papilla. The principal risk in either of these techniques is perforation, and thus precut sphincterotomy should be performed by experienced endoscopists and even then only sparingly, in cases with definite therapeutic indications.

B. Pancreatic Sphincterotomy

1. Perform a **biliary sphincterotomy** before pancreatic sphincterotomy to facilitate access to the pancreatic duct.

2. **Selective cannulation of the pancreatic duct.** We prefer the "short" position of the scope for access to the ampulla, but in some instances placing the endoscope in the "long" position can improve the cannulation angle for the PD. Insert a guidewire into the pancreatic duct and confirm position under fluoroscopy. Pass the sphincterotome over the wire into the orifice of the pancreatic duct.

3. **Cutting the pancreatic ductal septum and sphincter.** Depending on the variable anatomy, there may be a short or long septum between the pancreatic duct and the bile duct within the ampulla. There is an additional muscular sphincter specifically encircling the orifice of the pancreatic duct. In some cases, pancreatic septoplasty may be sufficient to allow free flow of pancreatic juice. In other cases, the cut must be extended further into the pancreatic ductal orifice to ablate the muscular sphincter. This is particularly true when the indication for pancreatic ductal sphincterotomy is papillary hypertension with recurrent pancreatitis as its clinical manifestation. Direct the sphincterotome in

an orientation toward the 1 o'clock position. Cutting proceeds as
described in Section A.

C. Minor Papilla Sphincterotomy

The minor papilla is amenable to the same techniques described earlier. This
structure is typically slightly proximal and to the right of the ampulla of Vater.
Cannulation can be achieved in the "short" position but often requires an endoscope in the "long" position for a favorable lineup.

D. Biliary Tract Stone Removal

In general, endoscopic stone retrieval via the ampulla should be done
after an adequate sphincterolysis. A forced passage of a stone through an
intact ampullary sphincter can be too traumatic, leading to postprocedure
obstruction from edema, which can be complicated further by cholangitis or
pancreatitis.

1. **Basket stone removal.** Stones may be removed from the bile ducts
   and intrahepatic biliary radicals using a standard stone basket.
   a. Insert the basket into the bile duct, open it, and engage the
       stone. The assistant can open and partially close the basket, while
       the operator jiggles the catheter to trap stones. The catheter can
       be withdrawn in the open position, and stones often will pop
       out.
   b. Larger stones can be individually engaged and removed after
       securing the basket around them.
   c. Apply traction in the axial direction of the bile duct in removing
       a stone so that the apex of the sphincterotomy is not further cut
       with the wire of the stone basket during stone extraction. Perfo-
       ration may result if the wire of the stone basket cuts the apex of
       the sphincterotomy (Figs. 64.3 and 64.4).
2. **Balloon stone extract removal.** For smaller stones, a balloon stone
   extractor can be used to pull stones through the sphincterotomy.
   a. Insert the balloon catheter through the sphincterotomy and inflate
       the balloon above the stone.
   b. As the catheter is retrieved, the stone is pulled into the
       duodenum.
3. As an alternative to sphincterotomy, **the sphincter can be dilated** first
   using a longitudinal hydrostatic dilating balloon, with balloon stone
   extraction of small stones following. While this method avoids sphincterotomy, it is associated with a higher incidence of pancreatitis and
   cannot be unequivocally recommended at this time. When we utilize
   ampullary balloon dilation, we place a predilation PD stent to lessen
   the risk inducing a pancreatitis.

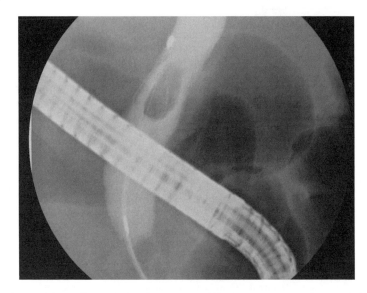

Figure 64.3. Radiograph showing common bile duct stone extraction using the basket.

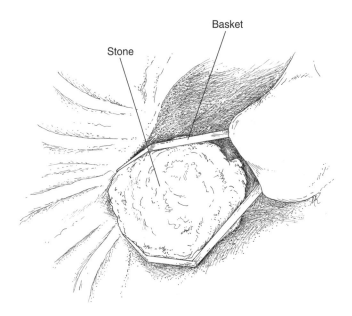

Figure 64.4. Endoscopic view of successful extraction of common bile duct stone with the basket.

4. **Mechanical lithotripsy.** For larger stones, lithotripsy is often necessary to fracture the stone before extracting it. Extracting a very large stone through the sphincterotomy risks either perforation or stone entrapment. If the stone becomes entrapped in the distal bile duct with the basket still around it, a surgical procedure may be necessary to disengage it. The mechanical lithotripter functions by using a hand crank to tighten the wire basket around the stone against a metal sheath.

5. **Electrohydraulic and candela laser lithotripsy.** When mechanical fracture of the stones is not successful, one may employ electrohydraulic or pulsed-dye laser techniques. In each of these approaches, a catheter is passed under direct vision into the bile duct and placed in direct contact or close proximity to the stone before applying the energy. The mother-daughter scope is often used for this, as it allows for direct vision of intrabiliary stones. Direct visualization with a daughter scope is necessary to reduce the risk of common bile duct injury from poor positioning of the catheter, particularly if the electrohydraulic lithotriptor is used. After the stone has been fractured, the pieces can be extracted using conventional techniques.

6. **Extracorporeal lithotripsy** has also been used for fracture of large common bile duct stones with some success. This is most often necessary for occlusive stones that do not allow passage of a basket or balloon. In these cases, if a guidewire can be passed above the stone, a stent may be placed to relieve obstruction. Treatment can then be performed with extracorporeal lithotripsy or gallstone dissolving agents prior to another ERCP attempt at stone extraction.

7. **Intrahepatic stones.** In many cases, intrahepatic stones may be extracted using stone basket or balloon stone extraction methods described earlier. When the stones are larger, a mother-daughter scope can be used with intrahepatic lithotripsy. For multiple, large intrahepatic stones, it is often better to use a percutaneous transhepatic approach. With this method, a percutaneous transhepatic tract is developed and dilated to the diameter of a choledochoscope with a working channel. Percutaneous choledochoscopy is then performed with fracture and extraction of intrahepatic stones. Electrohydraulic or candela laser lithotripsy is often necessary as an adjunct procedure for successful stone clearance in these cases.

E. Pancreatic Duct Stone Removal

Stones in the pancreatic duct should be removed when possible. In some cases, stones are a result rather than a cause of the disease process, and removing them may not always improve a patient's course of recurring pancreatitis. There are good data, however, that complete stone clearance improves patient outcome with regard to chronic pain.

1. Stones may be removed with a combination of stone basket and balloon. The stone basket is often necessary to fracture the stones, which are frequently soft, and the balloon can clear the fragments.
2. Some stones are embedded in the wall of the duct or are located at junctions or angulated curves in the duct, which makes them inaccessible to the basket or balloon.
3. Large stones often will obstruct the duct, making extraction impossible. In these cases, a guidewire should be passed above the stone and a 5-French (Fr) stent passed if at all possible. Extracorporeal lithotripsy can then be performed to fracture the stone followed by endoscopic stone fragment extraction.

F. Biliary Stenting

The choice of type and size of stent, as well as the duration of stenting and the use of accessory procedures (sphincterotomy or balloon dilation) are guided by the condition being treated or managed. An academic discussion of this topic is beyond the scope of this manual; the reader is directed to the literature cited in Section J.

1. **Stent selection.** Polyethylene stents are available in 7-, 10-, and 11.5-Fr diameters.
    a. For short-term stenting of 30 days or less or in cases of difficult access in which changing to a larger diameter working channel scope could compromise access, the 7-Fr stent is appropriate.
    b. For longer-term stenting, indications such as cancer, the 10 or 11.5 Fr is a better choice. These larger stents remain open significantly longer than the 7-Fr stents in randomized trials. There is no significant difference between the longevity of the 10- and 11.5-Fr stents.
    c. Metallic self-expanding stents are indicated for longer-term cancer stenting indications and last for a mean of approximately 1 year. These stents are nonremovable and may limit some treatment options later in the course of disease, and thus should be used selectively.
    d. Nasobiliary stents can be used for temporary stenting situations when repeat opacification of the biliary tract is desirable.
2. **Stent insertion.** For the 10- and 11.5-Fr stents, a wire-guided stent introducer is passed above the level of the stenosis over which the stent is pushed into position. The 7-Fr stents are placed directly over the guidewires and pushed into place. Metallic stents are initially 7 Fr prior to deployment and are positioned over a guidewire across the stenosis. They are released by retracting a plastic sleeve, which holds the stent in its stretched, compressed configuration. Upon release, the stent shortens and assumes its full diameter of 8 to 10 mm. Nasobiliary stents are introduced over a guidewire into the biliary tree above the level of obstruction and then are brought out through the nasopharynx (Fig. 64.5).

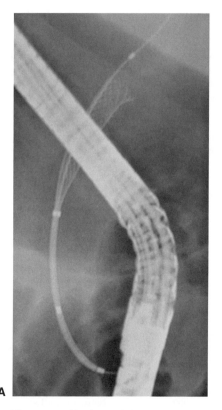

A

Figure 64.5. Metallic stent positioning and deployment in the common bile duct for malignant stricture. A. The stent is released initially. B. The stent is completely released. C. Endoscopic view of metallic stent at common bile duct orifice.

3. **Stent change.** Polyethylene stents can be changed electively every 3 to 4 months, or one can wait to change the stent until serum bilirubin and liver enzyme levels indicate impending obstruction. Stent exchange is usually a simple process, except in cases of long or very high level strictures. In those cases, it is wise to pass a guide-wire through the stent prior to removing it through the scope, using a stent retriever designed for this purpose. Polyethylene stents can be exchanged repeatedly over time, allowing the biliary system to remain patent indefinitely. Metallic stents when obstructed cannot be removed, but a second plastic or metallic stent can be passed through the center of the original stent restoring biliary patency. Newer metallic stent designs incorporating a Silastic sleeve over the mesh may reduce tumor and granulation tissue ingrowth, thus improving patency and facilitating recannulation (Fig. 64.6).

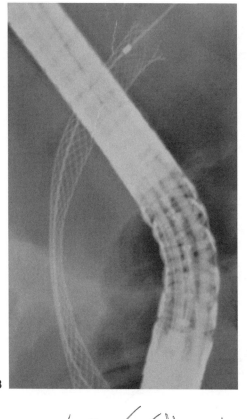

B

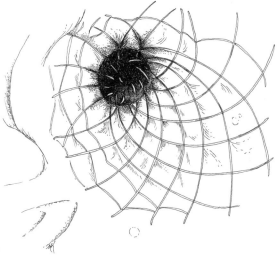

C

Figure 64.5. *Continued*

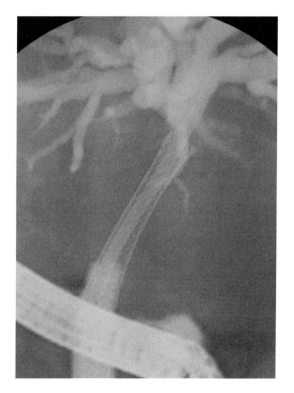

Figure 64.6. Radiograph shows a biliary polyethylene stent placed inside an obstructed uncovered metallic stent as a result of tumor overgrowth.

G. Pancreatic Duct Stenting

1. **Stent options.** Smaller (5- or 7-Fr) stents are used in the pancreatic ducts. These stents have multiple side holes and flanges and are more specifically designed to facilitate pancreatic duct drainage. Metallic stents have been used for benign pancreatic strictures, but their use in that clinical setting remains experimental.

2. **Stent insertion.** Stent insertion is accomplished over a guide wire that has been placed in the pancreatic duct. Balloon dilatation of strictures prior to stent placement may be necessary to allow stent placement. Stents are left in place for shorter intervals than in the biliary system. As noted earlier, simultaneous clearance of pancreatic duct stones improves long-term results.

H. Endoscopic Dilatation of Biliary Tree and Pancreatic Duct

High-pressure balloons and rigid dilators exist for benign or malignant strictures to relieve obstruction. Polyethylene balloons have been designed for the pancreas and biliary ducts in different sizes ranging from 4 to 10 mm. Each balloon inflates at a specific pressure and requires a minimum scope channel of 2.8 mm.

1. **Technique.** After the stricture has been demonstrated, a catheter and guidewire are advanced through the stricture. The catheter is exchanged for the balloon over the guidewire into the stricture. Radiopaque markers are located on the balloon to assist in positiong the balloon in the strictured duct. The balloon is inflated to its specific diameter with a 1:1 mixture of contrast medium and normal saline, so the process can be visualized on a monitor under fluoroscopic guidance. After dilatation, the balloon is deflated and retrieved through the scope channel, or if resistance is felt, the endoscope and balloon can be removed as one unit.

Rigid dilation also exists for pancreas and biliary ductal strictures. These dilators vary in size from 4 to 11.5 Fr and will allow dilatation of tight strictures by passage over a guidewire. Radiopaque control markers at 3 cm from the catheter tip help identify the position of the dilator relative to the stricture.

2. **Potential complications** occur at about the same frequency as with ERCP, and balloon dilatation does not seem to significantly increase the incidence of perforation, hemorrhage, or pancreatitis (Figs. 64.7 and 64.8).

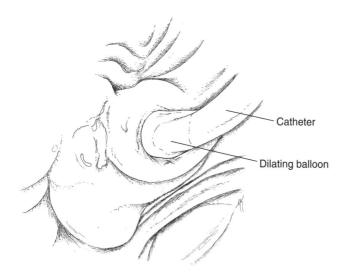

Figure 64.7. Balloon dilatation of accessory pancreatic duct orifice at minor papilla in a patient with pancreas divisum.

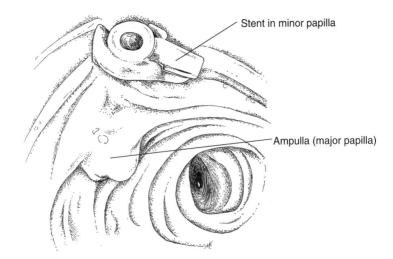

Figure 64.8. Stent placement at minor papilla in a patient with pancreas divisum.

I. Endoscopic Management of Pancreatic Pseudocysts and Endoscopic Cyst-Enterostomy

Pancreatic pseudocysts are classified as **communicating** if the lumen of the pseudocyst can be filled with contrast via the pancreatic duct at ERCP. These pseudocysts are amenable to pancreatic ductal stenting (decompression via the ampulla). Pancreatic duct stenting in these patients is done using the techniques described in Section G, Pancreatic Duct Stenting.

A **noncommunicating** pseudocyst lumen is not visualized at ERCP; the pancreatic ductal system and the lumen of the pseudocyst are disconnected. The endoscopic management of these pseudocysts is also termed internal drainage; this involves creating a fistula between the pseudocyst lumen and the alimentary tract (stomach or duodenum). The following is specific to this technique.

    1.   **Pseudocyst identification.** Location of the pseudocyst adjacent to the gastric or duodenal wall by CT imaging is essential. During endoscopy, indentation by the cyst of the gastric or duodenal wall confirms location. Adherence of the cyst wall to the gut decreases the incidence of perforation or leak. The procedure is contraindicated if adherence of these two structures is not present, a condition that should also raise suspicion of the possibility of a cystic neoplasm. Endoscopic ultrasound (EUS) can be used to further identify the pseudocyst if it is not obvious on the endoscopic view. Wall thickness is determined

from the CT scan or EUS and should be less than 1 cm to consider endoscopic drainage. Patients with associated masses in the pancreas or with pancreatitis of unclear etiology may have tumors such as pancreatic cancer with associated pancreatitis and pseudocyst, serous cystadenoma, or lymphoma. Adequate biopsy or a nonendoscopic operative approach is mandatory in these patients.

2. **Technique of endoscopic cyst-enterostomy**

   a. At the apex of the bulge of the cyst into the gastric or duodenal lumen, a small area of mucosa is coagulated with the precut knife.

   b. In the center of this area, a direct puncture of the cyst is made using cutting or blended current.

   c. A guidewire is passed into the cyst, an opacifying cannula is passed over the guidewire, and contrast is injected to confirm cyst size and position compared to the CT scan.

   d. A biopsy of the pseudocyst wall is taken at some point in the process of draining the cyst. A sphincterotome is then passed into the cyst, and the opening enlarged. Care is taken to use a combination of cutting and cautery to avoid bleeding at the site of the cyst-enterostomy.

   e. A polyethylene stent is placed into the cyst in selected cases. If the pseudocyst is in communication with the pancreatic duct, or if the duct is obstructed, a stent should be placed to allow longer-term drainage. Also, if the cyst wall is thick or if a small opening has been made due to risk of bleeding, a stent should be placed to ensure that the cyst-enterostomy remains open until the cyst resolves. The stent should remain in place until the cyst has resolved by CT and there is demonstration of a patent pancreatic duct. The stent may be left indefinitely if there is obstruction of the mid portion of the pancreatic duct with the tail of the pancreas draining into the stomach or duodenum via the stent. In younger, healthy patients operative intervention should be considered in cases of complete duct occlusion and recurrent/persistent cyst or pancreatitis following stent removal (Figs. 64.9–64.11).

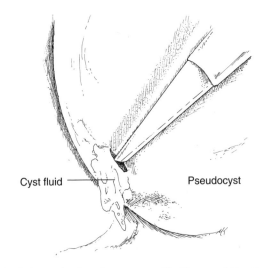

Cyst fluid ——————   Pseudocyst

Figure 64.9. Endoscopic view shows a precut knife coagulating the apex of the cyst bulge and fluid drainage into the stomach.

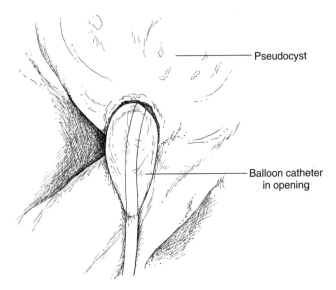

————— Pseudocyst

————— Balloon catheter
in opening

Figure 64.10. Enlargement of endoscopic cyst-gastrostomy opening with an 8-mm high-pressure balloon.

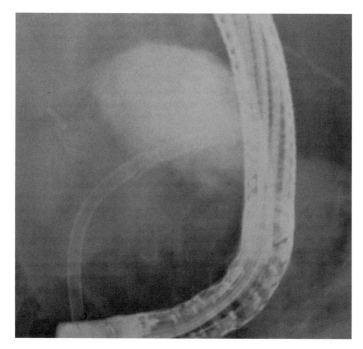

Figure 64.11. Radiograph shows a polyethylene stent placed into the cyst to ensure that the cyst-gastrostomy will remain open until the cyst resolves.

J. Selected References

Barkun AN, Barkun JS, Fried GM, et al. Useful predictors of bile duct stones in patients undergoing laparoscopic cholecystectomy. Ann Surg 1994;220:32–49.

Binmoeller KF, Soehendra N, Liguory C. The common bile duct stone: time to leave it to the laparoscopic surgeon? Endoscopy 1994;26:315–319.

DeIorio AV Jr, Vitale GC, Reynolds M, Larson GM. Acute biliary pancreatitis: the roles of laparoscopic cholecystectomy and endoscopic retrograde cholangiopancreatography. Surg Endosc 1995;9:392–396.

Fan TS, Lai ECS, Mok FPT, et al. Early treatment of acute biliary pancreatitis by endoscopic papillotomy. N Engl J Med 1993;328:228–232.

Freeman ML, Nelson DB, Sherman S, et al. Complications of endoscopic biliary sphincterotomy. N Engl J Med 1996;335:909–918.

Fulcher AS, Turner MA, Capps GW, Zfass AM, Baker KM. Half-Fourier RARE MR cholangiopancreatography in 300 subjects. Radiology 1998;207:21–32.

Grace PA, Williamson RCN. Modern management of pancreatic pseudocysts. Br J Surg 1993;80:573–581.

Huibregtse K. Complications of endoscopic sphincterotomy and their prevention [editorial]. N Engl J Med 1996;335:961–962.

Neoptolemos JP, Carr-Locke DL, London NJ, et al. Controlled trial of urgent endoscopic retrograde cholangiopancreatography and endoscopic sphincterotomy versus conservative treatment of acute pancreatitis due to gallstones. Lancet 1988:II:979–983.

Nowak A, Nowakowska-Dulawa E, Marek T, Rybicka J. Final results of the prospective, randomized, controlled study on endoscopic sphincterotomy versus conventional management in acute biliary pancreatitis [abstract]. Gastroenterology 1995; 108(Suppl):A380.

Pitt HA, Venbrux AC, Coleman J, et al. Intrahepatic stones. The transhepatic team approach. Ann Surg 1994;219:527–535.

Scholmerich J, Lausen M, Lay L, et al. Value of endoscopic retrograde cholangiopancreatography in determining the cause but not course of acute pancreatitis. Endoscopy 1992;24:244–247.

Segel. Techniques for Endoscopic Decompression of the Biliary Tree. In: Therapeutical Gastrointestinal Endoscopy. 2d ed. 1989;282–312.

Vitale GC. Advanced interventional endoscopy. Am J Surg 1997;173:21–25.

Vitale GC, George M, McIntyre K, et al. Endoscopic management of benign and malignant biliary strictures. Am J Surg 1996;171:553–557.

Vitale GC, Larson GM, Wieman TJ, Cheadle WG, Miller FB. The use of ERCP in the management of common bile duct stones in patients undergoing laparoscopic cholecystectomy. Surg Endosc 1993;7:9–11.

Vitale GC, Stephens G, Wieman TJ, Larson GM. The use of ERCP in the management of biliary complications following laparoscopic cholecystectomy. Surgery 1993;114: 806–814.

65. Complications of Endoscopic Retrograde Cholangiopancreatography

Morris Washington, M.D.
Ali Ghazi, M.D.

A. Pancreatitis

1. **Cause and prevention.** Pancreatitis is the most common complication following endoscopic retrograde cholangiopancreatography (ERCP). While hyperamylasemia may be seen in up to 60% of patients after ERCP, clinical pancreatitis occurs in approximately 5%. The incidence is the same for both diagnostic and therapeutic procedures. The severity of post-ERCP pancreatitis in the majority of cases is mild to moderate and self-limited. Unfortunately, however, fatal necrotizing post-ERCP pancreatitis is reported. Post-ERCP pancreatitis is more common in younger patients and has its highest incidence in patients having ERCP for suspected sphincter of Oddi dysfunction (19%).

   a. The exact **mechanism** that initiates post-ERCP pancreatitis is still unproven, but it is believed by most to be mechanical in nature, caused by an increase in pancreatic intraductal pressure with release of pancreatic enzyme from acini into the pancreatic parenchyma. This increased intraductal pressure may result from the following.

      i. Difficulty with cannulation leading to overmanipulation of the papilla of Vater, causing trauma and spasm of the sphincter of Oddi.

      ii. Repeated injection into the pancreatic ductal system in an attempt to access the bile duct.

      iii. Overzealous injection of contrast media into the pancreatic ductal system, resulting in a complete outline of the pancreas on x-ray known as acinarization.

      iv. Injury to the papilla of Vater from the electrocautery used during endoscopic sphincterotomy (ES).

      v. Placement of large endobiliary stents without an ES, causing obstruction of the pancreatic duct orifice.

   b. **Prevention.** Intuitively, better technique during cannulation and ES should lower the incidence of post-ERCP pancreatitis; however, this has been difficult to study and document. Nevertheless, the following technical considerations may be helpful in the prevention of post-ERCP pancreatitis.

    i. Selective cannulation to avoid injection into the pancreatic ductal system if a pancreatogram is not required.

    ii. Use only a few milliliters of contrast to fill the main pancreatic ducts of Wirsung and Santorini.

    iii. A 50-mL syringe to inject contrast media delivers less hydrostatic pressure than a syringe of lesser volume and thus may avoid inadvertent overfilling of the pancreatic ductal system.

    iv. If the initial cannulation of the bile duct has been difficult and therapeutics are required, then maintain access with the use of a guidewire.

    v. During ES, use more cutting than coagulation current to decrease the amount of edema and tissue injury.

    vi. Early precut sphincterotomy using a needle-knife sphincterotome on difficult bile duct cannulations is controversial and requires particular endoscopic skill.

    vii. There have been many attempts at pharmacologic prevention of post-ERCP pancreatitis using atropine, glucagon, calcitonin, steroids, and somatostatin, all of which have shown limited efficacy in experimental and clinical trials. Recently, however, Gabexate, a protease inhibitor, has been shown to decrease the severity of post-ERCP pancreatitis if given intravenously for 30 to 90 minutes prior to the procedure and continued for 12 hours thereafter. Additional clinical trials are needed to further document its efficacy prior to general use.

  2. **Treatment.** Most cases of post-ERCP pancreatitis are mild to moderate in severity and will resolve with modest treatment. Restriction of oral intake and intravenous fluids until the symptoms abate and the serum amylase and lipase normalize is usually all that is required. In a minority of patients the pancreatitis may be more severe, with the establishment of several Ranson's criteria and phlegmon development on imaging studies. Oral intake should be restricted in these patients, parenteral nutrition instituted, and serial sonograms obtained to assess the degree of pancreatic inflammation. Pseudocysts may develop in the acute phase and take several weeks to resolve. Avoid the temptation of starting oral intake prematurely, leading to an exacerbation. Sonographic evidence of resolution of the phlegmon or pseudocysts should be established prior to oral intake. Large pseudocysts that persist with therapy longer than 6 to 8 weeks will require internal drainage. This can be accomplished surgically via cystogastrostomy or cystojejunostomy. Persistent symptomatic cysts in the tail of the pancreas can be treated with resection. Some pseudocysts can be drained internally via an endoscopic approach (see Chapter 66). Endoscopic ultrasound may help to determine the feasibility of endoscopic drainage. Percutaneous drainage should be avoided because of the high incidence of prolonged catheter drainage.

  Death from post-ERCP pancreatitis is fortunately a rare occurrence. These patients develop necrotic pancreatitis frequently with infection. Dynamic CT scanning will demonstrate a large amount of devitalized pancreas. The patients appear severely toxic and frequently have positive blood cultures. Exploration with pancreatic debridement and necrosectomy will be required as a lifesaving measure. These patients often require repeated debridement as the inflammatory process progresses.

B. Cholangitis

1. **Cause and prevention.** The overall incidence of cholangitis following ERCP is low (0.1%). Cholangitis following ERCP in patients with nonobstructed biliary systems is exceedingly rare, and therefore antibiotic prophylaxis is not indicated in these patients. When cholangitis does occur following ERCP it almost always occurs in jaundiced patients with obstructed biliary systems. Patients at particular risk for cholangitis are those undergoing stenting for malignant biliary strictures, those having combined percutaneous endoscopic procedures, and those who have had failed biliary drainage. Antibiotic prophylaxis has been shown to lower the incidence of cholangitis in these patients following ERCP. Piperacillin, which is secreted in the bile, has been particularly effective.

Cholangitis following ERCP can be completely prevented by timely relief of the biliary obstruction. This can be accomplished using ERCP therapeutics or surgical intervention. If surgical intervention is chosen, prior coordination between endoscopist and surgeon is important to effect timely relief of the biliary obstruction.

2. **Treatment.** Once cholangitis has been established, immediate drainage is indicated. At this point the patient must be considered to have an undrained abscess, and therefore every hour counts. If the patient is allowed to progress to septic shock, then risk of mortality is high.

C. Hemorrhage

1. **Cause and prevention.** Clinically significant bleeding following ES is reported to occur in 2% of cases. Minor bleeding (oozing) is not uncommon and will stop spontaneously provided the patient has normal coagulation parameters. In patients with obstructive jaundice it is important that the prothrombin time (PT) be checked prior to ES, since these patients will frequently have elevation secondary to impaired vitamin K absorption. If ES can be delayed for a few days, the PT can be easily corrected with vitamin K given subcutaneously. If ES must be done urgently, fresh frozen plasma must be given until the PT is corrected. Patients who are taking antiplatelet medication (e.g., aspirin, persantine) should have them discontinued 7 to 10 days prior to ES. If ES cannot be delayed, bleeding time should be ascertained and, if abnormal, corrected with platelet transfusion.

While it is again difficult to document what role technique has in preventing clinically significant bleeding following ES, it has been reported that endoscopists who perform ES more frequently have a lower rate of complications. The following technical considerations may be helpful:

a.   ES should be made as close to the 12 o'clock position as possible to avoid duodenal vasculature.
b.   A blended cutting current should be used that has some cautery effect.
c.   ES should be made slowly in sequential steps instead of one uncontrolled cut.
d.   Tailor the size of the ES to the need (e.g., only a small ES is needed to extract small stones or insert large endobiliary stents).
e.   Do not forcefully extract large stones; use a mechanical lithotriptor.

2.   **Treatment.** As mentioned earlier, minor oozing after ES is not uncommon and will usually stop spontaneously with observation. Pulsatile (arterial) bleeding after ES is of more concern. If the bleeding is not so brisk as to impair endoscopic visualization, it may also stop spontaneously; or it can be treated by injection of the bleeding point with epinephrine solution. A few milliliters of 1 : 10,000 epinephrine solution delivered using a variceal injection device may be helpful.

Brisk arterial bleeding that obscures endoscopic visualization must be treated more aggressively. The patient should be admitted to the intensive cane unit for close monitoring. A baseline ratio of hemoglobin to hematocrit (Hgb/Hct) and type and cross-match should be obtained. Two large-bore intravenous catheters should be placed for infusion of crystalloid and blood products. An arterial line and a Foley catheter should be inserted. If there is evidence of brisk active bleeding manifested by tachycardia, hematemesis, hematochezia, and a falling Hgb/Hct, intervention is required. If an experienced interventional radiologist is available, celiac arteriography with selective embolization of the bleeding branch of gastroduodenal artery may avoid operative intervention. However, if embolization fails or is unavailable and the bleeding continues, operative intervention must be undertaken prior to the onset of hypovolemic shock. The patient should be explored through a midline incision and a full Kocher maneuver should be performed on the duodenum. A duodenotomy in the second portion of the duodenum will allow access to the papilla of Vater. The bleeding can be controlled with a suture ligature, being careful not to stenose the sphincterotomy. If the patient is stable, possibly then attention can be turned to surgical correction of the problem for which the ES was being done. Otherwise, a T-tube should be placed, the duodenotomy closed in two layers, and a drain placed.

D. Perforation

1.   **Cause and prevention.** Perforation following ES is uncommon and occurs in approximately 0.3% of cases. The patient frequently will complain of abdominal and back pain. There may be associated fever and leukocytosis. The perforation is usually retroperitoneal, and hence abdominal x-rays will demonstrate retroperitoneal air. Intraperitoneal (free) air is unusual, and suspicion of perforation in another area of the gastrointestinal tract should be entertained. The mistaken diagnosis of pancreatitis is sometimes made, leading to delay in recognition and management.

The following technical considerations may help to avoid this complication:

a. Use sphincterotomes with short cutting wire lengths (20–25 mm).
b. Do not extend the ES beyond the transverse duodenal fold that lies proximal to the papilla of Vater.
c. As mentioned earlier, tailor the length of ES to the need.

2. **Treatment.** If recognized early, perforations as a result of ES can be managed conservatively with good success. A nasogastric tube should be inserted and broad-spectrum antibiotics with adequate gram-negative coverage administered. The patient should be followed closely, and improvement should be expected in 12 to 24 hours. If the patient's condition fails to improve and signs of ongoing sepsis are present, operative intervention should be undertaken. The patient should be explored through a midline incision and the duodenum subjected fully to the Kocher maneuver, revealing the site of the perforation posteriorly. Depending on the degree of inflammation and induration of the tissues, either primary closure or an omental patch should be done. Depending on the adequacy of the repair, a pyloric exclusion procedure should be considered. This can be accomplished by performing a gastrotomy, closing the pylorus with absorbable suture, gastrojejunostomy, and T-tube drainage. A drain should be placed and consideration should be given to placement of a gastrostomy and feeding jejunostomy.

E. Rare Complications

There are rare complications of ERCP that can occur; some are unique to ERCP and others can occur with any endoscopic procedure targeting the upper gastrointestinal tract. They are listed here so that one may have a general knowledge of them.

1. Esophageal perforations
2. Mallory-Weiss tears
3. Hepatic and splenic hematomas
4. Bile duct perforations by guidewires
5. Stone extraction basket entrapment
6. Stent loss within the bile duct

G. Selected References

Arcidiacono R, Gambitta P, Rossi A, Grosso C, Bini M, Zanasi G. The use of long acting somatostatin analogue (octreotide) for prophylaxis of acute pancreatitis after endoscopic sphincterotomy. Endoscopy 1994;26:715–718.

Aronson N, Flamm CR, Bohn RL, Mark DH, Speroff T. Evidence-based assessment: patient, procedure, or operator factors associated with ERCP complications. Gastrointest Endosc 2002;56(6 Suppl):S294–S302.

Byl B, Deviere J, Struelens MJ, et al. Antibiotic prophylaxis for infectious complications after therapeutic endoscopic retrograde cholangiopancreatography: a randomized, double-blind, placebo-controlled study. Clin Infect Dis 1995;20:1236–1240.

Cavallini G, Tittobello A, Frulloni L, Masci E, Mariana A, DiFrancesco V. Gabexate for the prevention of pancreatic damage related to endoscopic retrograde cholangiopancreatography. N Engl J Med 1996;26:961–963.

Demols A, Deviere J. New frontiers in the pharmacological prevention of post-ERCP pancreatitis: the cytokines. Pancreas 2003;4:49–57.

Flemmer M, Oldfield EC 3d. Prophylax or perish? Am J Gastroenterol 1996;91: 1867–1868.

Freeman ML. Adverse outcomes of endoscopic retrograde cholangiopancreatography: avoidance and management. Gastrointest Endosc Clin North Am 2003;13:775–798.

Freeman ML. Understanding risk factors and avoiding complications with endoscopic retrograde cholangiopancreatography. Current Gastroenterol Rep 2003;5:145–153.

Freeman ML, Nelson DB, Sherman S, Haber GB. Complications of endoscopic biliary sphincterotomy. N Engl J Med 1996;335:909–918.

Ghazi A, Washington M. Endoscopic diagnosis and management of diseases of the pancreas and hepatobiliary tract. Curr Probl Surg 1990;7:161–174.

Lo AY, Washington M, Fischer MG. Splenic trauma following endoscopic retrograde cholangiopancreatography. Surg Endosc 1994;8:692–693.

Pasricha P. Prevention of ERCP-induced pancreatitis: success at last. Gastroenterology 1997;112:1415–1417.

Schneider J, Barkin J. Gabexate for prevention of pancreatic damage related to endoscopic retrograde cholangiopancreatography. Gastrointest Endosc 1997;45:447–448.

Tarnasky PR, Cunningham JT, Hawes RH, et al. Transpapillary stenting of proximal biliary strictures: does biliary sphincterotomy reduce the risk of postprocedure pancreatitis? Gastrointest Endosc 1997;45:46–51.

Flexible Endoscopy
V—Choledochotomy

66. Diagnostic Choledochoscopy

Bruce V. Macfadyen, Jr., M.D., F.A.C.S.

A. Intraoperative

1. **Indications.** Intraoperative choledochoscopy is performed at the time of laparoscopic or open cholecystectomy with common duct exploration, or when common duct exploration is performed as an isolated procedure. The major indications are listed in Table 66.1.
2. **Preparation, equipment, and room setup (laparoscopic)**
   a. When choledochoscopy is performed during laparoscopic biliary surgery, the standard laparoscopic cholecystectomy room setup, patient position, and trocar sites are used. Place an additional 5-mm trocar in the mid–right subcostal abdominal wall and use this for access into the common bile duct (CBD). A sixth 5-mm trocar is frequently inserted in the upper midline between the umbilical and subxiphoid ports to perform CBD exploration (CBDE) and choledochoscopy using a two-handed surgical technique.
   b. The surgeon stands at the patient's left side, and the video monitors are placed over the right and left shoulders as in laparoscopic cholecystectomy.
   c. A second camera is attached to the choledochoscope and using a video mixer, the monitor displays a simultaneous split image from the laparoscope and the choledochoscope.
   d. **Passing the scope (laparoscopic)**
   a. **Transcystic.** When the operative cholangiogram (performed through the cystic duct) indicates that choledochoscopy is required, first advance a 0.035-in. guidewire through the cholangiocatheter into the cystic duct, common bile duct, and into the duodenum.
      i. Remove the cholangiocatheter and advance a 5-mm trocar with a plastic seal (instead of a valve) over the guidewire into the right subcostal area.
      ii. Pass rigid or balloon dilators over the wire to dilate the cystic duct to 5 mm. Sometimes the valves of Heister prevent advancement of the wire or dilator into the bile duct. In this case, it may be necessary to make another 2-mm opening in the cystic duct 7 to 10 mm from its entry into the bile duct. However, in most cases, if the cystic duct can be dilated to 5 mm, passage of the choledochoscope easily occurs. The smaller flexible choledochoscope with an outside diameter of 3 mm and a 1.2-mm accessory channel is preferred for the transcystic approach.

Table 66.1. Indications for intraoperative choledochoscopy.

Indication	Purpose
• Filling defect(s) on operative cholangiogram	• Visualize and remove stone(s)
• Bile duct stricture on operative or preoperative cholangiogram	• Visualize and obtain biopsy/brush cytology samples
• Polypoid filling defect on cholangiogram	• Visualize and obtain biopsy/brush cytology samples
• Evaluate common duct after mechanical removal of CBD stones	• Assure completion of stone removal

    iii. Backload the 0.035-in. guidewire through the accessory channel of the choledochoscope, where a special dual valve is used on the exit port, thus allowing a pressurized saline solution to be infused through the choledochoscope channel to maximize bile duct visualization. At the same time, instruments can be advanced through the accessory channel for biopsy, stone removal, lithotripsy, and cytology.

  b. **Alternative technique via choledochotomy.** Another alternative is to open the CBD longitudinally for 5 mm at its midportion, thus eliminating the resistance from the valves of Heister. Direct access to the common bile duct is performed when CBD stones are greater than 5 mm in diameter, when visualization of the upper bile ducts is necessary, and when the choledochoscope cannot be advanced through the cystic duct. The length of the choledochotomy should be no longer than the diameter of the choledochoscope or the largest stone because significant leakage of the pressurized saline solution in the common bile duct can occur, thus decreasing visualization.

    i. Place a 5-0 Prolene stay suture on each side of the choledochotomy and use these to keep the incision open.

    ii. Pass a rubber-tipped grasper through the upper midline trocar and use this for manipulation of the endoscope into the bile duct. This type of grasper minimizes injury to the outer sheath of the choledochoscope.

    iii. Complete the common duct exploration as described earlier (see Chapter 19).

  e. **Passing the scope (open).** Perform a Kocher maneuver to allow the distal bile duct to be straightened. Insert the choledochoscope into the choledochotomy. Cross the stay sutures over the choledochoscope to allow the bile duct to distend with saline. Pass the scope proximal and distal under visual control. Generally the scope must be removed and reinserted to reverse the direction from proximal to distal or vice versa.

  f. **Technical points for performing choledochoscopy by either route.** The bile duct must be continuously flushed with saline during choledochoscopy. Saline provides distention and is the viewing medium. It also serves to flush away blood or debris.

a. Keep the lumen of the bile duct in the center of the field. If the picture becomes red, the scope may be impacted against the bile duct wall. Pull the scope back 1 to 2 cm and deflect the tip until the lumen is in the center of the screen.

b. In the transcystic technique, visualization of the distal bile duct can be readily performed but proximal duct visualization is only successful in 10% to 20% of the cases because of the angulation of entry of the cystic duct into the CBD. If proximal bile duct visualization is crucial, a choledochotomy should be performed.

B. Postoperative Choledochoscopy

Postoperative choledochoscopy is most commonly performed when retained common duct stones are seen on a postoperative cholangiogram. Possible routes of access to the common duct include percutaneous (through the **T**-tube tract), peroral (mother-daughter scope technique during endoscopic retrograde cholangiopancreatography [ERCP]), and transhepatic. Each will be described briefly here. Fluoroscopy is needed for all three methods.

1. **Percutaneous via T-tube tract**

   a. Insertion of the choledochoscope into the CBD can be performed percutaneously when the **T**-tube tract has matured for 5 to 6 weeks.

   b. Position the patient supine.

   c. The surgeon stands on the patient's right side, with the video monitor directly opposite.

   d. Prep and drape the right upper quadrant of the abdomen around the **T**-tube exit site in the standard manner. Intravenous sedation is given.

   e. Pass two 0.035-in. guidewires through the **T**-tube into the CBD and then into the duodenum under fluoroscopic guidance. One wire is the guiding wire and the second wire is a safety wire that can maintain access to the duct, should the first wire become dislodged.

   f. Remove the **T**-tube over the wires. Using one of the wires as a guide, insert a 5-mm dilating balloon and expand it to dilate the tract.

   g. After complete tract dilation, backload one 0.035-in. guidewire through the accessory channel of the choledochoscope and advance the endoscope into the CBD.

   h. Proximal CBD visualization can be accomplished by withdrawing the 0.035-in. wire and deflecting the endoscope tip toward the bifurcation of the common hepatic duct. Since the endoscope tip deflection ranges from 90 to 120 degrees, visualization of the upper bile ducts can be accomplished.

      i.   When choledochoscopy has been completed and the endoscope removed, reinsert a 12- to 14-French T-tube or straight catheter into the CBD over the wire and remove both wires.

2. **Peroral cholangioscopy**

     a.   This technique is performed using a therapeutic duodenoscope and a small "baby" scope inserted through the accessory channel of the duodenoscope using a fluoroscopic guidewire. There are two therapeutic duodenoscopes that can be used for this technique. The largest one has an outside diameter of 15 mm and an accessory channel of 5.5 mm, which allows the passage through its accessory channel of a 5-mm cholangioscope with an accessory channel in the "baby" scope of 2.2 mm. A smaller therapeutic duodenoscope has an outside diameter of 11.5 mm and an accessory channel of 4.2 mm and allows the passage of a 3-mm cholangioscope with a 1.2-mm accessory channel. The diagnostic and therapeutic accessories for the smallest cholangioscope are limited to a cytology brush, a four-wire helical basket, and an electrohydraulic lithotripsy (EHL) fiber.

     b.   The patient is sedated and the duodenoscope passed as described in Chapter 64, therapeutic ERCP.

     c.   The endoscope and fluoroscopic monitors are placed opposite the surgeon on the patient's left side in the prone position.

     d.   Visualize the papilla, and position it so that the longitudinal axis is in the center of the video monitor.

     e.   Insert a tapered papillotome through the duodenoscope channel into the papillary orifice at the 11 to 12 o'clock position to visualize the CBD. (If the papillotome is advanced into the papilla at the 3 o'clock position, the pancreatic duct will be injected.)

     f.   Perform a 7- to 10-mm papillotomy at the 11 to 1 o'clock position of the papilla, being careful not to cut through the transverse duodenal fold (which may produce perforation of the duodenum).

     g.   After this is done, advance a 0.035-in. guidewire through the papillotome, high into the biliary radicals. Withdraw the papillotome from the duodenoscope, leaving the wire in place.

     h.   Backload the guidewire through the 3-mm cholangioscope and advance the daughter scope through the duodenoscope accessory channel. This part of the procedure requires an assistant to hold the duodenoscope in position, and the surgeon advances the daughter endoscope over the wire. Take care not to cause sharp angulation of the daughter scope at the duodenoscope accessory port, which can cause breakage of the fiberoptic bundles. Additionally, to more easily advance the daughter scope, the duodenoscope should lie in the shortest route to the papilla.

     i.   As the choledochoscope exits the accessory channel, the elevator of the mother scope is left completely open so that the daughter scope can be advanced out of the mother scope into the duodenum and then into the CBD over the wire, thus avoiding breakage of the cholangioscope. In addition, any movement of the duodenoscope can cause potential breakage of the daughter scope.

j. When the daughter scope is in the CBD, remove the guidewire and use pressurized saline to irrigate the bile duct to maintain visualization. Since the daughter scope channel is small (1.2 mm), only a cytology brush, lithotriptor fiber, and a three- or four-wire spiral basket can be used. Biopsy forceps are not yet available for the smallest daughter endoscope.

k. Once the choledochoscope has been removed, use the papillotome catheter to obtain a completion cholangiogram for documentation.

3. **Transhepatic choledochoscopy**

a. Position the patient supine, give intravenous sedation, and inject local anesthesia into the skin for needle access into the right or left lobe of the liver.

b. Pass a needle into the ductal system under fluoroscopic guidance. For access to the right or left hepatic duct, the surgeon stands on the patient's corresponding left or right side and the TV and fluoroscopy monitors are facing the surgeon.

c. Dilate the tract to 5 mm using a dilating balloon. Tract dilatation can be done in one procedure or serially every 2 to 3 days over a 2-week period using Amplatz dilators.

d. Finally, a 22- to 24-French Amplatz dilator sheath is inserted to keep the liver tract open during the insertion of the choledochoscope. The same two-wire technique for **T**-tube tract access is used as for the **T**-tube tract technique, and the choledochoscope is advanced into the left or right hepatic and common hepatic ducts through the sheath. The left and right hepatic ducts, common hepatic and common bile ducts can be visualized.

C. Biopsy and Brush Cytology Techniques

The technique for biopsy and brush cytology is similar for the choledochoscope and cholangioscope except that there is not a biopsy forceps for the 3-mm cholangioscope.

1. It is important to visualize all the bile ducts that can be safely cannulated, to ensure completeness of examination. Bile duct tumors are frequently multicentric.

2. Note tumor size and length. In addition to biopsy and cytology samples, bacterial and fungal cultures may be appropriate.

3. Perform at least six biopsies of the tumor or stricture in all quadrants.

4. Perform brush cytology on the tumor and in all quadrants of a stricture after the biopsy has been done. Three to four passes of the brush over the tumor in different areas are necessary to ensure adequate sampling.

5. Obtaining a successful diagnosis in the bile duct using these techniques is only 60% to 80%, whereas in the stomach or colon, similar techniques are 95% accurate.

D. References

Cheung M-T. Postoperative choledochoscopic removal of intrahepatic stones via a T tube tract. Br J Surg 1997;84(9):1224–1228.

Cheung M-T, Wai S-H, Kwok P, C-H. Percutaneous transhepatic choledochoscopic removal of intrahepatic stones. Br J Surg 2003;90(11):1409–1415.

Csengeri A, Zwick M, Takacs GY. Intraoperative choledochoscopy as an alternative to intraoperative T-tube cholangiography in detecting retained stones in the biliary tree. Br J Surg 1998;85(Suppl 2):166.

Fernandez JM, Munoz J, Blasco F, Partida R, Tirapo J. Flexible choledochoscopy: technical improvements and indications. Br J Surg 1998;85(Suppl 2):197.

Giurgiu DI, Margulies DR, Carrol BJ, et al. Laparoscopic common bile duct exploration: long-term outcome. Arch Surg 1999;134(8):839–844.

Martin IJ, Bailey IS, Rhodes M, O'Rourke N, Nathanson L, Fielding G. Towards T-tube free laparoscopic bile duct exploration: a methodologic evolution during 300 consecutive procedures. Ann Surg 1998;228(1):29–34.

Ponchon Thierry, Genin G, Mitchell R, et al. Methods, indication, and results of percutaneous choledochoscopy: a series of 161 procedures. Ann Surg 1996;223(1):26–36.

Takada T, Uchiyama K, Yasuda H, Hasegawa H. Indications for the choledochoscopic removal of intrahepatic stones based on the biliary anatomy. Am J Surg 1996; 171(6):558–561.

67. Therapeutic Choledochoscopy and Its Complications

Raymond P. Onders, M.D.
Thomas A. Stellato, M.D.

A. Therapeutic Choledochoscopy

1. **Stone retrieval** (see also Chapter 18)
   a. The simplest method is to **flush** the stones through the ampulla under direct visualization. This is usually aided by the administration of 1 mg of glucagon given intravenously. By advancing the choledochoscope against the stones and directing the stone to the ampulla, bile duct stones can at times be forced through the ampulla and into the duodenum.
   b. The second method to remove stones that are visualized with the flexible choledochoscope is with the use of a straight **four-wire basket**.
      i. Advance the basket beyond the stone and then slowly withdraw it until the stone is in the basket.
      ii. Close the basket to entrap the stone. Visually verify stone capture.
      iii. Pull the basket up to the scope and withdraw scope, basket, and stone as a unit.
      iv. Repeat this process until all visualized stones have been removed and a completion cholangiogram shows a clear duct.
   c. When stones are larger than the junction between the cystic duct and the common bile duct, vigorous attempts to remove them can injure the duct. In these cases **lithotriptors**, introduced through the working port of the choledochoscope, can deliver an energy source to fragment the calculus. Mechanical lithotriptors are used to crush the stones but are difficult to use if a stone is adherent to the wall of the duct or is lodged in the ampulla. Electro-hydraulic and pulsed-dye laser lithotriptors deliver an energy beam to break up the stones when placed in direct contact with the stones. If inadvertent bursts of energy strike the bile duct wall instead of the stone, there may be damage to the tissue, causing perforation. It is important to make sure that the electrohydraulic lithotriptor is firmly in contact with the stone when power is

applied. After the stones are broken up, they can be removed by the previously mentioned techniques.

B. Complications of Choledochoscopy

1. **Bile leak**
    a. **Cause and prevention.** Bile may leak from the cystic duct stump, the choledochotomy site, or from an unrecognized injury to the common bile duct. If choledochoscopy was performed via the cystic duct, the cystic duct may have been dilated or damaged during instrumentation. In this situation, the closure of the cystic duct stump should not be performed with clips but rather with a suture loop or some other type of suture ligation. The most common reason for a leak is a partial or complete obstruction of bile flow across the ampulla because of a retained stone or edema.
    b. **Recognition and management.** If a closed suction drain was placed, the presence of bile in the drain would signify a biliary leak. The drain may be adequate to control the biliary fistula. In patients with a T-tube in which a biliary complication is suspected, a T-tube cholangiogram should be performed expeditiously. This may demonstrate a normal system (no leak), an obstruction without leakage, leakage without obstruction or a dislodged T-tube. In those patients without a T-tube, a hepatic 2,6-dimethyliminodiacetic acid (HIDA) scan is an easy and non-invasive way to confirm the presence of a leak. Once a leak has been recognized, the source of it needs to be identified. This can be done through endoscopic retrograde cholangiography (ERC). If the reason for the leak is a retained stone, this can then be removed endoscopically. If the leak is via the cystic duct stump, then an endoscopically placed transampullary biliary stent will allow for decompression and healing. Small bile leaks and collections recognized promptly will not require drainage if the leak is controlled with an endoprosthesis. If the collection is significant, it can be drained percutaneously by computed tomography or ultrasound guidance.
2. **Bleeding**
    a. **Cause and prevention.** Inflamed bile ducts can be quite friable, tending to bleed when manipulated. To prevent bleeding it is necessary to be as gentle as possible with guidewires, baskets, and the choledochoscope. Bleeding from the edges of the choledochotomy can be annoying but is rarely serious. Guy sutures at the site of the bleeding can control the bleeding and assist with access to the common bile duct. If there appears to be a fair amount of oozing during surgery, it would be better to place a T-tube for decompression and flushing in the postoperative period. A rare

complication is a fistula formation between the hepatic artery or portal structures and the bile duct secondary to perforation during the instrumentation by wires, baskets, and so on. To prevent this complication, the baskets, balloons, and guidewires all need to be visualized with the choledochoscope or with fluoroscopy while being manipulated.

b. **Recognition and management.** Bleeding can be recognized postoperatively as either a blood through the **T**-tube or as an upper or lower gastrointestinal tract hemorrhage. If the bleeding is significant, it can be localized to the biliary tract by blood from the **T**-tube or if endoscopy shows blood coming from the ampulla. Bleeding can be further localized and treated by angiography if a branch of the hepatic artery has fistulized to the biliary system.

3. **Perforation**

a. **Cause and prevention.** Manipulation of wires and baskets through the choledochoscope can result in perforations of the common bile duct or duodenum. Observing the baskets and wires through the choledochoscope or with fluoroscopy as they are being placed can prevent this problem. A second camera and a video mixer (picture in picture) allows the entire operating team to view the proceedings, which may decrease the risk of perforation or not recognizing that a perforation has occurred.

b. **Recognition and management.** The injury can be seen on completion cholangiogram, or it may present as a bile leak postoperatively. If the injury can be visualized, then it can be sutured. Small leaks from the common bile duct can be managed as described earlier. An injury to the duodenum that cannot be visualized laparoscopically will necessitate converting to an open operation for definitive repair.

4. **Pancreatitis**

a. **Cause and prevention.** Excessive and forceful flushing of contrast when the ampulla is obstructed can cause reflux into the pancreatic duct with resultant pancreatitis. This can also occur when high-pressure water is infused through the choledochoscope in an obstructed system. This complication cannot always be avoided, but the use of gentle manipulation of the distal common bile duct and avoiding unnecessary instrumentation of the ampulla can help decrease its incidence.

b. **Recognition and management.** The patient will present with excessive nausea and pain postoperatively and with elevated amylase and lipase values. The usual treatment regimen of bowel rest usually suffices, and this process will be self-limited. A more serious problem exists if the pancreatitis is secondary to a retained stone. This scenario should be considered if the pancreatitis fails to improve and/or if the hepatic enzymes progressively increase. In severe cases of pancreatitis secondary to a retained stone, an endoscopic retrograde cholangiopancreatography and stone removal may be indicated.

5. **Retained common bile duct stones**
   a. **Cause and prevention.** It is difficult to pass the choledochoscope into the proximal common hepatic and intrahepatic ducts, and therefore it is crucial to obtain a completion cholangiogram under fluoroscopy to prevent the retention of CBD stones.
   b. **Recognition and management.** If it is recognized intraoperatively, then the choledochoscope can be replaced to attempt further removal of the stones. If the stone is in the proximal ducts and the exploration was done via the cystic duct, it may be necessary to divide the cystic duct to better position the passage of the scope into the proximal ducts. This is usually the last maneuver because once the cystic duct has been divided it is very difficult to replace the scope. The other option for retained stones is to convert to a laparoscopic choledochotomy, which can allow a larger choledochoscope (4.5 mm) to be placed and a better angle for passing the scope into the proximal ducts. Postoperatively retained stones can present with pain, pancreatitits, cholangitis, or asymptomatic jaundice. If a T-tube was used, the stones can be removed percutaneously through the T-tube tract. A postoperative ERC can also be used to identify and treat most retained stones.

6. **Stricture of the common bile duct**
   a. **Cause and prevention.** Excessive manipulation of a small common bile duct with a large choledochoscope through a choledochotomy can result in a difficult to close choledochotomy with a T-tube. Common duct explorations are the leading causes of bismuth level I strictures. This can be prevented by preferentially using a transcystic method of exploration, not performing a choledochotomy on a small duct, not using electrocautery on the duct, and using meticulous suturing when closing the choledochotomy. If these precautions cannot be implemented, a postoperative ERC may be preferential to a bile duct exploration.
   b. **Recognition and management.** This difficult problem can be a late complication from laparoscopic CBDE and is recognized by elevated liver enzymes and diagnosed with ERC. The treatment includes endoscopic balloons, stent placement, and more definitive biliary enteric anastomosis.

7. **Damaging the choledochoscope**
   a. **Cause and prevention.** The manipulation of a fine and fragile choledochoscope across the peritoneal cavity can easily damage the scope, which can be quite expensive to repair. Care must be utilized in handling the scope with laparoscopic instruments and in placing the scope through a trocar. Many times it is better to place the scope through a separate port and use a long flexible "peel-away" sheath from a Cordis-type introducer set.
   b. **Recognition and management.** The damage is usually recognized when the scope is examined after the procedure and the protective sheath is noted to be cracked, which can limit its ability to be sterilized.

C. Selected References

Hunter JG, Soper NJ. Laparoscopic management of bile duct stones. Surg Clin North Am
1992;72:1077–1097.

Giurgiu DI, Margulies DR, Carrol BJ, et al. Laparoscopic common bile duct exploration:
long term outcomes. Arch Surg 1999;134:839–843.

Petlin JB. Laparoscopic approach to common duct pathology. Am J Surg 1993;165:
487–491.

Sandosal BA, Goettler CE, Robinson BA, O'Donnel JK, Adler LP, Stellato TA. Cho-
lescintigraphy in the diagnosis of bile leak after laparoscopic cholecystectomy. Am
Surg 1997;63:611–616.

Strasberg SM, Hertl M, Soper NJ. An analysis of the problem of biliary injury during
laparoscopic cholecystectomy. J Am Coll Surg 1995;180:101–125.

Wood T, Macfadyen BV. Diagnostic and therapeutic choledochoscopy. Semin Laparosc
Surg 2000;7:288–294.

Flexible Endoscopy
VI—Flexible Sigmoidoscopy

68. Flexible Sigmoidoscopy

John A. Coller, M.D.

A. Indications

The flexible sigmoidoscope is now the standard device for evaluation of the distal large bowel. Flexible sigmoidoscopy is used for screening of asymptomatic patients. When neoplastic polyps are found in the distal colon during **asymptomatic screening**, the entire colon must subsequently be examined. Flexible sigmoidoscopy may also be used to investigate symptoms referable to the distal large bowel, but it is not a substitute for complete colon evaluation (e.g., for workup of an iron deficiency anemia).

B. Instrumentation

Two principal 65-cm flexible sigmoidoscopic imaging systems are currently available.
1. The older style instrument is the **flexible fiberoptic sigmoidoscope**. A fiber bundle carries the illumination light down the shaft, and a second fiber bundle carries the image back to the eyepiece.
2. The second instrument is an electronic **videoscope**. The light is carried down by a fiber bundle, but the image is registered on a charge-coupled device chip at the tip of the scope. Although a great number of traditional fiberscopes remain, they are gradually being replaced by video technology. As with other endoscopes, the video system provides better image quality, reliability, image capture, annotation, and printing.
3. Both fiberoptic scopes and videoscopes require thorough mechanical cleansing and high-level disinfection of external surfaces and internal channels. A **sheathed videoendoscope system** has been developed that addresses some of the elements of scope cleansing. The use of a sheath may prolong examination time slightly, but it significantly decreases downtime.

C. Patient Preparation

Adequate bowel preparation is essential for more than simple accuracy reasons. Any residual material that is more substantive than a thin aspiratable liquid prolongs the examination, contributes to discomfort by requiring greater air insuflation, and adds to the risk of injury. Once adherent to the viewing lens, formed stool can be very tenacious, requiring blind removal of the instrument. Stool coating the mucosa obscures surface morphology and vasculature. A pool of opaque liquid between folds may be much deeper than is apparent and consequently may harbor a significant lesion beneath the surface. Fecal residue has a tendency to adhere to an abraded or demucosalized surface more readily than to the surrounding normal epithelium. Consequently, all stool-coated surfaces must be exposed if one is to clear the examined area with confidence.

Either cathartic, lavage, or enema preparation can be used for flexible sigmoidoscopy preparation. Preparation with a hypertonic sodium phosphate (Fleets, CB Fleet, Lynchburg, VA) enema is simple and safe in most patients. Symptomatic hyperphosphatemia and hypocalcemia can occur in children or patients with renal insufficiency.

Flexible sigmoidoscopy is an office procedure. Sedation is rarely needed.

D. Technique of Flexible Sigmoidoscopic Intubation

1. Flexible sigmoidoscopy does not require special positioning, but most right-handed physicians find the **left lateral decubitus** position most convenient.

2. Perform a **digital examination** with a well-lubricated gloved finger. This lubricates the anal canal and confirms that there are no lesions of the distal rectum. Carefully palpate the prostate (in male patients) and the posterior ampulla of the rectum, an area that may be difficult to visualize with the endoscope.

3. **Grasp the control housing** of the scope with the left hand, so that the thumb can manipulate the deflection controls and the second and third fingers can activate the air and suctions channels. Grasp the distal end of the scope with the right hand, apply lubricant to the shaft (not the lens).

4. Use the index finger of the right hand to **stabilize the deflection mechanism** (bendable tip). Gently insert the scope. The complete deflection mechanism, about 10 cm, must be inserted before the dial controls become effective.

5. After obtaining a view of the rectum, **position the right hand** on the shaft about 10 to 15 cm from the anal verge. Use the right hand to maintain shaft position, manipulating the deflection controls with the left hand. Greater speed and efficiency will be attained if the endoscopist avoids jumping the right hand back and forth between the shaft and the dials.

6. **Intubation** is performed using a combination of tip deflection, shaft torque, and shaft advancement/withdrawal, along with air insufflation and removal (see Chapter 48).

   a. Two concentric dials control **tip deflection**. The larger outer dial deflects the distal 10 cm of scope nearly 180 degrees in either the up or down direction. The smaller dial does the same in the left-right direction. When both dials are maximally applied, the tip of the scope will overdeflect, well beyond 180 degrees. Judicious use of tip deflection greatly facilitates finding the lumen. However, once 90 degrees of deflection has been applied, the deflection mechanism begins to impede forward advancement of the scope. The leading edge of the scope is no longer the tip of the scope but rather the sharply angled shaft of the deflection tip itself (see later: Fig. 68.1B), and the colon deforms rather than permitting scope passage. Severe tip deflection, when necessary, should be restricted to finding the lumen, flattening the angle as much as possible before further advancement.

b. **Shaft torquing** permits the partially deflected tip to press against a fold and ease into the lumen ahead. This is particularly useful when there is considerable circular muscular hypertrophy associated with diverticular disease in the sigmoid. When the full length of the scope has been inserted into a redundant sigmoid, **clockwise** torquing tends to straighten the loop, whereas **counterclockwise** torque usually accentuates the redundancy.

c. **Shaft advancement** is obviously necessary to obtain maximum intubation with the flexible sigmoidoscope. Incorporate torque and tip deflection as the scope is advanced. Rather than simply pushing the scope ahead, it is more effective to advance and withdraw the shaft in a repetitive rhythmic fashion covering 10 to 15 cm (**dithering**). This shortens the colon by reefing it back onto the shaft of the scope.

7. **Insufflate air** to visualize the lumen, but avoid excess insufflation. Unnecessary distention increases patient discomfort and accentuates the angulation between fixed loops of colon. Since there is continuous airflow to the control button, a lazy finger blocking the air vent can result in a great deal of unnecessary insufflation.

8. There are **three general approaches** to complete intubation using the flexible sigmoidoscope: intubation by elongation, intubation by looping, and intubation by dither-torquing.

a. **Intubation by elongation**, the most basic approach, simply means advancing the shaft of the scope until there is no longer any scope left to advance. In some circumstances, such as after anterior resection, when all left colon redundancy has been removed, it may be possible to maximally insert the scope with minimal manipulation of the control dials. More often, however, this approach will result in substantial stretching of the sigmoid colon into a large bow, with the tip of the scope reaching only the sigmoid-descending junction (Fig. 68.1).

   i. To advance further, direct the deflection tip of the scope proximally into the distal-descending colon lumen.

   ii. Reduce the elongated sigmoid by clockwise torquing while withdrawing scope shaft. The net result is to reef the sigmoid onto the shaft of the scope.

   iii. After reducing the sigmoid, advance the shaft while maintaining clockwise torque.

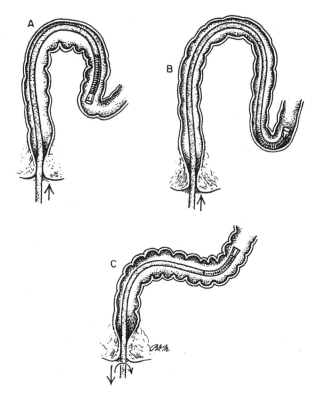

Figure 68.1. Intubation by elongation. A. The sigmoidoscope is advanced to the proximal sigmoid. B. Severe tip deflection prevents further advancement resulting in sigmoid elongation. C. Clockwise torquing and shaft withdrawal accordionizes the sigmoid.

b.   **Intubation by looping** takes advantage of a redundant sigmoid and manipulates it into position (Fig. 68.2).
    i.   Upon reaching the rectosigmoid, apply counterclockwise torque during shaft advancement. The proximal sigmoid will be directed toward the right side of the lower abdomen and pelvis.
   ii.   This creates an **alpha loop** (name derived from resemblance to Greek letter α). The sigmoid-descending junction can then be approached in a horizontal direction, thus flattening the angle that has to be negotiated with the deflection tip of the scope.
  iii.   Once the deflection tip has been positioned at the mid- or distal-descending colon, reduce the loop by **simultaneous clockwise torque and shaft withdrawal**. As the loop is

removed, the tip of the scope will extend more proximally as the colon accordionizes onto the scope even though some shaft is being withdrawn.

    iv.   When the sigmoid is straight, advance the shaft while maintaining clockwise torque.

  c.   Intubation by **dither-torquing** attempts to minimize stretching or deforming of the colon. The colon is shortened and reefed during intubation, rather than after a large loop has been produced. Synchronous use of a back-and-forth movement with the shaft while torquing left and right is very effective in showing the way to the lumen while encouraging the colon to accordianize onto the scope (Fig. 68.3). This avoids the development of a large and often uncomfortable loop. When the sigmoid is tightly nested in the

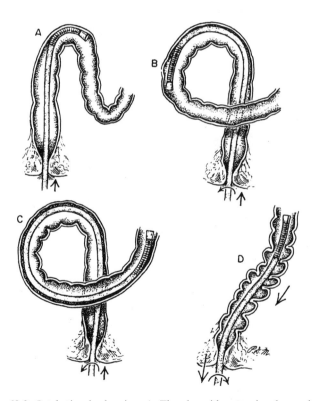

Figure 68.2. Intubation by looping. A. The sigmoidoscope is advanced to the distal sigmoid. B. Counterclockwise torquing during further advancement loops the proximal sigmoid in front of the distal sigmoid. C. The looped sigmoid flattens the angle at the distal-descending colon. D. Clockwise torquing and shaft withdrawal accordionizes the sigmoid.

712   J.A. Coller

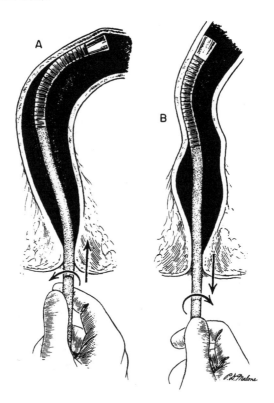

Figure 68.3. Intubation by dither-torquing. A. The shaft is torqued counter-clockwise while advancing the shaft 10 to 15 cm. B. The shaft is torqued clockwise while withdrawing the shaft 10 to 15 cm. Repetition of this cycle encourages the sigmoid to accordionize onto the sigmoidoscope.

pelvis, the dither-torquing method is usually the only way the intubation can be accomplished.

i. Move the right hand (on the shaft) in a figure-of-eight–like motion and apply clockwise torque during a few centimeters of withdrawal.

ii. Continue this repetitive motion, attempting to bring the colon down onto the scope rather than pushing the scope into the colon.

iii. Advance additional scope only when there is no further progress. Use gentle tip deflection toward the lumen. Severe deflection will prevent accordionization of the colon.

E. Biopsy

Biopsy forceps are used to obtain tissue specimens. The forceps can have either a simple cup for single specimen retrieval or a cup with a central spire upon which two or three specimens are gathered. **Avoid the use of electrocautery** (hot biopsy forceps, snare) in the absence of complete mechanical bowel preparation to reduce hydrogen and methane gas concentrations. Always ensure a clear view of the lumen when passing the biopsy forceps through the channel, to avoid perforation of the bowel wall (particularly in diverticular bowel).

F. Complications

Intubation may be difficult in the presence of extensive diverticulosis or pelvic adhesions. A dense population of large-diameter diverticular orifices in association with circular muscular hypertrophy can confuse identification of the lumen. Do not proceed with shaft advancement in the absence of a clear view of the lumen. If the next proximal fold cannot be clearly identified through the prospective opening, one is more likely peering into a diverticulum rather than the lumen.

Pelvic adhesions may severely limit the degree of manipulation that one can apply to the sigmoid and descending colon. Prior gynecologic surgery, a history of peritoneal sepsis, and radiation injury are often responsible for severe adhesive formation. If the colon between the rectosigmoid and the distal-descending colon is fixed into tightly nested loops, intubation may not be possible.

Persistence or the application of undue force may result in perforation. This complication is quite rare when proper technique is used.

G. Selected References

Coller JA. Technique of flexible fiberoptic sigmoidoscopy. Surg Clin North Am 1980; 60:465–479.

Harrington L, Schuh S. Complications of Fleet enema administration and suggested guidelines for use in the pediatric emergency department. Pediatr Emerg Care 1997;13(3):225–226.

Helikson MA, Parham WA, Tobias JD. Hypocalcemia and hyperphosphatemia after phosphate enema use in a child. J Pediatr Surg 1997;32(8):1244–1246.

Preston KL, Peluso FE, Goldner F. Optimal bowel preparation for flexible sigmoidoscopy—are two enemas better that one? Gastrointest Endosc 1994;40(4):474–476.

Rothstein RI, Littenberg B. Disposable, sheathed, flexible sigmoidoscopy: a prospective, multicenter, randomized trial. The Disposable Endoscope Study Group. Gastrointest Endosc 1995;41(6):566–572.

69. Therapeutic Flexible Sigmoidoscopy

Irwin B. Simon, M.D., F.A.C.S.

A. Polypectomy

Polypectomy is the major therapeutic maneuver performed at flexible sigmoidoscopy. Snare polypectomy is used for medium and large polyps. Small polyps (<4–5 mm) may be removed with the hot biopsy forceps. Identification of polyps during screening flexible sigmoidoscopy should prompt full colonoscopy to exclude the presence of other lesions above the reach of the flexible sigmoidoscope.

1. **Snare polypectomy.** Pedunculated polyps are ensnared at their stalk, and sessile polyps are ensnared within normal mucosa lateral to the polyp. The snare is tightened and monopolar electrocautery is used to coagulate and transect the polyp at the level of the snare.

   a. Push the snare out the distal tip of the sigmoidoscope.
   b. Open the snare well proximal to the lesion. Open the snare fully regardless of lesion size, to obtain better control for placement of the snare.
   c. Withdraw the snare to position the plastic sheath at the base of the polyp or lesion.
   d. Close the snare slowly until the tissue is visualized and felt to give resistance.
   e. Set the electrocautery to apply primarily coagulating current. Minimal if any cutting current should be required.
   f. Apply cautery slowly and in short bursts.
   g. When the polyp is large, minimize the risk of electrocautery complications by two means:
      i. Moving the snare tip slowly back and forth to avoid prolonged contact with the wall of the colon with concentration of current at one place.
      ii. Deliberately placing the broad surface of the polyp against the colon wall to maximize the surface area over which the electric current is distributed.

2. **The hot biopsy forceps** utilizes monopolar cautery to destroy the base of a minute polyp while preserving the architecture of the specimen within the biopsy jaws. The specimen may then be examined histologically.

B. Dilatation of Anastomotic Strictures and Control of Bleeding

1. **Anastomotic strictures** within reach of the flexible sigmoidoscope may be therapeutically dilated by use of pneumatic balloon dilators in a fashion identical to that of colonoscopy.

2. **Control of bleeding** has previously been less emphasized and felt to be impractical in flexible sigmoidoscopy and colonoscopy. More recent studies have shown that endoscopic evaluation of the lower gastrointestinal tract in the setting of acute bleeding is feasible and of value from a diagnostic as well as therapeutic standpoint.

   a. **Injection sclerotherapy** is most commonly used. Generally sodium tetradecol or ethanolamine oleate is used. Absolute alcohol injection is not recommended. This agent has caused full-thickness necrosis and perforation of the colon wall.

   b. **Monopolar cautery** may be cautiously applied in a short burst. The very tip of a closed snare may be extended beyond the plastic sheath to allow for a controlled application of current in a desired location.

   c. **Heater probe** may be used to apply heat directly over a source of bleeding. The technique is similar to application of a branding iron. It is best utilized in cases of small angiodysplasias.

   d. The **bicap** is a bipolar application of electrical current. It is generally considered safer than monopolar current. The current path flows between two electrodes, thus limiting stray current and the risk of full-thickness burn that may occur with monopolar electrocautery.

   e. **Lasers** may be utilized in a therapeutic fashion but are often not available in the office setting, where flexible sigmoidoscopy is most often performed. Lasers must be of a frequency that yields low depth of penetrance. They are best utilized in cases of bleeding angiodysplasia.

C. Removal of Foreign Bodies

Foreign body removal from the rectum and colon has become more common today. The embarrassed patient may give minimal history but usually knows the object is there. From 70 to 80% of swallowed foreign objects will pass spontaneously and do not require removal. In contrast, foreign objects that have been inserted through the anus frequently will not pass, owing to size and associated sphincter spasm, thus requiring endoscopic extraction.

First obtain an abdominal x-ray series to assess that the foreign body is within reach of the flexible sigmoidoscope and to rule out a perforation. Perforation changes the procedure to an operative procedure. If removal by flexible sigmoidoscopy is felt to be feasible:

1. First apply **topical anesthetic** to the anal sphincter to help break the reflexive sphincter spasm.
2. **Consider the size** of the object. Spinal anesthesia allows wide sphincter dilatation for removal of large or rounded objects.
3. Try to **obtain a duplicate** of the foreign object. Careful analysis may yield the solution as to what instrument will allow the best purchase and the most secure/safest orientation to remove the object.
4. A large snare is usually the best tool for sigmoidoscopic retrieval.
5. Use an overtube for multiple objects or objects with leading edges.
6. Turn sharp objects such that the leading edge becomes a trailing edge.
7. Repass the scope after foreign body removal to assess for injury such as bowel wall perforation or laceration that may have occurred during removal.

D. Complications of Flexible Sigmoidoscopy

1. **Missed diagnosis**
    a. **Cause and prevention.** The diagnosis may be missed as a result of failure to recognize the pathologic finding. Formal training and experience are key to avoiding this complication.
    b. **Recognition and management.** This is difficult because the complication is truly one of omission. The diagnosis may be missed owing to failure to recognize the indication and thus failure to perform the procedure. A classic example would be to attribute bright red blood per rectum to hemorrhoids, rather than doing the endoscopic evaluation needed to diagnose cancer of the rectum or sigmoid colon.
2. **Complications of the bowel preparation** may arise and include electrolyte imbalance and cardiac effects, hypovolemia, and solitary rectal ulceration resulting from enema insertion.
    a. **Cause and prevention.** Pay careful attention to the overall status of the patient. Avoid the 4-L polyethylene glycol solutions in patients with poor functional status. Such patients may require a 2- or 3-day prep to avoid fluid imbalance. For flexible sigmoidoscopy, most patients can be prepped with simple enemas. Even then, the patient and/or nurse must be attentive to technique to avoid local trauma.
    b. **Recognition and management.** Poor skin turgor, obvious dyspnea, or cardiac dysrhythmias signal fluid and electrolyte abnormalities. New onset of anorectal pain should prompt careful examination of the anorectal region during the procedure. Solitary rectal ulcers are managed by bulking agents, topical anesthetics, and careful hygiene.
3. **Anorectal trauma due to scope insertion**
    a. **Cause and prevention.** Anal injury may result in painful fissures. Causes include inadequate lubrication and reflexive sphincter spasm at scope insertion. Avoid this by careful and gentle digital

pressure on the perineal body just prior to and at the insertion of the scope. This causes reflex relaxation of the anal sphincter, minimizing the risk of trauma.

b. **Recognition and management.** Acute bleeding and pain with blood on the insertion tube should make this issue suspect. This should be followed by careful anorectal examination during the procedure. The management includes bulking agents, topical anesthetics, and keeping tissues dry to promote healing.

4. **Perforation** is the most common and most morbid complication of therapeutic flexible sigmoidoscopy.

   a. **Cause and prevention.** Immediate perforation may result from electrocautery injury, taking too large a bite with the snare or hot biopsy forceps, traction injury (excessive wall tension during scope manipulation), or blowout of a diverticulum. Delayed perforation occasionally results when wall necrosis from electrocautery is not obvious for several days.

   b. **Recognition and management.** Acute perforation is frequently easy to recognize. The view through the scope shows intra-abdominal organs rather than mucosa. Other signs include pain beyond that normally encountered, along with mild to moderate distention. The diagnosis is confirmed by free air on upright or left lateral decubitus film. Suspect delayed perforation in the appropriate setting when pain, leukocytosis, abdominal distention, and signs of peritonitis develop several days to even several weeks after flexible sigmoidoscopy. Acute perforations taken to surgery immediately may be managed without creation of a stoma. The amount of time since perforation, degree of spillage of colonic contents, and health status of the patient all factor into decisions to repair the perforation, resect the segment, or create a colostomy. The preparation for flexible sigmoidoscopy may be sufficient for primary repair if the perforation is recognized immediately and the patient taken to the operating room promptly, before much spillage occurs. Either an open or a laparoscopic approach may be used at the discretion of the surgeon.

5. **Hemorrhage** is generally recognized after the procedure is terminated.

   a. **Cause and prevention.** Immediate, visible bleeding is most often due to inadequate cauterization during polypectomy or biopsy. Immediate occult (internal) bleeding occasionally results from mesenteric or splenic capsule tears from overly aggressive endoscope manipulation. Delayed visible bleeding usually occurs around the eighth day when the eschar separates from coagulated site.

   b. **Recognition and management.** At times brisk bleeding is noted immediately, setting the endoscopist into therapeutic maneuvers. Otherwise, immediate bleeding may first be recognized by the passage of bright red blood per rectum in the recovery area or unfortunately, in the case of flexible sigmoidoscopy, by the patient at home. Tachycardia and hemodynamic symptoms are not always obvious. Splenic injury may be noticed by a frightening and rapid instability with possible expanding abdomen. However, it may also go unnoticed until the patient becomes unstable at home. Endoscopic interventions are most commonly applied to hemorrhagic complications. The most common setting would be in postpolypectomy bleeding. Even this is generally self-limited.

   i. If recognized at endoscopy, the bleeding polypectomy site may be immediately recauterized with monopolar cautery or bipolar cautery (bicap) instrumentations.

   ii. Intervention with injection sclerotherapy is also fast, safe, and strongly recommended. The agents most commonly utilized are sodium tetradecol and ethanolamine oleate. This technique does carry with it the risk of a full-thickness colonic wall necrosis. The volume of any agent utilized should be minimized. Use of absolute alcohol is not recommended owing to the significant risk for full-thickness necrosis after alcohol-induced desiccation.

   iii. Delayed postpolypectomy bleeding may be suspected in the patient who develops acute lower gastrointestinal bleeding at around 8 days postpolypectomy. The eschar separation classically occurs in this time frame. It is usually self-limited and may be managed with intravenous hydration and supportive care. In specific cases, endoscopic interventions as outlined earlier will usually be successful.

   iv. Surgery is rarely required for postpolypectomy bleeding. When surgery is required, localize the bleeding site accurately before laparotomy. It is rarely feasible to mark the bleeding site preoperatively with vital dye at endoscopy (although this is helpful when it can be accomplished). Colotomy with oversewing of the bleeding point is the simplest maneuver but is not always possible. The patient may need an anatomic resection to ensure that the site has been removed.

6. **Bacteremia and possible sepsis.** Bacteremia has been demonstrated after colonic manipulation. Antibiotic prophylaxis is recommended for high-risk patients (e.g., patients with artificial heart valves or other implanted prosthetic devices).

7. **Incomplete polypectomy** may be a technical error or deliberate in cases of large sessile polyps. Attention to detail of polypectomy technique is the best prevention. If snare placement does not seem appropriate, it is generally possible to regrasp the polyp, as long as electrocautery has not yet been applied. Reapplication of the snare to complete an adequate polypectomy prevents a clinical situation requiring repeat endoscopy. Mark polyps that are too large to completely remove with indigo carmine or other vital dyes to facilitate removal of the proper colonic segment at open or laparoscopic surgery.

8. **Explosion** is far less common with better methods of bowel preparation that prevent accumulation of hydrogen or methane gas. If the prep is not good, it may be prudent to defer use of electrocautery (sched-

uling a second procedure if necessary) until an adequate mechanical preparation has been attained.

9. **Glutaraldehyde-induced colitis** results from inadequate washing of endoscopes with ineffective flushing of biopsy/instrument channels. This iatrogenic colitis can be prevented by careful training of endoscopy personnel and attention to detail. Newer methods of endoscope cleansing avoid use of the inciting agent. The colitis generally presents less than 6 hours after flexible sigmoidoscopy. Management is supportive.

10. **Rare and unusual complications.** Though rare, the theoretical possibilities must be known and vigilant attention paid to avoid such occurrences as the following:
    a. Incarceration of bowel in a hernia
    b. Incarceration of the flexible sigmoidoscope in a hernia
    c. Aortic aneurysm rupture
    d. Creation of a sigmoid volvulus
    e. Pneumocystoides intestinalis
    f. Accidental removal of a ureterosigmoidoscopy stoma by mistaking it for a polyp

E. Selected References

Anderson ML, Pasha TM, Leighton JA. Endoscopic perforation of the colon: lessons from a 10-year study. Am J Gastroenterol 2000;95:3418–3422.

Hayashi K, Urata K, Munakata Y, Kawasaki S, Makuuchi M. Laparoscopic closure for perforation of the sigmoid colon by endoscopic linear stapler. Surg Laparosc Endosc 1996;6:411–413.

Jentschura D, Raute M, Winter J, Henkel T, Kraus M, Manegold BC. Complications in endoscopy of the lower gastrointestinal tract. Therapy and prognosis. Surg Endosc 1994;8:672–676.

Levin TR, Conell C, Shapiro JA, Chazan SG, Nadel MR, Selby JV. Complications of screening flexible sigmoidoscopy. Gastroenterology 2002;123:1786–1792.

Manier JW. Flexible sigmoidoscopy. In: Sivak MV, ed. Gastroenterologic Endoscopy. Philadelphia: WB Saunders, 1987;975–991.

Norfleet RG. Infectious endocarditis after fiberoptic sigmoidoscopy. With a literature review. J Clin Gastroenterol 1991;13:448–451.

Ponsky JL, Mellinger JD, Simon IB. Endoscopic retrograde hemorhhoidal sclerotherapy using 23.4% saline: a preliminary report. Gastrointest Endosc 1991;37:155–158.

Sanowski RA. Foreign body extraction in the gastrointestinal tract. In: Sivak MV, ed. Gastroenterologic Endoscopy. Philadelphia: WB Saunders, 1987;321–331.

Simon IB, Lewis RJ, Satava RM. A safe method for sedating and monitoring patients for upper and lower gastrointestinal endoscopy. Am Surg 1991;57:219–221.

Waye JD, Kahn O, Auerbach ME. Complications of colonoscopy and flexible sigmoidoscopy. Gastrointest Endosc Clin North Am 1996;6:343–377.

West AB, Kuan SF, Bennick M, Lagarde S. Glutaraldehyde colitis following endoscopy: clinical and pathological features and investigation of an outbreak. Gastroenterology 1995;108:1250–1255.

Williard W, Satava R. Inguinal hernia complicating flexible sigmoidoscopy. Am Surg 1990;56:800–801.

Flexible Endoscopy
VII—Colonoscopy

70. Diagnostic Colonoscopy

Bassem Y. Safadi, M.D.
Jeffrey M. Marks, M.D.

A. Indications

Generally accepted indications for diagnostic colonoscopy are summarized in Table 70.1. Colonoscopy has now become recognized as a screening tool for colorectal cancer in average-risk patients by the American Cancer Society. Only 30% of patients harbor risk factors for colorectal cancer, so the majority of patients are considered average risk. There is indirect evidence from the fecal occult blood testing trials that colonoscopy may reduce colorectal cancer mortality. The recommended interval for subsequent surveillance colonoscopy depends upon the number, size, and type of polyps previously removed. Colonoscopy is usually **not indicated** in patients with bright red rectal bleeding when a convincing anorectal source has been found on anoscopy or sigmoidoscopy and when there are no other symptoms suggesting a more proximal source of bleeding. It is also not necessary in upper gastrointestinal bleeding when a source proximal to the colon has been clearly identified. Colonoscopy is generally **not indicated** in the workup of metastatic carcinoma in the absence of symptoms related to the colon. Colonoscopy is indicated for evaluation of unexplained abdominal pain or change in bowel habits **only in select cases**. It is generally **not indicated** in patients with chronic stable abdominal pain or symptoms of irritable bowel in the absence of other indications for colonoscopy.

Contraindications to colonoscopy include peritonitis or suspected colorectal perforation, severe acute diverticulitis, fulminant colitis, and hemodynamic instability. **Relative contraindications** include large bowel obstruction and recent myocardial infarction or pulmonary embolus.

B. Preparation and Positioning of the Patient and Room Setup

1. **Bowel preparation** is essential; the entire colon should be cleansed of all fecal matter for an adequate exam and to decrease the risk for potential complications.
   a. Discontinue iron-containing medications or constipating agents.
   b. **Clear liquids** or other residue-free diets for 24 hours.

Table 70.1. Indications for diagnostic colonoscopy.

Evaluation of gastrointestinal bleeding
- Hemoccult positive stools
- Hematochezia when an anal or rectal source is not certain
- Melena after excluding an upper gastrointestinal tract source
- Unexplained iron deficiency anemia

Surveillance for colon neoplasia
- Following resection of carcinoma or neoplastic/adenomatous polyp
- When a cancer or neoplastic polyp has been found on screening sigmoidoscopy (provided the results will change treatment plan)
- In patients at high risk for cancer
  First-degree relatives or multiple family members with colon cancer, adenomatous polyps, or polyposis syndromes
  Cancer family syndrome
  Chronic ulcerative colitis with pancolitis greater than 7 years or left-sided colitis of greater than 10 years

Inflammatory bowel disease
- Determination of extent of disease
- Confirmation of diagnosis
- Cancer surveillance in chronic ulcerative colitis

Evaluation of
- Clinically significant abnormalities on barium enema
- Clinically significant diarrhea of unexplained etiology
- Suspected ischemic colitis

Intraoperative localization of lesions not apparent at surgery

c.   Beginning approximately 18 hours prior to the exam, 4 L of specially balanced electrolyte lavage solution (e.g., **polyethylene glycol electrolyte [PEG]**) U.S. given orally. Administer at a rate of 1 to 2 L per hour (8 oz every 10 minutes). Modifications include sulfate-free PEG lavage solution, which tends to be less salty, and various flavored PEG solutions. Sugars should not be added to the gut lavage because this may cause sodium retention or lead to production of potentially explosive gases. Reglan is occasionally given prior to the prep to prevent the associated nausea and vomiting.

d.   An alternative small-volume regimen of **oral sodium phosphate** (Fleet Phospho R-Soda). One 1.5-oz bottle is given orally, twice, the day before the colonoscopy. One **small-volume enema** (Fleet Enema) is given the morning of the examination. This regimen has been shown to be as effective, better tolerated, and less expensive than the PEG prep. This is a highly osmotic buffered saline laxative that stimulates the small bowel and therefore may cause dehydration and electrolyte imbalance, and transient hyperphosphatemia. Use cautiously in patients with symptomatic congestive heart failure, ascites, or renal insufficiency. Oral pill forms of sodium phosphate are now also available for bowel preparation.

e. Alternatively, the "traditional" bowel prep consists of **clear liquids** for 2 days and a purge with **oral magnesium** and **enemas** the day before the exam.

f. Do not use mannitol or other fermentable carbohydrates, which could be converted to explosive gases.

2. **The instruments.** The newer generation of colonoscopes that are predominantly used nowadays are **videoscopes**. Light signals pass through a wide-angle lens onto a charge-coupled device chip, which in turn transmits them into electronic signals to a video processing unit, where the image is reconstructed digitally. This is in contrast to **fiberoptic scopes**, where the image is a real image transmitted through the eyepiece via fiberoptics (see Chapter 47). Become familiar with the basic components of the endoscope and the video system. Always check the instrument before the examination.

3. **Patient preparation and positioning**

a. Before beginning any endoscopic procedure, review the procedure with the patient, answer questions, ease the patient's concerns, and obtain an informed consent.

b. For patients with high risk of developing infections from bacteremia such as patients with valvular heart disease and prosthetic valves, **endocarditis prophylaxis with antibiotics** is recommended.

4. **The basic room setup** is diagrammed in Figure 70.1. The patient is in the center of the room in the left lateral position with thigh and legs flexed. The endoscopist stands on the right side of the patient and the assistant on the left. The presence of two video monitors allows both endoscopist and assistant a comfortable view.

5. **Appropriate monitoring** includes continuous electrocardiogram, pulse rate, and pulse oximetry monitoring, and intermittent blood pressure recording. Most patients will need supplemental oxygen given via a nasal canula (see Chapter 49).

6. **Conscious sedation** is used for most patients. The most popular agents are a combination of a narcotic (e.g., Demerol or morphine sulfate) and a benzodiazepine (e.g., diazepam, midazolam). Titrate dose to effect and always have reversal agents (naloxone and flumenazil) available.

C. General Principles of Colonoscopy

After adequate sedation has been ensured, the exam should always start with a visual inspection of the anus and a digital rectal exam.

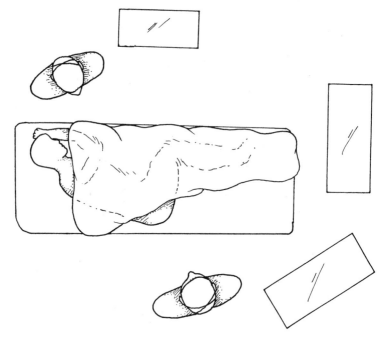

Figure 70.1. Patient position and room setup. A video monitor is placed in the direct line of sight of the endoscopist (at the back of the patient) and the assistant (who stands in front of the patient). Monitoring equipment for EKG, blood pressure, and oxygen saturation are positioned at the foot of the bed.

1. Place your index finger about an inch from the tip of the scope and **insert the scope** by sliding the tip across the perineal body and into the anus. This reduces trauma to the anal canal. Use plenty of lubricant on the endoscope, but not on the lens. Insert the scope straight without twists.
2. Use **air insufflation** to open the rectum and to visualize the lumen, and from there on advance the scope while keeping the lumen of the colon in view.
3. **General principles** to follow (see Chapter 48):
   a. To maintain maximal control during the colonoscopy, keep your right hand on the shaft of the scope and use the left hand to control the suction, irrigation, insufflation, and tip deflection.
   b. Use a combination of simultaneous moves to maneuver your way through the colon.

   c.   Torque with the right hand, moving clockwise and counterclockwise; push, pull, and jiggle and use the left hand to deflect the tip of the scope up and down, left and right.

   d.   Alternatively, a two-operator technique can be used: one operator controls scope deflection while the other advances and withdraws the scope.

4.   Pay attention to the following.

   a.   Avoid overinsufflation.

   b.   Minimize "loop" formation by periodically straightening the colon by jiggling and withdrawing the colonoscope. This facilitates the procedure (Fig. 70.2).

   c.   Always try to **keep the lumen in view** and avoid pushing the scope blindly or "sliding by" as this may increase the risk of perforation.

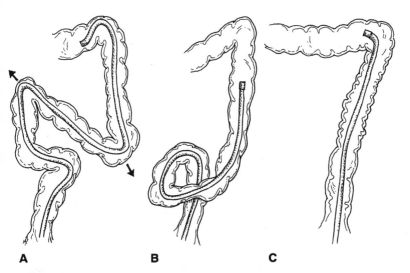

A   **B**   **C**

Figure 70.2 A. Formation of loops in the colon can cause patient discomfort, difficulty in advancing the scope, and may increase the risk of perforation. B. Here an alpha loop has been formed in the sigmoid colon, facilitating passage into the descending colon. Clockwise torque is sometimes necessary to derotate the loop. C. In the early phase of colonoscopy, try to keep the tip of the scope straight or only slightly bent. Use a combination of push, pull, jiggle, and torque to remove the loops and "straighten" the colon. This facilitates passage through the splenic flexure.

D. Passing the Colonoscope: Normal Anatomy

1. **The rectum.** The rectum is characterized by its valves of Houston, which will appear as semilunar folds as soon as you enter the rectal vault. In addition the rectal wall has a prominent submucosal venous plexus, and the rectal veins are larger than elsewhere in the colon.

2. **The sigmoid colon.** The sigmoid colon has a high muscular tone and can easily go into spasm. It is tortuous with a semilunar appearance of folds. Diverticula are common in this portion of the colon, and they may mimic the lumen, so be careful advancing. Passage of the scope may be particularly difficult in patients who have had prior pelvic surgery (e.g., hysterectomy) and in the elderly. In general, avoid overinsufflation and periodically straighten the scope and reduce loops as they form.

3. **The descending colon.** The descending colon has a straight, tubular shape with no haustral markings and has less musculature than the sigmoid colon. Although passage of the scope may be easier here, continue to periodically jiggle back and forth attempting to straighten the scope. "A straight sigmoid is the key to an easy splenic flexure" (Church, 1995).

4. **The splenic flexure.** The splenic flexure will appear as a turn at the end of the descending colon. It has a characteristic blue shadow reflecting the spleen and frequently a strong transmitted cardiac pulsation can be seen. Often, asking the patient to take a deep breath will help making the turn.

5. **The transverse colon.** The transverse colon has a characteristic triangular appearance.
   a. Difficulty in advancing the scope or complaints of pain from the patient are probably caused by a sigmoid loop.
   b. Try to "reduce" the loop in the scope by withdrawing to straighten the sigmoid colon.
   c. Sometimes it is possible to gently "push through the loop" to advance, but be careful, as force may cause tears and perforations in the sigmoid colon.
   d. Applying pressure to the left or lower abdominal wall or changing the patient's position may help (supine or prone).

6. **The hepatic flexure.** The hepatic flexure has a characteristic blue liver shadow, and there is usually a pool of liquid at the end of the transverse colon.

7. **The ascending colon and cecum.** The ascending colon is also triangular. The three colonic taeniae converge at the cecum, giving it its characteristic "Mercedes sign," where the appendiceal orifice can be found. The ileocecal valve will appear as a yellowish fold or may look polypoid, and occasionally may look flat. Flowing liquid stool or gas bubbles sometimes can be seen emerging from it. Advancing the scope beyond the hepatic flexure will often lead to a paradoxical movement (i.e., scope moves backward). Pull the scope back and use intermittent suctioning and that will most often push the tip of the scope forward toward the cecum (another paradox). Remember the suction channel

is at the 6 o'clock position on the screen, so tip the scope up as you apply suction to avoid catching the mucosa. Rotating the patient here can also be helpful in advancing the scope. It is very important to ascertain reaching the cecum by clearly identifying the appendiceal orifice and the ileocecal valve. Other maneuvers include transilluminating the right lower quadrant (RLQ) and seeing indentations on the cecal wall as the RLQ is palpated. The only way to verify with 100% confidence that the ileocecal valve has been reached is to intubate the terminal ileum and visualize ileal mucosa.

8. **Scope withdrawal.** After complete insertion, withdraw the colonoscope gradually, carefully inspecting the colonic mucosa circumferentially. If an area slips, readvance the scope to get a satisfactory exam. When the rectum is reached, "retroflexing" the scope will provide a view of the lower rectal ampula. After careful inspection straighten the scope, suction excess air in the lumen, and withdraw the scope.

E. Passing the Colonoscope: Postsurgical Anatomy

After colon resections, the colon is generally shorter and the colonoscopy is correspondingly easier and less time-consuming.

1. If the sigmoid colon has been resected, the colon will appear straighter.
2. Anastomoses are recognized by visualizing either a suture or a staple line with its characteristic whitish linear scar. Occasionally suture or staple material can be seen through the mucosa. Anastomoses may be end to end (one lumen), side to side (two lumina seen simultaneously), or end to side (one lumen and one blind end). It is very important to recognize the blind end and avoid forceful insertion, as this may lead to perforation. This is especially true in stapled low anterior resection anastomoses and stapled colostomy takedowns. A sharp turn is frequently noted in stapled side-to-side, functional end-to-end anastomoses.
3. **Passing scope via colostomy.** This is done with the patient in the supine position. Again, a careful visual inspection and digital exam to the level of the fascia is mandatory before introducing the scope. This will also help in gently dilating the stoma prior to introducing the scope. The remainder of the colonoscopy follows the above-mentioned principles. A problem particular to this situation is air leakage around the stoma, which could compromise insufflation. Applying mild pressure with a gauze around the scope at the stoma level may be helpful.

F. Biopsy

Colonoscopic biopsy samples are generally mucosal. Submucosal lesions cannot be subjected to biopsy using these conventional methods. The cecum and right colon are thin walled, and caution should be exercised when one is using the hot biopsy technique in that portion of the colon owing to increased risk of perforation.

1. **The indications for biopsy** are very broad and are guided by their clinical relevance to diagnosis and treatment. In general, biopsies are performed to check for neoplasia (e.g., carcinoma, adenoma, dysplasia, lymphoma) or colitis (e.g., eosinophilic, ischemic, radiation-induced, infectious, or inflammatory bowel disease).

2. **Introduce biopsy forceps** into the scope via the biopsy channel. This may be difficult when the scope is looped and is often facilitated by straightening the scope.

3. Because the forceps exit the scope at the 6 o'clock position, make an effort to **position the lesion at 6 o'clock** on the screen to facilitate the biopsy.

4. When **random biopsy samples** are needed (such as in ulcerative colitis) it is easiest to **obtain them from a fold**.

5. Direct the forceps to the target, open the forceps, push in, and close the forceps. Pull abruptly to obtain the specimen.
    a. There are numerous types of biopsy forceps.
    b. Biopsy forceps can be equipped with a spike that holds the first sample, allowing the forceps to be used for an immediate second biopsy.
    c. In general a **cold biopsy** refers to one done without the use of cautery.
    d. **Hot biopsy** uses cautery and is primarily used for removing small polyps (<5 mm).
        i. Advantages include the ability to obtain a sample suitable for histologic examination, destroy the residual polyp with the effect of the cautery, and achieve hemostasis.
        ii. Grasp the polyp with the biopsy forceps and pull it away from the bowel wall.
        iii. Push the forceps out until the tip of the insulating sheath is seen to avoid damage to the scope.
        iv. Use medium-strength coagulating current in short bursts until the polyp and 2 mm of surrounding mucosa turn white (coagulum).
        v. Pull the forceps and withdraw from the scope.

G. Endoscopic Ultrasound

1. **Indications for rectal endoscopic ultrasound (EUS).** EUS examination of the rectum has been primarily used for the following proposes.
    a. **Staging of rectal cancer.** It is useful for selecting tumors for local treatment, selecting patients for neoadjuvant therapy, and predicting patients who may need en bloc resection of other pelvic organs.
    b. **Follow-up of rectal cancer** to monitor local recurrence.

    c.   Delineating **perianal fistulas** and **abscesses** and their relationship to the sphincters.

    d.   Imaging internal and external sphincter in the evaluation of incontinence.

    e.   Identification of **submucosal** masses.

2.   **Indications for colonic EUS.** EUS in colon cancer staging and follow-up has not been as clinically relevant as in rectal cancer for several reasons. Generally, there is no role for neoadjuvant therapy in colon cancer (controversial in T4 lesions) and local recurrence is uncommon. In addition, EUS of the colon is technically more difficult. EUS **may** have a role in the following:

    a.   Guiding therapeutic plans on large sessile adenomatous polyps whether endoscopic, laparoscopic, or open removal is appropriate.

    b.   Differentiating between transmural colitis (Crohn's) and mucosal (ulcerative) colitis.

3.   **Equipment**

    a.   **Radial scanning** EUS scopes are the most popular. They give a circumferential ultrasonic image, producing cross-sectional anatomic sections. The longitudinal extent of the lesion can be determined by carefully moving the instrument in the proximal-distal direction.

    b.   **Linear scan** EUS scopes provide a longitudinal section, and this instrument must be rotated to delineate the entire circumference of the rectal wall. For acoustic interface, a water-filled balloon surrounds the transducer head. The frequency most commonly used is about 7.5 MHz. (The shorter the frequency, the greater the depth of penetration and the worse the resolution, and vice versa.)

    c.   **Rectal EUS probes** are either rigid, inserted blindly or via a proctoscope ($\leq$20 cm), or flexible.

    d.   The ultrasonic colonoscope is a flexible instrument, forward-viewing with a biopsy channel and a radial scanning method. Alternatively, miniature ultrasound scanners can be mounted on a probe that is inserted into the biopsy channel of an endoscope.

    e.   Newer scanners have the capability of imaging with color Doppler as well as ultrasound-guided needling. Future-generation probes will allow for three-dimensional intrarectal ultrasonography with computer-generated three-dimensional reconstruction using a continuous pull-through technique with the radial scanner.

4.   **General principles of EUS technique**

    a.   **Bowel prep.** For rectal EUS, bowel preparation with enemas is usually sufficient, whereas a routine bowel prep is necessary for colonic EUS.

    b.   Start with direct examination by proctosigmoidoscopy or total colonoscopy.

    c.   Identify the target lesion and determine its distance from the anal verge. Place the EUS probe at that level (for colonic EUS, fluoroscopy may help in localization). Some EUS scopes allow you to identify the lesion through an optical piece. Scanning begins proximal to the lesion.

d. Withdraw the probe slowly to assess the entire length of the gastrointestinal lumen. Repeat the exam two or three times. Optimal imaging is obtained by the combination of balloon insufflation and water instillation.

5. **Normal findings**
   a. Tissues with high levels of collagen (e.g., submucosa) or fat appear hyperechoic, whereas tissues with high water content (e.g., muscle) appear hypoechoic. Using a probe having a frequency of approximately 7.5 MHz allows visualization of five layers in the rectal wall (Fig. 70.3):
      i. Hyperechoic/hypoechoic (two layers)—mucosa
      ii. Hyperechoic—submucosa
      iii. Hypoechoic—muscularis propria
      iv. Hyperechoic—perirectal fat
   b. Occasionally seven layers can be delineated (separation of inner circular muscle layer and the outer longitudinal muscle layer of the muscularis propria).
   c. Normal rectal wall thickness is between 2 and 4 mm.
   d. Normal colonic wall is between 2 and 3 mm.

6. At a frequency of 7.5 MHz, the penetration depth of an ultrasound scan is about 3 to 4 cm; therefore, other structures could be visualized with rectal EUS: prostate and seminal vesicles in males, vagina and uterus in females. Urinary bladder can be shown in both sexes, especially if full. Valves of Houston may mimic lesions. Adjacent organs occasionally visualized in colonic EUS include parts of the left and right kidneys, liver, pancreas, and spleen.

7. **The staging of rectal cancers** follows the TNM classification. Depth of penetration determines the tumor (T) stage. In determining the node (N) state, any enlarged lymph node is suspicious. Generally inflammatory nodes are hyperechoic, elongated, and heterogeneous, and have

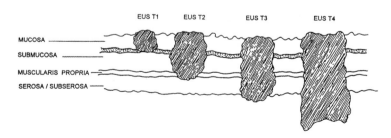

Figure 70.3. System of T tumor-staging of rectal cancers based upon endoscopic ultrasound appearance.

Table 70.2. EUS staging of rectal cancers.

T staging (Fig. 70.3)

    T1. Tumor confined to mucosa and/or submucosa
        Does not interrupt the middle hyperechoic layer
    T2. Invasion of muscularis propria
        Does not interrupt the outer hyperechoic area
    T3. Penetration through the muscularis propria into perirectal fat
        Through the outer hyperechoic area
    T4. Invasion of adjacent organs

Stages EUS3 and EUS4 are combined.

N staging

    N0. lymph nodes not visualized, or hyperechoic
    N1. lymph nodes hypoechoic or with mixed echo patterns

---

indistinct borders, whereas metastatic (M) nodes are hypoechoic, rounded, sharply demarcated, and homogeneous (Table 70.2).

8. **Results**

    a. Accuracy is approximately as follows: 88% to 92% in assessing the depth of invasion, 69% to 80% in assessing regional adenopathy, with a sensitivity of 70% to 80% and a specificity of 80% to 90%.

    b. Limitations

        i. It is difficult to evaluate obstructing lesions.

        ii. Small lymph nodes with micrometastases are difficult to differentiate from normal lymph nodes. Newer scopes with capability of EUS-guided needle biopsy of nodes may increase diagnostic yield.

    c. The **most common misinterpretation** of endosonographic tumor staging is caused by **overstaging**, specifically for T2 tumors. A peritumoral inflammation that appears hypoechoic on ultrasound may result in false prediction of a penetration through the wall (this may be seen following biopsy).

H. Selected References

ASGE. Policy and Procedure Manual for Gastrointestinal Endoscopy: Guideline for Training and Practice. May 1997.

ASGE. Preparation of patients for gastrointestinal endoscopy: guidelines for clinical application. Gastrointest Endosc 1988;34(3):32S.

ASGE. The role of colonoscopy in management of patients with colonic neoplasia. Gastrointest Endosc 1999;50:921–924.

Catalano MF. Normal structures on endoscopic ultrasonography: visualization measurement data and interobserver variation. Gastrointest Endosc Clin North Am 1995; 5(3):475–486.

Church JM. Endoscopy of the Colon, Rectum, and Anus. New York: Igaku-Shoin, 1995.

Golub RW, Kerner BA, Wise WE Jr, et al. Colonoscopic bowel preparations—which one? Dis Colon Rectum 1995;38(6):594–599.

Hildebrandt U, Feifel G. Importance of endoscopic ultrasonography staging for treatment of rectal cancer. Gastrointest Endosc Clin North Am 1995;5(4):843–849.

Mandel JS, Bond JH, Church TS, et al. Reducing mortality from colorectal cancer by screening for fecal occult blood. Minnesota Colon Cancer Control Study. N Engl J Med 1993;328:1365–1371.

Ponsky JL, ed. Atlas of Surgical Endoscopy. St. Louis: CV Mosby-Year-Book, 1992.

Romano G, Belli G, Rotondano G. Colorectal cancer: diagnosis of recurrence. Gastrointest Endosc Clin North Am 1995;5(4):831–841.

Rosch T, Lorenz R, Classen M. Endoscpic ultrasonography in the evaluation of colon and rectal disease. Gastrointest Endosc 1990;36(2):S33–S39.

Senagore AJ. Intrarectal and intra-anal ultrasonography in the evaluation of colorectal pathology. Surg Clin North Am 1994;74(6):1465–1473.

Silverstein FE, Tytgat GNJ, Hunter J, eds. Atlas of Gastrointestinal Endoscopy. 2d ed. New York: Gower Medical, 1991.

Van Outryve M. Endoscopic ultrasonography in inflammatory bowel disease, paracolorectal inflammatory pathology, and extramural abnormalities. Gastrointest Endosc Clin North Am 1995;5(4):861–867.

Winawer SJ, Fletcher RH, Miller RH, et al. Colorectal cancer screening:clinical guidelines and rationale. Gastroenterology 1997;112.

71. Therapeutic Colonoscopy and Its Complications

C. Daniel Smith, M.D.
Aaron S. Fink, M.D.
Gregory Van Stiegmann, M.D.
David W. Easter, M.D.

A. Introduction

Polypectomy is the commonest therapeutic maneuver performed at the time of colonoscopy. This technique is described in Chapter 69, which also discusses control of bleeding and removal of foreign objects. Here we describe decompressive colonoscopy for Ogilvie's syndrome, reduction of volvulus, band ligation of hemorrhoids, and complications of colonoscopy.

B. Decompressive Colonoscopy for Ogilvie's Syndrome

Acute colonic pseudo-obstruction (Ogilvie's syndrome) is a condition in which the colon becomes massively dilated without apparent mechanical obstruction. Commonly associated conditions are listed in Table 71.1. The cause is unknown but likely to be multifactorial.

The diagnosis is usually straightforward. The predominant clinical feature is abdominal distention developing over 3 to 4 days. Bowel sounds are variably present, and the abdomen is generally tense with mild tenderness. Fever and leukocytosis are common. Plain abdominal x-rays frequently reveal massive dilatation of the proximal colon with relatively normal colonic diameter from midtransverse colon to rectum. Contrast enema is necessary to exclude mechanical obstruction. Radiographic demonstration of perforation mandates urgent laparotomy.

Initial therapy includes cessation of oral intake, nasogastric decompression, and correction of fluid and electrolyte abnormalities. All potentially exacerbating medications (such as narcotics) should be discontinued. Prokinetic agents, epidural anesthesia, frequent positional change, or ambulation may promote motility. Serial abdominal examinations and daily abdominal x-rays should be used to monitor response or progression. The cecum is at greatest risk of perforation owing to the thin wall and greater circumference. When cecal diam-

Table 71.1. Conditions associated with Ogilvie's syndrome.

Nonabdominal surgery	• Orthopedic surgery
Blunt trauma	
Electrolyte abnormalities	• Hypokalemia
	• Hypomagnesemia
	• Hypophosphatemia
Chronic illness	• Renal failure
	• Diabetes mellitus
	• Malignancy
	• Autoimmune disorders
	• Hypothyroidism
Medications	• Anticholinergic agents
	• Narcotics
	• Phenothiazines
	• Tricyclic antidepressants

eter exceeds 12 cm, or if there is persistence or progression of colonic dilatation despite conservative measures, colonoscopic decompression is indicated.

1. Set up the room and position the patient as for routine colonoscopy.
2. Minimize air insufflation during endoscope passage. The pathologic distention usually facilitates endoscope passage, which is often surprisingly easy.
3. Irrigate frequently with small volumes (50 mL) of saline through the endoscope's suction channel to help maintain channel patency and a good view of the lumen.
4. It is not necessary to reach the cecum with the colonoscope to effect colonic decompression, especially if the colon is distended beyond the hepatic flexure.
5. Carefully inspect the mucosa during insertion and withdrawal. Cyanotic or ischemic mucosa may indicate the need for operative intervention. Sometimes bloody drainage is the only sign of proximal ischemia.
6. Use of an overtube for this purpose must be done with care, as the large size and stiff nature of this tube complicate endoscope insertion while increasing the risk of perforation or erosion.
7. After maximal insertion, apply intermittent suction as the endoscope is withdrawn until the colonic lumen collapses. Withdraw the scope in 4- to 5-cm increments, keeping the tip of the scope in the middle of the bowel lumen. This allows decompression of gas and liquid through the suction channel without trapping bowel mucosa.
8. Evaluate the success of decompression by serial abdominal physical and radiographic examination.
9. A nasogastric tube or long intestinal tube may be passed with the colonoscope and left in place after scope removal.

C. Decompressive Colonoscopy for Sigmoid Volvulus

Sigmoid volvulus occurs when a large bowel segment abnormally twists or folds on its mesentery. Volvulus produces a closed-loop obstruction with a high mortality unless treated. The diagnosis may be suspected on the basis of clinical presentation and plain abdominal films (which may be diagnostic). Contrast studies confirm the problem by showing the typical bird's beak deformity of the twisted segment.

In the absence of signs of gangrene, the safest initial treatment of sigmoid volvulus is sigmoidoscopic reduction and decompression. This provides assessment of mucosal viability, and more importantly, may decompress the dilated loop and reduce the volvulus. Urgent laparotomy is mandated for suspicion of colonic gangrene (elevated temperature, leukocytosis, abdominal tenderness with peritoneal signs, necrotic mucosa at endoscopy) or inability to reduce the volvulus.

In contrast to sigmoid volvulus, endoscopic reduction and decompression is not effective for cecal volvulus. Although both colonoscopic and barium-assisted reduction of cecal volvulus have been described, successes have been limited and associated with high morbidity owing to delays in definitive management. The mainstay of management for cecal volvulus remains prompt laparotomy, at which time the volvulus is reduced.

1. Begin preparing the patient for surgery, so that operative intervention will not be delayed if endoscopic treatment fails.
2. Position the patient in the prone jackknife position. This facilitates decompression by allowing the colon to fall away. The lateral decubitus position is acceptable if the patient cannot tolerate the jackknife position.
3. Because the twist is low in the sigmoid, it can generally be reached with a **rigid sigmoidoscope**. This instrument facilitates decompression, often resulting in a dramatic passage of gas and stool as the volvulus is entered and the segment is decompressed.
   a. Minimize air insufflation during insertion.
   b. Carefully insert the rigid sigmoidoscope until the site of torsion is seen. Thoroughly inspect the mucosa at this point for signs of ischemia or necrosis.
   c. If the mucosa appears intact, gently advance the sigmoidoscope beyond the point of torsion until there is an immediate return of gas and stool from the obstructed loop.
   d. Perform a further limited examination of the bowel mucosa to assure viability, then place a rectal tube well above the site of torsion, secure it to the perianal skin, and leave it for at least 48 hours. This will maintain decompression and facilitate subsequent bowel preparation or further evaluation.
   e. Alternatively, a soft, well-lubricated 40- to 60-cm rectal tube can be gently passed beyond the site of torsion under endoscopic vision to accomplish decompression. Obviously, endoscopic evaluation of mucosal viability may be limited with this tecnique.

4.   Points of axial rotation and obstruction beyond the reach of a rigid scope require use of a **flexible sigmoidoscope or a colonoscope**.
     a.   Suction and an assistant are critical to safe completion of endoscopic decompression and evaluation.
     b.   The colonoscope is passed through the site of torsion, often with gentle air insufflation, as the scope is passed beyond the site of obstruction.
     c.   Suction decompression may be facilitated by attaching an external suction device to the colonoscope's biopsy channel, or by attaching a long, soft, 14- to 16-French straight catheter to the colonoscope while advancing past the torsion and into the proximal colon. This tube is then left in place for subsequent decompression.
5.   Endoscopic decompression and detorsion is successful in 85% of cases of sigmoid volvulus. A high rate of recurrence argues in favor of elective resection of the redundant segment. Patients in whom endoscopic decompression fails, or in whom nonviable mucosa is seen on colonoscopy, require urgent surgery.

D. Endoscopic Band Ligation Treatment of Internal Hemorrhoids

Indications for treatment of internal hemorrhoids include bleeding and prolapse. Hemorrhoids of grade 1, 2, or 3 are suitable for endoscopic treatment. Band ligation treatment is usually preceded with a Fleet enema. Thorough examination of the anorectum, including anoscopy and flexible sigmoidoscopy/colonoscopy is indicated for most patients with such symptoms.

Patients with external hemorrhoids, some patients with large grade 3 hemorrhoids, and those with grade 4 hemorrhoids are **not suitable** for endoscopic therapy. Caution is indicated in patients who are neutropenic or have compromised immune function. These patients may have a higher risk of impaired healing or septic complications.

1.   Place the patient in the **Sims position** (left lateral decubitus with right knee flexed).
2.   Sedation is usually not necessary.
3.   Mount the ligating device on the endoscope and pass the endoscope just beyond the dentate line. When a "see-through" ligator is used, the dentate line is easily visualized as it passes by.
4.   Perform ligations 1 cm or more above the dentate line to avoid patient discomfort.
5.   The direct approach (Fig. 71.1) is simplest and best tolerated by most patients.
     a.   Identify the largest hemorrhoid.
     b.   Aspirate it into the ligating cylinder using endoscopic suction, and release the rubber band to produce ligation.

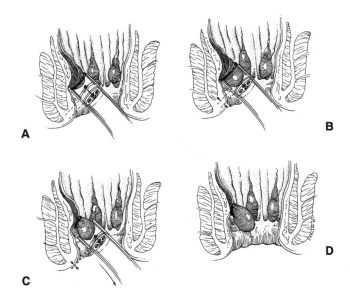

A

B

C

D

Figure 71.1. Direct endoscopic ligation of internal hemorrhoids. A. The endo-scopist positions the ligator in contact with the hemorrhoid about 1 cm above he dentate line. B. Endoscopic suction draws the hemorrhoid into the banding cylin-der. C. The elastic **O**-ring is ejected to ensnare the hemorrhoid. D. The ligated hemorrhoid.

c. Single-fire instruments require that the endoscope be removed and a second band loaded. Multifire devices do not require this maneuver.

d. Repeat the ligation for additional hemorrhoids. Up to three liga-tions are done at one sitting.

e. Patients with a short anal canal, such as female patients, may be more easily approached with the endoscope retroflexed.

   i. Insert the endoscope with the attached ligating device into the rectum.

   ii. Retroflex the endoscope within the rectum to visualize the region above the dentate line.

   iii. The cephalad view facilitates visualization and ligation when the anal canal is too short to permit a direct approach.

   iv. The retroflexed approach is best suited to endoscopic liga-tion done with a multifire device, which does not require removal and reloading. From one to three ligations are done at one sitting as described in item 5.d.

E. Complications of Colonoscopy

A sure way to compound any complication is to delay its recognition and treatment. Inexperienced endoscopists are more likely to produce complications—including both technical and judgmental errors. At both the beginning and end of each procedure, review any risks and unusual events specific to the individual patient and procedure. For example, is the patient on antiplatelet medications? Was any undue difficulty experienced during the procedure?

Instruct the patient and/or guardian of the common presenting symptoms and signs of complications that can follow an "uneventful" colonoscopy. These generally include pain, bleeding, sensorium changes, nausea, and abdominal distention. Any worrisome event should prompt urgent physician contact and an appropriate evaluation.

1. **Bleeding**
   a. **Cause and prevention.** Bleeding, the most common complication following colonoscopy, is usually a result of faulty hemostasis following biopsy. Resections of polyps exceeding 15 mm are at particular risk of continued or delayed bleeding. Rarely, bleeding can occur from trauma to hemorrhoidal veins, or from mucosal erosions caused by mechanical trauma. Very rarely, direct mechanical trauma results in splenic rupture. The best ways to prevent these injuries are to (1) anticipate potential problems, (2) correct coagulation disorders prior to <u>and</u> following any biopsy, (3) carefully inspect all biopsy sites minutes after manipulation, and (4) not overmedicate the patient (to the state of being unable to report undue pain).
   b. **Recognition and management.** Do not aggressively pursue self-limited bleeding from biopsy sites, to avoid me risk of perforation from the nonindicated use of excessive cautery. Less than 50% of biopsy sites will require additional cautery and/or the injection of 1:100,000 epinephrine. Delayed bleeding, which occurs between hours and 30 days following colonoscopy, requires immediate resuscitation, correction of any coagulating disorders, and, usually, repeat colonoscopy. As arterial embolization is largely contraindicated (the risk of perforation is already high), abdominal exploration must occur if bleeding sites cannot be promptly controlled. If, after replacement of fluids and coagulation deficits, the patient has clearly and decidedly stopped bleeding, one may elect to omit repeat colonoscopy to minimize the risk of perforation at the biopsy site(s). Unaltered, fresh blood per rectum should raise the suspicion of hemorrhoidal bleeding. Bleeding hemorrhoids require immediate banding, or unusually, open hemorrhoidectomy. Clinical fluid losses and/or shock without an obvious source should raise the concern of an occult splenic rupture. Emergency ultrasound of the abdomen (as for trauma patients) is indicated, and any free fluid should prompt an immediate laparotomy.

2. **Perforation**
   a. **Causes and prevention.** The incidence of perforation following routine diagnostic colonoscopy is approximately 0.8%. This rate doubles following therapeutic procedures. Prior surgery, diverticulitis, or any cause of preexisting intra-abdominal adhesions increase the difficulty of the procedure and enhance the possibility of a colon perforation. Causes include barotrauma from excessive insufflation, direct mechanical trauma from the scope or its instruments, and perforation from compromised biopsy sites. Oversedation can promote the creation of this deadly complication; that is, a reasonably alert patient can complain of overdistention and mechanical scope trauma. The rate of perforation increases with the size of any resected lesion and the amount of cautery used. Large lesions should prompt the consideration of staged, partial resections. Miscellaneous causes of perforation include overzealous dilation of strictures, excessive laser ablation, and inappropriate use of biopsy instruments. Manipulations should occur under visual control at all times, and patience and caution are the foundations of any therapeutic procedure.
   b. **Recognition and management.** If there has been any departure from a smooth and uneventful colonoscopy, it must be considered that a perforation might have occurred. This is particularly true when the patient complains of, or awakens with, unexpected discomfort. Escalating pain is a very worrisome sign, and should prompt urgent evaluation and abdominal radiographs. An elevated temperature, tachycardia, and/or a leukocytosis add to the specificity of diagnosis. Broad-spectrum antibiotics and fluid resuscitation should be considered at the first suspicion of perforation. Upright chest x-ray and left lateral decubitis films are the standards for detecting free intra-abdominal air. Computed tomography (CT) is more sensitive, but also more costly. Intraperitoneal air is absent in about 12% of perforations. Delayed recognition and gross soilage requires a diverting colostomy and washout of the abdomen (note: consider laparoscopy). Early suspicion and no free air on plain radiographs may be managed expectantly with broad-spectrum antibiotics in selected patients. Of note, patients who are "poor surgical candidates" are those who are least likely to survive continued fecal soilage. Whether employing laparoscopy, CT, or other means of diagnosis (e.g., contrast enemas if CT is not available), the decision tree should clearly anticipate what will be required with each finding. For example, if a "confined leak" will be treated expectantly, then CT plays a role. Likewise, if the results of laparoscopic diagnosis or treatment are untrusted, one should not utilize laparoscopy for this situation!

3. **Infection**
   a. **Causes and prevention.** The transmission of infectious material from one patient to another via colonoscopic equipment is certainly possible, but also, fortunately, a rare event. Proper atten-

tion to scope preparation, especially the mechanical scrubbing of all ports and instruments, is essential. Even the most hearty spore or virus is reliably rendered harmless with standard soaking protocols. That colonoscopy can and does produce a transient bacteremia is well known. Antibiotic prophylaxis should be given to patients with vascular prostheses or valvular abnormalities.

b. **Recognition and management.** Delayed presentation of vague or confusing symptoms following colonoscopy should prompt a careful history, physical, and review of symptoms. Awareness of this possible iatrogenic complication will facilitate appropriate recognition and management.

4. **Missed diagnosis**

a. **Causes and prevention.** A most serious "complication" is the failure to diagnose an existing condition that warrants prompt treatment. An inadequate bowel prep can certainly obscure significant colon and rectal neoplasia. The three anatomic "silent areas" of the colon are the cecum, the most distal rectum, and the splenic flexure. Even in experienced hands, the cecum is not adequately visualized in 5 to 10% of cases. Confirmation of reaching the cecum is verified using multiple criteria. Accuracy is nearly 100% when three of the following criteria are met: (1) transillumination of the cecum in the right lower abdomen, (2) convergence of the cecal haustra, (3) identification of the appendiceal lumen, (4) identification and/or cannulation of the terminal ileum, (5) exact recognition of the palpating hand in the right lower abdomen, or (6) the normal progression of intraluminal landmarks (e.g., hepatic flexure and capacious cecum). If doubt persists, fluoroscopy will confirm the exact location of the colonoscope. Careful attention to technique, with meticulous inspection of all potential blind spots including a retroflexed view of the anoderm junction, will minimize the chance of a missed lesion. If the preparation of the bowel is inadequate, thorough washing/irrigation of the retained feces is attempted via the colonoscope. If the visual inspection remains incomplete, then a second exam is indicated at a later date with a more vigorous preparation.

b. **Recognition and management.** Faulty judgment and pride can obscure the realization of an incomplete colonoscopy. Unless complications ensue, if a full diagnostic colonoscopy was initially indicated, then full screening must be accomplished. If necessary, repeat colonoscopy and/or double-contrast barium enema should be scheduled. Good relations and personal communication which radiology colleagues will often secure an "add-on" barium enema exam on the same day as the incomplete colonoscopy, thus sparing the patient a second bowel prep.

5. **Lost specimens**

a. **Causes and prevention.** It can be difficult at times to retrieve biopsy specimens. This is particularly true for small polyps resected with the snare loop. Careful cleansing of surrounding feces **prior** to polypectomy, and optimal patient positioning (e.g., rolling the patient on his or her side, abdomen, or back) will prevent many frustrating situations.

b. **Recognition and management.** If a specimen is not retrieved on initial attempts, a series of maneuvers can be employed. A suction trap is placed inline. Careful removal of all debris and fecal material with suction is essential to recovering small lost specimens. Often, the small polyp, when found, can be immobilized at the suction port, and the scope can be removed while constant suction is applied. If the desired specimen is not found upon removal of the scope (following all due diligence), the suction trap is first completely inspected, and second, the suction port of the scope is probed. Next, it is recommended that the diagnostic colonoscopy be completely repeated. Finally, the patient is instructed in the use of a collection "seat" for the home toilet and is encouraged to participate in the search by screening all fecal matter over the next 2 days. But clearly, the best hope of retrieving a lost specimen rests with the careful attempts of an experience endoscopist.

6. **Complications of endoscopic hemorrhoid ligation**
   a. **Pain**
      i. **Cause and prevention.** The most common complication of endoscopic ligation for hemorrhoid disease is pain. Severe pain immediately after ligation usually indicates that the site of ligation was too close to the dentate line.
      ii. **Recognition and management.** Recognition is usually easy. If severe pain occurs immediately following endoscopic ligation, an anoscope may be inserted and, using a pointed scissors, the elastic band divided and removed. Repeat endoscopic ligation may then be performed at a more cephalad site if the patient is willing.
   b. **Bleeding.** Limited bleeding that occurs from 3 to 6 days after endoscopic ligation treatment is common, and the patient should be advised to expect it. Occasionally, breakage or dislodgment of an elastic band in the first 24 to 48 hours following endoscopic ligation is associated with significant (>100 mL) bleeding, which may require repeat application of an elastic band or suture ligation via an anoscope to control. The latter complication is uncommon.
   c. **Thrombosis of external hemorrhoids** occasionally occurs following band ligation of internal hemorrhoids. Most cases can be managed conservatively with sitz baths and analgesics.
   d. **Pelvic sepsis**
      i. **Cause and prevention.** This **very** rare complication of band ligation has been reported most frequently in younger males and may be devastating. No specific preventive measures have been identified.
      ii. **Recognition and management.** The typical patient develops perineal pain, swelling, inability to urinate, and

may have cellulitis, perineal ulceration, or gangrene on examination. These symptoms mandate admission to hospital, computed tomography of the pelvis to rule out other pathology, intravenous antibiotics, examination under anesthesia, and possibly perineal debridement and colostomy. This complication has been reported in a small number of cases over the past two decades. It is wise to inform patients of both the symptoms associated with this complication as well as its rarity as part of the informed consent.

F. Selected References

Ballantyne GH. Review of sigmoid volvulus: history and results of treatment. Dis Colon Rectum 1982;25:494–501.

Ballantyne GH, Brandner MD, Beart RW Jr, Ilstrup DM. Volvulus of the colon: incidence and mortality. Ann Surg 1985;202:830–892.

Bat L, Melzer E, Koler M, Dreznick Z, Shemesh E. Complications of rubber band ligation of symptomatic internal hemorrhoids. Dis Colon Rectum 1993:36:287–290.

Berkelhammer C, Moosvi SB. Retroflexed endoscopic band ligation of internal hemorrhoids. Gastrointest Endosc 2002;55(4):532–537.

Branum GB, Fink AS. Ogilvie's syndrome. In Cameron JL, ed. Current Surgical Therapy. 6th ed. St Louis: CV Mosby-Year-Book, 1997.

Brothers TE, Strodel WE, Eckhauser FE. Endoscopy in colonic volvulus. Ann Surg 1987;206:1–4.

Geller A, Petersen BT, Gostout CJ. Endoscopic decompression for acute colonic pseudoobstruction. Gastrointest Endosc 1996;44:144–150.

Jetmore AB, Timmcke AE, Gathright JB, et al. Ogilvie's syndrome: colonoscopic decompression and analysis of predisposing factors. Dis Colon Rectum 1995;35:1135–1142.

Komborozos VA, Skrekas GJ, Pissiotis CA. Rubber band ligation of symptomatic internal hemorrhoids: results of 500 cases. Dig Surg 200;17(1):1–6.

MacRae HM, McLeod RS. Comparison of hemorrhoidal treatment modalities. A meta-analysis. Dis Colon Rectum 1995;38:687–694.

Rex DK. Colonoscopy and acute colonic pseudo-obstruction. Gastrointest Endosc Clin North Am 1997;7(3):499–508.

Smith CD, Fink AS. The management of colonic volvulus. In: Cameron JL, ed. Current Surgical Therapy. 6th ed. St Louis: CV Mosby-Year-Book, 1997.

Flexible Endoscopy
VIII—Pediatric Endoscopy

72. Pediatric Gastrointestinal Endoscopy

Thom E. Lobe, M.D.

A. Pediatric Esophagoscopy

1. **Indications**
   a. **Diagnostic esophagoscopy** is performed for the evaluation of caustic ingestion, gastroesophageal reflux, and the diagnostic of specific inflammatory or infectious problems.
   b. **Foreign body removal** by esophagoscopy is indicated whenever the foreign body has been present for more than 48 hours and cannot be removed by simple means such as Foley catheter extraction or advancing the foreign body into the stomach with insertion of a bougie.
   c. Strictures due to caustic ingestion or gastroesophageal reflux may need **dilatation**.
   d. **Sclerotherapy of esophageal varices** is performed for control of hemorrhage in patients with portal hypertension.
2. The examination may be performed with either a rigid or a flexible esophagoscope. General anesthesia is commonly used.
   a. **Rigid esophagoscopy** must be done under endotracheal general anesthesia. The patient lies supine on the operating table with the anesthesiologist to the left of the patient's head.
   b. **Flexible esophagoscopy** can be done under general endotracheal anesthesia with the patient supine and either straight or turned with the anesthesiologist sitting to the side of the patient's head (whichever seems most comfortable or convenient).
3. **Rigid esophagoscopy**
   a. Place a roll under the patient's neck to extend the neck and make it easier to pass the rigid scope.
   b. Use a laryngoscope to lift the endotracheal tube anteriorly and to expose the pharyngeal opening so that the esophagoscope can be introduced under direct vision.
   c. Take care to protect the patient during the introduction of the esophagoscope. Wrap the head with a towel to protect the face and eyes.
   d. Introduce the esophagoscope with the right hand while using the left hand to guide the esophagoscope and to protect the lips, gums, and teeth.

e. Never advance the esophagoscope blindly. Advance the scope only under direct vision and with caution, only as far as necessary to visualize the lesion.

f. Use suction liberally to ensure adequate vision.

4. **Flexible esophagoscopy under general anesthesia**

a. Use a mouth guard of an appropriate size for the patient (although this may be less necessary in the anesthetized child).

b. Confirm that the end of the scope is free to move in all directions during its introduction.

c. Use the index finger of the dominant hand to elevate the patient's tongue and mandible.

d. Introduce the endoscope into the pharynx and just into the esophagus with the nondominant hand.

e. Advance the endoscope gently under direct inspection with gentle insufflation of air. Never advance the esophagoscope blindly.

5. **Flexible esophagoscopy under conscious sedation**

a. Sedation may consist of Demerol, 1 to 2 mg/kg, and Versed 0.1 mg/kg, administered intravenously or the equivalent.

b. Monitoring may consist of assessing heart rate, blood pressure, respiratory rate, and oxygen saturation (by pulse oximetry), every 5 minutes during the procedure and every 30 to 45 minutes during the recovery time.

c. Position the patient supine. Use the appropriate size of mouth guard to protect the endoscope.

d. Passage of the scope proceeds in the same manner described for rigid esophagoscopy.

6. **Special considerations**

a. **Diagnostic esophagoscopy.** Inspect for mucosal abnormalities including hemangiomas and other vascular malformations, esophageal varices, esophagitis, or evidence of gastroesophageal reflux. If the child has ingested caustic material, do not advance the rigid esophagoscope beyond the first indication of injury. If a flexible scope is used, advance the scope through the injured esophagus with caution.

  i. If biopsy samples are needed, use a cup biopsy forceps to take superficial bites.

  ii. Multiple samples should be taken for histology, cultures, and any special studies.

b. **Stricture**

  i. Pass a balloon dilator (size depends upon age and size of child) through the stricture under direct vision until it is in the proper location. Introduce radiopaque contrast into the balloon and dilate the stricture under fluoroscopic and direct visual guidance. Steroid injections in conjunction with dilatation are favored by some and can be performed using a retractable sclerotherapy needle.

  ii. If the stricture is tight, it may be necessary to pass a string or a wire and create a gastrostomy. One end of the string is withdrawn through the nose and the other end through the gastrostomy. The two ends are tied and left in place. Dilators can then be passed serially to accomplish gradual dilatation.

c. **Foreign body removal**

    i. **Coins.** Use an alligator or rat-tooth grasper with teeth on the end of the instrument to catch the rim of the coin. Securely grasp the coin, edge on, and then remove the entire unit (scope, grasper, and coin) together.

    ii. **Sharp objects.** Grasp the object by the blunt end and withdraw it, or maneuver the sharp end of the object into the lumen of a rigid esophagoscope, withdrawing the scope, grasper, and object as a unit.

d. **Variceal sclerotherapy** is performed in a manner similar to that used for adults.

    i. Inject 1 to 3 mL of sclerosant into each varix at or just proximal to the esophagogastric junction.

    ii. Use a total of about 5 to 10 mL of sclerosant at each session.

    iii. Space sessions at 3- to 6-week intervals.

7. **Complications**

a. **Perforation**

    i. **Cause and prevention.** Rigid esophagoscopy beyond the cephalad margin of injury from caustic ingestion may result in perforation. Minimize the risk by not advancing the rigid scope beyond the first recognition of injury. Forceful dilatation of an esophageal stricture or forceful removal of a foreign body that has been present for more that 48 hours may result in perforation. The former can be prevented by not being too zealous in attempts at dilatation of tight strictures. The latter may not be preventable.

    ii. **Recognition and management.** Blood at the site of injury or stricture should make one suspect of a perforation. A two-view chest x-ray should be taken to search for mediastinal air or pneumothorax. If these images are suspicious, a contrast esophagram should be performed. Additional management of a perforation depends on the location. In most instances drainage will be required with or without repair of the perforation. A thoracoscopy or a thoracotomy may be required to accomplish this. Rarely, a gastrostomy and a cervical esophagostomy may be required to protect the area of injury. For perforation of the cervical esophagus, a cervical exploration with drainage may be necessary.

b. **Mucosal injury**

    i. **Cause and prevention.** Mucosal injury can occur from forceful dilatation, the removal of a foreign body, or the injection of esophageal varices. All these maneuvers should be carried out by experienced endoscopists and with care to prevent injury.

    ii. **Recognition and management.** When mucosal injury is apparent, radiographs should be taken to exclude the possibility of a perforation. In the absence of perforation, most of these injuries will heal without any specific therapy.

   c. **Extraesophageal injection of sclerotherapy solution**
     i. **Cause and prevention.** When sclerotherapy is performed, the possibility exists of injecting the solution outside the esophagus, rather than intra- or paravariceal.
     ii. **Recognition and management.** Failure to do a proper injection is immediately apparent. Either the varices blanch or the paravariceal esophageal mucosa swells and blanches to indicate a proper injection. If neither of these occurs, one should be suspicious of a transmural injection, and a two-view chest x-ray should be obtained to exclude perforation. In most instances, nothing need be done beyond observation.

B. Gastroduodenoscopy

1. **Indications**
   a. **Diagnostic gastroduodenoscopy** is indicated for the assessment of inflammatory conditions and suspected gastritis or peptic ulcer disease. Biopsy may be required for diagnosis of *Helicobacter pylori* or other infections.
   b. **Foreign bodies** such as coins or sharp objects such as pins or needles often need to be removed using endoscopic snares or graspers.
   c. **Hemorrhage** from the stomach and duodenum can best be assessed by endoscopy.
   d. Assessment of an upper gastrointestinal **mass** can be made by inspection and biopsy depending on the nature of the mass.
   e. **Percutaneous endoscopic gastrostomy** (**PEG**) tube placement is a useful alternative to open gastrostomy.
2. The examination may be performed under general anesthesia using the same patient position and room setup described earlier, or it may be performed under conscious sedation with appropriate monitoring. In this case, the patient is often placed in a lateral position starting with the left side down.
3. The initial part of the examination proceeds as described earlier for flexible esophagoscopy.
4. Upon entering the stomach, retroflex the endoscope to inspect the cardia of the stomach and the gastric side of the gastroesophageal junction.
5. Next, thoroughly inspect the body of the stomach, including the greater and lesser curvature.
6. In the small infant and child, the pylorus is quite high, at about at the level of the gastroesophageal junction. The best way to find this structure is by retroflexing the endoscope and maneuvering the scope back and forth on either side of the incisura.
7. With the pylorus in view, advance the endoscope toward the pyloric opening and into the duodenum.

Table 72.1. Causes of upper gastrointestinal bleeding
in children.

- Gastric varices
- Peptic ulcer disease
- Vascular malformations (rare)
- Mallory-Weiss tears (rare)
- Tumors (uncommon)
- Gastritis (common)

8. **Special considerations**
   a. Common causes of upper gastrointestinal bleeding are listed
      in Table 72.1. When gastritis is found, biopsy to evaluate for
      H. pylori.
   b. Most patients who are scoped for evaluation of pain will prove
      to have gastritis. Biopsy samples should be taken to evaluate for
      H. pylori.
9. Removal of foreign bodies from the stomach
   a. Coins may sit in the stomach for prolonged periods and often are
      adherent if they are multiple.
   b. Use forceps with teeth on the end. This allows the grasper to gain
      a firm grip on the raised edge of the coin.
   c. Remove sharp foreign bodies blunt end first, to avoid injuring the
      esophagus on the way out.
10. Percutaneous gastrostomy placement
    a. The techniques are essentially the same as those used in adults.
    b. Take care to avoid injury to colon or small intestine, and consider
       using laparoscopic visualization to minimize the danger of injury
       to adjacent viscera.
11. Complications
    a. The complications of **diagnostic gastroduodenoscopy** in chil-
       dren are the same as in adults.
    b. **Extragastric placement of PEGs**
       i. **Cause and prevention.** PEG tubes can be placed erro-
          neously in the adjacent colon or small bowel. Minimize the
          risk by considering alternate techniques in patients with pre-
          vious abdominal surgery, peritonitis, or tumors. Carefully
          distend the stomach and choose the site of the PEG tube
          carefully. When the stomach is distended and illuminated,
          look for a transverse shadow across the upper abdomen
          (which may represent a loop of small bowel or colon
          between the stomach and the abdominal wall). Avoid this
          problem completely by using a laparoscopic assisted
          technique.
       ii. **Recognition and management.** This complication may not
           be recognized immediately. Local peritonitis may develop,
           leading one to suspect the possibility. When gastrostomy

feedings result in severe abdominal cramping (with small bowel placement) or diarrhea (colon placement), perform a contrast study to document the position of the tube. If the complication is discovered late, then it may suffice to remove the tube and allow the tract to seal itself. If the complication is discovered early or if the contrast study suggests intraperitoneal extravasation, then a laparotomy may be required for repair of the injured bowel.

C. Sigmoidoscopy

1. **Pediatric sigmoidoscopy** can be used to assess bleeding or a suspected mass in the sigmoid colon. Just as with adults, biopsy or excision of polypoid masses can be performed.
2. In young children, sigmoidoscopy is often performed under general endotracheal anesthesia. Position the patient either in the lateral flexed position with the buttocks over the side of the table, or in the lithotomy position. Conscious sedation may be used in older children. In some children, it may be feasible to perform flexible sigmoidoscopy in the office without sedation.
3. A pediatric Fleet enema or its equivalent should be given to the child before sigmoidoscopy.
4. First introduce a finger into the anus to dilate it and to assess whether there exist any obstructing lesions.
5. **Rigid sigmoidoscopy.** Having established that the anus and distal rectum are clear of obstruction, introduce the sigmoidoscope with obturator into the anus. Remove the obturator, close the observation window, and gently introduce sufficient air into the rectum to visualize the lumen. Advance the scope in the direction of the lumen under direct vision. Never force the scope blindly. Inspect the mucosal surface through its entire circumference as the scope is withdrawn.
6. **Flexible sigmoidoscopy** (see Colonoscopy, Section D).
7. During sigmoidoscopy, search for fissures, arteriovenous malformations, foreign bodies, signs of trauma, or mass lesions. **Always remember the possibility of child abuse.**

D. Colonoscopy

1. **Indications.** As with adult patients, colonoscopy is performed for evaluation of suspected infectious or inflammatory colitis, bleeding, or mass lesion above the range of the flexible sigmoidoscope.
2. **Bowel preparation.** A bowel prep consisting of clear liquids the evening before (2 days in older children), and a cathartic the day before works well. Alternatively (although most children do not tolerate the

volume well), Go-Lytely (Braintree Laboratories, Braintree, MA) can be administered by mouth in a dose of 4 mL/kg/h for 4 hours the day preceding the examination, to be accompanied by a clear liquid diet to follow. The patient should be NPO for the examination. The duration of the NPO period is different for each age and may vary somewhat with the patient's condition to the extent that the patient's condition can alter gastric emptying. It is sufficient for infants less than six months of age, for example, to be NPO for 4 hours after which their stomachs will be empty. Children older than 5 or 6 years of age act more like adults and should be NPO for 6–8 hours before their endoscopy.

3. First introduce a finger into the rectum to be certain that no obstructing lesions are present.

4. Next, insert the colonoscope and advance in the direction of the lumen. The general technique is similar to that used in adults (see Chapter 70).

5. It may be helpful to have an assistant hold the scope at the anus and advance the scope as necessary while the endoscopist manipulates the scope.

6. Redirect the scope by palpating the patient's abdomen, or by repositioning the patient as necessary. Sometimes it is useful to jiggle the endoscope to aid in its advancement into the colon.

7. Occasionally, the endoscope will be difficult to advance, or remain in the same location despite insertion of significant additional length of scope. The scope may have formed a loop, or the bowel may have telescoped on itself. Withdraw the body of the scope until the end of the scope retracts. It should then be possible to resume advancing the scope. Advance the colonoscope to the cecum, and inspect 360 degrees of the mucosal circumference for each length of bowel as the scope is withdrawn.

8. **Biopsy** is best performed with a cup biopsy forceps to minimize tissue destruction. It may be advisable to send specimens for cultures or special studies in addition to routine histology.

9. Before performing **polypectomy**, carefully assess the nature of the polyp. Pedunculated polyps may be removed by snare with electrocautery. Sessile polyps may be sampled for histology, but removal may require operative resection.

10. **Sigmoid volvulus** may sometimes be reduced endoscopically (sigmoidoscope or colonoscope).
    a. Suspect the diagnosis from clinical presentation and abdominal x-rays, especially in mentally impaired patients or those with chronic constipation.
    b. If the passage of the sigmoidoscope fails to reduce the volvulus, flexible colonoscopy or operative reduction may be required.

11. **Severe constipation** occurs in some pediatric patients. Mechanical disimpaction under anesthesia may be required. This is particularly likely in the mentally impaired, in patients with undiagnosed Hirschsprung's disease, or following corrective surgery for Hirschsprung's disease or imperforate anus. Digital disimpaction

accompanied by irrigation may be necessary to make room for the sigmoidoscope, which is of limited use in the evaluation of this problem.

12. The **complications** of pediatric colonoscopy include bleeding and perforation. Measures of prevention, recognition, and management are similar to those used for the adult.

Part 3 Thoracoscopy for the Gastrointestinal Surgeon

73. Video-Assisted Thoracic Surgery: Basic Concepts

Rodney J. Landreneau, M.D.
Ricardo Santos, M.D.
Jason Lamb, M.D.

A. Indications

Video-assisted thoracic surgery (VATS) has come to be the primary operative approach for a wide variety of intrathoracic problems previously addressed through open thoracotomy. The primary uses of VATS approaches in general thoracic surgical practice today are listed in Table 73.1. Not all thoracic surgeons utilize the VATS approach for this entire range of intrathoracic problems. The majority of thoracic surgeons limit their use of VATS to the management of pleural pathologic conditions and wedge resection biopsy of peripheral lung lesions. Nevertheless, as experience and enthusiasm with minimally invasive surgical techniques grows, a growing number of thoracic surgeons completing their training are expanding their use of VATS.

This chapter details principles of perioperative patient management, instrument needs, and basic intercostal approach strategies crucial for a successful VATS intervention.

B. Anesthesia Issues Related to VATS

VATS is usually performed under general endotracheal anesthesia. Generally speaking, the physiologic derangements that occur during VATS are the same as those encountered during open thoracic surgery. Thus, it is critical that the anesthesia team be accomplished in the standard open incisional thoracic surgical management.

VATS requires ipsilateral pulmonary collapse. Without adequate collapse, pulmonary lesion localization is suboptimal and the risk of pulmonary injury significantly greater. Lung collapse may be obtained in one of several ways.

1. Occasionally, a patient with a large pleural effusion may have already sufficient collapse of the ipsilateral lung to allow pleural biopsy, breakdown of loculations, pleurodesis, and strategic chest tube placement to be done with a standard endotracheal tube. The lung rarely expands immediately after drainage of the effusion.

   a. It is important to examine the airway first to ensure that lung collapse is not due to bronchial obstruction.

Table 73.1. Uses of VATS in general thoracic surgery.

- Diagnosis and management of the idiopathic complex pleural effusive process and pleural-based masses
- Diagnosis of the peripheral indeterminate pulmonary nodule
- Diagnosis of idiopathic interstitial lung disease
- Thymectomy for myasthenia gravis and selective biopsy and/or resection of mediastinal masses
- VATS pulmonary lobectomy
- VATS management of spontaneous pneumothorax and lung volume reduction surgery for pulmonary emphysema
- VATS sympathectomy and splanchnicectomy for hyperhidrosis and pain syndromes
- Performance of the intrathoracic dissection as a part of minimally invasive esophagectomy
- Esophagomyotomy
- Resection of esophageal diverticulum

     b.   If central main stem bronchial obstruction is encountered, VATS should not be undertaken until airway obstruction has been overcome through endoluminal laser, stenting, or brachytherapy.

    2.   We believe that **double-lumen endotracheal tube** intubation is required for almost all VATS interventions, and this is the technique used by most surgeons.

    3.   An **endotracheal bronchus blocking approach** may be considered in lieu of a double-lumen tube if the anesthesia and thoracic surgical team have experience with this approach. This approach is often satisfactory, but occasional difficulty with lung isolation will be seen among patients with a short right main stem bronchus.

It is imperative that the thoracic surgeon evaluate the adequacy of the positioning the double-lumen tube or bronchus blocker. We also recommend a second bronchoscopic evaluation by the surgeon and anesthesia team after lateral positioning of the patient for the VATS procedure to ensure that the endotracheal tube or blocker has not become malpositioned during patient transfer.

Carbon dioxide insufflation is generally not used for VATS interventions. The exception is VATS to accomplish thoracodorsal sympathectomy for hyperhidrosis or upper extremity pain syndromes (see Chapter 78).

C. Patient Positioning for VATS

Most VATS interventions are accomplished in a near full lateral decubitus position. We tend to lean the patient slightly backward to provide additional access to the anterior intercostal spaces, which are wider. Access through these anterior spaces may reduce the risk of intercostal neurovascular or rib injury and resulting acute and chronic pain.

Exceptions to this generally lateral positioning approach occur for VATS thymectomy and thoracodorsal sympathectomy. For thymectomy we prefer to approach the patient from the right side at 45 to 60 degrees from the supine. This gives better access to the anterior mediastinum, by allowing gravity to produce dependent displacement of the collapsed lung.

For VATS bilateral sympathectomy, as mentioned in Chapter 78, we prefer to place the patient in a supine position with a roll beneath the shoulders and perform the bilateral intervention without repositioning of the patient. The operating table is established in a sharp reverse Trendelenburg position for VATS sympathectomy to allow for dependent displacement of the lungs during the apical thoracic VATS dissection.

For patients who are approached through a lateral decubitus position, ensure that the midsection is at the central break of the operating table. This allows flexing of the table to further open the intercostal spaces and to displace the patient's hip so that manipulation of instrumentation and videothoracoscopic camera unit is not impeded by it. We also establish the operating table in a reversed Trendelenburg position after lateral positioning of the patient to take advantage of gravity in overcoming the effects of the ipsilateral cephalad diaphragmatic displacement seen during contralateral single-lung ventilation.

A wide surgical preparation with anterior exposure to include the breast is important. This ensures the anterior disposition of the patient positioning, which is often forgotten in favor of the positioning and preparation that have been used for a posterolateral thoracotomy. Again, we stress that the positioning commonly used for posterolateral thoracotomy will result in inferior operative dexterity and the potential for increased postoperative pain syndromes.

D. VATS Instrumentation

VATS requires superior video-optics and intracavitary illumination. A variety of companies have developed three-chip video cameras that provide excellent visibility and image definition. Table 73.2 lists the basic instrumentation.

1. We prefer to use an "operating thoracoscope" for most of our VATS interventions. These 10-mm-diameter scopes have an inline 5-mm biopsy channel and a prismatic visual optic configuration that allows for a 45-degree offline orientation of the eyepiece–camera connection. With this scope, single intercostal access VATS can be readily accomplished for the biopsy, evaluation, and treatment of simple idiopathic pleural problems (i.e., pleural-based masses and simple pleural effusions). Since most VATS interventions are also conducted under open atmospheric conditions, the open biopsy channel also allows for an air entry site during intrathoracic suctioning, preventing a closed-space vacuum that can instantaneously result in expansion of the lung. For VATS sympathectomy and with smaller individuals, we routinely use 5-mm direct-viewing thoracolaparoscopes. In the case of thoracodorsal sympathectomy, we limit the intercostal access to two 5-mm sites. One is used for the scope–camera and the other is used for an endosurgical "duck bill" grasper and hook cautery suction device.

2. Trocar protection of the thoracoscope is another important instrument-related concern. For the most part, we choose reusable metal "ports" to protect the smudging of the optics during introduction into the chest.

Table 73.2. Basic instrumentation for VATS.

- "Three-chip" endoscopic video camera and high-definition television monitor
- Operating thoracoscope (with 5-mm biopsy channel)
- Three standard-length ringed forceps
- Suction-irrigation system 10 mm diameter
- Endoscopic hook cautery (5 mm) with trumpeted suction
- Standard electrocautery unit with extended tip for application through intercostal access site
- Landreneau "Masher" set
- Bulbed syringe (60 ml)
- Standard Metzenbaum scissors (10–12 in.)
- Standard University of Michigan Mixner clamp (10–12 in.)
- Standard-sized and pediatric Yankour metal suckers
- Standard 28-French chest tubes (straight and right angled) and closed drainage system

---

We will use a second port to protect the entry of the 10-mm endoscopic stapling device during the conduct of VATS wedge resection and lobectomy. Beyond these two trocars, we usually rely upon direct instrument entry through the sites of intercostal access. These trocar ports are not sealed and are open to the atmosphere. Two closed-system 5-mm disposable trocars are used during the VATS thoracodorsal sympathectomy, as this intervention is accomplished using a closed-chest preparation with low pressure (5–10 mm) carbon dioxide insufflation.

3. Appropriate hand instrumentation also is required for a successful VATS intervention.

    a. We will commonly use regular open surgical hand instrumentation during VATS. Long Metzenbaum scissors and long "University of Michigan" 60-degree Mizner forceps are helpful to begin VATS and to accomplish lysis of adhesions. We also find the "Stern" chest tube passing instrument with its alligator jaws and gently curved coaxial alignment to be useful in positioning chest tube and accomplishing pleural biopsy and pleurectomy. Standard-length straight and slightly curved gauze sponge holders, commonly limited to use for skin preparation prior to surgery, are also important standard hand instrumentation used during our VATS procedures for grasping and palpating the lung parenchyma. As with many other standard hand instruments, these tools cannot be passed into the chest through trocar access.

    b. The **Landreneau "mashers"** are a hybrid form of VATS and laparoscopic instrumentation incorporating the coaxial "feel" of standard hand instrumentation and the ability to traverse the intercostal space through small trocars access (Starr Medical, New York, and Pilling USA). These coaxial tools have also been designed for use in the laparoscopic surgical setting for the management of complex esophagogastric disorders. We have found these tools to be particularly useful during the conduct of VATS wedge resection and VATS. Once the location of the pulmonary lesion has been determined the "masher" clamp can be approximated beneath the proposed parenchymal margin of resection to permit estimation of the safety and adequacy of the site of the staple line. The lung parenchyma is grasped and effaced beneath the lesion with the "masher," and this is followed by introduction of the endoscopic stapling device along this line of proposed resection, estimated with the aid of the tissue compression by the "masher" forceps. These "masher" tools are also useful for the examination of the lung and for the performance of VATS lobectomy, as they give the surgeon the ergonomic "feel" of standard surgical tools and thus provide the proprioceptive feedback that the surgeon is familiar with.

c. In addition to the instrumentation mentioned, we recommend a good 10-mm suctioning and irrigation system (Davol, subsidiary of CR Bard, Murray Hill, NJ, USA) and a sturdy specimen retrieval bag (Pleatman Sac, ACMI Corporation, Southborough, MA, USA). We utilize a standard 60-mL bulbed syringe for distribution of sterile talc during the conduct of chemical pleurodesis.

E. Intercostal Access Strategies for Frequently Performed VATS Procedures

Although individual patient anatomic variation and peculiar location of intrathoracic lesions may require some thought to determine the most appropriate intercostal access, the following basic intercostal access strategies we what we generally recommend for frequently performed VATS procedures. Additional information for more complex procedures is given in the chapters that follow.

1. Idiopathic Loculated Extensive Pleural Effusion

Three sites of intercostal access are usually established in the anterior axillary, midaxillary, and posterior axillary lines. These are established approximately in the fifth, seventh, and eighth intercostal spaces, respectively. We usually start with the midaxillary seventh intercostal space access and work from there to obtain the remaining sites of access necessary to accomplish the procedure. Not infrequently, a fourth site of access is established in the midaxillary line at the third or fourth intercostal space to break down complex loculated processes or perform pulmonary decortication.

We have almost always been successful in managing such pleural problems when using this three- to four-intercostal-access approach. Pleural biopsy, evacuation of the effusion, pleurodesis, and decortication can usually be accomplished without problem. On rare occasion, conversion to thoracotomy is necessary to accomplish decortication. The three lower intercostal access sites will also be used for chest tube placement tube at the end of the VATS procedure.

2. Empyema and Contained Hemothorax

Empyema and contained hemothorax are pleural processes frequently associated with dense, broad pleural adhesions between the lung and the chest wall. In contradistinction to the management described earlier for more diffuse pleural fluid problems, it is critical to establish the initial intercostal access squarely in the middle of the fluid collection to prevent lung injury at the site of unsuspected adhesion. Once the principal cavity has been entered and its anatomic extent appreciated, other sites of intercostal access are established under direct thoracoscopic visibility. Dense adhesions are left undisturbed unless significant pulmonary restriction is present. Strategic chest tube placement is established under videoscopic guidance.

3. VATS Wedge Resection Biopsy of Indeterminate Interstitial Lung Disease

The use of VATS for the diagnosis of interstitial lung disease has for the most part made elective "open lung biopsy' an obsolete term. There is the potential for misuse of VATS when biopsy of diffuse interstitial infiltrates is needed for the ventilator-dependent patient in the intensive care unit. The primary advantage of VATS over limited anterolateral thoracotomy for lung wedge biopsy is in reducing perioperative morbidity for the "walking and talking" patient and in allowing for a panoramic assessment of the lung for directed biopsy in the setting of heterogeneous interstitial lung inflammation. When the patient is already on the ventilator and the pulmonary infiltrates are diffuse, the simplicity of a small inframammary thoracotomy approach with the avoidance of double-lumen intubation appears to be the most prudent course.

First, study the computed tomography scan closely to determine the principal target area of pathology. Evaluation of the volume of the ipsilateral pleural cavity is necessary because it is common for this volume to be reduced owing to the restrictive nature of the patient's disease. This reduced lung volume may alter the intercostal access site decisions for the patient. The initial site of intercostal access is usually in the midaxillary line at the seventh intercostal space. This location usually allows for the best panoramic image of the lung and pleural space. A second site of intercostal access is usually at the anterior axillary line near the inframammary crease. This is the usual site of introduction of the endoscopic mechanical stapling device used for pulmonary wedge resection. We are often able to accomplish wedge resection with these two intercostal sites only when an operating thoracoscope is used. The lung parenchyma can be grasped through the biopsy channel of the scope while the stapling device is applied from the other intercostal access site. More commonly, we will establish a third intercostal access site at the midaxillary line in the fourth intercostal space. This fourth intercostal space site usually establishes access near the confluence of the major and minor pulmonary fissures on the right and at the midpoint of the pulmonary fissure on the left. The ringed sponge forceps (minus the sponge) can be introduced through this intercostal access site to grasp the lung in the area of representatively diseased parenchyma for the proposed wedge resection.

At the completion of the VATS wedge resection, a single chest tube is positioned through the lower midaxillary line seventh interspace access site. The chest tube is connected to the standard underwater seal drainage system with intentions to remove the tube in the recovery room if there is no air leak, excessive drainage, or chest roentgenographic abnormality.

4. VATS for the Management of Spontaneous Pneumothorax

VATS has become the preferred approach for the surgical management of recurrent spontaneous pneumothorax. In our clinical practice we continue to utilize primary chest tube evacuation of first-time pneumothoraces. We are quick to move ahead with definitive VATS management if a persistent air leak or incomplete expansion of the lung is present in the setting of a properly positioned and functional chest tube. VATS management is routinely recommended for the recurrence of pneumothorax without intervening chest tube placement, if clinically safe and appropriate.

We routinely use three sites of intercostal access for this VATS intervention. An initial site of access is usually at the sixth or seventh intercostal space in the midaxillary line. A second site of access is at the third intercostal space in the midaxillary line at the axillary hairline. This is used for introduction of the ringed forceps to grasp and examine the apical segment of the lung and the superior segment of the lower lobe. After identification of the area of bullous disease, preparation for wedge resection of the lung to completely encompass the area of involvement is made. As is the case with lung wedge biopsy for interstitial lung disease, we prefer to utilize an anterolateral site of intercostal access at or near the level of the inframammary crease (usually at the fourth or fifth intercostal space). The interspace is usually wide here and the line of stapler application ideal for this wedge resection procedure. If no definitive area of bullous disease is discernible, we will perform a wedge of the apical segment the upper lobe and also perform an apical pleurectomy to reduce the known postoperative recurrence reported in this setting.

A single 28-French chest tube is introduced and secured through the lower axillary line access and positioned near the apex of the chest. Underwater seal drainage is employed for 2 to 3 days to enhance the likelihood of pleural symphysis.

F. Selected References

Chechani V, Landreneau RJ, Shaikh SS. Open lung biopsy for diffuse infiltrative lung disease. Ann Thorac Surg 1992;54:296–300.

d'Amato TA, Galloway M, Szydlowski G, Chen A, Landreneau RJ. Intraoperative brachytherapy following thoracoscopic wedge resection of stage I lung cancer. Chest 1998;114:1112–1115.

Ferson PF, Landreneau RJ. Thoracoscopic lung biopsy or open lung biopsy for interstitial lung disease. Chest Surg Clin North Am 1998;8:749–762.

Ferson PF, Landreneau RJ, Dowling RD, et al. Comparison of open versus thoracoscopic lung biopsy for diffuse infiltrative pulmonary disease. J Thorac Cardiovasc Surg 1993;106:194–199.

Kirby TJ, Mack MJ, Landreneau RJ, Rice TW. Lobectomy: video-assisted thoracic surgery versus muscle-sparing thoracotomy. A randomized trial. J Thorac Cardiovasc Surgery 1995;109:997–1001.

Landreneau RJ, Keenan RJ, Hazelrigg SR, Mack MJ, Naunheim KS. Thoracoscopy for empyema and hemothorax. Chest 1996;109:18–24.

Landreneau RJ, Mack MJ, Dowling RD, et al. The role of thoracoscopy in lung cancer management. Chest 1998;113:6S–12S.

Landreneau RJ, Mack MJ, Hazelrigg SR, et al. Video-assisted thoracic surgery: basic technical concepts and intercostal approach strategies. Ann Thorac Surg 1992;54:800–807.

Landreneau RJ, Mack MJ, Keenan RJ, Hazelrigg SR, Dowling RD, Ferson PF. Strategic planning for video-assisted thoracic surgery. Ann Thorac Surg 1993;56:615–619.

Landreneau RJ, Sugarbaker DJ, Mack MJ, et al. Wedge resection versus lobectomy for stage I (T1N0M0) non-small cell lung cancer. J Thorac Cardiovasc Surg 1997;113(4):691–700.

Landreneau RJ, Wiechmann RJ, Hazelrigg SR, Mack MJ, Keenan RJ, Ferson PF. Effect of minimally invasive thoracic surgical approaches on acute and chronic postoperative pain. Chest Surg Clin North Am 1998;8:891–906.

Mitruka S, Landreneau RJ, Mack MJ, et al. Diagnosing the indeterminate pulmonary nodule: percutaneous biopsy versus thoracoscopy. Surgery 1995;118:676–684.

Naunheim KS, Mack MJ, Hazelrigg SR, et al. Safety and efficacy of video-assisted thoracic surgical techniques for the treatment of spontaneous pneumothorax. J Thorac Cardiovasc Surg 1995;109:1198–1204.

Russo L, Wiechmann RJ, Magovern JA, et al. Early chest tube removal after video-assisted thoracoscopic wedge resection of the lung. Ann Thorac Surg 1998;66:1751–1754.

Santos R, Colonias A, Parda D, et al. Comparison between sublobar resection and [125]iodine brachytherapy after sublobar resection in high-risk patients with stage I non-small-cell lung cancer. Surgery 2003;134(4):691–697; discussion 697.

Yim APC, Landreneau RJ, Izzat MB, Fung ALK, Wan S. Is video-assisted thoracoscopic lobectomy a unified approach? Ann Thorac Surg 1998;66:1155–1158.

74. Exploratory Thoracoscopy for Staging of Malignancies

Alberto de Hoyos, M.D.
Peter F. Ferson, M.D.

A. Introduction

The role of video-assisted thoracic surgery (VATS) for pretreatment staging of intrathoracic malignances continues to evolve. As with other malignancies, precise staging allows more accurate prediction of survival, treatment planning, evaluation of results of therapy, exchange of information among cancer centers, and investigation of newer therapies.

Preoperative staging of lung cancer can be achieved by the use of imaging modalities such as computed tomography (CT) and positron-emission tomography (PET). These techniques however, do not provide histologic confirmation of tumor involvement and may underestimate or overestimate the true extent of tumor extension. Surgical staging for lung cancer was pioneered by Carlens and Pearson, who established mediastinoscopy as an important diagnostic tool for the preoperative assessment of lung cancer patients.

Lymph node metastases have been shown to be an important predictor of survival in lung and esophageal cancer patients, and their detection may allow prospective selection of patients who might benefit from neoadjuvant or preoperative chemotherapy or radiotherapy. Because treatment strategies and prognoses vary depending on the stage at the time of presentation, the need for more complete and accurate pathologic staging has become more clearly defined.

Accurate staging of thoracic malignancies typically begins with noninvasive techniques; however, definitive diagnosis and final staging still depend on pathologic specimens. Although noninvasive techniques (including percutaneous and endobronchial procedures) have been used and continue to improve, many patients still have suboptimal clinical staging compared with final pathologic staging, resulting often in poor results of surgical therapy. Until recently, the final determination of the true pathologic stage was made by direct surgical exploration at the time of the intended resection. With the introduction and refinements in minimally invasive techniques, most thoracic malignancies can now be accurately diagnosed and staged with minimal morbidity before definitive therapy. This chapter summarizes the recent experience with thoracoscopy in the staging of intrathoracic malignancies, with emphasis on lung and esophageal cancer.

B. Lung Cancer

From the perspective of the thoracic surgeon, the primary issue in the care of patients with non–small cell lung cancer (NSCLC) is a determination of the stage of their disease. Stage determines the treatment patients will receive and their prognoses.

Lung cancer staging often requires both noninvasive and invasive procedures to assess the extent of tumor involvement. Accurate preoperative staging is mandatory for a proper selection of patients to be included in a neoadjuvant treatment protocol. This allows proper clinical stratification to standardize inclusion criteria, which leads to valid and reproducible posttreatment results. Unnecessary thoracotomies are avoided by identifying unresectable disease.

The current staging system for NSCLC in large part centers on the size of the primary tumor (T) and on presence or absence of metastatic involvement of hilar and mediastinal lymph nodes (N).

1. **Cervical mediastinoscopy** remains the primary diagnostic approach for the evaluation of paratracheal and high subcarinal lymphadenopathy associated with a presumed or known lung cancer. Adenopathy located in the aorticopulmonary window, anterior mediastinum, or low subcarinal plane, however, is difficult or impossible to access through standard cervical mediastinoscopy, although accessible through an extended cervical mediastinoscopy.

2. The role of **VATS** is still limited but provides specific information often not obtainable by other diagnostic modalities. Currently, most centers do not perform routine VATS staging in patients with NSCLC and is reserved for patients with cytologically negative pleural effusion or patients with inferior mediastinal lymphadenopathy. VATS is particularly useful to do the following:

   a. Evaluate suspected contralateral lung metastases

   b. Exclude pleural effusion in otherwise operable patients

   c. Stage lymph node stations not easily accessible by mediastinoscopy; these include the subaortic (aortopulmonary window), nodes (level 5), paraortic (ascending aorta or phrenic) nodes (level 6), posterior subcarinal (level 7) nodes, paraesophageal (level 8) nodes, and pulmonary ligament nodes (level 9)

   d. Provide a panoramic exploration of the entire surface of the lung and pleura

   e. Employ as a first step on patients with undiagnosed peripheral lung nodules associated with lymphadenopathy

C. Esophageal Cancer

Most patients with esophageal cancer have a dismal prognosis, as most lesions are found to be full thickness (T3, T4) or to involve lymph nodes (N1) at the time of diagnosis. In the United States, approximately 20 to 30% of patients who have carcinoma of the esophagus have distant metastatic disease at the time of presentation. The most common visceral metastatic sites include, in decreasing order of prevalence, liver, lung, bone, and adrenal glands. Recently there has been renewed interest in preoperative or neoadjuvant therapy to decrease tumor volume, increase respectability, and improve survival.

Imaging modalities such as CT and endoscopic ultrasound (EUS) often fail to determine clearly whether an esophageal cancer is locally invading surrounding structures. As with lung cancer, size criteria alone are inaccurate in evaluating lymph node metastases in patients with esophageal cancer. Endoscopic ultrasound has been increasingly useful in detecting invasion of local structures but technical limitations prevent it from assessing accurately the invasion of the membranous wall of the trachea. Although EUS-guided fine-needle aspiration of suspicious lymph nodes has been performed with increasing success, the number of specimens that can be obtained usually is limited. Lymph nodes may be beyond the reach of the endoscopic needle. In addition, because of the possibility of specimen contamination by passage of the needle through the primary tumor, peritumoral nodes cannot be sampled accurately by EUS.

Recent additions to the armamentarium available to stage esophageal cancer include VATS and laparoscopy. VATS staging of esophageal cancer is especially useful in distinguishing between T3 and T4 tumors and in assessing mediastinal lymph node metastases. However, patients with esophageal carcinoma also have a high incidence of perigastric and celiac lymph node metastases. These nodes can be sampled accurately by laparoscopy. Thoracoscopic and laparoscopic techniques have been proposed as tools for staging esophageal cancer in patients with negative EUS or in patients who cannot undergo EUS (i.e., those with esophageal obstruction and those who have suspicious nodes on imaging modality such as CT scanning). Pretreatment lymph node biopsy samples obtained by these means allow further molecular biologic analysis to detect occult metastasis for more accurate lymph node staging. Recent studies have shown that pretreatment surgical lymph node staging can predict response and survival of patients with esophageal cancer receiving trimodality therapy (radiation, chemotherapy, and surgery).

D. Technique of VATS Staging

Generally, VATS staging for lung cancer is done on the side of involvement. Sampling of regional lymph nodes and inspection of pleural surfaces and superficial parenchyma can be performed on either side. Right thoracoscopy allows sampling of peritracheal, periesophageal, subcarinal, and inferior pulmonary ligament nodes. When aortic invasion or aortopulmonary window lymph node involvement must be ruled out, a left thoracoscopy is performed.

1. The patient is intubated with a single-lumen endotracheal tube.
2. First, perform a standard bronchoscopic examination of the main airways and lobar and segmental orifices.
3. Exchange the tube for a double-lumen endotracheal tube to achieve selective left lung ventilation. Confirm accurate positioning of the tube by bronchoscopic examination.

4. With the patient in full left lateral decubitus position, place the first trocar (11 mm) at the level of the eighth or ninth intercostal space anterior to midaxillary line. It is important to place this port anterior and low in the chest cavity to facilitate full exploration of the hemithorax.

5. Insert the thoracoscope and place two to three additional working ports (5 mm). Although position must be individualized, we prefer to place one port just inferior to the tip of the scapula and the other one at the fourth intercostal space anterior axillary line.

6. Inspect all pleural surfaces for any evidence of tumor implant or effusion. If effusion is present, aspirate and collect it for cytopathologic analysis.

7. Retract the lung anteriorly through the anterior port, incise the mediastinal pleura overlying the trachea or esophagus and continue the incision inferiorly to the level of the carina or inferior pulmonary vein. This incision can be carried down to the level of the inferior pulmonary ligament to include dissection of lymph nodes in this area.

8. Dissect meticulously with a grasper and harmonic scalpel to sample individual lymph nodes at each lymph node station. Take special care when working in the plane behind the right main stem bronchi and carina to avoid injury to the airway.

9. On the right, thorough sampling of the lower paratracheal lymph nodes on the right may be facilitated by dividing the azygos arch with a vascular endoscopic stapler. To allow sampling of the inferior pulmonary ligament node, divide the ligament with electrocautery or harmonic scalpel with the patient in steep Trendelenburg position.

10. Before partially mobilized lymph nodes are excised completely, use an endoscopic clip applier to secure the vascular pedicle. Meticulous hemostasis is important to avoid troublesome bleeding from the bronchial arteries and aortoesophageal branches.

11. Retrieve individual lymph nodes from the chest utilizing the cut finger of a surgical glove and label these appropriately. If necessary, mobilize the primary tumor to assess local invasion into surrounding structures.

12. At the end of the procedure, infiltrate the intercostal nerves with bupivacaine 0.25% and a place single chest tube posteriorly and superiorly toward the apex of the chest cavity. Gently allow the lung to reexpand and close the incisions in two layers.

13. The patient is then extubated in the operating room and a chest-x-ray obtained in the recovery room.

E. Technique of Laparoscopic Staging for Esophageal Cancer (see also Chapter 13)

1. Position, prepare, and anesthetize the patient as for exploratory laparoscopy. We prefer the Hasson cannula to the closed insertion of a Veress needle. Carefully evaluate patients who have had abdominal

procedures for alternative sites of placement of the initial port for establishing pneumoperitoneum. The Hasson trocar (11 mm) is typically placed midway between the xyphoid process and the umbilicus, 2 to 3 cm to the right of the midline.

2. Establish pneumoperitoneum and insert the laparoscope. The use of a high-resolution 10-mm, oblique-viewing laparoscope maximizes lighting and increases visual field and access to most areas of the peritoneal cavity.

3. Perform a thorough exploration of the abdomen, with special attention to the following.

   a. Carefully survey the hepatic, diaphragmatic, peritoneal, and omental surfaces for any evidence of tumor implants. These will appear as dense nodules, clearly distinguishable from the liver parenchyma and the shiny translucent appearance of the peritoneum or fatty surface of the omentum. Small occult metastases at these locations are not uncommon for esophageal cancer. These implants should be sampled if encountered, placing additional trocars for graspers and biopsy forceps.

   b. Place a 5-mm trocar in a mirror-image location with the first trocar. Then place bilateral subcostal 5-mm trocars at the anterior axillary line.

   c. If desired, place a liver retractor through a trocar inserted under laparoscopic guidance just below the edge of the liver to elevate the left lobe and expose the diaphragmatic hiatus.

   d. Aspirate any ascitic fluid and send it for cytologic examination.

   e. A laparoscopic ultrasound probe can also be utilized through a 10-mm port to examine the superior aspect of the liver for occult metastases. While certain ultrasonic features may be suggestive of malignancy, no ultrasonic image can confirm malignant versus benign hepatic parenchymal disease. In these situations, ultrasound-guided percutaneous biopsy is required.

   f. After adequate examination of the peritoneal cavity and the liver parenchyma, attention is turned to evaluating the perigastric and celiac lymph nodes.

   g. Divide the lesser omentum with the ultrasonic shears and retract the lesser curvature of the stomach laterally to the patient's left. The lymph nodes are then readily visualized and subjected to biopsy, utilizing the harmonic scalpel to achieve hemostasis.

   h. Additional lymph nodes may be encountered along the angle of His and splenic hilum and can be sampled if desired.

   i. Place each lymph node in a cut finger of a glove for retrieval from the abdominal cavity through the 11-mm port. Take care to avoid injury to the stomach and vascular structures.

   j. After achieving hemostasis, withdraw the retractor and instruments and close the port sites in the usual fashion.

F. Selected References

Brega Massone PP, Conti B, Magnani B, Lequaglie C, Cataldo I. Video-assisted thoracoscopic surgery for diagnosis, staging and management of lung cancer with suspected mediastinal lymphadenopathy. Surg Laparosc Endosc Percutan Techniques 2002;12:104–108.

Buenaventura P, Luketich JD. Surgical staging of esophageal cancer. Chest Surg Clin North Am 2000;10:487–497.

CALBG 9380. A prospective trial of the feasibility of thoracoscopy/laparoscopy in staging esophageal cancer. Ann Thorac Surg 2001;71;1073–1079.

Detterbeck FC, DeCamp MM Jr, Kohman LJ, Silvestri GA. American College of Chest Physicians. Lung cancer. Invasive staging: the guidelines. Chest 2003;123: 167S–175S.

Jiao X, Krasna MJ, Sonett J, et al. Pretreatment surgical lymph node staging predicts results of trimodality therapy in esophageal cancer. Eur J Cardiothorac Surg 2001;19: 880–886.

Jiao X, Sonett J, Gamliel Z, et al. Trimodality treatment versus surgery alone for esophageal cancer. A stratified analysis with minimally invasive pretreatment staging. J Cardiovasc Surg (Torino) 2002;43:531–537.

Krasna MJ. Minimally invasive staging for esophageal cancer. Chest 1991;112: 191S–194S.

Krasna MJ, Jiao X. Thoracoscopic and laparoscopic staginf for esophageal cancer. Semin Thorac Cardiovasc Surg 2000;12:186–194.

Krasna MJ, Jiao X, Mao YS, et al. Thoracoscopy/laparoscopy in the staging of esophageal cancer: Maryland experience. Surg Laparosc Endosc Percutan Techniques 2002;12:213–218.

Krasna MJ, Jiao X, Sonett JR, et al. Thoracoscopic and laparoscopic lymph node staging in esophageal cancer: do clinopathological factors affect the outcome? Ann Thorac Surg 2002;73:1710–1713.

Landreneau RJ, Hazelrigg SR, Mack MJ, et al. Thoracoscopic mediastinal lymph node sampling: useful for mediastinal lymph node stations inaccessible by cervical mediastinoscopy. J Thorac Cardiovasc Surg 1993;106:554–558.

Luketich JD, Schauer P, Landreneau R, et al. Minimally invasive surgical staging is superior to endoscopic ultrasound in detecting lymph node metastases in esophageal cancer. J Thorac Cardiovasc Surg 1997;114:817–823.

Passlick B. Initial surgical staging of lung cancer. Lung Cancer 2003;42:S21–S25.

Roberts JR, Blum MG, Arildsen R, et al. Prospective comparison of radiologic, thoracoscopic, and pathologic staging in patients with early non–small cell lung cancer. Ann Thorac Surg 1999;68:1154–1158.

Sebastian-Quetglas F, Molins L, Baldo X, Buitrago J, Vidal G. Spanish Video-Assisted Thoracic Surgery Study Group. Clinical value of video-assisted thoracoscopy for preoperative staging of non–small cell lung cancer. A prospective study of 105 patients. Lung Cancer 2003;42:297–301.

75. Minimally Invasive Esophagectomy

D. Mario del Pino, M.D.
Alberto de Hoyos, M.D.
James D. Luketich, M.D.

A. Indications

Esophagectomy has traditionally been performed by open methods. Recently, a review of mortality following esophagectomy in the United States showed that mortality rates ranged from 8% to as high as 22% depending on institutional experience and surgeon volume. Results from experienced centers specializing in esophageal surgery demonstrate better outcomes but still include significant morbidity, mortality rates in excess of 5%, and hospital stays frequently greater than 10 days. In an effort to lower morbidity, our group at the University of Pittsburgh Medical Center has developed a minimally invasive approach to esophageal resection.

Our early experience with minimally invasive esophagectomy (MIE) was limited to patients with Barrett's high-grade dysplasia or small tumors. This has evolved and now includes most patients with resectable esophageal cancer after evaluation with positron-emission tomography (PET), endoscopic ultrasound (EUS), and computed tomography (CT) including those with limited nodal involvement. Neoadjuvant chemoradiation is not a contraindication for a minimally invasive approach. If the EGD, EUS, or CT scan findings suggest gastric extension, T4 local extension, or possible metastases, we perform a staging laparoscopy or a thoracoscopy or both. We perform an on-table esophagogastroduodenoscopy (EGD) to make a final assessment of the tumor's location and the gastric conduit's suitability for reconstruction. If there is histologic evidence of node-positive disease and the patient is a candidate for chemotherapy, we encourage participation in a neoadjuvant trial. In our recent report of 222 patients undergoing MIE in a single institution, we reported a shorter hospital stay, lower mortality rate, and more rapid recovery to full activity compared with the results of most open series. A prospective, multicenter trial is now under way to more rigorously assess the results of MIE in our own institution and others with significant minimally invasive surgical expertise (Eastern Cooperative Group Trial E2202). In addition to esophageal carcinoma, we have successfully performed MIE for other esophageal disorders including end-stage achalasia, lymphoma, perforation, and tracheoesophageal fistula.

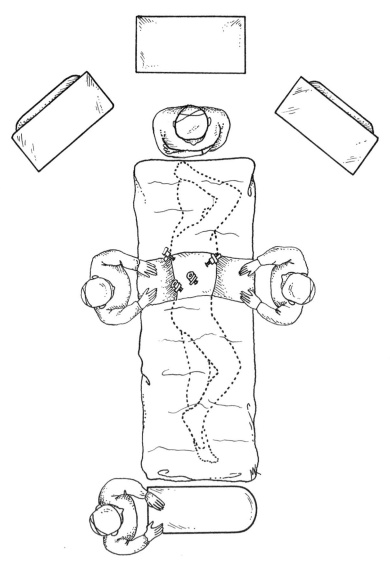

Figure 75.1. Room setup for thoracoscopic esophageal mobilization.

B. Room Setup, Initial Patient Position, and Port Placement for Thoracic Phase of Operation

1. The operating room setup is illustrated in Fig. 75.1.
2. The surgeon stands on the right and the assistant on the left.
3. After completion of the esophagogastroduodenoscopy, the patient is intubated with a double-lumen tube for single-lung ventilation. An arterial line and a urinary catheter are inserted.
4. The thoracic phase of the operation is performed first.
5. The right lung is deflated as soon as the patient is placed in a left lateral decubitus position.
6. Optimal port placement is crucial to facilitate the technical aspects of the esophageal dissection and mobilization. Four thoracoscopic ports are used, placed as shown in Fig. 75.2.

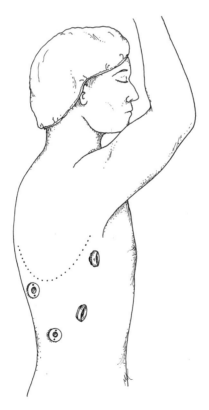

Figure 75.2. Port placement for thoracoscopic esophageal mobilization.

7. Place a 10-mm port at the eighth or ninth intercostal space, anterior to the mid axillary line, and pass the thoracoscope.
8. Place a 5-mm port at the eighth or ninth intercostal space, posterior to the posterior axillary line, for the ultrasonic coagulating shears (U.S. Surgical, Norwalk, CT).
9. Place a third port (5 or 10 mm) anterior to the axillary line at the fourth intercostal space. This port is used for the assistant to provide retraction of the lung anteriorly and assist the surgeon.
10. Place the fourth port (5 mm) just posterior to the tip of the scapula, for use by the operating surgeon to place instruments for traction and countertraction.
11. If the diaphragm is elevated, interfering with esophageal exposure, a single retracting suture (0-Endostitch, U.S. Surgical, Norwalk, CT) is placed at the central tendon of the diaphragm and brought out through the lower costal margin through a 1-mm skin incision. This will provide downward traction on the diaphragm, allowing good exposure of the distal esophagus.

B. Thoracoscopic Esophageal Mobilization

1. Gently retract the lung anteriorly with the fan retractor to expose the inferior pulmonary ligament.
2. Begin the esophageal dissection by dividing the pulmonary ligament up to the inferior pulmonary vein using the ultrasonic shears coagulator.
3. Divide the mediastinal pleura overlying the esophagus to the level of the azygos vein, preserving the pleura intact above the vein, to the level of the thoracic inlet, as shown in Figure 75.3. This may help seal the plane around the gastric tube at the thoracic inlet, preventing potential extension of a cervical leak into the mediastinum.
4. Circumferentially dissect the azygos vein. Divide it with a vascular stapler (Endo-GIA II; U.S. Surgical, Norwalk, CT).
5. Next, circumferentially mobilize the esophagus with lymph node dissection from the diaphragm up to 1 to 2 cm above the carina for lower one-third tumors, taking care to include all surrounding lymph nodes including the subcarinal lymph node packet, periesophageal fat, and areolar tissue along the pericardium, aorta, and contralateral mediastinal pleura. Also take care to avoid injury to the thoracic duct, and apply endosurgical clips liberally to aortoesophageal vessels and branches of the thoracic duct prior to division.
6. Place a Penrose drain around the esophagus to facilitate traction and exposure. As the esophageal mobilization proceeds toward the thoracic inlet, keep the dissection plane near the esophagus to avoid trauma to the membranous trachea and recurrent laryngeal nerves.
7. Near the diaphragm, take care to avoid violating the peritoneum, which would result in difficulty in maintaining adequate pneumoperitoneum during the abdominal portion of the procedure. Prior to moving to the

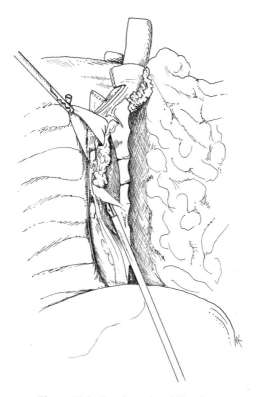

Figure 75.3. Esophageal mobilization.

laparoscopic port, the entire thoracic esophagus and surrounding lymph nodes should be mobilized.

8. Insert a single 28-French-chest tube through the lower, anterior thoracoport and infiltrate the intercostal nerves with 1 to 2 mL of 0.5% bupivacaine with epinephrine at each interspace. Gently inflate the right lung and check the membranous airway for potential air leaks.

9. Withdraw the ports and scope and close the incisions.

C. Gastric Mobilization and Tubularization

1. Turn the patient to the supine position with the neck slightly turned to the right, with the patient prepped and draped from chin to pubic symphisis and laterally down to the posterior axillary lines. The room setup is shown in Figure 75.4.

2. With the surgeon standing on the right and the assistant on the left, insert five abdominal ports utilizing a similar approach as for laparo-

scopic fundoplication (Fig. 75.5). In general, these ports are placed slightly lower toward the umbilicus compared with our antireflux surgery ports.

3. Insufflate the abdomen and maintain an intra-abdominal pressure of 15 mm Hg. We have on many occasions operated with pressures in the

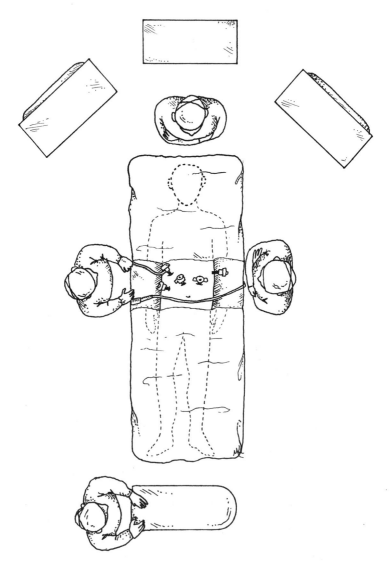

Figure 75.4. Room setup for gastric mobilization and tubularization.

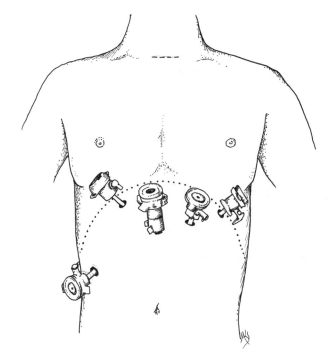

Figure 75.5. Port placement for gastric mobilization and tubularization.

6 to 8 mm Hg range with good visualization if the blood pressure is labile with higher insufflating pressures.

4. Insert the camera and explore the abdomen for evidence of metastatic disease.

5. Place the patient in steep reverse Trendelenburg position.

6. Retract the left lobe of the liver upward to expose the esophageal hiatus, using a Diamond flex retractor (Genzyme, Tucker, GA) held in place with a self-retaining system (Mediflex, Velmed, Wexford, PA).

7. Divide the gastrohepatic ligament with the endoshears above the hepatic branch of the vagus nerve.

8. Dissect the right crus of the diaphragm, taking care to preserve the phrenoesophageal membrane to avoid entry into the mediastinum and loss of pneumoperitoneum, which would lead to pneumothorax and technical difficulties.

9. Begin gastric mobilization by dividing the gastrocolic omentum 2 cm away from the stomach, to avoid injury to the right gastroepiploic arcade. Extreme care must be taken to avoid trauma to the gastric tube.

10. Divide the short gastric vessels using the ultrasonic coagulating shears taking care to avoid injury to the spleen. Clip and divide larger branches.

11. Next, retract the stomach superiorly and divide the left gastric artery and vein using the Endo-GIA stapler with a vascular load.

12. Dissect the left crus of the diaphragm to complete the hiatal mobilization.

13. Mobilize the first portion of the duodenum. Performing a full Kochermaneuver of the duodenum is usually not necessary.

14. Next, perform a pyloroplasty (Fig. 75.6), using the ultrasonic shears to open the pylorus for a distance of approximately 2 cm. The pylorus is then closed transversely using the Endo-stitch loaded with 2-0 sutures (U.S. Surgical, Norwalk, CT) (Fig. 75.7).

15. Construct the gastric tube constructed by dividing the stomach with the 4.8 mm stapler (Endo-GIA II, U.S. Surgical, Norwalk, CT) (Fig. 75.8). Position the stapler along the lesser curve, preserving the right gastric artery, and direct it toward the fundus (Fig. 75.9). The characteristics of the tumor will determine, to a point, the configuration of the gastric tube. If gastric tumor extension is significant, we prefer to resect more proximal stomach and may need to perform an intrathoracic anastomosis depending on the length of the gastric tube. In our experience, excessively narrow gastric tubes (<3–4 cm) had a higher incidence of gastric tip necrosis and anastomotic leaks with extension into the chest. It is our current practice to keep the gastric tube wider (5–6 cm).

16. Minimize manipulation and trauma to the tubularized stomach during its mobilization.

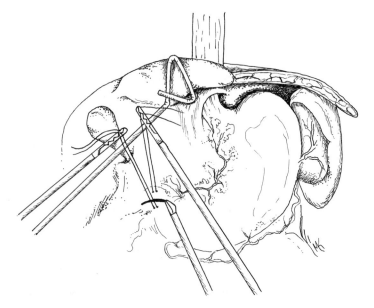

Figure 75.6. Pyloroplasty: opening of the pylorus.

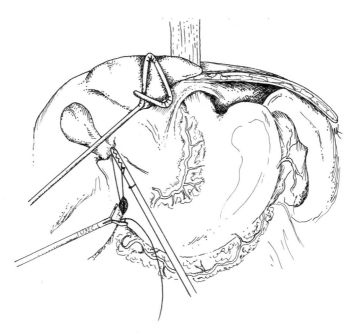

Figure 75.7. Pyloroplasty: closure of pylorus.

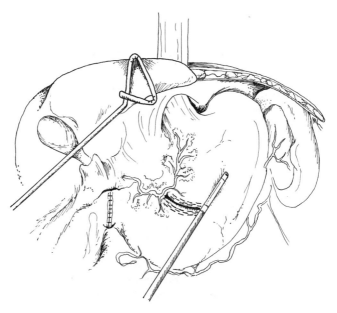

Figure 75.8. Construction of the gastric conduit.

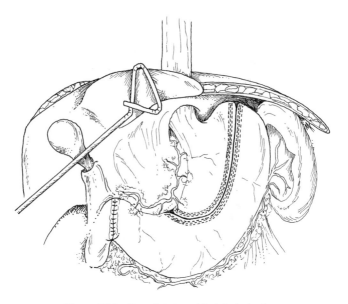

Figure 75.9. Completed gastric tubularization.

17. Next, attach the most cephalad portion of the gastric tube to the divided esophageal and gastric specimen using two figure-of-eight Endo-sutures (Fig. 75.10).
18. An additional superficial stitch may be placed on the anterior gastric tube to facilitate orientation and to prevent twisting as the tube is guided into the mediastinum to the neck.
19. A feeding jejunostomy is then placed by first attaching a limb of proximal jejunum (25 cm distal to the ligament of Treitz) to the anterior abdominal wall in the left midquadrant using the Endo-stitch. In most cases this is facilitated, by placing an additional 10-mm port in the right lower quadrant of the abdomen.
20. A needle catheter kit (Compact Biosystems, Minneapolis, MN) is placed percutaneously into the peritoneal cavity. Under direct laparoscopic vision, the needle is placed into the loop of jejunum and the guidewire advanced gently. The needle is withdrawn and the catheter advanced over the wire. The loop of jejunum adjacent to the entry site of the catheter is secured to the anterior abdominal wall with Endo-stitches for a distance of several centimeters to avoid twisting (see also Chapter 29).
21. With the stomach fully mobilized and prepared for delivery into the mediastinum, divide the phrenoesophageal membrane and partially incise the right and left crura to avoid gastric tube outlet obstruction. Take care to maintain orientation of the greater curvature towards the left crus (Fig. 75.11).

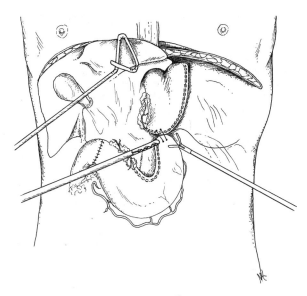

Figure 75.10. Attaching the esophageal and gastric tube prior to mobilization.

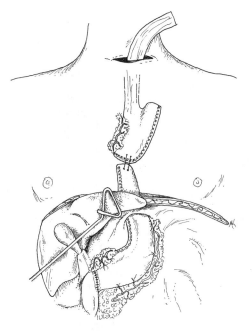

Figure 75.11. Mobilization of the gastric tube.

D. Cervical Esophagogastric Anastomosis

1. Make 4- to 6-cm horizontal incision just above the suprasternal notch.
2. Continue careful dissection along the anterior border of the sternocleidomastoid muscle. Identify the tracheoesophageal groove and encircle the esophagus with a Penrose drain.
3. To avoid injury to the left laryngeal recurrent nerve, no retractors are placed.
4. The degree of neck dissection is minimal owing to the high intrathoracic dissection performed well into the thoracic inlet during the thoracoscopic portion of the case. Generally, this plane is very easily entered, and we then pull up the Penrose drain that was left around the esophagus and pushed up into the inlet during the last video-assisted thorncic surgery step. This facilitates delivery of the mobilized esophagus into the neck.
5. Divide the cervical esophagus after applying the autopurse-string device and pull the esophagogastric specimen out of the neck incision. The autopursestring device is used only if we are planning to perform the anastomosis with the end-to-end device. There are many options for neck anastomosis, but end-to-end anastomosis (EEA) has proved to be a good option in our experience. We do believe the esophagus should be divided quite high, just below the cricopharyngeus. This high division minimizes any residual Barrett's mucosa and also tends to leave the anatomosis lying very high and near the cervical neck incision. Other anastomotic techniques may leave additional length to the cervical esophagus, and if excessive length is left at this point, the anastomosis tends to lie well into the thoracic inlet. Owing to the thoracoscopic mobilization of most of the mediastinal pleura, leaks in this location tend to drain into the chest.
6. As traction is applied to the specimen in the neck, the assistant guides the gastric tube in proper orientation into the mediastinum and into the neck. Separate the specimen from the gastric tube and remove it from the field. Inspect the gastric tube for ischemia or vascular congestion.
7. The anastomosis is then constructed. In most cases, as stated above, we use the EEA, 25 mm diameter. Place the anvil into the proximal esophagus (1–2 cm below the cricopharyngeus) and secure the pursestring. Next, deliver the gastric tube well into the neck to achieve at least 5 to 6 cm of length. If this length is not achievable, it may be technically difficult to perform the EEA anastomosis in this fashion. Open the gastric tube near the tip of the fundus and insert the EEA stapler. We then direct the EEA point out through the posterolateral wall of the gastric tube and dock it with the EEA anvil placed previously in the proximal esophagus. Careful alignment is made and the device is fired. Examine the rings for completeness, and oversew any areas of concern.
8. Next a nasogastric tube is passed from above and guided into the gastric tube to a point near the lower chest. Resect the open tip of the fundus with the Endo-GIA II stapler and copiously irrigate the area with warm antibiotic solution. Next, reinsufflate the abdomen and

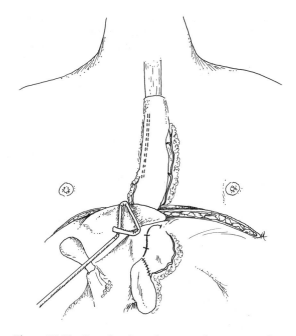

Figure 75.12. Completed esophago gastric reconstruction.

apply gentle downward traction on the pyloroantral area to reduce any redundant gastric tube to the abdomen. Perform this pull only until the assistant at the neck observes the tube beginning to be pulled down at the level of the anastomosis. Taking care to preserve the right orientation of the gastric tube at the diaphragmatic hiatus, place three tacking sutures to prevent subsequent thoracic herniation.

a.   Place one stitch between the left crus and the stomach just anterior to the greater curve arcade.

b.   The second stitch is placed on the right side of the gastric tube between the area just above the right gastric vessels and the right crus.

c.   The third stitch is placed anteriorly between the stomach and the diaphragm.

9.   Inspect the incisions for hemostasis and close them.

10. The completed reconstruction is shown in Figure 75.12.

E. Early Complications

1.   Cervical anastomotic leak
     a.   **Cause and prevention.** Ischemia and necrosis of the proximal part of the gastric tube will cause breakdown and leakage of the

cervical anastomosis. Careful manipulation and atraumatic grasping of the stomach are of utmost importance to prevent this complication. Prior to performing the esophagogastric anastomosis, the gastric tube should be thoroughly inspected, and ischemic or necrotic tissue must be resected. In our recent experience, excessive narrowing of the gastric tube to less than 4 cm resulted in an increase in anastomotic leaks.

b. **Recognition and management.** Presence of erythema and drainage at the neck wound suggests a cervical leak. Intrathoracic extension must be ruled out. Generally, we perform a barium esophagogram to assess the path of the leak and the requirement for drainage. Open drainage of the neck wound is indicated, and if extension of the leak into the right chest occurs, additional drainage procedures may be required.

2. Gastric tube necrosis

a. **Cause and prevention.** Inadequate vascularization of the stomach secondary to venous congestion or poor arterial blood supply can cause necrosis of the gastric tube. Technical considerations to prevent this complication include preservation of the right gastric vessels and preservation of the right gastroepiploic arcade during dissection of the gastrocolic ligament. Twisting of the gastric tube as the conduit is brought up to the neck must be avoided by direct laparoscopic inspection. In the postoperative period, hemodynamic stability must be maintained to achieve adequate gastric perfusion. Nasogastric decompression prevents distention of the stomach and venous congestion. Construction of a narrow conduit may impair vascularization of the stomach.

b. **Recognition and management.** A protracted course with hemodynamic instability should raise suspicion for gastric tube necrosis. If major necrosis is confirmed, takedown of the anastomosis may be required, with return of the gastric tube to the abdomen and construction of a cervical esophagostomy.

3. Mediastinal abscess

a. **Cause and prevention.** Downward extension of a cervical anastomotic leak or a missed gastric perforation can cause a mediastinal abscess. Careful gastric mobilization and intraoperative recognition and repair of a perforation will avoid this problem. Prevention of a cervical leak is as described earlier. In addition, construction of a wider gastric tube (providing more bulk at the thoracic inlet), preservation of the mediastinal pleura above the azygos vein, and a very high anastomosis just below the level of the cricopharyngeus muscle may prevent mediastinal contamination if a cervical anastomotic leak does occur.

b. **Recognition and management.** Fever, leukocytosis, and the presence of a cervical leak suggest the possibility of a mediastinal abscess. Confirmation by CT mandates drainage by right thoracoscopy or thoracotomy.

4. Recurrent laryngeal nerve injury

a. **Cause and prevention.** Inadvertent injury or excessive traction of the recurrent laryngeal nerve can be avoided by gentle blunt and sharp dissection of the cervical esophagus. Retractors should not be used. Care is taken to stay near the esophagus during its mobilization, as the dissection proceeds toward the thoracic inlet.

b. **Recognition and management.** Hoarseness, dysphagia, or aspiration suggests injury to the recurrent nerve. Laryngoscopy confirms the diagnosis. Treatment options include observation and vocal cord injection with polytetrafluoroethylene (Teflon).

5. Chylothorax

a. **Cause and prevention.** Dissection of the posterior esophagus in the area of the thoracic duct, which can lead to a thoracic duct leak, can be prevented by the liberal use of endosurgical clips.

b. **Recognition and management.** Persistent and unexpected large chest tube drainage should raise suspicion. Initially, treatment is conservative by closed drainage and diet. If this is unsuccessful, surgical intervention is indicated.

6. Right main stem bronchi injury

a. **Cause and prevention.** While dissecting at the level of the subcarinal nodes, care is taken to stay near the esophagus and continous attention must be paid to avoid injuring the main stem bronchi.

b. **Recognition and management.** Injury to the airway can be identified by direct visualization at the time of surgery or postoperatively by the presence of an air leak. Conservative management or operative repair is indicated.

7. Bleeding

a. **Cause and prevention.** To date we have not had bleeding complications. The ultrasonic coagulating shears save time and avoid the tedium of clipping and dividing, or tying. The left gastric vessels are safely and rapidly divided using the endoscopic stapling device with a vascular load. No clips are placed on the gastric side of the short gastric vessels to avoid potential displacement during the gastric pull-through. Care is taken to clip any aortoesophageal vessels posteriorly during mobilization of the esophagus.

b. **Recognition and management.** Clinical evidence of bleeding requires identification of the source of bleeding. Conservative or surgical management is indicated.

F. Late Complications

1. Delayed gastric emptying

a. **Cause and prevention.** In our early experience, two patients who had an initial pyloromyotomy developed persistent delayed gastric emptying (DGE) requiring pyloroplasty with good results. Therefore, pyloroplasty is now part of our standard MIE. DGE has also been caused by obstruction of the gastric tube at the level of the crura. Therefore, we partially divide the right and left crura routinely. We place tacking sutures between the gastric tube and the diaphragm to prevent hiatal herniation.

    b.   **Recognition and management.** Contrast studies confirm the diagnosis and level of obstruction. Pyloric dilatation or reoperation will be necessary to relieve the obstruction.

2.   Anastomotic stricture

    a.   **Cause and prevention.** Avoidance of cervical anastomotic leaks.

    b.   **Recognition and management.** Presence of progressive dysphagia confirmed with barium swallow. Strictures resolve with endoscopic balloon dilation.

G. Selected References

Birkmeyer JD, Stukel TA, Siewers AE, et al. Surgeon volume and operative mortality in the United States. N Engl J Med 2003;349:2117–2127.

Fernando HC, Luketich JD, Buenaventura PO, et al. Outcomes of minimally invasive esophagectomy (MIE) for high-grade dysplasia of the esophagus. Eur J Cardiothorac Surg 2002;22:1–6.

Litle VR, Luketich JD. Minimally invasive esophagectomy. In: Ferguson MK, ed. CTSNet Experts' Techniques 2002. http://www.ctsnet.org/doc/6762#PATIENT

Luketich JD, Alvelo-Rivera M, Buenaventura PO, et al. Minimally invasive esophagectomy (MIE): outcomes in 222 cases. Ann Surg 2003;238(4):486–494.

Luketich JD, Friedman DM, Weigel TL, et al. Evaluation of distant metastases in esophageal cancer: 100 consecutive positron emission tomography scans. Ann Thorac Surg 1999;68:1133–1137.

Luketich JD, Schauer P, Landrenau R, et al. Minimally invasive surgical staging is superior to endoscopic ultrasound in detecting lymph node metastases in esophageal cancer. J Thorac Cardiovasc Surg 1997;114:817–823.

Luketich JD, Schauer PR, Christie NA, et al. Minimally invasive esophagectomy. Ann Thorac Surg 2000;70:906–912.

Nguyen N, Follette DM, Wolfe BM, et al. Comparison of minimally invasive esophagectomy with transthoracic and transhiatal esophagectomy. Arch Surg 2000;135:920–925.

Perry Y, Petrick A, Luketich JD. Minimally invasive esophagectomy. In: Putnam JB, Franco KL, eds. Advanced Therapy in Thoracic Surgery. BC Decker, Hamilton, Ontario, Canada 2005.

Pierre AF, Luketich JD. Technique and role of minimally invasive esophagectomy for premalignant diseases of the esophagus. Surg Oncol Clin Noth Am. 2002;11:337–350.

76. Thoracodorsal Sympathectomy and Splanchnicectomy

Rodney J. Landreneau, M.D.
Ricardo Santos, M.D.
Christopher Baird, M.D.

A. Sympathectomy

1. Indications

Thoracodorsal sympathectomy is primarily used today for the surgical management of intractable facial blushing/sweating, upper extremity hyperhidrosis (hand and axilla), vasospastic disorders of the hand, and upper extremity pain syndromes (causalgia). The video-assisted thoracic surgery (VATS) approach to thoracodorsal sympathectomy is preferred because it combines limited incisional morbidity with exceptional videoscopic exposure of the upper thoracic sympathetic chain.

The extent of sympathectomy required depends upon the anatomic involvement of the syndrome. We recommend a T2-T3 sympathectomy for facial manifestations. We primarily perform a T3 sympathectomy for patients with palmar hyperhidrosis and vasospastic disorders of the hand (Raynaud's syndrome, Beurger's syndrome). Axillary hyperhidrosis and/or bromidism will lead us to include the T4 ganglia with the T3 sympathectomy. For upper extremity chronic pain syndromes (causalgia), we recommend a T2 through T4 ganglionectomy.

The clinical results of VATS thoracodorsal sympathectomy vary depending upon the nature of the problem being addressed. Good results are consistently seen in over 90% of patients approached for palmar hyperhidrosis. Improvement is also consistently seen for patients undergoing sympathectomy for vasospastic syndromes. The long-term benefits of thoracodorsal sympathectomy for axillary symptoms are less consistent; however, most series report long-term benefit in greater than 70% of patients. The most variable results with thoracodorsal sympathectomy are seen among patients approached for chronic pain (causalgia) syndromes. Results vary from one third to over 70% of patients benefiting from sympathectomy. In this latter group, it is appreciated that the benefit may be longer to mature clinically than for other syndromes and also that delay in the diagnosis and treatment of the disorder lessens the general effectiveness of sympathectomy.

2. Operative Approach for VATS Thoracodorsal Sympathectomy

   a.   Position the patient supine.

   b.   After general anesthesia and double-lumen endotracheal tube intubation have been accomplished, place a roll between the patient's shoulders. We usually have both arms extended laterally to ensure adequate exposure to the anterior chest and axilla.

   c.   Bronchoscopically confirm proper position of the endotracheal tube.

   d.   Prep and drape the entire chest axilla and inner aspect of the upper arms within the operative field. Radial arterial pressure monitoring is not usually necessary. Place the operating table in a 45-degree reverse Trendelenburg position to allow the lung to fall away from the operative field.

   e.   We usually begin a bilateral VATS intervention on the right side but will start on the left if that is the patient's dominant upper extremity. We routinely utilize two sites of intercostal access. The operating table is rolled away from the surgeon to enhance operating space and for improved dexterity with the endosurgical instrumentation. Sealed laparoscopic ports (5mm) are used, and carbon dioxide insufflation to an intracavitary pressure of 5 to 8mmHg is established once videoscopic confirmation of entry into the pleural space has been assured.

       i.   The first site of intercostal access is at the inframammary crease in the anterior axillary line at the level of the fifth interspace. We routinely tunnel the trocar through the subcutaneous tissues and over the rib for actual entry into the chest through the interspace above the skin incision. A 5-mm-diameter, 30-degree-lens thoracoscope is introduced into the chest through the port and carbon dioxide insufflation begun.

      ii.   The second site of intercostal access is in the anterior axillary line just lateral to the belly of the pectoralis muscle. This port is directed apicomedially toward the apex of the chest through the third intercostal space. A trumpeted endoscopic suction device with a hook cautery attachment is introduced through the upper port.

     iii.   Count the rib level with the tip of the suction device to identify the location of the third rib. This will be the central point for the future dissection.

     iv.   Score the pleura over the lateral aspect of the third rib head with the hook cautery and ablate the pleura over the rib head to the lateral origin of the musculature of the intrathoracic fascia. This will result in a line of pleural ablation over the proximal third rib of approximately 6cm. This maneuver is done to ensure division of any accessory sympathetic fibers of "Kuntz" located in this region.

     v.   Then elevate the pleura over the third rib head and extend the pleural incision medially to expose the sympathetic chain. Take care to avoid injury to intercostal venous tributaries in this region.

   vi.   Divide the communicating sympathectic fibers coming in perpendicularly with the main sympathetic trunk with the hook cautery at the primary sympathetic level of concern. After dividing these fibers, sharply excise the cord of the sympathetic chain at the level of therapeutic interest with endoscopic scissors and submit it for pathologic review.

  vii.   Ensure hemostasis, and place a 14-French red rubber catheter into the chest through the upper trocar, with the outer aspect of the catheter submerged in a basin fulled with saline. Confirm apical positioning of the catheter tip under videoscopic guidance. Desufflate the chest through the underwater sealed red rubber catheter while the anesthesia team gently reinflates the lung. When the lung is completely inflated, remove both trocars and the red rubber catheter and seal the 5-mm wounds with Steri-Strips.

f.   The steps of the intervention are then initiated and completed on the left side. Chest tubes are avoided.

g.   The patient is usually admitted for overnight observation; however, a significant percentage of patients can be discharged to home the same evening of surgery. Postoperative pain control is accomplished with intravenous ketorolac (30 mg every 6 hours) and oral narcotic agents.

3. Complications

a.   The primary complication associated with thoracodorsal sympathectomy is injury to the stellate ganglion resulting in "Horner's syndrome" of varying degrees. In most series, the incidence of partial or full Horner's syndrome is reported to occur in less than 1% of patients after sympathectomy.

b.   The development of "compensatory" truncal hyperhidrosis involving the small of the back, groins, and periumbilical area is noted in over one half of patients. This is usually a mild phenomenon; however, it may be considered significant in a minority of patients.

B. Splanchnicectomy

1. Indications and Results

Chronic upper abdominal pain resulting from chronic pancreatitis or infiltrating carcinoma of the stomach, gastroesophageal junction, or pancreas is a difficult management problem. A number of surgical investigators have seen a benefit from splanchnic denervation. The VATS approach is particularly suited for this intervention. The anatomic variability of the intrathoracic splanchic nerves is becoming increasingly appreciated. It is now recognized that an extensive pleurotomy over the course of the T4 through the T12 levels is important to ablate the fibers of the greater splanchnic nerve (usually T6–T9 but sometimes ranging to T4), the lesser splanchnic nerve (usually T10–T11) and the least splanchnic nerve (T10–T12). Less than satisfactory results with splanchnicectomy may be explained by incomplete ablation of the full extent of the thoracic splanchnic innervation.

The splanchnic nerve communication to the celiac plexus involved with pancreatic, perinephric, and gastric innervation is predominantly left sided. Accordingly, the left chest is usually approached first to accomplish VATS splanchnicectomy. If only partial relief of symptoms is obtained following the left VATS approach, and the residual pain is located predominantly on the right, consideration of a right-sided ablation is reasonable if the patient's functional status allows.

The addition of thoracic truncal vagotomy with thoracic splanchnicectomy has been variably advocated in the past. The theoretical benefit of vagotomy results from reduction gastric acid stimulation of pancreatic secretion and the pain associated with this stimulation. The additive benefit of this vagotomy maneuver has been hard to quantitate, and the risk of important gastric emptying problems related to vagal denervation of the stomach can be seen in nearly a quarter of patients. Accordingly, we do not advocate the addition of transthoracic truncal vagotomy at this time.

The results of spanchnicectomy have been variably good, with nearly 70% of patients noting a reduction in upper abdominal pain and requirements for narcotic pain medicine.

2. Technique of VATS Splanchnicectomy

a.   Establish and confirm general anesthesia and double-lumen endotracheal tube position as noted for VATS thoracodorsal sympathectomy (Section A.2.b).

b.   Place the patient in a right lateral decubitus position with a 15-degree forward tilt. The table is placed in a moderate reverse Trendelenburg position and rotated toward the right to aid in exposure to the posterior aspect of the thoracic cavity. The surgeon usually stands on the patient's right side for the upper aspect of the splanchnicectomy and then switches to the left to continue the dissection inferiorly.

c. We presently utilize 5-mm closed endosurgical ports so that modest carbon dioxide insufflation can be accomplished for optimal lung collapse and thoracoscopic exposure of the splanchnic nerves.

d. We establish intercostal access for the 5-mm thoracoscope and camera at the seventh intercostal space in the posterior axillary line. Three other intercostal access sites are established in the midaxillary line of the third interspace (for left hand grasping tool), the fifth or sixth intercostal space midaxillary line (trumpeted suction device with hook electrocautery attachment), and the ninth intercostal space midaxillary line (for lung and diaphragmatic retraction).

e. Create an extended pleurotomy medial to the sympathetic chain, from the T4 level through the T12 level. During the conduct of this extrapleural exposure, numerous fibers will be seen coalescing from an oblique plane to form the greater, lesser, and least splanchnic nerves. All these fibers must be ablated during this extended extrapleural dissection.

f. Postoperative tube thoracostomy drainage is employed owing to the extent of the extra-pleural dissection. This tube is usually removed within 48 hours of surgery.

3. Complications

Complications related to the procedure are generally like those common to other thoracoscopic explorations. Chronic intercostal pain is uncommon with the use of smaller trocar access. Patients who have not had previous surgical interventions related to their primary upper abdominal pathology appear to do better than previously operated patients. VATS splanchnicectomy seems to be a reasonable minimally invasive surgical approach to pain management of the patient with a reasonable functional status who has upper abdominal pain.

C. Selected References

Berguer R, Smit R. Transaxillary sympathectomy (T2 to T4) for relief of vasospastic/sympathetic pain of upper extremities. Surgery 1981;89(6):764–769.

Chapuis O, Sockeel P, Pallas G, Pons F, Jancovici R. Thoracoscopic renal denervation for intractable autosomal dominant polycystic kidney disease-related pain. Am J Kidney Dis 2004;43(1):161–163.

Chester M, Hammond C, Leach A. Long-term benefits of stellate ganglion block in severe chronic refractory angina. Pain 2000;87(1):103–105.

de Campos JR, Kauffman P, Werebe Ede C, et al. Quality of life, before and after thoracic sympathectomy: report on 378 operated patients. Ann Thorac Surg 2003;76(3): 886–891.

De Giacomo T, Rendina EA, Venuta F, et al. Thoracoscopic sympathectomy for symptomatic arterial obstruction of the upper extremities. Ann Thorac Surg 2002; 74(3):885–888.

Doolabh N, Horswell S, Williams M, et al. Thoracoscopic sympathectomy for hyperhidrosis: indications and results. Ann Thorac Surg 2004;77(2):410–414; discussion 414.

Drott C. Results of endoscopic thoracic sympathectomy (ETS) on hyperhidrosis, facial blushing, angina pectoris, vascular disorders and pain syndromes of the hand and arm. Clin Auton Res 2003;13(Suppl 1):126–130.

Drott C, Claes G, Gothberg G, Paszkowski P. Cardiac effects of endoscopic electrocautery of the upper thoracic sympathetic chain. Eur J Surg Suppl 1994;(572):65–70.

Gossot D, Galetta D, Pascal A, et al. Long-term results of endoscopic thoracic sympathectomy for upper limb hyperhidrosis. Ann Thorac Surg 2003;75(4):1075–1079.

Hashmonai M, Kopelman D. History of sympathetic surgery. Clin Auton Res 2003;13(Suppl 1):16–19.

Leksowski K. Thoracoscopic splanchnicectomy for the relief of pain due to chronic pancreatitis. Surg Endosc 2001;15(6):592–596.

Makarewicz W, Stefaniak T, Kossakowska M, et al. Quality of life improvement after videothoracoscopic splanchnicectomy in chronic pancreatitis patients: case control study. World J Surg 2003;27(8):906–911.

Moodley J, Singh B, Shaik AS, Haffejee A, Rubin J. Thoracoscopic splanchnicectomy: pilot evaluation of a simple alternative for chronic pancreatic pain control. World J Surg 1999;23(7):688–692.

Naidoo N, Partab P, Pather N, Moodley J, Singh B, Satyapal KS. Thoracic splanchnic nerves: implications for splanchnic denervation. J Anat 2001;199(Pt 5):585–590.

Olak J, Gore D. Thoracoscopic splanchnicectomy: technique and case report. Surg Laparosc Endosc 1996;6(3):228–230.

Pohjavaara P, Telaranta T, Vaisanen E. The role of the sympathetic nervous system in anxiety: is it possible to relieve anxiety with endoscopic sympathetic block? Nord J Psychiatry 2003;57(1):55–60.

Rizzo M, Balderson SS, Harpole DH, Levin LS. Thoracoscopic sympathectomy in the management of vasomotor disturbances and complex regional pain syndrome of the hand. Orthopedics 2004;27(1):49–52.

Singh B, Moodley J, Shaik AS, Robbs JV. Sympathectomy for complex regional pain syndrome. J Vasc Surg 2003;37(3):508–511.

Stone HH, Chauvin EJ. Pancreatic denervation for pain relief in chronic alcohol associated pancreatitis. Br J Surg 1990;77(3):303–305.

Welch E, Geary J. Current status of thoracic dorsal sympathectomy. J Vasc Surg 1984;1(1):202–214.

Worsey J, Ferson PF, Keenan RJ, Julian TB, Landreneau RJ. Thoracoscopic pancreatic denervation for pain control in irresectable pancreatic cancer. Br J Surg 1993;80:1051–1052.

Yoon do H, Ha Y, Park YG, Chang JW. Thoracoscopic limited T-3 sympathicotomy for primary hyperhidrosis: prevention for compensatory hyperhidrosis. J Neurosurg 2003;99(Suppl 1):39–43.

77. VATS Management of the Indeterminate Pulmonary Nodule

Jason Lamb, M.D.
Gintas Antanavicius, M.D.
Rodney J. Landreneau, M.D.

A. General Considerations

An indeterminate pulmonary nodule (IPN) is any radiologically described parenchymal pulmonary lesion of unknown histology that is less than 3 cm. In diameter without associated atelectasis or adenopathy. More than 150,000 patients with indeterminate pulmonary nodules are newly identified each year in the United States, with greater than 90% of these found incidentally in unrelated diagnostic workups. This number continues to increase as the widespread use of computed tomography identifies many small, previously nondetectable nodules. While the majority of IPNs will be benign, approximately 40% to 45% of patients will be found to have malignant lesions; 75% of the malignant lesions represent primary lung carcinoma. With 5-year survival of up to 75% following resection of early lung cancer and the relative late presentation of lung cancer clinically, the discovery of IPNs creates a diagnostic dilemma.

1. Benign lesions that present as IPNs include the following:
    a. Intrapulmonary lymph nodes
    b. Hamartomas
    c. Granulomas, teratomas
    d. Sarcoidosis
    e. Rheumatoid nodules
    f. Arteriovenous malformations, traumatic lesions
    g. Congenital lesions
2. Malignant lesions include the following:
    a. Primary lung cancers including non–small cell and small cell types
        i. Found in approximately 35% of IPNs.
        ii. Predictors of malignancy include advanced age, history of cigarette smoking, increased lesion size, and nodule growth.
    b. Pulmonary metastases from other primary malignancies. In patients who have previously been diagnosed with cancer, any pulmonary lesion may potentially represent metastatic disease, and solitary metastases can account for 20% of IPNs. The most common metastatic pulmonary metastases are from lung primary carcinomas followed by breast and colorectal malignancies.

Obtaining tissue is often mandatory in this group as the impact on future therapeutic intervention may be great. The presence of pulmonary metastases may lead to an abandonment of a planned local procedure and initiation of systemic therapy. Alternatively, possible metastatic lung nodules proven to be benign allow more aggressive local therapies and potentially longer survival.

B. Diagnostic Workup

IPNs are most commonly discovered incidentally by plain chest radiograph (CXR) or computed tomography (CT) of the chest during diagnostic workup for unrelated problems. Less commonly, they are found on follow-up surveillance for prior malignancy or during screening of at-risk populations. Both CXR and chest CT have been shown to accurately predict the presence of malignancy in up to 60% of lesions based on morphologic characteristics and tissue density, though a substantial proportion of solitary pulmonary nodules remain indeterminate. Confirmatory tissue diagnosis is usually required, as the consequences of an undiagnosed malignancy are life threatening and therapies aimed at malignant conditions usually demand histological confirmation.

1. Chest X-Ray

The two findings on CXR that most heavily predict benign histology are calcification pattern and chronicity.
   a.   Benign calcifications are described as a diffuse, central, "popcorn," or laminar pattern.
   b.   Stippled and eccentric calcifications are indeterminate, as they are seen in benign and malignant conditions.
   c.   The absence of growth over a 2-year time period suggests benign etiology. In patients with an IPN identified by CXR, all previous CXRs should be reviewed. No further investigation is needed if the lesion is unchanged over 2 more years or.
   d.   Other criteria that may be helpful include margins of lesion, size, presence of cavitations, and presence of satellite nodules, though none of these have been consistently accurate in differentiation of benign and malignant nodules.

2. Computed Tomography

Spiral CT with intravenous contrast has become the imaging test of choice in the evaluation of IPNs.
   a.   Chest CT better characterizes the nodule in respect to location, surrounding structure involvement, mediastinal involvement, and

additional nodule identification, and even allows staging of the liver and adrenal gland.

b. CT is more sensitive in detecting calcification within a pulmonary nodule allowing indeterminate noncalcified nodules on CXR to be further assessed for benign calcifications.

c. An irregular border on chest CT is strongly suggestive of malignancy, as 84% to 90% of spiculated lung nodules are malignant.

d. CT is also particularly helpful in detection of fat within a pulmonary nodule, another indicator of benign disease most often seen in hamartoma.

e. CT provides a much more accurate estimate of size and growth than CXR. CT is typically reliable to approximately one millimeter. Size conveys importance in malignancy risk, as the vast majority of nodules greater than 2 cm by CT are malignant and 42% of nodules between 1 and 2 cm are proven malignant. In smaller IPNs, the lack of significant growth on chest CT over a 2-year period implies a doubling time of over 730 days, strongly correlated with benign behavior.

f. Contrast enhancement of the pulmonary nodule on CT provides additional prognostic information. Blood flow in malignant pulmonary nodules is increased compared with benign pulmonary nodules, and the degree of enhancement is directly related to vascularity. With sensitivity of 98% and specificity of 73%, nodules that enhance to greater than 20 Hounsfield units have been found to be predictive of malignancy, while those less than 15 Hounsfield units are characteristically benign.

3. Positron-Emission Tomography (PET)

PET is a newer imaging technique that uses 18-fluorodeoxyglucose (FDG) as a radiotracer taken up by active cells in glycolysis but bound within the cell. Metabolically active cells are typically neoplastic or inflammatory. A meta-analysis of the use of PET in pulmonary nodules and masses demonstrated an overall sensitivity of 96.8% in diagnosing malignancy and sensitivity of 96% in diagnosing benign nodules. Unfortunately, two barriers to PET exist. First, owing to the uptake of radiotracer into active, nonneoplastic inflammatory cells, the specificity is 77% in malignant nodules and 88% in benign nodules. Second, the current resolution of PET is approximately 8 mm, and results in lesions less than 1 cm are unreliable. The indications for PET are currently debated and need further investigation.

4. Magnetic Resonance Imaging (MRI)

MRI has a very limited role in the evaluation of IPNs. It may be used in patients who cannot tolerate intravenous contrast medial. Although MRI is superior to CT in the evaluation of nerve root, brachial plexus, and vertebral body involvement in some lung neoplasms, for most purposes CT is less costly and just as accurate.

C. Options for Management

After thorough radiologic analysis of an IPN, approximately one third of the initial pulmonary nodules will remain indeterminate. In the management of these nodules, many factors must be considered, including the patient's concern for definitive diagnosis, general state of health, age, smoking history, and medical history. Current options in the evaluation and management of indeterminate solitary pulmonary nodules include observation, bronchoscopy, transthoracic needle aspiration (TTNA), video-assisted thoracic surgery (VATS), and thoracotomy. Each will be considered here, with special emphasis on VATS.

1. Observation

As many IPNs discovered on radiology evaluation are benign, "watchful waiting" can be a reasonable option in certain clinical situations. Observation is usually favored in individuals without a tissue diagnosis but with low probability for malignancy secondary to age, smoking history, and/or tumor characteristics on imaging. Observation may also be the only option for patients who are high-risk candidates for interventions because of poor lung function or associated cardiovascular disease, regardless of their probability for malignancy.

Close, responsible follow-up with serial chest CT should be the mainstay during observation of low-risk, but potentially malignant, IPNs. Though few objective data exist, current recommendations include an initial CXR with serial CT scanning at 3, 6, 12, and 24 months. A solitary pulmonary nodule should be considered benign if it remains unchanged during a 2-year period of observation, and tissue diagnosis should be pursued for nodules increasing in size or demonstrating malignant tendencies on imaging.

2. Tissue Diagnosis

When tissue diagnosis is required, several options exist.
   a.   Bronchoscopy is commonly implemented in the diagnosis of large, central, or advanced-stage lung neoplasms with mediastinal involvement, though its role in the management of IPNs is quite limited. Though it is a safe, minimally invasive procedure, a definite diagnosis is obtained in less than 10% of patients with nodules less than 2 cm in size. Bronchoscopy has been shown to have no preoperative

measurable benefit to the patient and is not currently recommended in the management of IPNs.

b. Transthoracic needle aspiration offers tissue diagnosis through a minimally invasive outpatient procedure. Typically performed by interventional radiology with CT- guidance, a diagnosis can be established in 90% to 95% of nodules larger than 2 cm. The yield falls to 60% or less for malignant nodules less than 2 cm in size, and nodules less than 1 cm are exceedingly hard to diagnose via TTNA. Nondiagnostic TTNA is not uncommon, especially in benign disease, as the diagnostic yield is between 12% and 68%. This yield can be improved some what by use of core needle biopsy and on-site pathology evaluation for adequacy of specimen. TTNA is a generally safe procedure, though pneumothorax occurs in approximately 25% patients, with 5% to 10% requiring tube thoracostomy. Hemoptysis and pulmonary hemorrhage may be seen in up to 10% of patients. TTNA avoids the need for subsequent surgery only in about 10% of patients who are physiologically able to undergo surgical resection. Additionally, high false negative rates are unacceptable, as many patients may have potentially curable early-stage lung cancer. Often nonspecific benign diagnoses are not believed and surgical excisional biopsy may be employed regardless of findings. Accordingly, for the treatment of patients who are good surgical risks with a new indeterminate peripheral pulmonary nodule, VATS should be considered as a first diagnostic approach in directing the patient's treatment.

3. IPNs of Unknown Etiology

VATS with thoracoscopic wedge resection is often the initial step in IPNs of unknown histology. Indications include unknown nodules peripheral in location with a size greater than 10 mm and within 10 mm of the pleural surface. Probability of detection of the nodule using VATS alone decreases to 63% in cases with nodules less than 10 mm and more than 5 mm from the pleural surface. Nodules less than 10 mm in size and more than 10 mm from the pleural surface are often undetectable with VATS alone. In multivariate analysis, distance to the pleural surface has been shown to be the most significant factor, with tumor size of borderline significance. To assist in the localization of deeper lesions for VATS resection, various preoperative localization techniques have been reported, including CT-directed percutaneous guidewire, injection of methylene blue dye, coil insertion, or injection of contrast media with intraoperative fluoroscopy. Though true indications are lacking, certainly nodules less than 10 mm in diameter or more than 5 mm from the pleural surface may be more easily resected with VATS techniques if preoperative localization is employed. Despite these efforts, the conversion to thoracotomy or minithoracotomy for localization of lesion in larger series is between 21% and 54%.

Frozen-section analysis should be used at the time of VATS resection for definitive tissue diagnosis. In patients suitable for lobectomy, a diagnosis of non–small cell lung carcinoma (NSCLC) should warrant complete oncologic resection by lobectomy and mediastinal lymph node dissection (MSLND). The approach consisting of VATS lobectomy and MSLND has been described and is favored by some authors, though it has not gained widespread acceptance and is relatively unproven pertaining to long-term survival to date. Traditionally, thoracotomy has been employed to accomplish complete oncologic resection with 5-year survival rates of 65% to 80% for stage IA and 50% to 60% for stage IB NSCLC. In patients with pulmonary function prohibitive for lobectomy, wedge resection or segmentectomy is acceptable, though local recurrence rates have been shown to be significantly higher with prospective data. Brachymesh with ^{125}I has been placed via VATS or thoracotomy at the time of limited resection to decrease local recurrence rates with yet unproven long-term success. In more than half of those undergoing VATS resection for IPN, the frozen section reveals a benign histology. The operation is completed following placement of a tube thoracostomy.

D. Contraindications and Complications Associated with VATS

Even with localization techniques, initial VATS wedge resection approaches to IPNs more than 2.5 cm from the periphery of the lung become difficult. Failure to include the lesion within a deep wedge resection becomes more common with central nodules. Additional complications, including air leaks, pulmonary arterial bleeding, and parenchymal bleeding, become much more likely as tissue thickness exceeds the stapling device capabilities, resulting in inadequate staple lines. Many central IPNs require lobectomy or segmentectomy and therefore often incorporate thoracotomy. As the definition of the IPN includes only nodules less than 3 cm, size alone is not usually a contraindication to VATS resection. Conversion to thoracotomy for reasons not associated with depth or size of the lesion is seen in about 15% and most commonly is due to pleural adhesion.

E. Selected References

Ginsberg MS, Griff SK, Go BD, Yoo H, Schwartz LH, Panicek DM. Pulmonary nodules resected at video-assisted thoracoscopic surgery: etiology in 426 patients. Radiology 1999;213:277–282.

Leef JI 3rd, Klein IS. The solitary pulmonary nodule. Radiol Clin North Am 2002; 40:123–143.

Mack MJ, Hazelrigg SR, Landreneau RJ, Acuff TE. Thoracoscopy for the diagnosis of the indeterminate solitary pulmonary nodule. Ann Thorac Surg 1993;56:825–832.

Mack MJ, Shennib H, Landreneau RJ, Hazelrigg SR. Techniques for localization of pulmonary nodules for thoracoscopic resection. J Thorac Cardiovasc Surg 1993;106:550–553.

Mitruka S, Landreneau FJ, Mack MJ, et al. Diagnosing the indeterminate pulmonary nodule: percutaneous biopsy versus thoracoscopy. Surgery 1995;118:676–684.

Tan BB Flaherty KR, Kazerooni EA, Iannettoni MD. The solitary pulmonary nodule. Chest 2003;123:89S–96S.

78. Pleural Disease

Alberto de Hoyos, M.D.
Peter F. Ferson, M.D.

A. Indications

The most common indications for video-assisted thoracic surgery (VATS) for pleural disease are as follows:
  Undiagnosed pleural effusion
  Treatment of spontaneous pneumothorax
  Drainage, debridement, and decortication of early empyema
  Chemical and mechanical pleurodesis for benign and malignant effusions
  Evacuation of traumatic and postoperative hemothorax
  Biopsy of pleural-based lesion
  Excision of primary lesions of the pleura

B. Anesthesia and Lung Isolation

1. VATS requires single-lung ventilation for facilitation of the procedure.
2. Lung isolation is achieved with a double-lumen endotracheal tube or a single-lumen tube with the selective placement of a bronchial blocker in the operative side.
3. In collaboration with the anesthesia team, the surgeon performs a fiberoptic bronchoscopy to confirm correct placement of the double-lumen tube or bronchial blocker.
4. On occasion, if the patient does not tolerate single-lung anesthesia, periods of apnea after hyperventilation will allow sufficient time to perform short diagnostic and therapeutic interventions.
5. Most patients also require electrocardiographic monitoring, pulse oximetry, arterial line, and if necessary, central venous pressure monitoring.

C. Patient Position and Room Setup

1. Position the patient in full lateral decubitus position with the operative side up on a beanbag.

2. Protect all pressure points with gel or foam pads to protect against nerve compression or tissue ischemia.
3. The arms need to be placed in a neutral position (i.e., prayer position) to avoid hyperextension injury of neurovascular structures.
4. Place the hips of the patient aligned with the angle of the table to allow flexion at that level.
5. Elevate the head of the bed slightly (reverse Trendelenburg) to a comfortable position for the operating team.
6. Secure the patient well to the table.
7. The surgeon generally stands in front of the patient, and the assistant and scrub nurse in the back.
8. Place the monitors at the head of the table.

D. Trocar Position and Choice of Thoracoscope

1. General concepts
    a. Place the initial intercostals access site at a distance from the lesion to achieve a panoramic view and provide full visibility of additional instruments.
    b. Avoid instrument crowding ("fencing").
    c. Avoid mirror image by positioning instruments and thoracoscope within the same 180-degree arc. That is, approach the lesion from the same general direction with instruments and camera.
2. For fluid collections, place the first port at the center of the fluid collection as x-ray and computed tomography scans. On occasion, aspiration of fluid with a small needle may aid in localizing a fluid collection.
3. For pneumothorax or general inspection of the pleural space, place the first port anteriorly and low in the hemithorax (i.e., eighth or ninth intercostal space), just in front of the anterior axillary line. This will provide a wide range of maneuvering without undue pressure on intercostal structures.
4. When the skin incision is made (1.5 cm), carefully dissect over the top of the rib to enter the pleural space. Insert a finger gently to corroborate entry into the pleural space. On occasion, adhesions will be present that can be cautiously disrupted with the finger to allow safe placement of the thoracoscope.
5. In general, three to five ports are necessary for most procedures. On occasion, if utilizing the operating thoracoscope, two ports will suffice.
6. The 10-mm 0- or 30-degree scope is preferred for most procedures.
7. Select optimum placement of the additional ports based on the initial assessment of the pleural space problem at hand. Most working ports can be 5 mm and converted to 10 mm if necessary, as for stapling devices.

E. Performing the Exploration and Intervention

1. If fluid is present, aspirate and send it for culture, cytology, and chemical studies as necessary. A large trap will provide enough samples for most studies.

2. If the patient has a large long-standing effusion, we prefer to place a pigtail catheter the day before to drain some fluid over a few hours to decrease the risk of reexpansion pulmonary edema. The pigtail is removed at the time of VATS.

3. Perform a general inspection of the pleural space, including the diaphragm and pericardium, then take biopsy samples of any abnormal areas on the pleural or lung surfaces. Most parietal pleural biopsies can be performed with a sponge stick holder or thoracoscopic graspers.

4. Aspirate thick fluid or retained clotted hemothorax with a large-bore suction device, taking care not to injure the lung parenchyma or mediastinal structures.

5. Divide adhesions from the visceral to the parietal pleura with electrocoagulating shears to avoid troublesome bleeding, which makes visualization more difficult.

6. Disrupt fluid loculations with blunt-tipped suction devices, digital manipulation, sponge stick holder or Metzenbaum scissors. The goal is complete and adequate visualization of all structures and full mobilization of the lung to allow full reexpansion.

7. Early empyemas entrapping the lung can be debrided by gently stripping off the exudates from the surface of the lung, taking care to avoid injury to the lung and potential air leaks. Entry into the appropriate plane of dissection is at times facilitated by partially reinflating the lung with small tidal volumes.

8. Apical bullae responsible for pneumothoraces are easily accessible for resection with endoscopic gastrointestinal anastomosis stapling devices.

9. Mechanical abrasion for pleurodesis can be done with sponges, cotton-tipped applicators, electrocautery, or pleurectomy.

10. Chemical pleurodesis is achieved by insuflation of talc (3–5 g) or doxycycline (500 mg in 100–250 mL of normal saline solution).

11. At the conclusion of the procedure, insert a 28-French chest tube and direct it posteriorly and apically for pneumothorax or malignant effusions. For empyemas or hemothorax, strategically positioned, multiple large-bore (32–36 Fr) chest tubes are preferred.

12. After pleurodesis the chest tubes are connected to continuous suction (20–40 cm H_2O) for 48 to 72 hours and removed after an additional 24 hours on water seal. If an air leak is present, continue suction until 24 hours after resolution of the air leak.

13. Chest tubes for drainage of empyema are typically left in place for 2 to 4 weeks. The tubes can be opened to air and connected to a drainage system after a few days if the lung remains expanded while the tube is open. These tubes can later be withdrawn a few centimeters every 2 to 3 days until removed.

F. Complications

1. **Persistent air leak**
   a. **Cause and prevention.** This complication is usually secondary to inadvertent injury to the lung parenchyma in the process of mobilizing the lung or performing the decortication for empyema. Occasionally it is also seen after stapled resection of apical blebs in patients with emphysematous lungs. To an extent, utilizing staple line reinforcement or buttressing with GoreTex or Vicryl strips can prevent this.
   b. **Recognition and management.** The patient will develop air bubbles in the water seal chamber of the pleural drainage system. The air leak can be graded from small to large depending on the amount of bubbles generated with quiet or forced exhalation. Most leaks are small and require only continuous suction for 2 to 3 additional days. If the air leak persists, the suction can be lowered or discontinued (water seal) as long as the lung remains expanded. Rarely a persistent air leak after a VATS procedure requires reoperation.

2. **Hemorrhage**
   a. **Cause and prevention.** This complication is usually secondary to intercostal vessel injury, hilar injury, or overly aggressive pleurectomy or decortication with bleeding from the chest wall or lung parenchyma, respectively. Gentle manipulation of tissues, attention to planes of dissection, and thorough hemostasis are required to prevent this complication.
   b. **Recognition and management.** Intrathoracic bleeding is most often recognized by excessive postoperative chest tube output. In general, over 100 mL/h for 3 or more consecutive hours requires close observation and possibly reexploration. A chest x-ray should be obtained to rule out the possibility of an underlying retained hemothorax. Persistent bleeding or a retained hemothorax is an indication for reexploration with VATS. If one is unable to resolve the bleeding with this approach, a thoracotomy may become necessary.

3. **Inadequate drainage of empyema**
   a. **Cause and prevention.** This is usually secondary to incomplete disruption of all loculations and failure to achieve full mobilization of the lung with creation of a unilocular pleural cavity. Gentle and meticulous disruption of all loculations should be the goal of VATS for drainage of empyema. Attention should also be directed at draining any fluid accumulated in the interlobar fissures, or paravertebral or diaphragmatic recesses. Strategic placement of large-bore, straight, and or right-angle chest tubes may decrease the incidence of this complication.
   b. **Recognition and management.** Before concluding the VATS procedure, the surgeon should be satisfied with the accomplished results. Suboptimal results usually will require reoperation. Postoperatively, the patient may persist with fever, leukocytosis, or

pleural densities representing residual undrained fluid collections. Management usually requires VATS or open thoracotomy. On occasion, administration of fibrinolytics (recombinant tissue plasminogen activator, 5–6 mg) through the chest tube may allow one to avoid reoperation.

G. Selected References

Landreneau RJ, Keenan RJ, Hazelrigg SR, et al. Thoracoscopy for empyema and hemothorax. Chest 1996;109:18–24.

Landreneau RJ, Mack MJ, Hazelrigg SR, et al. Video-assisted thoracic surgery: basic technical concepts and intercostal approach strategies. Ann Thorac Surg 1992;54: 800–807.

Ng C, et al. Paradigm shift in surgical approaches to spontaneous pneumothorax: VATS. Thorax 2003;58:39–52.

Ukale V, et al. Pleurodesis in recurrent pleural effusions: a randomized comparison of a classical and currently popular drug. Lung Cancer 2004;43:323–328.

Appendix: SAGES Publications

SAGES issues and periodically revises **guidelines**, **statements**, **and standards** on a variety of subjects related to endoscopy, laparoscopy, and education. **Patient education information** brochures are also available for selected laparoscopic procedures. Documents may be viewed or downloaded from the World Wide Web at **www.sages.org**. They are also available from:

SAGES
11300 W. Olympic Blvd., Suite 600
Los Angeles, GA 90064
Phone: (310) 437-0544
Fax: (310) 437-0585
email: sagesweb@sages.org

A. SAGES Guidelines, Statements, and Standards

1. Statement on Concentration in General Surgery Residency
2. Position Statement on Advanced Laparoscopic Training
3. Integrating Advanced Laparoscopy into Surgical Residency Training
4. Video Production Guidelines
5. Guidelines for the Surgical Practice of Telemedicine
6. Statement of First Assistants
7. Global Statement on New Procedures
8. Granting of Ultrasonography Privileges for Surgeons
9. Guidelines for Laparoscopic Surgery During Pregnancy
10. Guidelines for Diagnostic Laparoscopy, Clinical Application
11. Guidelines for the Clinical Application of Laparoscopic Biliary Tract Surgery
12. Guidelines for Surgical Treatment of Gastroesophageal Reflux Disease (GERD)
13. Statement on Policy, Laparoscopic Appendectomy
14. Guidelines for Collaborative Practice in Endoscopic/Thoracoscopic Spinal Surgery for the General Surgeon
15. Guidelines for Granting of Privileges for Laparoscopic and/or Thoracoscopic General Surgery
16. Framework for Post-Residency Surgical Education and Training
17. Granting of Privileges for Gastrointestinal Endoscopy by Surgeons
18. Summary Statement on Surgical Endoscopic Training and Practice
19. Guidelines for Office Endoscopic Services
20. Guidelines for General Surgery Resident Education in Gastrointestinal Endoscopy
21. Guidelines for Training in Diagnostic and Therapeutic Endoscopic Retrograde Cholangiopancreatography (ERCP)

Index